RECENT ADVANCES
IN MEDICINE

D. N. BARON

MD DSc FRCP FRCPath

Professor of Chemical Pathology,
The Royal Free Hospital School of Medicine,
London

NIGEL COMPSTON

MA MD FRCP

Physician, The Royal Free Hospital,
Royal Masonic Hospital, and
King Edward VII Hospital for Officers,
London

A. M. DAWSON

MD FRCP

Physician, St Bartholomew's Hospital and
King Edward VII Hospital for Officers, London,
Physician to the Royal Household

RECENT ADVANCES IN MEDICINE

EDITED BY

D. N. BARON
NIGEL COMPSTON
A. M. DAWSON

NUMBER SEVENTEEN

CHURCHILL LIVINGSTONE
Edinburgh London and New York
1977

CHURCHILL LIVINGSTONE
Medical Division of Longman Group Limited

Distributed in the United States of America by
Longman Inc., 19 West 44th Street, New York,
N.Y. 10036, and by associated companies,
branches and representatives throughout
the world.

© LONGMAN GROUP LIMITED 1977

First published 1977

ISBN 0 443 01316 0 (cased)
ISBN 0 443 01650 X (limp)

Library of Congress Cataloging in Publication Data
Baron, Denis Neville.
  Recent advances in medicine, No. 17
  Includes index.
  1. Medicine — Addresses, essays, lectures.
I. Baron, Denis Neville.   II. Compston, Nigel.
III. Dawson, Anthony Michael.   IV. Title DNLM:
1. Diagnosis.   2. Therapeutics.   WB300 R294
R111.B313   1977   610   77–3899

Printed in Great Britain by
T. & A. Constable Ltd., Edinburgh

PREFACE

The editors have continued the pattern which proved successful in the previous three editions, and have interpreted medicine broadly. The practice has been maintained of a complete change of subjects and contributors.

The selection of chapters from all those topics in which there have been major advances in the last five years has, as always, had to be arbitrary. We have tried to cover a wide range of interests, and have aimed at the postgraduate student, or at the consultant who is trying to keep up to date outside his own specialty. However, the book should have continued value for the senior medical student and general medical reader.

We wish to thank Churchill Livingstone for their pleasant collaboration, and for their patience.

D. N. BARON
NIGEL COMPSTON
A. M. DAWSON

September 1977

CONTRIBUTORS

G. M. BESSER BSc MD FRCP
Professor of Endocrinology, St Bartholomew's Hospital, London

J. D. BLAINEY MD FRCP
Professor of Renal Medicine (MRC External Staff), Queen Elizabeth Hospital, Birmingham

S. R. BLOOM MA MB BChir MRCP
Lecturer in Clinical Endocrinology, Royal Postgraduate Medical School, London

W. BRUMFITT PhD MD FRCP FRCPath
Professor of Medical Microbiology, Royal Free Hospital, London

D. P. BURKITT CMG MD DSc FRCS FRCSI FRS
Senior Research Fellow, St Thomas's Hospital Medical School, London

I. D. COOKE MB BS DGO FRCOG
Professor of Obstetrics, Jessop Hospital for Women, Sheffield

D. CROWTHER PhD MB MRCP
Professor of Medical Oncology, Christie Hospital, Manchester

R. GOLDSMITH BA MB BChir
Professor of Physiology, Chelsea College, London

J. M. T. HAMILTON-MILLER MA PhD MRCPath
Senior Lecturer in Medical Microbiology, Royal Free Hospital, London

J. R. W. HARRIS MB BCh BAO MRCP DTM&H
Consultant Venereologist, St Mary's Hospital, London

E. J. L. HEATHCOTE MD MRCP
Lecturer in Medicine, Royal Free Hospital, London

K. W. HEATON MA MD FRCP
Senior Lecturer in Medicine, Bristol Royal Infirmary, Bristol

E. W. HORTON DSc PhD MB ChB FRCP
Professor of Pharmacology, University of Edinburgh, Edinburgh

M. S. R. HUTT MD FRCP FRCPath
Professor of Geographical Pathology, St Thomas's Hospital Medical School, London

D. A. LEIGH MB BS MRCS LRCP
Consultant Microbiologist, Wycombe General Hospital, High Wycombe, Bucks.

B. LEWIS PhD MD FRCP MRCPath
Professor, Department of Chemical Pathology and Metabolic Diseases, St Thomas's Hospital, London

M. S. LIPSEDGE MPhil MRCP MRCPsych
Consultant Psychiatrist, City and Hackney Health District, London, Honorary Lecturer in Psychological Medicine, St Bartholomew's Medical College

J. S. MALPAS DPhil BSc MB BS FRCP
Director ICRF Medical Oncology Unit, St Bartholomew's Hospital, London

C. H. MORTIMER MB ChB MRCP
Lecturer in Endocrinology, St Bartholomew's Hospital, London

J. K. OATES MB FRCP(E)
Physician-in-charge of the Venereology Department, Westminster Hospital, London, and Addenbrooke's Hospital, Cambridge

J. K. ROSS MS FRCS
Consultant Cardiac Surgeon, Wessex Cardiac and Thoracic Centre, Southampton, Hants

J. H. SCARFFE MB MRCP
Lecturer in Medical Oncology, Christie Hospital, Manchester

A. K. THOMAS, MB BS MRCOG
Research Registrar, Department of Obstetrics and Gynaecology, Jessop Hospital for Women, Sheffield

H. E. WEBB MA DM FRCP
Consultant Neurologist and Senior Lecturer in Medicine, Neurovirology Unit, The Rayne Institute, St Thomas's Hospital, London

CONTENTS

1
EPIDEMIOLOGY OF CANCER

M. S. R. Hutt   D. P. Burkitt

'In studying the causes of disease we can seek information in three ways: we may devise experiments in the laboratory using animals or isolated tissue as our basic material; we may experiment directly on man; or we may observe and record what happens to man in the course of his ordinary life.'

Sir Richard Doll, 1975

The association between a specific environment and the development of certain tumours has been recognised since Percival Pott described the occurrence of scrotal cancer in chimney sweeps in 1775. During the last 50 years there has been a steady accumulation of data concerning the incidence rates of different tumours from cancer registries throughout the world (Doll, Payne and Waterhouse, 1966; Doll, Muir and Waterhouse, 1970). When corrections are made for the different age structures of the populations it is clear that the majority of human tumours show some variation in incidence in different geographical areas or in different groups of people living in the same area. Some tumours also show changes in incidence with the passage of time. Studies of migrants have shown that when population movement is associated with distinct changes in the biological, physical or human environment, some change is usually seen to have occurred in the pattern of tumours in the migrant group (Buell and Dunn, 1965; Wynder et al, 1969). This evidence has led to the suggestion that environmental factors are responsible for 85 per cent or more of all human cancers. The striking epidemiological feature of most cancers in man is that the incidence rates increase geometrically with age (Hammond, 1974).

All human populations are exposed to a variety of carcinogenic or cocarcinogenic factors in their particular environment and it is probable that the agents responsible for most common tumours have been widespread for centuries. An increasing incidence of any tumour over a period of time suggests that a new carcinogenic factor has been introduced into the environment. If the tumour is common it is likely that the causal factor will be found in some widespread social or cultural factor as in the association between lung cancer and cigarette smoking. On the other hand an increase in frequency of a rare tumour, such as angiosarcoma of the liver or adenocarcinoma of the vagina in children, is more likely to be due to an occupational or iatrogenic factor. Therapeutic hazards of the latter type are usually easier to identify as fewer people are exposed to the agent and it may be possible to recognise a cause and effect relationship. It is more difficult to identify the causal agents of the commoner tumours that have afflicted man for centuries, particularly as the experimental induction of tumours in animals demonstrates that the aetiology is often multifactorial. The production of tumours by specific chemical carcinogens can be influenced by cocarcinogens and by the metabolic, hormonal, immunological and nutritional state of the animal at the time of exposure. Such observations can, of course, equally apply to the development of other disease processes. Nevertheless, epidemiological studies have greatly enhanced our knowledge of the causes of many common tumours. The classical observations of Doll and Hill (1953) on the relationship between cigarette smoking and lung cancer were based initially on case/control studies and subsequently on prospective cohort studies. They identified cigarette smoking as an important factor in the development of this tumour. Evidence of a close relationship between the level of cigarette consumption and tumour incidence increased the probability of a causal effect, but the most impressive and ultimately the vital evidence in the epidemiology of this tumour was the observation in a defined group of doctors that stopping smoking decreased their risk of developing lung cancer (Doll and Hill, 1964).

Variations in the incidence rates of a tumour in a population exposed to an apparently uniform carcinogenic insult, such as heavy concentrations of cigarette smoke, require some explanation. These may be due to differences in smoking habits which influence effective dose or to other factors. Selikoff, Hammond and Churg (1968) found that insulation workers who smoked and were also exposed to asbestos dust had a much greater risk of dying of bronchial carcinoma than individuals exposed to only one of these two factors. A synergistic effect is also seen between cigarette smoking and exposure to uranium in mine workers in the USA (Lundin et al, 1969). On the other hand, cigarette smoking has no demonstrable effect on the incidence of mesothelioma which is also caused by asbestos.

The dominant role of environmental factors in the aetiology of cancer has led some workers to suggest that constitutional or genetic factors play no part in the genesis of most common tumours. It is clear, however, that environmental factors cannot explain the range of susceptibility of individuals in a population exposed to a similar carcinogenic agent. Susceptibility or resistance may depend on as yet undetermined genetic influences operating at enzymatic level, or on variations in immune response which may be determined by genetic or other environmental experiences. The low incidence of Burkitt's lymphoma in Africans with haemoglobin genotype AS is an example of a genetic influence on the development of a tumour. This is due to the protection conferred by the sickle cell gene against malaria, which appears to be an important aetiological factor in the development of this lymphoma in high incidence areas (Kafuko and Burkitt, 1970).

CARCINOMA OF THE OESOPHAGUS

Although carcinoma of the oesophagus occurs in all parts of the world, there are few other tumours which show such marked variations in incidence in different regions. Moreover, the areas of unusually high frequency are often of clearly limited geography and may show sharp gradients in incidence over short distances.

In Europe there is an unusually high incidence in Brittany and Normandy chiefly involving men (Tuyns and Massé, 1973, 1975). Within this region there are localised areas, such as Ille-et-Villaine, where the age-specific mortality rate for men is as high as 22.95; whereas the corresponding rate for women is only 1.44. Tuyns (1970) has shown a close relationship between oesophageal cancer and both alcoholism and cirrhosis of the liver in France, though it is generally accepted that alcohol is not, per se, carcinogenic. The high rates in Brittany are found particularly in rural areas and it has therefore been suggested they may be related to the consumption of apple cider distillates (Tuyns and Massé, 1975).

In South Africa Burrell (1957, 1962) first drew attention to the very high rate of oesophageal cancer in the Transkei. High incidence rates of this tumour have also been reported from other parts of South Africa, Cape Province, Johannesburg and Durban (Bradshaw and Schonland, 1974), and also from Bulawayo in Rhodesia and from southern Malawi and western Kenya (Cook, 1971). Examination of earlier records suggest that in Southern Africa the prevalence has been increasing over the last 40 years and that the more northerly areas were affected later than the more southerly regions (Keen, 1971). As in Brittany, and most other parts of the world, there is in Africa a strong male dominance though there is evidence that the rate in women is now increasing. Most authors have related these high rates either directly or indirectly to the consumption of alcoholic beverages. It has, in this connection, been suggested that a variety of carcinogens might be introduced during the illicit brewing of drinks, or that associated nutritional factors may play a role (Oettlé, 1964; McGlashan, 1969). More recently, Cook (1971) has suggested that the geographical pattern of high frequency in Africa might be related specifically to the use of maize for the brewing of local beers. Bradshaw and Schonland (1974), however, considered that the relationship between alcoholism and carcinoma of the oesophagus in Johannesburg was only a reflection of the relationship between smoking and alcohol and they concluded that it was the pipe smoking which was of greater importance; nor did they find any relationship with the consumption of maize beer.

Some of the highest rates of oesophageal carcinoma have been reported from northern Iran, along the south-east coast of the Caspian Sea and extending into the adjacent states of Soviet central Asia (Kmet and Mahboubi, 1972; Mahboubi et al, 1973). In this region, the highest rates are found along the eastern side of the Caspian and they decline sharply towards the west. In striking contrast to all other high incidence areas the tumour occurs with equal or greater frequency in women. The people of this area are Moslems and there is no evidence that either alcohol or smoking play a role in the aetiology. Ecologically, the high incidence area is characterised by semidesert conditions with a predominantly saline soil, but no specific aetiological factors have yet been identified (Hormozdiari et al, 1975).

Recently, a further high incidence area has been identified in northern China, in the southern parts of the Taihan mountains. The age-adjusted mortality rates in Linhsien, the area of highest frequency, are nearly 100 times greater than those in the south. Mortality rates over a 25-year period have shown little change, suggesting that the aetiological factors are to be sought in the geographical, rather than the cultural environment. A high concentration of nitrosamines, secondary amines, nitrites and nitrates were found in foodstuffs in the high incidence areas where there is also a deficiency of molybdenum in the soil (Coordinating Group for Research on the Etiology of Esophageal Cancer in North China, 1975). The possible association between nitrosamines and oesophageal cancer has been a subject of investigations since Magee and Barnes (1967) showed that oesophageal cancer could be induced by these substances in animals. Recently Reuber (1975) has induced carcinomas of the oesophagus by feeding a diet containing diethyl nitrosamine. Burrell, Roach and Shadwell (1966) suggested that there was in the Transkei an association between the place of residence of patients with the disease and molybdenum deficiency in the soil. This particular deficiency leads to an accumulation of nitrates in plants and it was suggested that these might combine with secondary amines to produce nitrosamines. It is difficult, however, to account for the sex ratios on this basis and nitrosamines have not been detected in drinks in other areas (Cook, 1971).

It is, perhaps, surprising that in the case of a tumour which shows such distinct epidemiological features, more definitive evidence should not have been forthcoming to indicate aetiological factors. It seems probable that the aetiology is multifactorial and that the responsible factors vary in different parts of the world. The association with smoking and drinking which is found in many areas may be an indirect relationship since neither of these factors can account for the high frequency in other places or regions.

GASTROINTESTINAL CARCINOMA

Carcinoma of the Stomach

Carcinoma of the stomach is an important cause of mortality from cancer in Europe and the USA but in both these areas the incidence and mortality rates are slowly decreasing. Cohort mortality rates show that in England and Wales this decline is more marked in women. One of the few known aetiological associations of this tumour is pernicious anaemia in which the risk of developing gastric cancer is some four to five times higher than in the general population (Blackburn, Callender and Dacie, 1968). It has been suggested that this association might be related to the increased frequency of blood group A, which occurs in both conditions, but it now seems unlikely that tumour frequency is dependent on blood groups (Callender et al, 1971).

The possible significance of some of these observations has been assisted by studies of the incidence of gastric carcinoma in different geographical areas. Incidence rates are very high in Japan, Finland and neighbouring territories of the USSR, Colombia and some other parts of eastern South America. There also appears to be a relatively high frequency in parts of the Nile–Congo watershed which include eastern Zaire, around Lake Kivu, the countries of Rwanda and Burundi and the West Lake Province of Tanzania (Gigasse, Clemmensen and Maisin, 1962). This tumour is also common in the environs of Mount Kilimanjaro. These high incidence areas contrast with the rest of Africa where rates are relatively low. The distribution of gastric carcinoma is entirely different from that of oesophageal or colon carcinoma. The importance of environmental factors in these high incidence areas has been demonstrated by studies on migrant groups. The incidence rates in Japanese who have migrated to the USA decreases in the first generation, but even in the second generation the rates are slightly higher than those in Americans of European descent (Haenszel and Kurihara, 1968; Haenszel, 1958). A similar decline in incidence has been shown in Japanese who migrate to Hawaii (Haenszel, 1961). In 1965, Lauren emphasised that there were two main types of gastric carcinoma, a diffuse (D) and an intestinal or adenocarcinomatous variety (I). It was suggested that these two types might be caused by different aetiological factors and that the intestinal type might be associated with chronic atrophic gastritis and intestinal metaplasia. Munoz et al (1968), who studied high and low incidence areas in Colombia and Mexico, concluded that the intestinal type occurred predominantly in high risk areas, whereas the diffuse type was more frequent in low risk areas. However, a comparison of the histology of gastric carcinomas in 800 Japanese and 627 American cases suggested that the age of the patient was a more important determinant (Kubo, 1971), the intestinal type of carcinoma being more common in both countries in patients over the age of 50. In Japan, younger patients were predominant and there was therefore a high proportion of diffuse carcinomas. Studies on Japanese migrants to Hawaii (Correa et al, 1973) showed, however, that the decline in overall incidence of gastric carcinoma after migration was due to a decrease in the intestinal type of gastric carcinoma. They also found that the association between blood group A and this tumour was limited to the diffuse variety.

In Colombia, South America, the highest incidence of gastric carcinoma occurs in the mountainous southern region around Narino. In contrast, the incidence in the coastal belt is low. Studies on the gastric mucosa from routine necropsies in Cali showed that intestinal metaplasia associated with chronic gastritis was present in 58.4 per cent of those people who originated from the high incidence areas but in only 21.3 per cent of those from the coastal belt (Correa, Cuello and Dugue, 1970). An association between chronic atrophic gastritis and a high frequency of gastric carcinoma has also been reported from Finland (Siurala, Varis and Wiljasalo, 1966) where 9 of 116 patients with atrophic gastritis, diagnosed by gastric biopsies, eventually developed gastric carcinoma. In contrast, only 1 of 261 subjects who originally had a normal mucosa developed cancer and this one developed an atrophic gastritis before the tumour appeared (Siurala et al, 1966). The association between atrophic gastritis and gastric carcinoma raises the question as to whether the development of the tumour is due to two or more factors or whether a single factor causes both conditions. There is also evidence from studies in Finland that there is a higher frequency of chronic atrophic gastritis in the relatives of patients with gastric carcinoma. This suggests that there may be a genetic component in the gastritis–carcinoma relationship (Kekki et al, 1973).

Investigations of aetiological factors that might be responsible for gastric cancer have lagged behind descriptive epidemiological observations. The high nitrate content of the soil in the high incidence areas of Colombia (Correa et al, 1970) is consistent with the suggestion that nitrosamines might be implicated in gastric carcinoma (Hill, Hawksworth and Tattersall, 1973). A recent report from Chile (Armijo and Coulson, 1975), where stomach cancer accounts for 30 per cent of deaths from malignant neoplasms, throws some new light on possible carcinogenic factors. Within the country there are high and low risk areas. Those provinces of highest risk are agricultural and a strong correlation was found between death rates and cumulative per capita exposure to nitrogen fertilisers which have been extensively used in the last 30 years. There was no correlation with several socioeconomic conditions.

In Japan, it has been suggested that ingestion of rice coated with talc (carcinogenic silicates) may play a role in the aetiology of carcinoma of the stomach (Matsudo, Hodgkin and Tanaka, 1974). It seems more likely that the high incidence is due to some general features of the Japanese diet. A relationship has been reported between the consumption of salted fish and gastric cancer. Fish preserved by the use of crude salt may contain nitrate, which can be reduced to nitrite (Weisburger and Raineri, 1975). The high level of methylguanidine in fish may, upon ingestion, result in the formation of the carcinogens, methylnitrosocyanamide and methylnitrosourea (Endo et al, 1974). Whatever factor, or factors, that are present in the Japanese diet and account for the high incidence of gastric carcinoma, it is evident that the change to a more Western type of diet is associated with a fall in the incidence in Japan (Oiso, 1975).

Carcinoma of the Large Bowel

In contrast to the curious focal geographical patterns of oesophageal and gastric carcinoma the incidence of carcinoma of the large bowel can be correlated very closely with the degree of Western civilisation of a country or area. The highest rates are found in the USA and UK and the lowest rates in the rural areas of developing countries (Doll, 1969; Burkitt, 1971). Japan is an exception in the sense that it is an affluent, urbanised country, but it has significantly lower rates than Europe. Migration to high incidence areas is associated with an increasing rate (Buell and Dunn, 1965; Burkitt, 1971). It is of particular significance that the incidence in black and white Americans today is closely comparable.

In regions where large bowel cancer is rare, adenomatous polyps are almost unknown. Bremner and Ackerman (1970) found only six in a 12-year survey of all surgical biopsies in a 2000 bed hospital in Johannesburg and in a series of 14 000 autopsies at the same hospital no polyps were found. Hutt and Templeton (1971) found only one adenomatous polyp of the large bowel in over 40 000 surgical specimens from Africans in Uganda and they are also uncommon in Nigerians (Williams et al, 1975). In these populations polyps are less frequent than cancers of the bowel (Hutt and Templeton, 1971). Benign and malignant tumours of the bowel are not only related in their geographical distribution but also in their anatomical distribution within the colon and rectum (Bockus et al, 1961). This suggests that they may share common aetiological factors.

It is now generally agreed that dietary factors are predominantly responsible for these tumours, but it seems likely that the carcinogen is not ingested, or at least not in an active form. Taking into account the enormous preponderance in mucosal surface of the small bowel relative to the large bowel, the latter is over

10 000 times more likely to develop tumours. This suggests that some carcinogen is formed or activated in the colon. Moreover, the fact that experimentally induced tumours do not develop when the animals are kept in a sterile environment suggests that faecal bacteria play a role in the aetiology of large bowel cancer (Spjut and Spratt, 1965). Hill et al (1971), Hill and Aries (1971) and Hill and Drasar (1974) have shown that certain anaerobic bacteria, in particular *Clostridia paraputrificum*, are more prevalent in faeces from areas of high, as compared with those of low, prevalences of bowel cancer and that this is associated with higher faecal bile acid concentrations. They have also demonstrated a relatively increased frequency of these organisms and high faecal bile acid concentrations in patients with large bowel cancer (Crowther et al, 1976), and have shown that these organisms can dehydrogenate the steroid nucleus of the bile salts to produce an active carcinogen. Since the latter are closely related chemically to known powerful carcinogens, it seems reasonable to suspect that certain products of bacterial action in the bowel might be carcinogenic (Hill and Drasar, 1974).

It is still not clear which factors in a Western type of diet are responsible for the unusual flora and high concentration of bile acids in faecal contents. The role of fibre in bowel physiology and in the aetiology of large bowel carcinoma has been emphasised by Burkitt (1971, 1975). An increase in the fibre content of the diet is associated with an increase in stool bulk and a more rapid bowel transit time. There is also evidence that some forms of fibre will reduce the concentration of faecal bile acids by increasing their excretion. This combination of effects might lower the concentration of any carcinogen formed and decrease its activity on the mucosa. The relative role of different types of fibre, which is chemically complex, is now being investigated. It has been shown that the amount of fat in the diet plays an important role in determining both bowel flora and bile acid concentration (Hill, 1971, 1975; Reddy et al, 1975). There is also a close epidemiological relationship between the incidence of carcinoma of the large bowel and other diseases associated with high dietary fat and low dietary fibre. These include ischaemic heart disease, cholelithiasis, and diverticular disease (Burkitt and Trowell, 1975).

Other workers have emphasised the possible role of a high protein diet. In a recent survey of large bowel cancer in Cali, Colombia, a marked social class gradient was found with the upper socioeconomic groups having the highest incidence. The main dietary differences between the groups were in the protein intake which was much higher in the richer section of the population (Haenszel, Correa and Cuello, 1975). There is also evidence that American Seventh Day Adventists who follow a lacto-ovo-vegetarian diet have a lower incidence of large bowel cancer than other Americans; this diet has a relatively low content of meat protein (Phillips, 1975). However, Mormons also have a lower incidence of colon carcinoma and there are no general restrictions on their consumption of meat (Lyon et al, 1976).

The complex interrelationships between various aspects of diet in relation to the aetiology of large bowel carcinoma are still not clear. More detailed studies of specific groups with unusual dietary patterns in otherwise homogeneous populations may unravel some of these problems.

CARCINOMA OF THE LIVER

Liver Cell Carcinoma

Age-specific incidence rates for primary liver cell carcinoma show marked differences throughout the world (Doll et al, 1966; 1970). High rates are found in the indigenous populations throughout the greater part of sub-Saharan Africa and large areas of the Far East (Hutt, 1971; Gibson, 1971). The highest rate is found in men in Mozambique where it reaches 98.2 per 100 000 per year (Prates and Torres, 1965). Examination of the records of admissions to the first mission hospital to be established in Uganda in 1897 shows that liver cell carcinoma was a common tumour at that time (Davies et al, 1964). In all high incidence areas epidemiological evidence suggests that the responsible factors lie in the rural environment and that poverty is a contributory factor (Alpert, Hutt and Davidson, 1968). The incidence decreases in Africans who have moved into an urban environment (Robertson, Harrington and Bradshaw, 1971).

No discussion of the aetiological factors responsible for liver cell carcinoma is possible without first considering its relationship to hepatic cirrhosis. There is no doubt that in both low and high incidence areas of liver cell carcinoma, those with cirrhosis have an increased risk of developing cancer. However, this risk appears to be greater in high incidence areas, a fact that may be related to the morphological type of cirrhosis or to its aetiology. Malignant change occurs more frequently in macronodular than in micronodular cirrhosis and the variants of the former predominate in Africa and the Far East (Steiner and Davies, 1957; Anthony et al, 1972). This close association with macronodular cirrhosis may explain why liver cell carcinoma is not common in France where the common cirrhosis due to alcoholism is micronodular. There is some evidence to suggest, however, that with improved treatment for alcoholic cirrhosis a macronodular pattern develops, and this is associated with an increased frequency of liver cell carcinoma (MacSween and Scott, 1974). In considering the aetiological agents that might be responsible for liver cell carcinoma in high incidence areas it must be recognised that the tumour may develop in the absence of cirrhosis in young people, suggesting that a large dose of carcinogen may induce tumour formation without producing chronic liver damage.

There is little evidence to suggest that either childhood or adult malnutrition play an important role in the development of cirrhosis in high incidence areas. During recent years attention has been increasingly focused on two agents, both of which are present in tropical environments and may affect man. In areas with a high incidence of primary liver cell carcinoma the carriage rate for hepatitis B surface antigen (HB_sAg) in the general population is high and may exceed 5 per cent (Williams et al, 1972). In such areas the frequency of HB_sAg in cases of cirrhosis or liver cell carcinoma is high and may reach 50 to 60 per cent (Vogel et al, 1970; Prince et al, 1970; Bagshawe, Parker and Jindani, 1971; Lowenthal et al, 1973). Maupas et al (1975) have shown that antibody to hepatitis B core antigen (anti-HBc) is found more frequently in patients with liver cell carcinoma than in controls. In Asia and Africa anti-HBc was shown to be present in 70 to 95 per cent of patients with liver cancer and in 20 to 69 per cent of controls; in the USA the corresponding figures were 24 and 4 per cent. This evidence has led to the suggestion that primary liver cell carcinoma may arise in a cirrhotic liver following hepatitis due to HBAg, though it is also possible that the virus itself may have oncogenic properties (*British Medical Journal*, 1975). In Uganda, Anthony, Vogel and Barker (1973) have also shown a relationship between liver cell dysplasia in cirrhotics and the presence of HBAg.

The discovery of the aflatoxins, metabolites of the fungus, *Aspergillus flavus*, opened up a new line of investigation of the aetiology of liver cell carcinoma. The carcinogenic activity of toxic groundnut meal was first shown in rats by Lancaster, Jenkins and McPhilip (1961). Since that time liver cell carcinomas have been induced by aflatoxins, particularly aflatoxin B_1, in a variety of animal species. The use of repeated small doses in primates has produced cirrhosis with hepatoma developing in some survivors (Lin, Lin and Svoboda, 1974). In 1962, Le Breton, Frayssinet and Boy suggested that contamination of dietary staples could be an important aetiological factor in human liver cell carcinoma. Keen and Martin (1971) found a very high incidence of liver cell carcinoma in immigrant Shangaans living in Swaziland and observed that their food storage and dietary customs increased the opportunities for the ingestion of aflatoxin-contaminated groundnuts. In Uganda, Alpert et al (1971) demonstrated a relationship between the incidence of liver cell carcinoma in different areas and the degree of contamination of market samples of food from these areas. Although most commonly associated with groundnuts, aflatoxin has also been demonstrated in a wide range of foods (Loosmore et al, 1964). A close association between the amount of aflatoxin in food samples and the incidence of liver cell carcinoma was demonstrated by Peers and Linsell (1973) in three areas of different altitude in the Muranga district of Kenya. The tumour incidence and the degree of contamination were greater in the lower altitude areas character-ised by a hot humid climate. In Thailand, Shank, Gibson and Wogan (1972) studied three randomly chosen villages from three areas in which the aflatoxin contamination of food had been estimated. The incidence of liver cell carcinoma in the village where concentration of aflatoxin was the highest was three times as high as that in the one where it was the lowest. A very high aflatoxin consumption has also been demonstrated in the Inhambane district of Mozambique where there is a uniquely high incidence of liver cell carcinoma (Van Rensburg, van der Watt and Purchase, 1974). These data indicate that there is a definite correlation between the degree to which foodstuffs are contaminated with aflatoxin and the incidence of liver cell carcinoma in an area. Although such relationships do not prove causation they are sufficiently strong, when taken with other evidence, to suggest that measures should be taken to reduce the contamination of cereals by toxin-producing fungi in tropical areas.

In the three areas of the Maranga district of Kenya investigated for aflatoxin levels by Peers and Linsell, there was no significant difference in the frequency of HBAg between the high and low altitude areas (Bagshawe et al, 1975). It is clear, nevertheless, that the population in all high incidence areas of liver cell carcinoma is exposed to both agents which may act synergistically. Urbanisation is likely to decrease the exposure to both and this could explain the falling incidence in the urban African population of Johannesburg.

The possible complex interrelationships of HB-antigenaemia, mycohepatotoxins, particularly aflatoxin B_1 and other cofactors are discussed by Coady (1976). He suggests that not only are these hepatotoxic agents common in areas of high incidence, but that either, or both, may affect immunological responses which may, in turn, affect the degree of liver damage or persistence of antigenaemia. The host responses may also be influenced by genetic and other environmental factors such as specific nutritional deficiencies or plant toxins.

Adenoma of the Liver and Oral Contraceptives

In 1973, Baum and her colleagues described the occurrence of benign hepatic adenomas in seven women who had been taking oral contraceptives. During the following six months four other case-reports were published. In 1974, O'Sullivan and Wilding described three cases of tumour-like lesions in women who had been on contraceptives for long periods. The histological features of these lesions were abnormally arranged nodules of liver tissue separated by fibrous trabeculae, associated with bile duct proliferation; thin-walled vascular channels were also a prominent feature. The authors originally described these lesions as liver hamartomas, but the term 'focal nodular hyperplasia' is more generally used (O'Sullivan, 1976). Over 50 cases of benign liver nodules have now been reported in women who have taken oral contraceptives. While some have been found incidentally at laparotomy, several have presented with haemoperitoneum as a result of haemorrhage from surface vessels, and some patients have died from this complication. There seems to be little doubt that there has been a true increase in the frequency of hepatic adenomas during the period of time that women have been on the contraceptive pill, as this tumour was extremely rare. Focal nodular hyperplasia has been recognised for many years but there are more reports of this condition in the last 20 years. It is still too early to be certain that there is a direct cause-effect relationship between oral contraceptives and these two conditions and the possible risk does not appear to be a contraindication to their use.

Of more concern are two reports of the development of liver cell carcinoma in women on the pill (Davis et al, 1975; Thalassinos et al, 1974), and one of hepatoblastoma (Meyer, LiVolsi and Cornog, 1974). The administration of anabolic steroids, which are closely related to synthetic progestogens, has also been associated with the development of nodular hyperplasia (Sweeney and Evans, 1976), adenoma (Bruguera, 1975) and liver cell carcinoma (Sherlock, 1975). The need for careful registration of all cases of nodular hyperplasia and adenomas of the liver is apparent; only by this means will the risks of hormonal therapy be adequately evaluated and the relationship of the association understood.

Liver Tumours Associated with Industrial Hazards

During the last 25 years there has been an increasing recognition of the carcinogenic hazards associated with various occupations. These are discussed by Doll (1975); only one will be considered in this chapter, vinyl chloride and angiosarcoma of the liver.

Although it has been recognised for some years that workers exposed to vinyl chloride may develop toxic effects such as acre-osteolysis and Raynaud's phenomenon, it was not until 1974 that Creech and Johnson reported three cases of hepatic angiosarcoma in men working with this substance. Since then further cases have been reported from the United States and Europe (Heath, Falk and Creech, 1975; Lange et al, 1974; Lee and Harry, 1974). The length of exposure to vinyl chloride monomers, which are used in the production of polyvinyl chloride, ranged from 12 to 19 years and all the tumours occurred in men exposed to these substances.

MALIGNANT LYMPHOMAS

Although questions of nomenclature and classification still present problems to the epidemiologist studying these tumours, one systematic international study has been done in which uniform diagnostic criteria were used (Correa and O'Conor, 1973). This study draws attention to marked differences in relative frequencies of lymphoreticular tumours in different parts of the world. As a result of this study the authors suggested that the countries involved could be placed into five categories.

(a) Nigeria and Papua–New Guinea: There is a high frequency of Burkitt's lymphoma. Hodgkin's disease is unusually common in children and does not show an incidence peak in young adults; in Nigeria there is a high frequency of histological types with a poor prognosis.

(b) Peru, Colombia, and El Salvador: Burkitt's lymphoma is rare. Hodgkin's disease has a similar pattern to Nigeria. Lymphosarcoma has a high frequency in children.

(c) Egypt, Singapore, Brazil, and Israel: Burkitt's lymphoma is rare. There is a high proportion of Hodgkin's disease in children and a rise in young adults with a relatively high proportion of the nodular sclerosing subtype in both age groups.

(d) Norway (characteristic of Europe and USA): Lymphomas of all types are rare in children. Hodgkin's disease has a bimodal age-specific rate and a predominance of nodular sclerosing subtypes.

(e) Japan: There is a low frequency of Hodgkin's disease and a high frequency of reticulum cell sarcoma (histiocytic or large cell lymphoma).

These authors also drew attention to the peculiar syndrome of Mediterranean lymphoma (vide infra). The complex environmental factors which underlie these differences in geographical incidence are yet to be resolved and only those associated with Mediterranean lymphoma, Hodgkin's disease and Burkitt's lymphoma will be considered.

Primary Intestinal Lymphoma (So-called Mediterranean Lymphoma)

Although it has been known for many years that various histological types of lymphoma may involve the gastrointestinal tract, either primarily or in association with lymphoma elsewhere, it is only recently that a geographically distinct type of upper small intestinal lymphoma has been described (Haghighi and Nasr, 1973).

Azar (1962) reviewing lymphomas seen in Beirut, Lebanon, found that 8.6 per cent originated in the gastrointestinal tract and that the majority of these started in the small bowel. The high frequency of upper intestinal lymphoma in Israel was reported by Ramot, Shakin and Bubis (1975) and Eidelman, Parkins and Rubin (1966), who observed that these cases were often associated with malabsorption. Similar cases were described in Iran by Nasr et al (1970) and the high frequency in several Middle Eastern countries resulted, perhaps unfortunately, in the use of the term Mediterranean lymphoma. Three cases have been reported in Italy but similar cases may be seen elsewhere and there is no evidence that the whole Mediterranean area is affected.

The condition is characterised clinically by abdominal pain and diarrhoea associated with malabsorption. The lymphoma is usually confined to the upper part of the small intestine and may be infiltrative, ulcerative or nodular (Ramot et al, 1965; Haghighi and Nasr, 1973); the mesenteric lymph nodes are often involved. Histologically the cell type is usually lymphoblastic or reticulum cell though plasmacytoid types have also been reported. In 1968, Seligmann et al described a young Syrian woman with this condition, a plasmacytoid cell in the tumour infiltrate, and α-1-heavy chain related to the Fc fragment in the serum. Cases of α-chain disease, as it is now called, have also been reported from Iran (Ala and Kodadoust, 1972), Israel (Ramot, 1972) and Lebanon (Shahid et al, 1974).

The epidemiological and geographical features of this disease show a high frequency in a relatively localised area of the Middle East and it involves two distinct ethnic groups, Jews and Arabs. The frequent occurrence of the condition in young adults suggests that causal factors should be sought in early life. The affected individuals in all populations tend to come from the underprivileged in terms of nutrition and hygiene. Both of these factors are associated with a high incidence of gastroenteritis in children and this leads to changes in the upper small intestinal mucosa and to secondary malabsorption. In Iran and other parts of the Middle East jejunal biopsies performed on apparently normal villagers from affected areas show villous atrophy (Haghighi and Nasr, 1973), and autopsies on children dying with diarrhoea and marasmus show structural abnormalities in the small intestine (Dutz et al, 1971). These authors have also demonstrated marked depression of humoral immunity in the marasmic infants and it has been postulated that these profound changes occurring at an early stage of life may predispose to lymphomatous change in later life. Alternatively the abnormal small gut may be more susceptible to unidentified carcinogenic agents.

Hodgkin's Disease

Although there is general agreement that Hodgkin's disease is a malignant neoplasm of lymphoid tissue, the clinical and histological features indicate a complex host–tumour reaction and this has suggested that an infectious agent might be involved. The broad epidemiological features that have already been described show variations in the age-incidence and histological subtypes in different parts of the world (Correa and O'Conor, 1973). This suggests that environmental factors, possibly acting from an early age, play an important role in the aetiology. Some authors (MacMahon, 1957, 1966) have suggested that the bimodal distribution found in some areas may reflect two entities, but at the moment it would seem better to regard Hodgkin's disease as one disease with varying manifestations.

The possibility that a transmissable agent is involved was brought to the fore by the observations that the condition may occur in 'epidemics' (Vianna, Greenwald and Davies, 1971b, c, Vianna et al, 1972). They found that an unusual number of cases had occurred in a group of close friends attending a high school in Albany, New York State, and in other individuals who had had contact with them. During a period of two decades there were 31 cases who could be linked in this way, though in eight this was through a healthy contact. This suggested that members of the original group might transmit the disease without being affected. These authors also found that the incidence of Hodgkin's disease in Albany County was significantly higher than in the rest of New York State over a period of eight years and that this was followed by a low incidence rate with a rise in the mean age at the time of diagnosis.

Vianna and Polan (1973) later observed that in five out of eight public schools in New York State, with an index case of Hodgkin's disease, further cases developed in the next quinquennium. In 16 matched schools there were no cases during this period.

An increased mortality from Hodgkin's disease among doctors and dentists has also been reported from New York State (Vianna et al, 1974), but this has not been found in a British study (Smith, Kinlen and Doll, 1974).

The possibility that Hodgkin's disease may be due to a virus of low-grade virulence and infectivity, which enters the host via the oral–respiratory tract was suggested by Vianna, Greenwald and Davies (1971a). They found a significantly higher frequency of previous tonsillectomy in cases, as compared with controls. Although this relationship has not been evident in all studies (Ruuskanen, Vanha-Perttula and Koubalainen, 1971) further analysis of the original data suggests that tonsillectomy is associated with an increased liability to Hodgkin's disease. There has been some speculation that EB virus, a possible aetiological agent in Burkitt's lymphoma, may play a role in the aetiology. However, there appears to be no difference between antibody titres in cases and age-matched controls (Goldman and Aisenberg, 1970) and it seems unlikely that EB virus is a direct aetiological agent.

Studies of Hodgkin's disease in families have shown a greater similarity in the time of onset than in the age of onset and also that the time interval between cases is shorter when the two individuals lived in the same household (MacMahon, 1966; Vianna et al, 1974). These observations point to an environmental, rather than a genetic factor. However, the similarity of Rye histological subtypes in familial pairs and the association of Hodgkin's disease with certain histocompatibility antigens suggests that genetic factors may play a role in determining the host reaction to the aetiological agents (Honeymoon and Meneer, 1974).

Although recent epidemiological investigations of Hodgkin's disease have not indicated any clear-cut aetiological factors, the differences in pattern of the disease between the Western world and Africa suggests environmental influences. It is of interest that the mortality rates of African and Asian born Jews living in Israel is higher than that of Jews born in Europe (Abramson, Avitzour and Peritz, 1975). Detailed epidemiological investigations on such immigrant populations may help to unravel the nature of this controversial tumour.

Burkitt's Lymphoma

This tumour was first described as a clinical syndrome with a variety of different presentations by Burkitt in 1958. It was later shown by O'Conor and Davies (1960) that the different clinical manifestations were all due to identical pathological tissue, and that the tumour was a form of lymphoma. Subsequently Wright (1963) demonstrated that it could be distinguished from other forms of lymphoma on histological and cytological criteria.

This tumour usually affects young children over the age of two years, with a maximum frequency in the middle of the first decade. Patients frequently present with tumours in one or more quadrants of the jaw, but the initial lesion may be in other sites such as the ovaries in young girls. It is the commonest childhood neoplasm in much of sub-Saharan Africa and in Papua–New Guinea; the tumour is occasionally seen in non-tropical areas (Burkitt, 1967) and may have an intermediate frequency in parts of Brazil and Malaysia. In both high incidence areas the tumour is limited to well-defined geographical areas; these are related to climatic factors and consist of regions within which the temperature does not fall below approximately 60°F (16°C) and the annual rainfall exceeds 20 in. (51 cm) (Burkitt and Wright, 1970). It is now believed that the distribution of the tumour is related to conditions in which there is intense infection with *Plasmodium falciparum* malaria (Dalldorf et al, 1964; Burkitt, 1969). The role of EB virus (Epstein–Barr virus), which was originally isolated from a tissue culture of Burkitt lymphoma cells (Epstein, Achong and Barr, 1964) is still under investigation. This virus is now known to be the cause of infectious mononucleosis, a self-limiting lymphoproliferative disease which is rarely seen in areas where Burkitt's lymphoma is common. In these areas infection is widespread in children but they do not show the clinical manifestations of infectious mononucleosis. Patients with Burkitt's lymphoma all have antibodies against EB virus, often to very high titres (Epstein and Achong, 1973; Klein, 1972). The likelihood of EB virus as a possible causative agent has been increased by observations that it can transform normal white cells into permanently growing lymphoblasts and that these in vitro transformed cells, as well as Burkitt lymphoma cells, have EB specific antigens (Epstein and Achong, 1973; Reedman and Klein, 1973).

The possible role of malaria as a cofactor in the aetiology of Burkitt's lymphoma was demonstrated by the observation that the oncogenic potential of a virus is enhanced by prior infection with malaria; this effect appears to be due to immunodepression (Wedderburn, 1970), though the effects of malaria in the lymphoreticular and immunological systems are very complex. Our current knowledge of the epidemiology of this tumour can be best explained by the hypothesis that EB virus infection in a population exposed to endemic *P. falciparum* infections will result in tumour formation in a proportion of the population (Burkitt, 1969).

CARCINOMA OF THE BREAST

The incidence of breast cancer has a very similar picture to that of large bowel cancer. It is the commonest malignant tumour in women in the Western world and has a much lower incidence in developing countries, particularly among the poor. In Bombay, the age-adjusted rates for breast cancer are much higher in Parsi women than in the general population (Jussawalla et al, 1970); the social and cultural pattern of Parsi life is recognised as being more 'European' than other Indian groups. In Uganda, the incidence of breast carcinoma in Europeans is high and that in indigenous Africans is low, with the Indian community having an intermediate frequency. In all communities there appears to be a close relationship between the frequency of cancer and of fibroadenosis of the breast suggesting that similar factors operate in their aetiology. Studies on Japanese women, who have a relatively low incidence of breast carcinoma, show that there is an increased rate in women who have migrated to America; this is evident in the second generation but does not reach American rates (Buell, 1973). These geographical and ethnic differences in incidence have been attributed to genetic, hormonal and dietary factors. The occurrence of families with a high incidence of breast cancer has been known for many years (Lilienfeld, 1963) and it has been suggested that this may be dependent on patterns of steroid hormones which may be, in part, genetically determined. In high incidence populations, such as Britain, breast cancer is more common in the unmarried and in the upper socioeconomic groups. It was originally thought that these associations might be related to parity and to breast feeding, both of which offered protection. It was subsequently shown that the association with parity was secondary to an association with the age of the woman at the time of their first pregnancy (MacMahon, Cole and Brown, 1973). The breast cancer risk for women having their first baby under the age of 20 in different parts of the world is about half that for nulliparous women (MacMahon et al, 1970a, b). There does not appear to be any direct association with lactation.

In the United States, epidemiological studies have shown a significantly increased risk of breast cancer in both maternal and paternal aunts. In the mothers of breast cancer patients the age at the time of first delivery and the age at the time of the menopause were greater than in controls (Henderson et al, 1974); these authors also suggested that the increased risk in these families may be related to their pattern of oestrogen secretion or metabolism.

Craig, Comstock and Geiser (1974) examined risk factors in a cross-section of American women. They suggested that early onset breast cancer (before 45 years) was associated with a positive family history and the experience of first childbirth, and that late onset cases were associated with lactation as a risk factor. Hems and Stuart (1975) in a study of single (never-married) women were unable to find any evidence that dietary factors play a role in the aetiology of breast cancer.

The role of hormones in the aetiology has assumed an increased importance with the prolonged administration of oral contraceptives and replacement oestrogen therapy after the menopause. There appears to be conclusive evidence that long-term administration of contraceptive pills is associated with a decrease in the incidence of benign fibroadenosis of the breast (Kelsey, Lindfors and White, 1974).

Prolonged postmenopausal hormonal treatment appears to be associated with a decreased risk of breast cancer (Henderson et al, 1974). Case-control studies in Britain have produced no evidence to suggest that women on the contraceptive pill have an increased risk and breast cancer in Britain is not increasing in frequency (Vessey, Doll and Jones, 1975). Another possible iatrogenic factor was raised by the observations of the Boston Collaborative Drug Surveillance Programme (1974), that breast cancer was more common in women who were being treated for hypertension with Rauwolfia. This risk has since been noted in studies in the Oxford region (Armstrong. Stevens and Doll, 1974) and in Finland (Heinonen et al, 1974). Further studies are required to assess the factors which determine this risk.

The complex interplay of genetic and environmental factors are well illustrated by these epidemiological observations on breast cancer and the mechanisms by which these factors operate are still imperfectly understood.

CONCLUSIONS

Although not all of the epidemiological studies considered in this chapter have led to an elucidation of the causal factors for each particular tumour, all have increased our knowledge of the aetiology and pathogenesis of tumours. In certain instances, such as the association between cigarette smoking and lung cancer, sufficient evidence is available on which to base a preventive campaign; intervention studies might also be initiated to reduce the incidence of liver cell carcinoma in the tropics by reducing aflatoxin contamination of foods, and the possibility of widescale prophylaxis of malaria in areas where Burkitt's lymphoma is common might be considered. Apart from these immediate applications to the problem in man, epidemiology has provided the data on which hypotheses can be erected. Such hypotheses can then be examined in laboratory models and by investigations in man. Our present knowledge of viral oncogenicity has resulted, at least in part, from the studies of Burkitt's lymphoma, and of the role of bacteria as producers of carcinogens from studies of the epidemiology of large bowel cancer. Nature's experiments in the field of tumours may provide the necessary clues on which new hypotheses can be formulated and tested (Hutt, 1973).

REFERENCES

Abramson, J. H., Avitzour, M. & Peritz, E. (1975) Mortality from lymphomas in Israel, 1950–71: the possible role of environmental factors. *International Journal of Epidemiology,* **4**, 321–329.
Ala, F. A. & Khodadoust, J. (1972) Alpha-chain disease in Iran. *Third Pahlavi Medical Congress,* Shiraz, Iran.
Alpert, M. E., Hutt, M. S. R. & Davidson, C. S. (1968) Hepatoma in Uganda: a study in geographic pathology. *Lancet,* **1**, 1265–1266.
Alpert, M. E., Hutt, M. S. R., Wogan, G. N. & Davidson, C. S. (1971) Association between aflatoxin content of food and hepatoma frequency in Uganda. *Cancer,* **28**, 253–260.
Anthony, P. P., Vogel, C. L., Sadikali, F., Barker, L. F. & Peterson, M. R. (1972) Hepatitis-associated antigen and antibody in Uganda: correlation of serological testing with histopathology. *British Medical Journal,* **1**, 403–406.

Anthony, P. P., Vogel, C. L. & Barker, L. F. (1973) Liver cell dysplasia a premalignant condition. *Journal of Clinical Pathology*, **26**, 217–223.

Armijo, R. & Coulson, A. H. (1975) Epidemiology of stomach cancer in Chile — the role of nitrogen fertilisers. *International Journal of Epidemiology*, **4**, 301–309.

Armstrong, B., Stevens, N. & Doll, R. (1974) Retrospective study of the association between use of Rauwolfia derivatives and breast cancer in English women. *Lancet*, **2**, 672–675.

Azar, H. A. (1962) Cancer in Lebanon and the Near East. *Cancer*, **15**, 66–78.

Bagshawe, A. F., Parker, A. M. & Jindani, A. (1971) Hepatitis-associated antigen in liver disease in Kenya. *British Medical Journal*, **1**, 88–89.

Bagshawe, A. F., Gacengi, D. M., Cameron, C. H., Dorman, J. & Dane, D. S. (1975) Hepatitis Bs antigen and liver cancer. A population based study in Kenya. *British Journal of Cancer*, **31**, 581–584.

Baum, J. K., Holtz, F., Bookstein, J. J. & Klein, E. W. (1973) Possible association between benign hepatomas and oral contraceptives. *Lancet*, **2**, 926–929.

Blackburn, E. K., Callender, S. T. & Dacie, J. V. (1968) Possible association between pernicious anaemia and leukaemia: a prospective study of 1625 patients with a note on the very high incidence of stomach cancer. *International Journal of Cancer*, **3**, 163–170.

Bockus, H. L. Tschdjian, V., Ferguson, L. K., Mouhran, Y. & Chamberlain, C. (1961) Adenomatous polyp of colon and rectum: its relation to carcinoma. *Gastroenterology*, **41**, 225–232.

Boston Collaborative Drug Surveillance Programme (1973) *Lancet*, **1**, 1399–1404.

Boston Collaborative Drug Surveillance Programme (1974) *Lancet*, **2**, 669–671.

Bradshaw, E. & Schonland, M. (1974) Smoking, drinking and oesophageal cancer in African males in Johannesburg, South Africa. *British Journal of Cancer*, **30**, 157.

Bremner, C. G. & Ackerman, L. V. (1970) Polyps and carcinoma of the large bowel in the South African Bantu. *Cancer*, **26**, 991–999.

British Medical Journal (1975) Leading article: more on the aflatoxin–hepatoma story. **2**, 647.

Bruguera, M. (1975) Hepatoma associated with androgenic steroids. *Lancet*, **1**, 1295.

Buell, P. (1973) Changing incidence of breast cancer in Japanese and American women. *Journal of the National Cancer Institute*, **51**, 1479–1483.

Buell, P. & Dunn, J. E. (1965) Cancer mortality among the Japanese Issei and Nissei of California. *Cancer*, **18**, 656–664.

Burkitt, D. P. (1967) Burkitt's lymphoma outside the known endemic areas of Africa and New Guinea. *International Journal of Cancer*, **2**, 562–565.

Burkitt, D. P. (1969) Etiology of Burkitt's lymphoma — an alternative hypothesis to a vectored virus. *Journal of the National Cancer Institute*, **42** (1), 19–28.

Burkitt, D. P. & Wright, D. H. (1970) *Burkitt's Lymphoma*. London: E. and S. Livingstone.

Burkitt, D. P. (1975) Large bowel cancer: an epidemiologic jigsaw puzzle. *Journal of the National Cancer Institute*, **54**, 3–6.

Burkitt, D. P. (1971) Epidemiology of cancer of the colon and rectum. *Cancer*, **28**, 3–13.

Burkitt, D. P. & Trowell, H. C. (1975) *Refined Carbohydrate Foods and Disease. Some Implications of Dietary Fibre*. London, New York, San Francisco: Academic Press.

Burrell, R. J. W. (1957) Oesophageal cancer in the Bantu. *South African Medical Journal*, **31**, 401–409.

Burrell, R. J. W. (1962) Oesophageal cancer among the Bantu in the Transkei. *Journal of the National Cancer Institute*, **28**, 495.

Burrell, R. J. W., Roach, W. A. & Shadwell, A. (1966) Esophageal cancer in the Bantu of the Transkei associated with mineral deficiency in garden plants. *Journal of the National Cancer Institute*, **36**, 201–209.

Callender, S., Langman, M. J. S., MacLeod, I. N., Mosbech, J. & Rahtkens Nielsen, K. (1971) ABO blood groups in patients with gastric carcinoma associated with pernicious anaemia. *Gut*, **12**, 465–467.

Coady, A. (1976) Tropical cirrhosis and hepatomas. *Journal of the Royal College of Physicians*, **10**, 133–143.

Cook, P. (1971) Cancer of the oesophagus in Africa: a summary and evaluation of the evidence for the frequency of occurrence and a preliminary indication of the possible associations with the consumption of alcoholic drinks made from mazie. *British Journal of Cancer*, **25**, 853–880.

Coordinating Group for Research on the Etiology of Esophageal Cancer of North China (1975) The epidemiology of esophageal cancer in North China and preliminary results in the investigation of its etiological factors. *Scientia Sinica*, **18**, 131–148.

Correa, P., Cuello, C. & Dugue, E. (1970) Cancer and intestinal metaplasia of the stomach in Colombian migrants. *Journal of the National Cancer Institute*, **44**, 297.

Correa, P. & O'Conor, G. T. (1973) Geographic pathology of lymphoreticular tumors: summary of survey from the Geographic Pathology Committee of the Internation Union Against Cancer. *Journal of the National Cancer Institute*, **50**, 1609–1617.

Correa, P., Sasano, N., Stemmermann, G. N. & Haenszel, W. (1973) Pathology of gastric carcinoma in Japanese populations: comparisons between Miyagi Prefecture, Japan and Hawaii. *Journal of the National Cancer Institute*, **51**, 1449–1457.

Craig, T. J., Comstock, G. W. & Geiser, P. B. (1974) Epidemiologic comparison of breast cancer patients with early and late onset of malignancy and general population controls. *Journal of the National Cancer Institute*, **53**, 1577–1581.

Creech, J. L. & Johnson, M. N. (1974) Angiosarcoma of liver in the manufacture of polyvinyl chloride. *Journal of Occupational Medicine*, **16**, 150–151.

Crowther, J. S., Drasar, B. S., Hill, M. J., MacLennan, R., Magnin, D., Peach, S. & Teoh-Chan, C. H. (1976) Faecal steroids, bacteria and large bowel cancer in Hong Kong by socio-economic groups. *British Journal of Cancer*, **34**, 191.

Dalldorf, G., Linsell, C. A., Barnhart, F. E. & Martyn, R. (1964) An epidemiological approach to the lymphomas of African children. *Perspectives of Biological Medicine*, **7**, 435–449.

Davies, J. N. P., Elmes, S., Hutt, M. S. R., Mtimavalye, L. A. R., Owor, R. & Shaper, L. (1964) Cancer in an African community 1897–1956. An analysis of the records of Mengo Hospital, Kampala, Uganda. *British Medical Journal*, **1**, R58–264, 336–341.

Davis, M., Portman, B., Searle, M., Wright, R. & Williams, R. (1975) Histological evidence of carcinoma in a hepatic tumour associated with oral contraceptives. *British Medical Journal*, **4**, 496–498.

Doll, R. (1969) The geographical distribution of cancer. *British Journal of Cancer*, **23**, 1.

Doll, R. (1975) Pott and the prospects for prevention. *British Journal of Cancer*, **32**, 263–272.

Doll, R. & Hill, A. B. (1953) Bronchial carcinoma: incidence and aetiology. *British Medical Journal*, **2**, 505–506.

Doll, R. & Hill, A. B. (1964) The mortality of doctors in relation to their smoking habits. *British Medical Journal*, **1**, 1451–1452.

Doll, R., Payne, P. & Waterhouse, J. A. H. (1966) *Cancer Incidence in Five Continents Vol. I.* Berlin, Heidelberg, New York: UICC, Springer-Verlag.

Doll, R., Muir, C. S. & Waterhouse, J. A. H. (1970) *Cancer Incidence in Five Continents, Vol. II.* Berlin, Heidelberg, New York: UICC, Springer-Verlag.

Dutz, W., Asvadi, S., Sadri, S. & Kohout, E. (1971) Intestinal lymphoma and sprue: a systematic approach. *Gut*, **12**, 804–809.

Eidelman, S., Parkins, R. A. & Rubin, C. E. (1966) Abdominal lymphoma presenting as malabsorption: a clinico-pathologic study of nine cases in Israel and a review of the literature. *Medicine (Baltimore)*, **45**, 111–137.

Endo, H., Takahaski, K., Kinoshiba, N. & Bala, T. (1974) Production of gastric and oesophageal tumours in rats by methylnitrosocyanamide, a possible candidate of etiological factors for human gastric cancer. *Proceedings of the Japan Academy*, **50**, 497–502.

Epstein, M. A., Achong, B. G. & Barr, Y. M. (1964) Virus particles in cultured lymphoblasts from Burkitt's lymphoma. *Lancet*, **1**, 702–703.

Epstein, M. A. & Achong, B. G. (1973) The EB virus. *Annual Review of Microbiology*, ed. Starr, M. P., Ingraham, J. L. & Raffel, S., 413–436. *California Annual Reviews Inc.*

Gibson, J. B. (1971) *Parasites, Liver Disease and Liver Cancer.* IARC Scientific Publications, No. 1, p. 42. Lyon.

Gigasse, P., Clemmensen, J. & Maisin, J. (1962) Report to the University of Louvain, Belgian Congo.

Goldman, J. M. & Aisenberg, A. C. (1970) Incidence of antibody to EB virus, herpes simplex and cytomegalovirus in Hodgkin's disease. *Cancer (Philadelphia)*, **26**, 327–331.

Haenszel, W. (1958) Variation in incidence of and mortality from stomach cancer with particular reference to the United States. *Journal of the National Cancer Institute*, **21**, 213–262.

Haenszel, W. (1961) Cancer mortality among the foreign-born in the United States. *Journal of the National Cancer Institute*, **26**, 37–132.

Haenszel, W. & Kurihara, M. (1968) Study of Japanese migrants. I. Mortality from cancer and other diseases among Japanese in the United States. *Journal of the National Cancer Institute*, **40**, 43–68.

Haenszel, W., Correa, P. & Cuello, C. (1975) Social class differences among patients with large-bowel cancer in Cali, Colombia. *Journal of the National Cancer Institute*, **54**, 1031–1035.

Haghighi, P. & Nasr, K. (1973) Primary upper small intestinal lymphoma (so-called Mediterranean lymphoma). *Pathology Annual* 1973, ed. Sommers, S. C. New York: Appleton-Century-Crofts; Educational Division Meredith Corporation.

Hammond, E. C. (1974) The epidemiological approach to the etiology of cancer. *Cancer*, **35**, 652–654.

Heath, C. M., Falk, H. & Creech, J. L. (1975) Characteristics of cases of angiosarcoma of the liver among vinyl chloride workers in the United States. *Annals of the New York Academy of Science.*

Heinonen, O. P., Shapiro, S., Tuominen, L. & Turunen, M. I. (1974) Reserpine used in relation to breast cancer. *Lancet,* **2,** 675–677.

Hems, G. & Stuart, A. (1975) Breast cancer rates in populations of single women. *British Journal of Cancer,* **31,** 118–123.

Henderson, B. E., Powell, D., Rosarie, I., Keys, C., Hanisch, R., Young, M., Casagrande, J., Gerkins, V. & Pike, M. C. (1974) An epidemiologic study of breast cancer. *Journal of National Cancer Institute,* **53,** 609–614.

Herbst, A. L. & Scully, R. E. (1970) Adenocarcinoma of the vagina in adolescence. A report of seven cases including six clear-cell carcinomas (so-called mesonephromas). *Cancer,* **25,** 745–757.

Herbst, A. L., Poskanzer, D. C., Robboy, S. J., Friedlander, L. & Scully, R. E. (1975) Prenatal exposure to Stilbestrol: a prospective study. *New England Journal of Medicine,* **292,** 334–339.

Hill, M. J. (1971) The effect of some factors on the faecal concentration of acid steroids, neutral steroids and urobilins. *Journal of Pathology,* **104,** 239–245.

Hill, M. J. (1975) Metabolic epidemiology of dietary factors in large bowel cancer. *Cancer Research,* **35,** 3398–3402.

Hill, M. J. & Aries, V. C. (1971) Faecal steroid composition and its relationship to cancer of the large bowel. *Journal of Pathology,* **104,** 129–139.

Hill, M. J., Drasar, B. S., Aries, V. C., Crowther, J. S., Hawkesworth, G. M. & Williams, R. E. O. (1971) Bacteria and aetiology of cancer of the large bowel. *Lancet,* **1,** 95–100.

Hill, M. J., Hawkesworth, G. & Tattersall, G. (1973) Bacteria, nitrosamines and cancer of the stomach. *British Journal of Cancer,* **28,** 562–567.

Hill, M. J. & Drasar, B. S. (1974) Bacteria and the aetiology of cancer of the large bowel. In *Anaerobic Bacteria,* ed. Balows, A., De Haan, R. M., Dowell, U. R. & Guze, L. B. Springfield, Illinois: Charles C. Thomas.

Honeymoon, M. C. & Menser, M. A. (1975) Ethnicity is a significant factor in the epidemiology of rubella and Hodgkin's disease. *Nature,* **251,** 441–442.

Hormozdiari, H., Day, N. E., Aramesh, B. & Mahboubi, E. (1975) Dietary factors and oesophageal cancer in the Caspian Littoral of Iran. *Cancer Research,* **35,** 3493–3498.

Hutt, M. S. R. (1971) Epidemiology of human primary liver cancer. *Liver Cancer,* IARC Scientific Publications, No. 1, p. 21. Lyon.

Hutt, M. S. R. (1973) Nature's experiments and medical research. *Pathologica et microbiologica,* **39,** 167–176.

Hutt, M. S. R. & Templeton, A. C. (1971) The geographical pathology of bowel cancer and some related diseases. *Proceedings of the Royal Society of Medicine,* **64,** 962–964.

Jussawalla, D. J., Deshpande, V. A., Haenszel, W. & Natekar, M. V. (1970) Differences observed in the site of incidence of cancer, between the Parsi community and the total population of Greater Bombay: a critical appraisal. *British Journal of Cancer,* **24,** 56–66.

Kafuko, G. W. & Burkitt, D. P. (1970) Burkitt's lymphoma and malaria. *International Journal of Cancer,* **6,** 1.

Keen, P. (1971) *International Seminar on Epidemiology of Oesophageal Cancer, Bangalore, India,* Monograph No. 1.

Keen, P. & Martin, P. (1971) The toxicity of fungal infestation of foodstuffs in Swaziland in relation to harvesting and storage. *Tropical Geographical Medicine,* **23,** 35–43.

Kekki, M., Ihamaki, T., Varis, K. & Siurala, M. (1973) Age of gastric carcinoma patients and susceptibility to chronic gastritis in their relatives. A mathematical approach using Poisson's process and scoring of gastric state. *Scandinavian Journal of Gastroenterology,* **8,** 673–679.

Kelsey, J. L., Lindfors, K. K. & White, C. (1974) A case control study of the epidemiology of benign breast diseases with reference to oral contraceptive use. *International Journal of Epidemiology,* **3,** 333–340.

Kinlen, L. J., Badaracco, M. A., Moffet, J. & Vessey, M. P. (1974) A survey of the use of oestrogens during pregnancy in the UK and of the genito-urinary cancer mortality and incidence rates in young people in England and Wales. *Journal of Obstetrics and Gynaecology of the British Commonwealth,* **81,** 849–855.

Klein, G. (1972) Herpes viruses and oncogenesis. *Proceedings of the National Academy of Science, U.S.A.,* **69,** 1056–1064.

Kmet, J. & Mahboubi, E. (1972) Oesophageal cancer in the Caspian Littoral of Iran. *Science,* **175,** 846–853.

Kubo, T. (1971) Histologic appearances of gastric carcinoma in high and low mortality countries: comparison between Kyushu, Japan, and Minnesota, USA. *Cancer,* **28,** 726–734.

Lancaster, M. C., Jenkins, F. P. & McPhilip, J. (1961) Toxicity associated with certain samples of groundnuts. *Nature (London)*, **192**, 1095.

Lancet (1975) Leading article: Prenatal oestrogen — continued. **1**, 960–961.

Lange, C. E., Juhe, S., Stein, G. & Veltman, G. (1974) Further results in polyvinyl chloride production workers. *Annals of the New York Academy of Sciences*, **246**, 18–21.

Lauren, P. (1965) The two histological-main types of gastric carcinoma — diffuse and so-called intestinal type carcinoma. An attempt at a histo-clinical classification. *Acta pathologica et microbiologica scandinavica*, **64**, 31–49.

Le Breton, E., Frayssinet, C. & Boy, J. (1962) Sur l'apparition d'hepatomes 'spontanes' chez le rat Wistan. Role de la Toxine de l'*Aspergillus flavus*. Interet en pathologie, humaine et cancerologie experimentale. *Comptes rendus hebdomadaires des séances de l'Académie des sciences: D. Sciences naturelles*, **255**, 784.

Lee, F. L. & Harry, D. S. (1974) Angiosarcoma of the liver in a vinyl-chloride worker. *Lancet*, **1**, 1316–1318.

Lilienfeld, A. M. (1963) Epidemiology of breast cancer. *Cancer Research*, **23**, 1503–1513.

Lin, J. J., Liu, C. & Svoboda, D. J. (1974) Long-term effects of aflatoxin B1 and viral hepatitis on marmoset liver. A preliminary report. *Laboratory Investigations*, **30**, 267–278.

Loosmore, R. M., Allcroft, R., Tutton, E. A. & Carhaghan, R. B. A. (1964) The presence of aflatoxin in a sample of cottonseed cake. *Veterinary Record*, **76**, 64.

Lowenthal, M., Banatvala, J. E., Chrystie, I. L., Jones, I. G. Nag, J., Mohlesky, V. & Hutt, M. S. R. (1973) Australia antigen in liver disease in Zambia. *Tropical Geographical Medicine*, **25**, 39–44.

Lundin, F. E., Lloyd, J. W., Smith, E. M., Archer, V. E. & Holaday, D. A. (1969) Mortality of uranium miners in relation to radiation exposure, hard rock mining and cigarette smoking — 1950 through September 1957. *Health Physics*, **16**, 571–578.

Lyon, J. L., Klauber, M. R., Gardner, J. W. & Smart, C. R. (1976) Cancer incidence in Mormons and non-Mormons: Utah 1966–1970. *New England Journal of Medicine*, **294**, 129–133.

McGlashan, N. D. (1969) Oesophageal cancer and alcoholic spirits in Central Africa. *Gut*, **10**, 643–650.

MacMahon, B. (1957) Epidemiological evidence on the nature of Hodgkin's disease. *Cancer*, **10**, 1045–1054.

MacMahon, B. (1966) Epidemiology of Hodgkin's disease. *Cancer Research*, **26**, 1189–1200.

MacMahon, B., Lin, T. M., Lowe, C. R., Mirra, A. P., Ravnihar, B., Salber, E. J., Trichopoules, D., Valaoras, V. G. & Yussa, S. (1970a) Lactation and cancer of the breast. *Bulletin of the World Health Organisation*, **42**, 185.

MacMahon, B., Cole, P., Lin, T. M., Lowe, C. R., Mirra, A. P., Ravnihar, B., Salber, E. J., Valaoras, V. G. & Yussa, S. (1970b) Age at first birth and breast cancer risk. *Bulletin of the World Health Organisation*, **43**, 209.

MacMahon, B., Cole, P. & Brown, J. (1973) Etiology of human breast cancer: a review *Journal of the National Cancer Institute*, **5**, 21–42.

MacSween, R. N. M. & Scott, A. R. (1974) Hepatic cirrhosis. A clinicopathological review of 520 cases. *Journal of Clinical Pathology*, **26**, 936–942.

Magee, P. N. & Barnes, J. M. (1967) Carcinogenic nitroso compounds. *Advances in Cancer Research*, **10**, 163.

Mahboubi, E., Kmet, J., Cook, P. J., Day, N. E., Ghadirian, P. & Salmasijadeh, S. (1973) Oesophageal cancer studies in the Caspian Littoral of Iran. *British Journal of Cancer*, **28**, 197–214.

Matsudo, H., Hodgkin, N. N. & Tanaka, A. (1974) Japanese gastric cancer: potentially carcinogenic silicates (talc) from rice. *Archives of Pathology*, **97**, 366–368.

Maupas, P., Werner, B., Larouze, B., Millman, I., London, W. T., O'Connell, A., Blumberg, B. S., Saimot, G. & Payet, M. (1975) Antibody to hepatitis-B core antigen in patients with primary hepatic carcinoma. *Lancet*, **2**, 9–10.

Meyer, P., LiVolsi, V. A. & Cornog, J. L. (1974) Hepatoblastoma associated with an oral contraceptive. *Lancet*, **2**, 1387.

Munoz, N., Correa, P., Cuello, C. & Dugue, E. (1968) Histologic types of gastric carcinoma in high and low risk areas. *International Journal of Cancer*, **3**, 809–818.

Nasr, K., Haghighi, P., Bakshandeh, K. & Haglshenas, M. (1970) Primary lymphoma of the upper small intestine. *Gut*, **11**, 673–678.

O'Conor, G. T. & Davies, J. N. P. (1960) Malignant tumours in African children. *Journal of Paediatrics*, **56**, 526–535.

Oettlé, A. G. (1964) Cancer in Africa, especially in regions south of the Sahara. *Journal of the National Cancer Institute*, **33**, 383–439.

Oiso, T. (1975) Incidence of stomach cancer and its relation to dietary habits and nutrition in Japan between 1900 and 1975. *Cancer Research,* **35**, 3254-3258.

O'Sullivan, J. P. (1976) Oral contraceptives and liver tumours. *Proceedings of the Royal Society of Medicine,* **69**, 351-353.

O'Sullivan, J. P. & Wilding, R. P. (1974) Liver hamartomas in patients on oral contraceptives. *British Medical Journal,* **3**, 7-10.

Peers, F. G. & Linsell, C. A. (1973) Dietary aflatoxin and liver cancer — a population-based study in Kenya. *British Journal of Cancer,* **27**, 473.

Phillips, R. L. (1975) Role of life-style and dietary habits in risk of cancer among Seventh Day Adventists. *Cancer Research,* **35**, 3513-3522.

Phillips, M. J., Langer, B., Stone, R., Fisher, M. M. & Ritchie, S. (1973) Benign liver cell tumours classification and ultrastructural pathology. *Cancer,* **32**, 463-470.

Prates, M. D. & Torres, F. O. (1965) A cancer survey in Lourenco Marques, Portuguese East Africa. *Journal of the National Cancer Institute,* **35**, 729.

Prince, A. M., Leblanc, L., Krohn, K., Masseyeff, R. & Alpert, M. E. (1970) Serum hepatitis antigen and chronic liver disease. *Lancet,* **2**, 717-718.

Ramot, B. (1972) The relationship between intestinal lymphoma and heavy chain of IgA. *Abstracts of the Third Pahlavi Medical Congress,* Shiraz, Iran, p. 100.

Ramot, B., Shakin, N. & Bubis, J. J. (1965) Malabsorption syndrome in lymphoma of small intestine. A study of 13 cases. *Israel Journal of Medical Science,* **1**, 221-226.

Reddy, B. S., Narisawa, T., Maronpot, R., Weisburger, J. H. & Wynder, E. L. (1975) Animal models for the study of dietary factors and cancer of the large bowel. *Cancer Research,* **35**, 3421-3426.

Reedman, B. M. & Klein, G. (1973) Cellular localisation of an Epstein–Barr virus (EBV)-associated complement-fixing antigen in producer and non-producer lymphoblastoid cell lines. *International Journal of Cancer,* **11**, 499-517.

Reuber, M. D. (1975) Carcinomas of the esophagus in rats ingesting diethyl-nitrosamine. *European Journal of Cancer,* **11**, 97-99.

Robertson, M. A., Harrington, J. S. & Bradshaw, E. (1971) Cancer pattern in Africans at Baragwanath Hospital, Johannesburg. *British Journal of Cancer,* **25**, 378.

Ruuskanen, O., Vanha-Perttula, T. & Kouvalainen, K. (1971) Tonsillectomy, appendectomy and Hodgkin's disease. *Lancet,* **1**, 1127-1128.

Sartwell, P. E., Arthes, F. G. & Tonascia, J. A. (1973) Epidemiology of benign breast lesions: lack of association with oral contraceptive use. *New England Journal of Medicine,* **288**, 551-554.

Seligmann, M., Danon, F., Jurez, D., Mihaesco, E. Preud'homme, J. L. & Rambaud, J. C. (1968) Immunochemical studies in four cases of alpha-chain disease. *Journal of Clinical Investigations,* **48**, 2374.

Selikoff, I. J., Hammond, E. C. & Churg, J. (1968) Asbestos exposure, smoking and neoplasia. *Journal of the American Medical Association,* **204**, 106-112.

Shahid, M. J., Alami, S. Y., Nassar, V. H., Balikan, J. B. & Salem, A. A. (1974) Primary intestinal lymphoma with paraproteinemia. *Cancer,* **35**, 848-858.

Shank, R. C., Gibson, J. B. & Wogan, G. N. (1972) Dietary aflatoxins and human liver cancer. I. *Food and Cosmetics Toxicology,* **10**, 51.

Sherlock, S. (1975) Hepatic adenomas and oral contraceptives. *Gut,* **16**, 753-756.

Siurala, M., Varis, K. & Wiljasabo, M. (1966) Studies of patients with atrophic gastritis: a 10–15 year follow-up. *Scandinavian Journal of Gastroenterology,* **1**, 40.

Smith, P. G., Kinlen, L. J. & Doll, R. (1974) Hodgkin's disease mortality among physicians. *Lancet,* **2**, 525.

Spjut, H. J. & Spratt, J. S. (1965) Endemic and morphological similarities existing between spontaneous neoplasma in man and 3:2-dimethyl-4-aminodiphenyl induced colonic neoplasma in rats. *Annals of Surgery,* **161**, 309-324.

Steiner, P. E. & Davies, J. N. P. (1957) Cirrhosis and primary liver carcinoma in Ugandan Africans. *British Journal of Cancer,* **11**, 523.

Sweeney, E. C. & Evans, D. J. (1976) Hepatic lesions in patients treated with synthetic anabolic steroids. *Journal of Clinical Pathology,* **29**, 626-633.

Thalassinos, N. C., Lymberatos, C., Hadjioannou, J. & Gardikas, C. (1974) Liver-cell carcinoma after long-term oestrogen-like drugs. *Lancet,* **1**, 270.

Tuyns, A. J. (1970) Cancer of the oseophagus; further evidence of the relation to drinking habits in France. *International Journal of Cancer,* **5**, 152.

Tuyns, A. J. & Massée, L. M. F. (1973) Mortality from cancer of the oesophagus in Brittany. *International Journal of Epidemiology,* **2**, 241-245.

Tuyns, A. J. & Massé, G. (1975) Cancer of the oesophagus in Brittany. An incidence study in Ille-et-Villaine. *International Journal of Epidemiology,* **4**, 55-59.

Van Rensburg, S. J., van der Watt, J. R. & Purchase, I. F. (1974) Primary liver cancer rate and aflatoxin intake in a high cancer area. *South African Journal of Medicine*, **48**, 2508A–2508D.

Vessey, M. P., Doll, R. & Jones, K. (1975) Oral contraceptives and breast cancer. *Lancet*, **1**, 941–944.

Vianna, N. J., Greenwald, P. and Davies, J. N. P. (1971a) Tonsillectomy and Hodgkin's disease: the lymphoid tissue barrier. *Lancet*, **1**, 431–432.

Vianna, N. J., Greenwald, P. & Davies, J. N. P. (1971b) Nature of Hodgkin's disease agent. *Lancet*, **1**, 733–735.

Vianna, N. J., Greenwald, P. & Davies, J. N. P. (1971c) Extended epidemic of Hodgkin's disease in high-school students. *Lancet*, **1**, 1209–1211.

Vianna, N. J., Greenwald, P., Brady, J., Polan, A. K., Maure, J. & Davies, J. N. P. (1972) Hodgkin's disease: cases with features of a community outbreak. *Annals of Internal Medicine*, **77**, 169–180.

Vianna, N. J. & Polan, A. K. (1973) Epidemiologic evidence for transmission of Hodgkin's disease. *New England Journal of Medicine*, **289**, 499–502.

Vianna, N. J., Keogh, M. D., Polan, A. K. & Greenwald, P. (1974) Hodgkin's disease mortality among Physicians. *Lancet*, **2**, 131–133.

Vianna, N. J., Polan, A. K., Davies, J. N. P. & Wolfgang, P. (1974) Familial Hodgkin's disease: an environmental and genetic disorder. *Lancet*, **2**, 854-857.

Vogel, C. L., Anthony, P. P., Mody, N. & Barker, L. F. (1970) Hepatitis-associated antigen in Ugandan patients with hepatocellular carcinoma. *Lancet*, **2**, 621–624.

Wedderburn, N. (1970) Effect of concurrent malarial infection on development of virus-induced lymphoma in BALB/C mice. *Lancet*, **2**, 1114–1116.

Weisburger, J. H. & Rameri, R. (1975) Dietary factors and the aetiology of gastric cancer. *Cancer Research*, **35**, 3469–3474.

Williams, A. O., Williams, A. I., Buckels, J. & Fabiyi, A. (1972) Carrier state prevalence of hepatitis associated antigen AU-SH in Nigeria. *American Journal of Epidemiology*, **96**, 227-230.

Williams, O., Chung, E. B., Agbata, A. & Jackson, M. A. (1975) Intestinal polyps in American Negroes and Nigerian Africans. *British Journal of Cancer*, **31**, 485–491.

Wright, D. H. (1963) Cytology and histochemistry of the Burkitt's lymphoma. *British Journal of Cancer*, **18**, 50–55.

Wynder, E. L., Kajitani, T., Ishikawa, S., Dodo, H. & Takano, A. (1969) Environmental factors of cancer of the colon and rectum. *Cancer*, **23**, 1210–1220.

2
THE MANAGEMENT OF HODGKIN'S DISEASE

J. H. Scarffe   D. Crowther

Hodgkin's disease has over the last two decades created an interest and acquired an importance out of all proportion to its frequency. The careful study of this disease and its treatment has shown that progress can be made through the collaboration of the pathologist, surgeon, radiotherapist, and chemotherapist, working closely together in special centres. This interdisciplinary approach is emerging as a successful model which may well help in the management of some of the more common and difficult malignant diseases of man. Despite advances, there remain many important problems to solve. The intensive radiotherapy and chemotherapy which is responsible for improved clinical results is demanding, both on the patient, doctor, and hospital facilities. New approaches are required to reduce the morbidity of the staging procedure and treatment.

PATHOLOGY

Thomas Hodgkin's original paper (1832) described the clinical histories and gross postmortem findings in a series of patients studied at Guy's Hospital, London. The histological separation of Hodgkin's disease from other lympho-proliferative disorders has been based upon the presence of large binucleate or multinucleated cells, now universally known as 'Reed–Sternberg cells', after their description by Sternberg (1898) and Dorothy Reed (1902). This is despite these cells having been previously observed by Langhans (1872) and Greenfield (1878). The 'Reed–Sternberg cells' and their mononuclear counterparts are seen amidst morphologically benign and reactive elements in a distinctive histo-pathological setting. Two important observations, the first by Rosenthal (1936) that the survival of patients with Hodgkin's disease was longer the larger the lymphocyte to abnormal cell ratio, and the second by Smetana and Cohen (1956) that patients with sclerosis in their biopsy formed a favourable group, was used by Lukes (1963) to put forward a new classification which was later simplified to form the Rye Classification (1966). The Rye Classification (Table 2.1) is now widely used and accepted*.

The nodular sclerosis category shows characteristic bands of collagen which divide the node into nodules of cellular tissue, in which there is often found 'the large cytoplasmic variants' of 'Reed–Sternberg cells', both mononuclear or multilobated, within clear spaces (lacunae) due to artefactual retraction of their cytoplasm, which is only found in formalin-fixed tissues. Lukes and Butler

* Supported by the Cancer Research Campaign, 2 Carlton House Terrace, London SW1Y 5AR.

(1966) first described a cellular presclerotic phase of nodular sclerosis in which numerous 'lacunae' cells are present in nodular aggregates without the presence of sclerosis. Strum and Rappaport (1971) reported the progression of a patient from the 'cellular' presclerotic phase to typical nodular sclerosis in sequential biopsies. Often patients with the cellular phase pathology have been shown by staging laparotomy to have classical nodular sclerosis in other biopsy sites (Dorfman, 1971). Necrosis accompanied by a neutrophil infiltration may also occur.

Table 2.1   Rye classification (1966)

	Relative frequency (%)
Lymphocyte predominance	10–15
Nodular sclerosis	20–50
Mixed cellularity	20–40
Lymphocyte depletion	5–15

In the lymphocyte predominant type the neoplastic elements are always in the distinct minority. In some cases the nodal architecture is partially preserved and Hodgkin's disease can be identified only in the paracortical regions between and subjacent to germinal centres. Other cases show effacement of nodal architecture by a diffuse or nodular proliferation of lymphocytes, benign histiocytes, and occasional abnormal cells with large vesicular lobated nuclei and prominent nucleoli. Multiple sections may be necessary to identify 'Reed–Sternberg cells'.

Abnormal mononuclear and multilobed cells are more numerous and classical 'Reed–Sternberg cells' can be readily identified in the mixed cellularity type. In association with this increase in malignant cells there is a reduction in number of normal histiocytes and lymphocytes. There is usually diffuse replacement of the nodal architecture although partial preservation of the normal pattern is occasionally observed. Eosinophils and plasma cells are often present. Diffuse or focal fibrosis may be seen and irregular foci of necrosis may be present.

As the name implies, lymphocyte-depleted Hodgkin's disease shows paucity of lymphocytes and benign histiocytes with relatively increased numbers of abnormal cells and 'Reed–Sternberg cells', or increased fibrosis and necrosis. Two types of lymphocyte depletion can be recognised. 'Diffuse fibrosis' in which the tissue is hypocellular and largely replaced by disorderly fibrous tissue, and a 'reticular' form where the process is hypercellular and malignant cells may be both more numerous and more bizarre. Patients with the 'reticular' type tend to have bulky disease and death appears to be a direct result of the proliferative capacity of the tumour in vital organs. Patients with the 'diffuse fibrosis' type may present with a febrile, wasting illness, with little or no peripheral node enlargement and die due to a variety of causes, including infection in an immunodeficient host (Neiman, Rosen and Lukes, 1973).

CLINICAL AND PATHOLOGICAL STAGING

Accurate staging in patients with Hodgkin's disease is important in deciding the optimum form of treatment for an individual patient, in predicting prognosis, and it also enables series of patients treated in different ways to be compared.

Staging classification

The staging classification now in common use is the Ann Arbor classification (Table 2.2). This classification makes a strong distinction between clinical staging and pathological staging. Pathological staging refers to any form of histological identification of tumour in sites other than the initial biopsy, for example, a bone marrow biopsy, a liver biopsy, or a laparotomy specimen. The clinical staging will refer only to the initial biopsy, physical examination, radiological procedures, and blood studies.

The other major change in staging has been that solitary extranodal extension into extralymphoid areas no longer makes the patient stage IV, but is designated with an 'E'. For example, a patient with mediastinal nodes with localised lung involvement is not stage IV but is clinical stage (CS) I_E. If, at laparatomy, he was found to have a positive spleen, the patient would become pathological stage (PS) III_{SE}.

The Ann Arbor classification is still subdivided into 'A' and 'B' categories, 'B' for those with symptoms defined as unexplained weight loss of more than 10 per cent of the body weight in the six months before admission, unexplained fever with temperatures above 38°C or night sweats. Pruritus alone is no longer considered a significant systemic symptom (Tubiana et al, 1971; Carbone, 1971).

When a patient is first seen, a careful history with special care spent on enquiring about 'B' symptoms, pruritus and alcohol intolerance is required. The physical examination must be thorough with special emphasis placed on peripheral lymph nodes, liver, spleen and any bony tenderness.

Table 2.2   The Ann Arbor classification

Stage	Extent
I	Nodal involvement within one region
IE	Single extralymphatic organ or site
II	Nodal involvement within two or more regions, limited by the diaphragm
IIE	Localised extranodal site and nodal involvement within one or more regions, limited by the diaphragm
III	Nodal involvement of regions above and below the diaphragm
IIIE	Nodal involvement of regions above and below the diaphragm with localised extralymphatic site
IIIS	Nodal involvement of regions above and below the diaphragm with spleen involvement
IIIES	Nodal involvement of regions above and below the diaphragm with localised extralymphatic site and spleen involvement
IV	Diffuse or disseminated involvement of one or more extralymphatic organs or tissues, with or without lymph node involvement

SYSTEMIC SYMPTOMS

A or B denotes the absence or presence, respectively, of documented unexplained fever above 38°C, night sweats, or unexplained weight loss of more than 10 per cent in six months. (*N.B.* Pruritus alone no longer qualifies for B classification.)

Clinical stage (CS) will be determined by history, physical examination, radiological studies, scans, laboratory tests and initial biopsy results.

Pathological stage (PS) will be determined if more tissue than the initial biopsy has been examined. The site or sites of the subsequent biopsies will be identified as follows:

N	Lymph node	H	Liver	S	Spleen
L	Lung	M	Bone marrow	P	Pleura
O	Osseous	D	Skin		

Staging investigations

Laboratory tests should include haemoglobin, white cell count, differential, platelet count, reticulocyte count, erythrocyte sedimentation rate, biochemical assessment of liver and renal function, serum calcium, uric acid, and alkaline phosphatase.

If a routine chest x-ray shows any abnormality, tomography is usually carried out. A bipedal abdominal lymphogram is performed in all patients except those with obvious intra-abdominal or stage IV disease. Care should be taken in assessing respiratory function in patients with severe respiratory disease before a lymphogram, since there is a small but reversible fall in gas transfer 24 to 48 h after the injection of the contrast medium. This change in respiratory function is due to the oil-based contrast medium embolising into the lungs after passing up the thoracic duct. It is advisable to allow one week for this to clear before a general anaesthetic is given for a staging laparotomy (White et al, 1973). Lymphograms are useful in identifying suspicious nodes for the surgeon to biopsy at laparotomy, to assist the radiotherapist to set up his treatment field, and for follow-up of the patient's response to treatment. When the lymphogram is positive an intravenous pyelogram is often performed to detect ureteric obstruction and to help the radiotherapist plan his treatment field. Other specialised investigations such as inferior vena cavagrams (Lee, Nelson and Schwarz, 1964), splenic arteriography (Castellino et al, 1972) and radioisotopic scans of liver and spleen (Silverman et al, 1972; Lipton et al, 1972) have been shown not to be sensitive enough for routine staging. Gallium-67 lymph node scans have not proved as reliable in staging procedures as conventional radiographs and surgical techniques (Glatstein and Goffinet, 1974). The new EMI total body scanner has yet to be evaluated as an aid to staging. A study has been started in Manchester where patients will have an EMI total body scan prior to staging laparotomy.

Bone skeletal surveys have a very low pick-up rate and are usually only done in the presence of bone symptoms. Radioisotopic bone scans may pick up bony deposits some weeks before lesions become apparent on the radiograph (MacDonald, 1973).

In the patient who presents with neurological signs in the legs, a myelogram is necessary as an emergency to localise any deposit causing spinal cord compression, before immediate treatment.

Bone marrow infiltration is often only focal in Hodgkin's disease. For this reason, aspiration is inadequate and a bone marrow trephine biopsy by a Westerman–Jenson needle or a Jamshidi needle is preferred. Open biopsy with a Stryker saw allows more bone marrow to be examined and increases the number of positive findings on trephine by approximately 5 per cent (Radin et al, 1971).

Percutaneous liver biopsy is only of limited value in assessing liver involvement. Bagley et al (1973) reported a study of 47 patients who were thought to have a high risk of liver disease in that they had 'B' symptoms, abdominal node involvement and/or splenomegaly. Percutaneous liver biopsy by the Menghini technique was positive in 5 of the 34 patients studied. The remaining 42 patients in the study were biopsied at peritoneoscopy, six needle biopsies being taken through right and left subcostal skin sites. These biopsies were positive in 6 of the 42 patients. In five of these six patients, a prior percutaneous liver biopsy had been negative and in one a percutaneous biopsy was not done. The positive patients could not be predicted by liver size, liver-function tests, 'B' symptoms, or histological type. There was a tendency for patients with positive percutaneous biopsies to have larger livers and higher alkaline phosphatase values, but the differences were not significant. A more recent study (Spinelli et al, 1975) has shown that liver biopsy at peritoneoscopy is as accurate as a wedge biopsy taken at laparotomy, but needle biopsy of the spleen taken at the same time only picked up 38 per cent of the positive spleens found at laparotomy.

Laparotomy

Staging laparotomy is now accepted at most centres as the only accurate method of staging patients with Hodgkin's disease, after patients with obvious stage IV disease have been excluded. The operation itself varies from series to series, from simple splenectomy and palpation of the lymph node areas to splenectomy and dissection of the para-aortic nodes en bloc. Irving (1975) describes a standard operation with a long incision from the xiphoid process to 5 cm above the symphysis pubis. After careful examination of the abdominal viscera and nodes, the spleen and splenic nodes are removed. Representative samples of any obviously enlarged nodes or nodes that appear suspicious on the lymphogram are taken. Lymph nodes are also routinely taken from the following areas, whether suspicious or not:

1. both external iliac nodes,
2. right and left paraortic nodes,
3. nodes at the root of the small bowel mesentery,
4. coeliac axis node.

The biopsy sites are marked with tantalum clips, as are the lateral borders of the ovaries after they have been fixed in the midline behind the uterus. The clips enable the exact sites of the biopsies to be seen on plain abdominal radiography and the position of the ovaries in relation to the radiation field, if it is required. A biopsy is taken from any obviously involved area of the liver. In the absence of an obvious lesion, a wedge biopsy is taken from the edge of the left lobe of the liver and a needle biopsy from the right. The vermiform appendix is routinely removed. After closure of the abdomen, an open bone biopsy of the left iliac crest is taken with a Stryker saw.

In a personal series of 150 laparotomies using the operation described above, Irving (personal communication) has had no mortality. The mortality rate estimated by Gazet (1973) from the published results of 1558 laparotomies for staging lymphomas from 24 centres was just over 1 per cent. There were the expected complications of extensive abdominal surgery such as chest infection, wound infection, subphrenic abscess, deep venous thrombosis, ileus and haemorrhage, but the complication rate was usually acceptable. Thrombotic complications were surprisingly low despite the thrombocytosis that follows splenectomy. Many authorities anticoagulate patients with a platelet count greater then 1000×10^9/litre. Splenectomy in children may be complicated by overwhelming infection in approximately 5 per cent of cases (Eraklis et al, 1967) In a recent study of 200 children with Hodgkin's disease who had undergone splenectomy, 20 had episodes of septicaemia or meningitis. The infective spisode was fatal in 11 of the 20 cases (Chilcote and Baehner, 1975). These infections occurred on average 16 months after splenectomy, and were not associated with leucopenia. Splenectomy in children should not be undertaken lightly.

A diligent search by the pathologist in examining the specimens is required if the small foci of disease are to be found. For example, the spleen should be serially sliced every 2 mm and histological sections made of any suspicious areas.

The results of laparotomy are very similar in most published series. Crowther et al (1974) reported the results of 111 patients with Hodgkin's disease who had staging laparotomies as described by Irving (1975). Twenty out of 49 patients (41 per cent) presenting with stages I and II disease above the diaphragm were found to have histological evidence of Hodgkin's disease at laparotomy. The incidence of unsuspected disease in the abdomen was greater in patients with poor histology (mixed cellularity and lymphocyte depletion). Of the 24 patients with poor histology, 18 had a positive laparotomy compared with 22 out of 48 with better histology (nodular sclerosing and lymphocyte predominance). Lymphography results did not correlate well for a number of reasons. Firstly, the spleen was involved in one-half of the patients with abdominal disease and this organ cannot be shown on lymphography. Secondly, splenic hilar nodes and coeliac nodes were important sites of involvement not revealed by lymphography. Six per cent of patients had a coeliac axis node as the only site of intra-abdominal disease. Thirdly, mistakes can be made even when the nodes do opacify. Sixteen per cent of patients with positive lymphograms were not found to have histological evidence of Hodgkin's disease at laparotomy whereas 13 per cent of patients with negative lymphograms were found to have histological evidence of disease. The spleen size was of little value in predicting involvement unless the spleen was massively enlarged. The liver was involved in 12 per cent, always in association with disease in the spleen. The reverse association was not true. Seven out of nine patients presenting with disease only in the right neck had unsuspected disease in the abdomen. This contradicted Kaplan (1972) who found that right neck node disease was only rarely associated with abdominal disease. The British National Lymphoma Investigation Group (1975b) found that 56 per cent of their patients with right neck disease had abdominal disease.

If the therapeutic plan is to use radiotherapy only to known sites of disease in clinical stage I and II disease above the diaphragm, then a staging laparotomy is indispensable for accurate assessment of the extent of the disease. If the therapeutic plan is to include the abdomen in the radiotherapy fields even in the absence of identified abdominal disease, then the surgical procedure has only the limited value of identifying the few patients with liver involvement. Chemotherapy may also be used in clinically staged patients where radiotherapy is only used to areas of known disease above the diaphragm since it treats inapparent disease both in the nodes and in extralymphatic sites.

Staging laparotomies are usually performed at present, but hopefully in the future we will have adequate curative treatment of inapparent disease in the abdomen and surgical staging will become unnecessary.

Surgical removal of the spleen allows the radiotherapist to limit his fields to the identified splenic pedicle, so eliminating radiation pneumonitis and pleuritis of the left lung base and radiation damage to the left kidney can be minimised (Rosenberg and Kaplan, 1970). In the occasional patient who presents with hypersplenism, splenectomy is necessary to increase the blood count before treatment. Even the average patient will demonstrate significant increases in the white blood cell and platelet count following splenectomy. This increase in blood count has been reported to improve tolerance to wide-field radiotherapy (Salzman and Kaplan, 1971). Similar increased tolerance to chemotherapy has been reported (Prosnitz, Fischer and Vera, 1972; Rosenberg and Kaplan, 1970) but this was not confirmed in a recent study by Ihde et al (1975).

TREATMENT

The treatment of Hodgkin's disease is best carried out by combined teams of experienced radiotherapists and chemotherapists in specialised centres.

Stages I and II

Radiotherapy

In stages I and II the primary treatment is radiotherapy. Care should be taken to distinguish between pathological stage (PS) I and II and clinical stage (CS) I and II disease. In clinically staged patients the treatment must take into account the 30 to 40 per cent of patients with inapparent disease in the abdomen.

An important factor in the development of current radiotherapy techniques has been the introduction of megavoltage equipment. The fine focus and sharp beam-edge provide good protection for structures outside the main beam, but scattered irradiation inevitably reaches some shielded structures. The skin sparing effect of these energies means that there is usually little more than erythema at the end of treatment, although there may be some more marked reactions in the axillae and supraclavicular fossae.

Kaplan and Rosenberg (1975) recommend a tumouricidal dose of 3500 rad (35 Gy) in three and a half weeks to 4400 rad (44 Gy) in four weeks with a boost up to 5000 rad (50 Gy) in five to six weeks to exceptionally large or slowly regressing lymph node masses. These dose recommendations are made on the finding that the local recurrence rate is inversely related to dose. Falling from a level of 60 to 80 per cent local recurrence with doses of 1000 rad (10 Gy) or less, to a rate of approximately 4 per cent for the dose range of 3500 to 4000 rad (35–40 At the dose level of 4400 rad (44 Gy) delivered in four and a half weeks, the recurrence rate is only 1 to 2 per cent (Kaplan, 1972). Many centres do not treat using the very high dose of 4400 rad (44 Gy) in four and a half weeks, but give a minimum tumour dose of 3500 rad (35 Gy), employing a dose rate of 1000 rad (10 Gy) per week. Peckham (1973) reported eight (6 per cent) recurrences within an apparently adequately irradiated area out of 127 patients. The majority of these patients had received 3500 rad (35 Gy) to a 'mantle' field over four or five weeks. The increase in local recurrence rate at the lower dose range must be balanced against the increased toxicity to normal tissues when higher doses are employed.

The field irradiated in stage I and II disease is either the 'involved' field only, that is the areas of clinically evident disease, or 'extended' field. 'Extended' field refers to the increased number or size of field needed to encompass all contiguous lymphatic structures to which microscopic spread of disease is likely to have occurred. In pathological stages I and II, the field is usually extended to cover contiguous spread on the side of the diaphragm involved. In disease above the diaphragm, the 'mantle' field is commonly used, where large anterior and posterior opposed fields encompass the cervical, axillary, and mediastinal node areas. The 'inverted Y' field is commonly used for disease below the diaphragm, treating the para-aortic, pelvic, and inguinal nodes, and splenic hilar region. In clinically staged patients account must be taken of the high risk of abdominal disease and the 'mantle' field may be followed after an interval of four weeks by the 'inverted Y' field to complete what is known as the 'total nodal' field. These large fields must be carefully shaped to the contours of the lymph node chains with lead blocks to protect normal tissues, such as lungs, kidneys, right lobe of liver, and gonads. Meticulous care is taken at the junction between fields to ensure the spinal cord is not overdosed but that nodes are adequately irradiated.

Despite the increase in accuracy of staging and improved radiotherapy techniques, approximately 20 per cent of PS I and II patients will relapse in the first five years after 'mantle' field irradiation (Peckham et al, 1975). Since effective chemotherapy is now available, it is an attractive idea to use it to eradicate any disease not adequately treated by irradiation. This would, however, lead to many potentially cured patients being treated unnecessarily. It may be equally efficacious to leave further treatment with either chemotherapy or radiotherapy till the patient relapses.

Combined radiotherapy and chemotherapy

The optimum irradiation field in patients who have undergone staging laparotomy and in whom combination chemotherapy is to be used is not known. There appear therefore to be six main alternatives in the treatment of PS I–II$_B$ Hodgkin's disease.

1. 'Involved' field irradiation only followed by chemotherapy or radiotherapy at the time of any subsequent relapse.
2. 'Involved' field irradiation followed immediately by chemotherapy to eliminate residual disease.
3. 'Mantle' or 'inverted Y' field irradiation only, followed by chemotherapy or radiotherapy at the time of any subsequent relapse.
4. 'Mantle' or 'inverted Y' field irradiation followed immediately by chemotherapy to eliminate residual disease.
5. 'Total' nodal field irradiation only, followed by chemotherapy ± radiotherapy at the time of any subsequent relapse.
6. 'Total' nodal field irradiation followed immediately by chemotherapy to eliminate residual disease.

The role of chemotherapy as an adjunct to radiotherapy has been difficult to assess in many trials because of inadequate staging, suboptimal irradiation, the use of relatively ineffective chemotherapy, and poor randomisation of patient groups. Patients with pathological stage I, II and III disease who received adjuvant chemotherapy had a significant increase in disease-free survival when compared with those who received radiotherapy alone in a study at Stanford (Rosenberg and Kaplan, 1975). However, no difference in survival was found between the two groups at this time. In France a group of patients with stage I–II disease who received chemotherapy for three months before their radiotherapy have had significantly less relapses than those who received irradiation alone (Bernard et al, 1974).

A trial has recently been started in Manchester to study the effect of combination chemotherapy (MVPP) as an adjunct to 'mantle' field irradiation in pathological stage I and II with supradiaphragmatic disease. The long-term value of such treatment from these and other studies of adjuvant chemotherapy will not be known for some years. Such trials are important for a proper assessment of recurrence rates, survival and morbidity following treatment in these modern studies of adjuvant combination chemotherapy.

Chemotherapy may also be used in the early stage of the disease for rapid relief of pressure on a vital structure such as the superior vena cava, major airways, or spinal cord, before definitive treatment with radiotherapy. In patients with large mediastinal masses, chemotherapy may be of advantage to reduce the volume to be irradiated and so protect as much lung tissue as possible.

Stage III

Patients with pathological stage IIIA disease are usually treated with 'total nodal' radiotherapy. Studies are however in progress to assess the role of adjuvant chemotherapy or chemotherapy alone. Chemotherapy is the primary treatment most commonly used for pathological stage IIIB. However, Kaplan prefers to give 'total nodal' irradiation as primary treatment followed, after a gap of eight weeks, by chemotherapy (Rosenberg and Kaplan, 1975).

In a study of relapses after chemotherapy, 88 per cent were at sites of previous disease (Young et al, 1975). This raises the possibility of using radiotherapy to previously involved areas in patients with advanced disease treated primarily using chemotherapy in an attempt to prevent recurrence. Several trials are in progress to assess this.

Stage IV

The treatment of pathological stage IV disease has been revolutionised by the introduction of combination chemotherapy. Until the introduction of combination chemotherapy, single agents, usually cyclophosphamide or chlorambucil, were given continuously until a relapse occurred. Treatment was then changed to a drug of another class such as procarbazine or vinblastine. Complete remission was obtained in less than one quarter (Fairley, Patterson and Scott, 1966) although 60 to 70 per cent had a partial response. Remissions were short.

The median survival of patients treated in this way was less than two years.

Lacher and Durant (1965) introduced the combination of vinblastine and chlorambucil which gave a complete remission rate of 63 per cent. De Vita and his colleagues (De Vita, Serpick and Carbone, 1970) obtained a complete remission rate of 81 per cent in 43 patients using the MOPP combination of nitrogen mustard, vincristine, procarbazine and prednisolone (Table 2.3) for six courses. The majority of these patients had stage IV disease. These results have since been confirmed by many workers and MOPP has become the standard form of chemotherapy used throughout the world.

Table 2.3 The 'MOPP' combination

Drug	Dosage
Nitrogen mustard	6 mg/m^2 i.v. on days 1 and 8
Vincristine (Oncovin)	1.4 mg/m^2 i.v. on days 1 and 8
Procarbazine	100 mg/m^2 orally on days 1 to 14 inclusive
Prednisone[a]	40 mg/m^2 orally on days 1 to 14 inclusive

Six courses are given with two weeks' rest between the end of one course and the beginning of the next

[a] Prednisone is only given with the first and fourth courses

Table 2.4 The 'MVPP' combination

Drug	Dosage
Nitrogen mustard	6 mg/m^2 i.v. on days 1 and 8
Vinblastine[a]	6 mg/m^2 i.v. on days 1 and 8
Procarbazine	100 mg/m^2 orally on days 1 to 14 inclusive
Prednisone[b]	40 mg orally on days 1 to 14 inclusive

A four week gap is left between courses

[a] The original MVPP regime (Nicholson et al, 1970) included an injection of vinblastine on day 14. This has been abandoned due to the development of transient leucopenia in many patients on day 14

[b] A total dose of 40 mg per adult patient is given. This dose is never exceeded but may be reduced in children

In Britain a similar regime to MOPP known as MVPP (Table 2.4) has been developed by Hamilton-Fairley and his colleagues at St Bartholomew's Hospital (Nicholson et al, 1970, McElwain, 1973). Vinblastine was preferred to vincristine because of its reduced incidence of peripheral neuropathy and alopecia, although it has more bone marrow toxicity. A lower dose of prednisone was given with every course, and an interval of one clear month was left between the courses. The MVPP regime obtained a complete remission rate of 74 per cent in 49 previously untreated patients and 93 per cent of 42 patients who had relapsed after previous radiotherapy (Sutcliffe, personal communication).

Most authorities feel that prednisone in these combinations has little direct action on the tumour, but may help to relieve the systemic symptoms and have some marrow protective effect. It was somewhat surprising that when it was omitted from the MOPP combination (report from the British National Lymphoma Investigation Group, 1975a) the remission rate fell from 80 to 44 per cent.

More recently, Bonnadonna et al (1975) have published results using a new regime ABVD (Table 2.5) which consists of six courses of adriamycin, bleomycin, vinblastine, and imidazole carboxamide. This regime gives a complete remission rate of 75 per cent and shows no cross resistance with MOPP. ABVD is, therefore, a useful regime in MOPP failures, or in sequential chemotherapy with MOPP.

After complete remission has been induced there is no clear evidence that chemotherapy maintenance is of value. Frei et al (1973) reported that 77 per cent of a group who were maintained for 18 months after complete remission with courses of MOPP every two months were disease free at three years compared with 46 per cent for an unmaintained group. Another study, however, showed no significant difference in first remission length between patients randomised to one of three regimes; no additional treatment, intermittent therapy with MOPP,

Table 2.5 The 'ABVD' combination

Drug	Dosage
Adriamycin	25 mg/m^2 i.v. on days 1 and 14
Bleomycin	10 mg/m^2 i.v. on days 1 and 14
Vinblastine	6 mg/m^2 i.v. on days 1 and 14
Imidazole carboxamide (DTIC)	150 mg/m^2 i.v. daily days 1 to 5 inclusive

Six courses are given with two weeks' rest between the end of one course and the beginning of the next one

Table 2.6 The 'CAVe' combination

Drug	Dosage
CCNU	100 mg/m^2 orally on day 1
Adriamycin	60 mg/m^2 i.v. on day 1
Vinblastine	5 mg/m^2 i.v. on day 1

Nine courses are given every six weeks

or intermittent therapy with BCNU (1-bis(2-chloroethyl)-1-nitrosourea). Complications and infections were more frequently seen in the patients receiving maintenance therapy, and particularly in those receiving BCNU (Young et al, 1973). The projected median remission duration of patients receiving no maintenance therapy in the study was greater than 48 months and is longer than in a previous study, reported from the National Cancer Institute at Bethesda of 36 months (De Vita et al, 1970). One possible explanation for this was that approximately 25 per cent of patients in the second series received more than the initially proposed six cycles of therapy before a solid complete remission was achieved, whilst in the original study treatment was stopped at six cycles. The management of the patients who are resistant to either MOPP or MVPP can be difficult but drugs such as the alternative Vinca alkaloid, adriamycin, a nitrosourea or bleomycin can be used singly or in combination with useful effect in such patients. The ABVD regime of Bonadonna may prove useful in this regard although bone marrow depression may entail reduction in dosage or omission of drugs with troublesome bone marrow toxicity. Kaplan and Rosenberg (1975) have described the CAVe regime utilising the nitrosourea CCNU in combination with adriamycin and vinblastine (Table 2.6), which give about a 50 per cent response rate in MOPP failures. In patients with poor bone marrow reserve, caused by prior treatment or bone marrow infiltration, a combination of vincristine and bleomycin is often effective palliation since this combination is of low marrow toxicity.

COMPLICATIONS OF TREATMENT

Both radiotherapy and chemotherapy are potentially dangerous treatments. The utmost care must be taken and attempts made to design treatment regimes that do least harm to the patient whilst ensuring eradication of the disease. These toxic effects can be considered as those of radiotherapy and chemotherapy alone, and those of the combined modalities.

'Mantle' treatment is remarkably well tolerated (Peckham, 1973); temporary epilation occurs in the posterior cervical region, dryness and soreness of the throat and radiation oesophagitis are not uncommon towards the end of the treatment. There is often a fall in platelet and white cell counts, but not severe enough to interrupt treatment. Tolerance to the 'inverted Y' field tends to be poorer since there is a greater volume of irradiated marrow. A fall in white count and platelet count may necessitate interruption of treatment for a few days. Nausea and vomiting may also necessitate reducing the daily dose level or temporarily interrupting treatment. With 'total nodal' field irradiation, bone marrow suppression is common, but if a rest period of two to four weeks between 'mantle' and 'inverted Y' fields is allowed, the suppressive effects are minimised. Great care should be taken if chemotherapy is required after 'total nodal' irradiation because of the risk of inducing a severe pancytopenia.

Radiation pneumonitis in patients who have had 'mantle' irradiation is typically seen two to three months after the completion of treatment. The mediastinal silhouette becomes less well defined and irregular strands of shadowing appear in the paramediastinal pulmonary parenchyma in the irradiated field. The patient may be asymptomatic, or complain of cough and shortness of breath which usually lasts for two to four months. The pneumonitis usually clears, leaving behind only slight fibrotic changes seen on the chest x-ray. Severe cases may progress to widespread fibrotic change. Kaplan (1972) reports 16 cases of pneumonitis out of 248 patients at risk, the pneumonitis was fatal in one patient. The role of steroids in the management of pneumonitis is controversial, and Kaplan (1972) warns of severe exacerbations if they are suddenly withdrawn.

Radiation injury to the heart most commonly manifests itself as acute pericarditis, often associated with pericardial effusion and, occasionally, signs of tamponade. This complication occurs in approximately 5 per cent of patients irradiated to a dose of 4000 to 4400 rad (40–44 Gy) in four weeks (Kaplan, 1972). Smithers (1973) reports having seen only one patient with a pericardial effusion at the lower radiation dose of 3500 rad (35 Gy) in four weeks.

Transverse myelitis following accidental overlapping of fields is, fortunately, very rare, with the meticulous care used in the setting up of the radiation fields. Lhermitte's syndrome may complicate irradiation of the spinal column. The patient complains of tingling, electric shock-like sensations, and numbness in arms, legs, and lumbar region, which may be produced or intensified by flexion of the neck. It is self-limiting and the patient requires no treatment beyond reassurance.

Attempts are made to protect the gonads from the effects of irradiation, but these are only partially effective. If the ovaries are routinely moved and fixed in the midline at staging laparotomy, menstruation will persist in approximately half of the patients, and some of them may conceive and achieve a normal pregnancy, even after a long period of amenorrhoea following 'inverted Y' field irradiation (Baker et al, 1972). The testes receive some irradiation by scatter, which can be reduced by the use of testicular shields (Smithers, 1973). In a small group of male patients followed for up to 40 months, aspermia was found in all specimens examined after 'inverted Y' irradiation (Spieser, Rubin and Casarett, 1973).

Hypothyroidism is a long-term complication that has an incidence that varies from 2 per cent (Peckham, 1973) to 10 per cent (Glatstein et al, 1971). This difference is probably due to the higher dose of radiotherapy given to the series Glatstein studied. Three cases of acute myeloid leukaemia were described following radiotherapy for Hodgkin's disease by Ezdinli et al (1969). Since then a number of other cases have been reported but the incidence is low, even in patients receiving combined chemotherapy and radiotherapy.

Table 2.7 Major drug toxicities

Drug	Toxicity
Nitrogen mustard	Nausea, vomiting, bone marrow
Vincristine	Neuropathy
Vinblastine	Bone marrow
Procarbazine	Bone marrow, nausea
Adriamycin	Bone marrow, alopecia, cardiomyopathy
Bleomycin	Febrile reactions, pulmonary fibrosis, skin changes
Nitrosourea (CCNU and BCNU)	Nausea, vomiting: bone marrow (nadir four to five weeks)
Imidazole carboxamide (DTIC)	Nausea, vomiting: bone marrow, flu-like syndrome

The major toxicities of the drugs used in the treatment of Hodgkin's disease are shown in Table 2.7. Nitrogen mustard, the Vinca alkaloids, adriamycin, and imidazole carboxamide all cause severe tissue necrosis if allowed to leak outside the vein. For this reason it is advisable to inject the drugs into a fast-running saline drip. If there is any sign of extravasation or pain the injection should be stopped immediately and an attempt made to aspirate as much of the drug as possible. Local injection of hyaluronidase and the application of warmth to the injection site may help minimise tissue damage. The extravasated drug may cause severe pain, tissue necrosis and ulceration.

Nitrogen mustard causes severe vomiting a few hours after injection and many patients are admitted overnight for the first injection of the course, but often tolerate the second injection better and can be treated as an outpatient. Sedation with chlorpromazine before the injection will help reduce the nausea and vomiting and give a night's rest before discharge the following morning.

Severe depression of the blood count may occur, particularly in patients who have had previous chemotherapy, irradiation, or have bone marrow involvement.

A full blood count should be done before each injection, and the dose of drugs modified accordingly. The long-term effects of MOPP chemotherapy were reported by De Vita et al (1972). They found no long-term impairment of immunocompetence or bone marrow function. Eight out of ten patients treatment with MOPP for six months were found to have aspermia or very low sperm counts. Six of these had only Sertoli cells present within the seminiferous tubules in their testicular biopsies. This feature was associated with raised levels of follicle stimulating hormone. A $3\frac{1}{2}$-fold increase in second malignant tumours was found in 425 patients treated with MOPP as compared with the normal population. A 29-fold increase in risk of a second malignant tumour was found in 35 patients treated with both intensive chemotherapy and intensive radiotherapy. Studies at other centres, however, have fortunately not shown such a high incidence of second malignancies and a study of the use of adjuvant chemotherapy at Stanford showed no increase in second malignancies (Rosenberg and Kaplan, 1975).

The effect of chemotherapy on the fertility of women is not so clear. Amenorrhoea is common but fertility may persist, and certainly, in our experience, pregnancies have occurred both during and after chemotherapy. Contraceptive advice is therefore important to prevent interruption of treatment and the risk of damage to the fetus.

The toxic effects of combined radiotherapy and chemotherapy are now being reported more frequently as combined modality treatment for malignancy becomes more common. Ruckdeschel, Martin and Byhardt (1975) reported 25 pericardial effusions in 81 stage I–II patients with Hodgkin's disease treated by 'mantle' field radiotherapy. In this group of pericardial effusions 14 were transient and 11 persistent. Nine of the eleven persistent pericardial effusions were in patients who have received MOPP as adjuvant chemotherapy. This is considerably higher than the 5 per cent incidence described for high-dose radiotherapy alone (Kaplan, 1972).

Bleomycin used with radiotherapy appears to have a much higher risk of pulmonary fibrosing alveolitis than when used alone (Skarkin et al, 1975). Other side effects such as skin and mucosal reactions following radiotherapy may also be increased if bleomycin is also given. Work in animals has shown increased cardiotoxicity when adriamycin and radiotherapy were used together (Tokita et al, 1975). The augmentation of radiation reactions by the concomitant administration of chemotherapeutic agents is now a well-recognised phenomenon in man. This augmentation has recently been described in four patients treated with adriamycin. Two of these patients demonstrated recall of a quiescent radiation reaction by the subsequent administration of adriamycin (Cassady et al, 1975). This 'recall' phenomenon was first described with the antitumour antibiotic actinomycin D (D'Angio, Farber and Maddock, 1959).

Clearly, as more treatment regimes are used, combined drug toxicities and drug–radiation interaction will need to be looked at very carefully.

Within each stage subgroups with a worse prognosis may be found. Peckham et al (1975) have defined a group with stage II disease who present with multiple node involvement, often of the nodular sclerosing type, particularly associated with infraclavicular nodes that have a high relapse rate.

Lymphocyte predominant and nodular sclerosing histologies have a more favourable outlook than mixed cellularity and lymphocyte depletion. In part this is related to the fact that patients with unfavourable histology often present with more advanced disease.

Females tend to do better than males at all stages of the disease (Smithers, 1973). This is, in part, a reflection of the large proportion of females who have the nodular sclerosing form of the disease with a good prognosis. The over-40 age group have a poorer survival rate than the younger patient, and this is associated with an increased instance of stage III and IV disease in this group.

A number of haematological prognostic factors have been studied of which the erythrocyte sedimentation rate (ESR) is the one with the greatest prognostic value. There is no correlation between ESR and histological type or between ESR and clinical stage. The ESR is, however, strongly correlated with loss of weight and fever (Tubiana et al, 1971). It is clear that many factors of prognostic importance are related and this makes analysis difficult.

The prognostic factors in patients treated with chemotherapy seem to differ from those based on the results of radiotherapy alone. McElwain (1973) found that the age of the patient, histological type, and the presence of 'B' symptoms had no significant influence on the complete remission rate obtained with MVPP. The length of first remission was, however, shorter in patients who were elderly, had 'B' symptoms, or had bone marrow involvement in a series of 81 patients treated with MOPP (Moore et al, 1973).

PROGNOSIS

The prognosis for patients with Hodgkin's disease has improved greatly over the last 50 years. Prior to the work of Dr René Gilbert long-term survival of patients was rare. Gilbert (1939) reported an increase in average survival time from 20 months in 1917 to 42 months in 1937. In the 1940s and 1950s, Dr Vera Peters (Peters, 1961) reported 30 to 40 per cent of patients surviving five years and 15 to 25 per cent, 10 years.

Easson and Russell in 1963 published an important paper entitled 'The cure of Hodgkin's disease'. They reported in patients, with localised disease, an age corrected survival rate of 50 per cent at five years, 42 per cent at 10 years, and 40 per cent at 15 years. They argued that the patients could be considered cured since between 10 and 15 years after treatment their death rate ran parallel to that of an age-matched control population.

Modern methods of investigation and treatment, as previously described, have again increased the prognosis considerably, especially in the more advanced cases. In a recent analysis of 504 patients of all stages, 61 per cent were relapse free, and 81 per cent had survived five years after treatment (Kaplan and Rosenberg, 1975). At 10 years, the curve for the relapse-free survival has flattened out at about 50 per cent, suggesting that at least 50 per cent of all cases may now be permanently cured of their once inevitably fatal disease. Even in stage IIIB and IV patients, who have the worst prognosis of all, the outlook is improving. Results from the late Professor Hamilton Fairley's unit at St Bartholomew's Hospital, London, show that of 91 patients who had not received prior chemotherapy, 80 per cent obtained a complete remission and the probability is that 50 per cent will be in their first remission, and over 70 per cent surviving at five years (Sutcliffe, personal communication).

CONCLUSION

Great strides have been made in the management of Hodgkin's disease, clearly demonstrating the benefit of collaboration between the pathologist, surgeon, radiotherapist, and chemotherapist, working together in special centres. Many important questions remain unanswered, such as the role of adjuvant chemotherapy in early stage disease, and of irradiation of areas of bulk disease after chemotherapy in advanced cases. Many trials in various parts of the world are in progress to answer these questions in order that we may improve our management of patients with Hodgkin's disease, and use this experience to benefit patients suffering from more common malignancies.

REFERENCES

Bagley, C., Thomas, L. B., Johnson, R. E., Chretien, P. B. & De Vita, V. T. (1973) Diagnosis of liver involvement by lymphoma. Results in 96 consecutive peritoneoscopies. *Cancer*, **31**, 840–847.
Baker, J. W., Morgan, R. L., Peckham, M. J. & Smithers, D. W. (1972) Preservation of ovarian function in patients requiring radiotherapy for para-aortic and pelvic Hodgkin's disease. *Lancet*, **1**, 1307–1308.
Bernard, J., Boirom, M., Teillet, C., Weisgerder, C., Thiedaud, N., Dama, M. & Jacquillat, C. (1974) Intensive chemotherapy combined with extended field radiotherapy in treatment of stage I and II Hodgkin's disease. *Abstract, XI International Cancer Congress*, pp. 1–270.
Bonadonna, G., Zucali, R., Monfardini, S., De Lena, M. & Uscenchi, C. (1975) Combination chemotherapy of Hodgkin's disease with adriamycin, bleomycin, vinblastine and imidazole carboxamide versus MOPP. *Cancer*, **36**, 252–259.
British National Lymphoma Investigation Group Report (1975a) Value of prednisone in combination chemotherapy of stage IV Hodgkin's disease. *British Medical Journal*, **3**, 413–414.
British National Lymphoma Investigation Group (1975b) The value of laparotomy and splenectomy in the management of early Hodgkin's disease. *Clinical Radiology*, **26**, 151–157.
Carbonne, P. (1971) Report of the committee on Hodgkin's disease staging classification. *Cancer Research*, **31**, 1860–1861.
Cassady, J. R., Richter, M. P., Piro, A. J. & Jaffe, M. (1975) Radiation–adriamycin interactions, preliminary clinical observations. *Cancer*, **36**, 946–949.
Castellino, R. A., Silverman, J. F., Glatstein, E., Blank, N. & Wexler, L. (1972) Splenic arteriography in Hodgkin's disease. A radiologic–pathologic study of 33 consecutive untreated patients. *American Journal of Roentgenology*, **114**, 453–454.
Chilcote, R. R. & Baehner, R. L. (1975) The incidence of overwhelming infection in children staged for Hodgkin's disease. *Abstract 1013*. American Society of Clinical Oncology and American Association for Cancer Research meeting.
Crowther, D., Hamilton Fairley, G., Irving, M. H., Wrigley, P. F. M., Smyth, J. F. & Stansfield, A. (1974) Changing concepts in the management of patients with Hodgkin's disease — staging laparotomy. *Quarterly Journal of Medicine*, **43**, 620.
D'Angio, G. J., Farber, S. & Maddock, C. L. (1959) Potentiation of x-ray effects by actinomycin D. *Radiology*, **73**, 175–177.
De Vita, V. T., Serpick, A. A. & Carbonne, P. P. (1970) Combination chemotherapy in the treatment of advanced Hodgkin's disease. *Annals of Internal Medicine*, **73**, 881–895.
De Vita, V. T., Arseneau, J. C., Sherins, R., Canellos, G. P. & Young, R. C. (1972) Intensive chemotherapy for Hodgkin's disease: long-term complications. *National Cancer Institute Monograph*, No. 36.
Dorfman, R. F. (1971) Relationship of histology to site in Hodgkin's disease. *Cancer Research*, **31**, 1786–1793.

Easson, E. C. & Russell, M. H. (1963) The cure of Hodgkin's disease. *British Medical Journal,* 1, 1704–1707.

Eraklis, A. J., Kevy, S. V., Diamond, L. R. & Gross, R. F. (1967) Hazard of overwhelming infection after splenectomy in childhood. *New England Journal of Medicine,* 276, 1225–1229.

Ezdinli, E. Z., Sokal, J. E., Aungst, C. W., Rim, A. & Sandberg, A. A. (1969) Myeloid leukaemia in Hodgkin's disease: chromosomal abnormalities. *Annals of Internal Medicine,* 71, 1097–1104.

Fairley, G. H., Patterson, M. & Scott, R. B. (1966) Chemotherapy of Hodgkin's disease with cyclophosphamide, vinblastine and procarbazine. *British Medical Journal,* 2, 75–78.

Frei, E., III, Luce, J. R., Gamble, J. F., Coltman, C. A., Constanzi, J. L., Talley, R. W., Monto, R. W., Wilson, H. E., Hewlett, J. S., Delaney, F. C. & Gehan, E. A. (1973) Combination chemotherapy in advanced Hodgkin's disease — induction and maintenance of remission. *Annals of Internal Medicine,* 79, 376–382.

Gazet, J. C. (1973) Laparotomy and splenectomy. In *Hodgkin's Disease,* ed. Smithers, D. W., pp. 190–200. Edinburgh: Churchill Livingstone.

Gilbert, R. (1939) Radiotherapy in Hodgkin's disease (malignant granulomatosis): anatomic and clinical foundations: governing principles: results. *American Journal of Roentgenology,* 41, 198–241.

Glatstein, E., McHardy-Young, S., Brast, M., Eltringham, J. R. & Kriss, J. P. (1971) Alterations in serum thyrotropin (TSH) and thyroid function following radiotherapy in patients with malignant lymphoma. *Journal of Clinical Endocrinology and Metabolism,* 32, 833–841.

Glatstein, E. & Goffinet, D. R. (1974) Staging of Hodgkin's disease and other lymphomas. *Clinics in Haematology,* 3, 77–90.

Greenfield, W. S. (1878) Specimens illustrative of the pathology of lymphadenoma and leucocythaemia. *Transactions of the Pathological Society of London,* 29, 272–304.

Hodgkin, T. (1832) On some morbid appearances of the absorbent glands and spleen. *Medico-Chirurgical Transactions,* 17, 68–114.

Ihde, D. C., De Vita, V. T., Canellos, G. P., Chabner, B. A. & Young, R. C. (1975) Effect of splenectomy on tolerance to combination chemotherapy in patients with lymphoma. *Abstract 1037.* American Society of Clinical Oncology.

Irving, M. (1975) The role of surgery in the management of Hodgkin's disease. *British Journal of Surgery,* 62, 853–862.

Kadin, M. E., Glatstein, E. & Dorfman, R. F. (1971) Clinicopathologic studies of 117 untreated patients subjected to laparotomy for the staging of Hodgkin's disease. *Cancer,* 27, 1277–1294.

Kaplan, H. S. (1968) Prognostic significance of the relapse free interval after radiotherapy in Hodgkin's disease. *Cancer,* 22, 1131–1136.

Kaplan, H. S. (1972) *Hodgkin's Disease.* Cambridge: Harvard University Press.

Kaplan, H. S. (1973) Hodgkin's disease. Modern radiotherapeutic techniques and their results. *Series Haematologica,* 6, 139–151.

Kaplan, H. S. & Rosenberg, S. A. (1975) The management of Hodgkin's disease. *Cancer,* 36, 796–803.

Lacher, M. J. & Durant, J. R. (1965) Combined vinblastine and chlorambucil treatment of Hodgkin's disease. *Annals of Internal Medicine,* 62, 468–476.

Langhans, T. (1872) Das maligne Lymphosarkom (pseudoleukämie). *Virchow's Archiv für pathologische Anatomie und Physiologie,* 54, 509–537.

Lee, B. J., Nelson, J. H. & Schwarz, G. (1964) Evaluation of lymphgraphy, inferior vena cavography and intravenous pyelography in the clinical staging and management of Hodgkin's disease and lymphosarcoma. *New England Journal of Medicine,* 271, 327–337.

Lipton, M. J., De Nardo, G. L., Silverman, S. & Glatstein, E. (1972) Evaluation of the liver and spleen in Hodgkin's disease. I. The value of hepatic scintigraphy. *American Journal of Medicine,* 52, 356–362.

Lukes, R. J. (1963) Relationship of histologic features to clinical stage in Hodgkin's disease. *American Journal of Roentgenology,* 90, 944–955.

Lukes, R. J. & Butler, J. J. (1966) The pathology and nomenclature of Hodgkin's disease. *Cancer Research,* 26, 1063–1081.

MacDonald, J. S. (1973) Bone involvement. In *Hodgkin's Disease,* ed. Smithers, D. W., pp. 128–136. Edinburgh: Churchill Livingstone.

McElwain, T. J. (1973) The chemotherapy of Hodgkin's disease. *British Journal of Hospital Medicine,* 9, 451–456.

Moore, M. R., Jones, S. E., Bull, J. M., William, L. A. & Rosenberg, S. A. (1973) MOPP chemotherapy for advanced Hodgkin's disease. Prognostic factors in 81 patients. *Cancer,* 32, 52–60.

Neiman, R. S., Rosen, P. J. & Lukes, R. J. (1973) Lymphocyte-depletion Hodgkin's disease. A clinicopathologic entity. *New England Journal of Medicine*, **288**, 751–754.

Nicholson, W. M., Beard, M. E., Crowther, D., Stansfeld, A., Varton, C., Malpas, J., Fairley, G. H. & Scott, R. B. (1970) Combination chemotherapy in generalised Hodgkin's disease. *British Medical Journal*, **3**, 7–10.

Peckham, M. J. (1973) The radiotherapy of Hodgkin's disease. *British Journal of Hospital Medicine*, **9**, 457–468.

Peckham, M. J., Ford, H. T., McElwain, T. J., Harmer, L. L., Atkinson, K. & Austin, D. E. (1975) The results of radiotherapy for Hodgkin's disease. *British Journal of Cancer*, **32**, 391–400.

Peters, M. V. (1961) The place of irradiation in the control of Hodgkin's disease. In *Proceedings of the 4th National Cancer Conference, 1960*, pp. 571–584. Philadelphia: Lippincott.

Peters, V., Brown, T. & Rideout, D. (1973) Prognostic influences and radiation therapy according to pattern of disease. *Journal of the American Medical Association*, **223**, 53–59.

Prosnitz, L. R., Fischer, J. J. & Vera, R. (1972) Hodgkin's disease treated with radiation therapy: follow-up data and the value of laparotomy. *American Journal of Roentgenology, Radium Therapy and Nuclear Medicine*, **114**, 583–590.

Reed, D. M. (1902) On the pathological changes in Hodgkin's disease, with especial reference to its relation to tuberculosis. *Johns Hopkins Hospital Report*, **10**, 132–196.

Rosenberg, S. A. & Kaplan, H. S. (1970) Hodgkin's disease and other malignant lymphomas. *California Medicine*, **113**, 23–38.

Rosenberg, S. A. & Kaplan, H. S. (1975) The management of stage I, II and III Hodgkin's disease with combined radiotherapy and chemotherapy. *Cancer*, **35**, 55–63.

Rosenthal, S. R. (1936) Significance of tissue lymphocytes in the prognosis of lymphogranulo-matosis. *Archives of Pathology*, **21**, 628–646.

Rye Classification (1966) *Cancer Research*, **26** (6), 1.

Ruckdeschel, J., Martin, R. G. & Byhardt, R. W. (1975) Non-radiotherapeutic factors in the development of radiation-related pericardial effusions in patients treated for Hodgkin's disease. *Abstract 1069*. American Society of Clinical Oncology.

Salzman, J. R. & Kaplan, H. S. (1971) Effect of prior splenectomy on haematological tolerance during total lymphoid radiotherapy of patients with Hodgkin's disease. *Cancer*, **27**, 471–478.

Silverman, S., DeNardo, G. L., Glatstein, E. & Lipton, M. (1972) Evaluation of the liver and spleen in Hodgkin's disease. II. The value of splenic scintigraphy. *American Journal of Medicine*, **52**, 362–366.

Skarkin, A., Lokich, J., Goodman, R., Chaffey, J. & Frei, E., III (1975) Combined intermittent chemotherapy and radiotherapy in oat cell carcinoma of the lung. *Abstract 1171*. American Society of Clinical Oncology.

Smetana, H. F. & Cohen, B. M. (1956) Mortality in relation to histologic type in Hodgkin's disease. *Blood*, **11**, 211–224.

Smithers, D. (1973) *Hodgkin's Disease*. Edinburgh: Churchill Livingstone.

Speiser, B., Rubin, P. & Casarett, G. (1973) Aspermia following truncal irradiation in Hodgkin's disease. *Cancer*, **32**, 692–698.

Spinelli, P., Beretta, G., Bajetta, E., Tancini, G., Castallani, R., Rilke, F. & Bonadonna, G. (1975) Laparoscopy and laparotomy combined with bone marrow biopsy in staging Hodgkin's disease. *British Medical Journal*, **4**, 554–556.

Sternberg, L. (1898) Über eine eigenartige unter dem Bilde der Pseudoleukämie verlaufende Tuberculae des Lymphatischen Apparates. *Zeitschrift für Heilkunder*, **19**, 21–90.

Strum, S. B. & Rappaport, H. (1971) Interrelations of the histologic types of Hodgkin's disease. *Archives of Pathology*, **91**, 127–134.

Tokita, M., Gilladoga, A., Madhu, J., Hahn, E. & D'Angio, G. (1975) Increased cardiotoxicity in rabbits given radiation and adriamycin. *Abstract 1020*. American Society of Clinical Oncology.

Tubiana, M., Attie, E., Flamant, R., Gerard-Marchant, R. & Hagat, M. (1971) Prognostic factors in 454 cases of Hodgkin's disease. *Cancer Research*, **31**, 1801–1810.

White, R. J., Webb, J. A. W., Tucker, A. R. & Foster, R. M. (1973) Pulmonary function after lymphography. *British Medical Journal*, **4**, 775–777.

Young, R. C., Canellos, G. P., Chabner, B. A., Schein, P. S., & De Vita, V. T. (1973) Maintenance chemotherapy for advanced Hodgkin's disease in remission. *Lancet*, **1**, 1339–1343.

Young, R. C., Canellos, G. P., Chabner, B. A. & De Vita, V. T. (1975) Pattern of relapse after complete remission in Hodgkin's disease treated with MOPP chemotherapy. *Abstract 114*. American Society of Clinical Oncology and American Association for Cancer Research meeting.

3
THE MANAGEMENT OF LYMPHOMAS OTHER THAN HODGKIN'S DISEASE

D. Crowther   J. H. Scarffe

Malignant diseases of the lymphoreticular system not classified as Hodgkin's disease form a protean group. They are widely varied in histological pattern and clinical features. As in Hodgkin's disease, the cell type forming the tumour cell population is not clearly defined in many cases and this means that the classification of these diseases is complex and appears confusing. It is not surprising, therefore, that at present the problems of evaluation and treatment in these diseases is one of the most controversial in the field of clinical oncology.

PATHOLOGY

One of the most important requirements for a useful pathological classification is that it should have prognostic significance within a defined clinical group. There are two main features defined on histological examination which have been shown to have prognostic significance; the degree of nodularity and the degree of tumour cell differentiation. In 1956, Rappaport, Winter and Hicks

Table 3.1   Histopathological classification based on Rappaport (1966)

Relatively 'good' prognostic group
  Well-differentiated diffuse lymphocytic
  Well-differentiated nodular lymphocytic
  Poorly differentiated nodular lymphocytic
  Mixed lymphocytic/histiocytic nodular
  Histiocytic nodular

Relatively 'bad' prognostic group
  Poorly differentiated diffuse lymphocytic (including lymphoblastic)
  Mixed lymphocytic/histiocytic diffuse
  Histiocytic diffuse
  Undifferentiated diffuse (including Burkitt-like)

proposed a classification of all lymphomas incorporating these principles and later defined the classification of lymphomas other than Hodgkin's disease more clearly (Rappaport, 1966). A classification based on these observations has now been used at several major clinical centres and retrospective analysis has shown a useful correlation with prognosis. The classification is shown in Table 3.1*. The terms lymphosarcoma and reticulum cell sarcoma should no longer be applied to these lymphomas since they are misleading.

* Supported by the Cancer Research Campaign, 2 Carlton House Terrace, London SW1Y 5AR.

Unfortunately, the classification suggested by Rappaport and his colleagues is by no means perfect and is to some extent misleading but it is, at present, the best working classification since its relation to prognosis is reasonably well defined.

One of the main problems is the difficulty, using histology alone, in defining the cell type involved in the malignant process. Attempts are now being made to identify the cell by other methods. It is reasonable to expect that lymphoid cell malignancies could involve not only the basic cells of the thymic-dependent and the bursa-equivalent lymphoid systems but also varyingly differentiated cells within these systems. Lukes and his colleagues have attempted to relate a histological classification to the cell types defined in this way but it remains difficult to categorise the cell type using histology alone (Lukes and Collins, 1975). For this reason many centres are now attempting to improve classification by identification of the cell type in terms of cell surface properties.

Table 3.2   T cell malignant disease

Acute lymphoblastic leukaemia (T cell variant) = 25 per cent
Chronic lymphocytic leukaemia (T cell variant) — rare
Thymic lymphoma
Some nodal lymphomas
Mycosis fungoides
Sézary syndrome

Table 3.3   B cell malignant disease

Myeloma
Chronic lymphocytic leukaemia (nearly all cases)
Waldenström's macroglobulinaemia
Well-differentiated and nodular lymphomas (most cases)
Burkitt's African lymphoma
Burkitt-like lymphoma/leukaemia outside tropics
Hairy cell leukaemia (controversial)

Sheep red cells tend to aggregate round T cells in vitro and this rosetting test forms a convenient way of identifying a T cell membrane marker on malignant cells. The mechanism involved in rosette formation is unknown. B cells possess surface immunoglobulin, and immunofluorescence tests are capable of identifying the immunoglobulin and providing evidence for a monoclonal proliferation of B cells in some malignant lymphomas. Using these methods, some malignant diseases of the lymphoreticular system can be defined as involving T or B cells and these are listed in Tables 3.2 and 3.3.

Using these tests and other cytological features, the cells forming the neoplastic mass of some patients classified as histiocytic lymphoma can be shown to be of lymphoid rather than histiocytic origin. Clearly these tests, used in conjunction with the histological classification, are providing an improved classification which should help the clinician in defining his groups for appropriate treatment.

Hairy cell leukaemia is a disease of insidious onset and slow course characterised by progressive splenomegaly and the presence of abnormal cells in the spleen, blood and bone marrow. Under phase microscopy the malignant cell has long cytoplasmic villi and these give a hairy appearance in fixed preparations.

The disease may be confused with chronic lymphatic leukaemia or malignant lymphoma. The difference is important since the disease has a slow course and the patient may be helped by splenectomy.

The Sézary syndrome is a rare condition characterised by chronic skin lesions associated with a mononuclear infiltrate and the appearance of large numbers of abnormal mononuclear cells in the peripheral blood. The classical features of the disease are usually confined to the skin and consist of infiltrative lesions with pruritus and erythroderma. The morphological and staining characteristics of the cells suggest they are of lymphoid origin, and the response to phytohaemag-glutinin and surface properties indicate they are of T cell type. Other lymphoid malignancies of T cell type may also have skin involvement and it is possible that these may be related to the surface properties of T cells.

CLINICAL AND PATHOLOGICAL STAGING

A most important feature in assessment of malignant lymphomas is the clinical presentation and the sites of involvement at the time treatment is started. Careful staging is mandatory if all the disease is to be eradicated in all detectable sites. If treatment is designed to be merely palliative, then extensive staging procedures are not required.

Unfortunately, there is no clear correlation between clinical types and pathological features, and there is also considerable overlap of clinical features from one group to another. A patient with a diffuse histiocytic lymphoma, for example, may present in exactly the same way as a patient with a well-differentiated lymphocytic lymphoma. The distinction between a leukaemia and a lymphoma is made on a staging procedure and the definition of acute leukaemia includes diffuse infiltration of the bone marrow with blast cells identified on bone marrow examination. The presence of blast cells in the blood is not necessary in this definition. The distinction between acute leukaemia and lymphoma becomes blurred in those patients with patchy marrow infiltration and in those with a small percentage of diffusely infiltrating cells. A further difficulty is seen in the group of patients who, after careful staging, are found to have a single deposit showing the histological features of a diffuse poorly differentiated lymphoblastic lymphoma who develop all the features of acute lymphoblastic leukaemia within a few months of apparently adequate local treatment. Indeed, this state of affairs is so common in children that many leading paediatric oncology centres use a therapeutic regime similar to that used for acute leukaemia in these patients (Pinkel, Johnson and Aur, 1975). Patients with chronic lymphocytic leukaemia (CLL) would be reported as well-differentiated lymphocytic lymphomas from lymph node biopsy by a histologist who has no knowledge of the blood or marrow findings. The blood and marrow may not be detectably involved initially in patients with well-differentiated lymphocytic lymphomas, but the disease may gradually pass into a condition indistinguishable from CLL with extensive blood and marrow involvement.

An additional problem is that the site of presentation and bulk of disease may vary enormously between different patients with the same histological classification but the appropriate treatment and prognosis may be quite different. A patient with bulky disease involving para-aortic and mesenteric lymph nodes will require different considerations from a patient with less bulky disease above the diaphragm, even though both patients have stage II disease. A convenient staging classification for these lymphomas involves similar procedures to those used in Hodgkin's disease (HD), but the site of disease must be taken into account in these lymphomas since the manifestations are more varied than in HD. It is convenient to group together patients with HD of the same stage, although there is a reservation that different sites of presentation may carry a different prognosis. This problem, however, is much more important in patients with other lymphomas because abdominal and extranodal involvement more frequently constitutes the main clinical problem. For these reasons it is unwise to group together all patients with a certain stage of non-Hodgkin lymphomas; their outlook may well vary considerably depending upon the site of disease. Classifications involving histology, cytological properties, clinical presentation, and staging must therefore be taken together for appropriate groupings to be made.

After a careful history and physical examination, initial investigations should include a full blood count, including platelet count and reticulocyte count, a Coombs' test, and a needle biopsy with aspiration of bone marrow. Biochemical assessment should include tests of hepatic and renal function, serum protein analysis with immunoglobulin levels, and serum calcium and uric acid estimations. Radiological studies should include chest x-ray (with tomography, if indicated), x-rays of the postnasal space and sinuses (if indicated on clinical examination), a skeletal survey and abdominal lymphography (patients with obvious intra-abdominal nodal disease or stage IV disease do not require lymphography). Isotope scanning of liver, spleen, and bone may also prove useful, but its value is at present under investigation. Some authorities advocate the use of inferior vena cavagrams and gallium-67 scans for the detection of lymph node disease but again their role is still under investigation. It is quite possible that in the not too distant future the EMI total body scanner may play a major part in clinical staging. Others advocate laparotomy but its value in staging is controversial.

Not infrequently the meninges are involved in patients with diffuse lympho-blastic, histiocytic, or undifferentiated lymphomas. This complication is more difficult to treat than CNS leukaemia in ALL of childhood and its prevention requires different measures from those used in childhood leukaemia. It is advisable to study the CSF in patients presenting with histology of poor prognostic type (Table 3.1). Careful investigation of these CNS problems and the development of appropriate treatment for their prevention is a most important challenge for the future.

Other investigations alluded to previously are proving useful in delineating groups of patients for special consideration. These tests include cell membrane marker assessment (T and B classification), morphological analysis using lymph node imprints, and proliferation studies but at the present time, these analyses are restricted to special centres where these diseases can be studied in detail.

Certain investigations will be discussed in further detail.

Bone marrow examination

The bone marrow is much more likely to be involved than in patients with Hodgkin's disease. In a prospective series of 109 patients studied routinely with bone marrow biopsy, the overall incidence of involvement was 41 per cent (Rosenberg, 1975). In the nodular lymphocytic, poorly differentiated group, 28 of 33 patients (85 per cent) had bone marrow involvement. Thirty-four of the 45 positive marrows were diagnosed by an aspiration biopsy. In the remaining 11 patients, marrow infiltration was identified with the use of a Stryker saw biopsy (1 cm open trephine). In six of these the results of aspiration were equivocal and in two patients a needle biopsy was not done. In only three cases was a positive trephine biopsy obtained after a definitely negative needle biopsy. These investigations suggest that biopsy using the Stryker saw technique is not mandatory.

The histiocytic lymphomas have a low incidence of bone marrow involvement whereas lymphomas with a predominance of lymphocytic cells have a higher incidence in both nodular and diffuse varieties. In spite of this, the survival rate of patients with histiocytic lymphoma without marrow involvement is far worse than that of those with nodular, poorly differentiated lymphocytic lymphomas in spite of an extremely high incidence of marrow involvement.

If the treatment planned involves an attempt to eradicate tumour from all sites of involvement, bone marrow biopsy is essential. A Westerman–Jensen or Jamshidi needle are appropriate for this purpose.

Staging laparotomy

The role of a staging laparotomy has not been clearly established in patients with lymphomas other than Hodgkin's disease. The large number of histological subgroups and the protean clinical manifestations makes analysis of its value difficult. In addition, the procedure is more hazardous than in HD, since the patients are usually in an older age group, they may have impairment of humoral immunity and complications such as tumour involvement of the laparotomy scar are more common. In some patients presenting with abdominal disease the procedure would be followed by a second operation.

A large group of patients present with nodal abdominal disease but no evidence of involvement above the diaphragm, and they require an appropriate technique for staging disease within the thorax, which should be non-invasive.

Rosenberg, Dorfman and Kaplan (1975) have described the results of bone marrow biopsy and laparotomy with splenectomy in a series of 127 consecutive untreated patients with non-Hodgkin lymphoma. The stage of patients with diffuse lymphoma under the age of 20 and the majority (86 per cent) of those under the age of 40, was not altered by laparotomy. Of the four patients whose stage was changed, three had less disease than suspected and one patient advanced from stage III to IV. In this group of patients a staging laparotomy would therefore not seem to be necessary for most treatment programmes.

In the same study, more than half the patients with diffuse histiocytic lymphoma were found to have pathological stage I or II but as will be shown later, the relapse rate in this group of patients suggests that disease was present but remained undetected by laparotomy. In contrast with this, 17 out of 24 patients with diffuse lymphoma of other histological types and 10 out of 11 with clinical stage III disease were found to have pathological stage IV disease. In practice, when careful staging procedures are employed, clinical stage III disease is uncommon and nearly all patients suspected of having clinical stage III disease, have evidence of extension of stage IV on pathological examination at laparotomy. Nodular poorly differentiated lymphocytic lymphomas nearly always present with stage IV disease, which was found in approximately one-third of patients with nodular mixed lymphocytic, histiocytic or nodular histiocytic lymphomas.

Although laparotomy is the most accurate way of staging patients with these lymphomas, it still tends to underestimate the extent of the disease. It seems very likely that nearly all nodular poorly differentiated lymphocytic lymphomas as well as diffuse lymphomas other than the histiocytic variety, are generalised at the time of diagnosis and the treatment programme should bear this in mind. In contrast with HD, the mesenteric nodes are involved in more than 50 per cent of those biopsied and this has important connotations in the choice of radiation field if curative radiotherapy programmes are envisaged.

In summary, it is clear from these and other laparotomy studies (Johnson et al, 1975; Hass et al, 1971; Hanks et al, 1972; Veronesi et al, 1974; Moran et al, 1975) that the majority of patients presenting with a non-Hodgkin lymphoma have generalised disease. This is quite unlike the findings in HD and indicates that the treatment should involve systemic measures in most cases if the aim of treatment is eradication of the disease, and not merely palliation.

These studies have, however, also shown important differences which may be a reflection of variation in different geographic areas. The distribution of histological types and staging features were rather different in the series reported from Italy by Veronesi and his colleagues (1974). It remains to be seen whether these differences are merely due to different techniques and interpretations or to rather more fundamental issues.

Central Nervous System Involvement

Disease within the central nervous system (CNS) may complicate the course of non-Hodgkin lymphomas. The CNS is involved most frequently in patients with ALL and diffuse lymphoblastic lymphomas and may also complicate diffuse histiocytic lymphomas. CNS disease is much less common in the nodular and well-differentiated lymphocytic lymphomas.

An early paper by Rosenberg reported the incidence of CNS complications in 1290 cases of non-Hodgkin lymphomas and indicated the need to consider this in planning appropriate treatment (Rosenberg et al, 1961). In this series, 14.7 per cent of patients had CNS involvement and this figure agrees fairly well with other reported series (Williams et al, 1959; Law et al, 1975). Nervous system complications may be of several varieties and not all are associated with infiltration by tumour; some are vascular in origin, others are infective or may be due to paramalignant disease in the CNS. The pathological incidence of CNS involvement with malignant disease is not clearly documented for the different histological subtypes of non-Hodgkin lymphomas and more information on this is urgently required.

There is an increasing awareness that CNS involvement may be detected early in the disease in a proportion of adult patients with ALL and undifferentiated diffuse lymphomas. In a series reported from St Bartholomew's Hospital (Lister et al, 1976), 5 out of 28 patients with ALL had blast cells in the CSF at the time of apparent complete remission. A further four patients subsequently relapsed with CNS disease, two of whom initially had had equivocal CSF findings. There are suggestions in the literature that some forms of non-Hodgkin lymphoma may be associated with a particularly bad prognosis and a high incidence of CNS disease. Of five patients with undifferentiated leukaemia of the Burkitt type in the St Bartholomew's Hospital series, all developed CNS involvement early in the course of the disease. A further five cases were classified as undifferentiated lymphomas of Burkitt type (<30 per cent blast cells in marrow) and in three the CNS became involved.

Patients with diffuse histiocytic lymphoma also have a relatively high incidence of CNS disease. In the St Bartholomew's Hospital series, 4 out of 17 with stage III and IV disease developed CNS involvement (three of these during remission induction therapy). Most patients with diffuse histiocytic lymphoma with CNS involvement tend to develop CNS manifestations early in the disease, CSF studies are therefore of great importance in planning treatment (Griffin et al, 1971; Law et al, 1975). It appears that most patients developing CNS disease have initial bone marrow involvement.

There is conclusive evidence that cranial irradiation (2400 rad (24 Gy) in three weeks) and intrathecal methotrexate (five doses during the period of irradiation at a dose of 12 mg/m^2) is highly effective in preventing CNS disease in children with ALL (Aur, 1974). The treatment was pioneered during many years of careful experimental work by the Memphis group at St Jude's Hospital and has been well substantiated by several groups in other countries (e.g. British MRC Report, 1973).

Several centres have adopted a policy of CNS prophylactic treatment in adults with ALL and certain groups of non-Hodgkin lymphomas with a bad prognosis. Unfortunately, there is a higher incidence of CNS relapse in adult patients treated with prophylactic cranial irradiation and intrathecal Methotrexate than in the ALL group of childhood. This complication is also more difficult to treat in adults than in children with ALL. In the St Bartholomew's Hospital series, several CNS relapses have occurred following CNS treatment using cranio-spinal irradiation (3000 rad (30 Gy) cranium, 1500 rad (15 Gy) whole spine in three weeks) and five intrathecal injections of methotrexate (8 mg/m^2) plus five of intrathecal cytosine arabinoside (30 mg/m^2) using a twice weekly schedule. Clearly, new methods for the treatment and prophylaxis of this distressing complication are required for the adult group of ALL and non-Hodgkin lymphomas.

PROGNOSIS

An important prerequisite for planning therapy in patients with lymphomas is a reasonably accurate appreciation of their prognosis. Several large retrospective studies have recently been published in which prognosis was evaluated following the conventional treatment of the time.

Patients with diffuse lymphomas tend to fare less well than those with nodular forms. For example, in one series of 100 patients with nodular lymphomas (stages I to IIIE) treated with radiotherapy with curative intent, the median survival was 7.5 years, compared with 2.6 years in 98 patients with diffuse

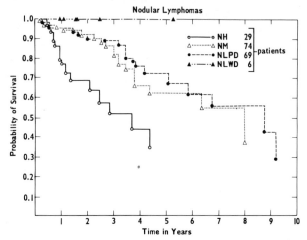

Figure 3.1 Survival curves for nodular lymphomas at Stanford Medical Center. NH, nodular histiocytic; NM, nodular mixed; NLPD, nodular lymphocytic poorly differentiated; NLWD, nodular lymphocytic well differentiated. (Reproduced with permission from Jones et al, 1973)

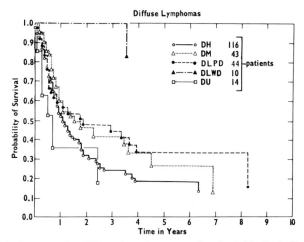

Figure 3.2 Survival curves for diffuse lymphomas at Stanford Medical Center. DH, diffuse histiocytic; DM, diffuse mixed; DLPD, diffuse lymphocytic poorly differentiated; DLWD, diffuse lymphocytic well differentiated; DU, diffuse undifferentiated. (Reproduced with permission from Jones et al, 1973)

lymphomas of similar stage and treatment (Jones et al, 1973). Several other series support this conclusion (e.g. Brown et al, 1975). Furthermore, the superior survival of the nodular types over the diffuse was sustained for each cell type and stage of disease.

The cell type and degree of differentiation have also been shown to be of immense importance in prognosis (Jones et al, 1973). Figure 3.1 shows the varying prognosis within the nodular group, and Figure 3.2 within the diffuse group. With the exception of the diffuse lymphocytic well-differentiated lymphoma, diffuse lymphomas have a poor prognosis unless quite localised.

Another most important factor determining prognosis is the stage of disease; this has been well documented in several series using different methods of histological classification (e.g. Freeman, Berg and Cutler, 1972; Jones et al, 1973). Localised involvement (stages I, IE, and II, IIE) is seen in about one-third of patients, the incidence of localised extranodal disease is much higher than it is

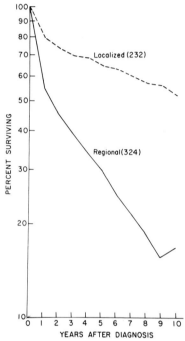

Figure 3.3 Survival curves for extranodal 'lymphosarcoma'. (Reproduced with permission from Freeman et al, 1972)

in patients with HD. A wide range of extranodal sites may be involved such as the gastrointestinal tract, Waldeyer's ring, gonads, thyroid and skin, etc. The prognosis is better when the lymphoma is localised to the extranodal site (IE) than if adjacent nodes are involved in addition (IIE regional). The series from the National Cancer Institute (Freeman et al, 1972), using the old-fashioned pathological classification, illustrates this quite well (Fig. 3.3, 3.4). Clearly, these two groups with and without nodal involvement, should be analysed separately in any new trial. It is noteworthy that the median survival of patients with stage II and IIE and diffuse pathology (but not well-differentiated lymphocytic) is less than two years (Jones, 1974). The survival of patients with stage IV diffuse lymphoma is significantly worse. In the worst prognostic group (diffuse histiocytic), patients with stage II and IIE disease have a median survival

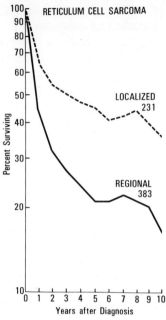

Figure 3.4   Survival curves for extranodal 'reticulum cell sarcoma'. (Reproduced with permission from Freeman et al, 1972)

of approximately one year following radiotherapy, whereas the median survival is less than a year in patients with stage III or IV disease.

TREATMENT

The studies previously described have given valuable information regarding the planning of treatment. A significant proportion of patients with stages IE, I, IIE and II relapse following radiotherapy alone. The Toronto group, for example, found that out of 44.6 per cent of patients with apparently localised disease who achieved a complete remission following radiotherapy alone, 40.8 per cent relapsed with a recurrence outside the treated fields (Brown et al, 1974); thus local therapy is inadequate for the control of a significant proportion of these patients. This statement is true even for those staged after laparotomy. The patients with a particularly high risk of relapse can be identified using careful histopathological assessment; the death rate is high in some 'bad' histological groups and these patients require further treatment in addition to local radiotherapy to the site of disease.

Radiotherapy with doses at or above 3000 rad (30 Gy) gives at a rate of approximately 1000 rad (10 Gy) per week results in few relapses in the irradiated area in patients with nodular lymphoma (Fuks and Kaplan, 1973). Using these doses, relapses are more common in the irradiated area in diffuse disease; indeed, in the diffuse histiocytic group, recurrences within the irradiated area may occur at doses of 5000 rad (50 Gy) or greater. These facts have important connotations in planning radiotherapy in patients with lymphomas.

The time of relapse is different in the various histological subtypes. Histiocytic lymphomas tend to relapse during the first year following radiotherapy or not at all, whereas nodular lymphomas and those of well-differentiated lymphocytic type show a continuing pattern of relapse and are at prolonged risk for late relapse. Clearly, the follow-up procedure should be designed with this in mind. It is of some interest that a similar pattern of relapse in relation to duration of first remission is seen following chemotherapy for more advanced disease (see later). There is also a tendency for the diffuse lymphomas to relapse at extranodal sites and in this group, systemic therapy in addition to radiotherapy is advisable if such relapses are to be prevented.

Apparently localised lymphomas (stage I, IE, II and IIE) are conventionally treated using 'high-dose' radiotherapy to the regions involved. Additional fields are sometimes included if a subsequent relapse in a contiguous area might prove difficult to treat with further radiotherapy for technical reasons. In nodal disease of nodular pathology, the disease-free survival rate is high and if the disease does relapse, further treatment using radiotherapy or chemotherapy can greatly prolong survival. In view of this further therapy following radiotherapy in this group of patients must be considered, because such treatment could be hazardous. Studies are at present in progress to see whether extended field irradiation or 'total nodal' irradiation is better than radiation of the involved areas only, in prolonging disease-free survival and total survival. Total nodal irradiation is potentially hazardous and must be extensive (more so than for HD), in view of the relatively high risk of 'distant' node involvement such as the epitrochlear, popliteal, and mesenteric nodes. Certainly this is not a form of therapy to be advocated at present and the trials already in progress will take several years before an appropriate analysis can be made. Our own view is that systemic chemotherapy is more likely to succeed in prolonging disease-free survival and total survival, but the choice of therapy must be carefully made to avoid morbidity and mortality in a group of patients with an overall good prognosis. Treatment at the time of relapse may be just as effective as prophylactic therapy and a control arm should be included in any study of this sort.

The localised group with histology of poor prognostic omen presents different problems; the death rate, for example, in the diffuse histiocytic lymphomas (stages II and IIE) is very high (median survival approximately one year). The relapses frequently involve extranodal sites, the majority of relapses in the diffuse lymphomas following radiotherapy occur during the first year of follow-up, and the risk progressively diminishes with each subsequent year of disease free observation. This is especially true of patients with diffuse histiocytic lymphoma in whom 95 per cent of the actual relapses occur during the first year of follow-up. A salient feature is that, following relapse, retreatment using additional radiotherapy or palliative single agent chemotherapy is of only transient value since the survival curves and disease-free survival curves are roughly parallel (Jones, 1974). In view of these data, there is much to be said for following radiotherapy with adjuvant systemic chemotherapy using cytotoxic drugs known to be effective in treating extensive disease. The type of chemotherapy most likely to be effective is controversial and studies are in progress to analyse this. In Manchester, the Lymphoma Group is randomising patients with supradiaphragmatic stages I, II and IIE lymphomas of poor prognosis between two forms of adjuvant chemotherapy following radiotherapy. One arm involves an approach similar to that used in acute leukaemia with six to eight weeks' treatment involving vincristine, adriamycin, and prednisolone followed by 6-mercaptopurine, methotrexate, and cyclophosphamide maintenance for two years. The other arm involves an antilymphoma type of approach using CMOPP as described by De Vita et al (1975). This combination involves cyclophosphamide, vincristine, procarbazine, and prednisolone.

There are no published studies concerning the value of involved field, extended field or total nodal therapy for localised nodular lymphomas using randomised prospective studies. A retrospective analysis has suggested that disease-free survival may have been superior for the patients who received wide field treatment but the difference was not significant at the 5 per cent level. No difference in total survival was found (Jones et al, 1973). There was no evidence that 'high-dose' extended field irradiation was of greater value than high-dose involved field irradiation in the other histological types but the analysis was retrospective and the relevant subgroups were rather small.

Evidence presented previously has shown that patients with clinical stage III lymphoma are usually found to have stage IV disease using careful staging procedures, including lymphography, bone marrow examination, laparoscopy or laparotomy (Johnson et al, 1975). The high incidence of relapse with extranodal disease and involvement of nodes outside the usual nodal areas of involvement by HD, means that systemic treatment will be required if cures are ever to be achieved in these groups. This raises the question of whether a 'curative' approach is the best method of treatment in all groups of lymphomas. Indeed, there is no other branch of oncology where the treatments used are so varied and controversial.

If we consider the well-differentiated lymphocytic lymphomas first, it is apparent that patients with generalised disease have a varied outlook, although the group as a whole has a reasonably good prognosis. Some patients do well for months or even years without specific therapy, others require urgent treatment and have a short survival. There are no established staging or histopathological criteria which can distinguish these groups; accordingly, in one centre the treatment may involve a 'wait and see' policy followed by radiotherapy to troublesome areas or single agent chemotherapy (e.g. chlorambucil or cyclophosphamide). Other centres recommend an attempt at remission induction using single agent or combination chemotherapy, extensive irradiation, or combined radiotherapy and chemotherapy. There is a very great danger of overtreating these patients and high dose total nodal irradiation with or without combination chemotherapy, which is being tested in some centres, may prove to be dangerous. Clearly, the quality in addition to the quantity of life needs analysing in these studies and this is a long-term project.

The use of combination chemotherapy in stage III and IV disease has resulted in increased remission rates compared with single agent chemotherapy but 'good' and 'bad' pathology groups behave in a different manner. Several forms of combination chemotherapy has been recommended for the 'good' group; one of the most popular is the CVP regime suggested by the chemotherapy group at the National Cancer Institute, the schedule is as follows:

Cyclophosphamide	400 mg/m^2 by mouth daily, days 1 to 5
Vincristine	1.4 mg/m^2 (maximum 2 mg) intravenously, day 1
Prednisolone	100 mg/m^2 orally daily, days 1 to 5

A reduced dose of prednisolone has been used in some series. The apparent complete remission rate following CVP is in the order of 60 per cent which is better than the remission rate previously reported after the use of a single agent. Following remission induction, however, there is a pattern of continuing relapse and, unlike the diffuse histiocytic group, late relapses are common. It is unknown whether some form of 'maintenance' or remission chemotherapy will prevent these relapses and improve the disease-free survival. The Manchester Lymphoma Group is studying this problem by testing the role of intermittent chlorambucil following remission induction with a modified CVP regime. The group at St Bartholomew's Hospital is randomising their stage III and IV 'good' pathology patients between CVP and a less intensive regime using chlorambucil in order to answer the important question of quantity and quality of survival in groups treated with the single agent and those treated using the more intensive combination chemotherapeutic regime. At the Stanford Medical Center similar patients are being randomised between CVP combined with total nodal irradiation, CVP alone, and single agent chemotherapy. Hopefully, studies such as these will provide useful information regarding the most appropriate treatment for this group of patients.

The problems raised in treating patients with generalised lymphomas of 'poor' pathology require urgent consideration since the median survival is so short. It is salutary to remember that the median survival of this group is no better and probably worse than that of adult ALL. There are a great number of drug combinations in use for such patients, and only a few will be discussed.

The chemotherapy group at the National Cancer Institute in Bethesda have introduced two useful drug combinations for diffuse histiocytic lymphoma. Twenty-seven patients with generalised histiocytic lymphoma were treated with combination chemotherapy using mustine hydrochloride (or cyclo-phosphamide), vincristine, procarbazine, and prednisone (CMOPP), 11 (41 per cent) achieved a complete remission and only one of these had a recurrence of tumour at the time of publication (De Vita et al, 1975); the remaining 10 were free of all evidence of tumour 26 to 105 months from the end of treatment. This suggests that unlike other histological subgroups of lymphoma, a long-term disease-free survival can be achieved in this group and the pattern of relapse is quite different. It is clearly of great importance to achieve a complete remission in this group of patients since all the non-responders and partial responders died, mostly within one year. Their second suggested drug combination for patients with diffuse histiocytic lymphomas also seems to be of value (Schein et al, 1975); this involves a combination of bleomycin, adriamycin, cyclophosphamide, vincristine, and prednisone (BACOP).

Several other regimes have also been suggested in which adriamycin is one of the key drugs. A combination of vincristine, adriamycin, and prednisolone has been shown to be of value in remission induction and several centres are investigating its use. Only appropriate randomised trials will show which drug combination is best.

Once remission induction has been successful, the question of the type of maintenance therapy and its duration must be considered. Would a late intensification procedure be of value at six months to one year after presentation? How common is CNS disease and should an attempt be made to prevent this? Clearly, there are many problems to be answered and trials have only recently been evolved to study them.

New Therapeutic Approaches

Whole body irradiation

The use of whole body irradiation as a systemic measure for the treatment of widespread malignant disease is not new; it was first used only 12 years after Roentgen's publication of the discovery of x-rays in 1896. Following the development of chemotherapy, its use fell from favour until Johnson and his colleagues at the National Cancer Institute presented further data (Johnson, O'Connor and Levin, 1970). Subsequently, a group in Boston have also reported suggesting that the method may be useful in treating patients with generalised lymphomas (Chaffee et al, 1975); Hellman et al, 1975). The dose rates used were in the order of 15 rad twice weekly to a total of 150 rad using a 4 MeV linear accelerator.

Figure 3.5 shows the results of treating generalised lymphocytic lymphomas using whole body irradiation compared with CVP in a trial conducted at the National Cancer Institute (Cannellos et al, 1975). Most of the patients in both the National Cancer Institute and Boston studies were of nodular type but a great deal more work is required before a definite role for whole body irradiation can be delineated. The treatment is potentially dangerous and severe thrombocytopenia can occur at some dose rates; nevertheless, the results look interesting and illustrate the potential role of **radiotherapy as** a form of systemic therapy for

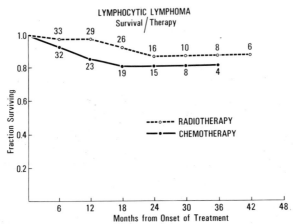

Figure 3.5 Survival curves for lymphocytic lymphoma comparing total body irradiation with combination chemotherapy. (Reproduced with permission from Canellos et al, 1975)

residual disease. The possible mechanisms behind the antitumour activity are also of great interest and studies in the future may be of value in formulating new plans for treating these malignant diseases.

Immunotherapy

The possibility of using methods to improve any antitumour immunity or host resistance in general against the growing tumour remains an attractive concept. Several studies involving the use of immunotherapy in its widest sense have been started but, as yet, no definitive results have been reported. Most controlled trials of 'immunotherapy' for malignant disease in man have involved the use of non-specific adjuvants such as BCG or *Corynebacterium parvum*, sometimes in conjunction with immunisations using irradiated tumour cells. These studies have not shown as yet that such techniques are really useful, although some prolongation in survival has been suggested in some trials with acute myelogenous leukaemia. Gorer and his colleagues showed in the late 1950s the potential use of antibody in some experimental leukaemias and lymphomas, and it is time that the possible use of antibody in these lymphomas should be reappraised. Soluble mediators produced by leucocytes could also prove to be of value in the future but work is required to characterise and assay the factors involved.

Certainly, the immunologist has an immense challenge here and his enthusiasm must not be curbed by undue pessimism. Lymphomas form a most useful research model, not only for clinical research, but also for more basic scientific research. Tumour material is easily available and the frequency of complete remissions means that normal small lymphocytes and other lymphoid cells may be relatively easily obtained for control purposes. It is pleasing to note that many major centres are now concentrating on this topic and undoubtedly the treatment of this group of conditions will rapidly improve during the next few years.

REFERENCES

Aur, R. J. A. (1974) Management of acute lymphoblastic leukaemia in children. In *Advances in Acute Leukaemia*, ed. Cleton, F. J., Crowther, D. & Malpas, J. S., p 95. ASP Biological and Medical Press BV (North-Holland Division).

British Medical Research Council Report (1973) Treatment of acute lymphoblastic leukaemia: effect of 'prophylactic' therapy against central nervous system leukaemia. *British Medical Journal*, 2, 381–384.

Brown, T. C., Peters, M. V., Bergsagel, D. E. & Reid, J. (1975) A retrospective analysis of the clinical results in relation to the Rappaport histological classification. *British Journal of Cancer*, 31, 174–186.

Canellos, G. P., De Vita, V. T., Young, R. C., Chabner, B. A., Schein, P. S. & Johnson, R. E. (1975) Therapy of advanced lymphocytic lymphoma: a preliminary report of a randomised trial between combination chemotherapy (CVP) and intensive radiotherapy. *British Journal of Cancer*, 31, 474–480.

Chaffey, J. T., Rosenthal, D. S., Pinuus, G. & Hellman, S. (1975) Advanced lymphosarcoma treated by total body irradiation. *British Journal of Cancer*, 31, 441–449.

De Vita, V. T., Canellos, G. P., Chabner, B., Schein, P., Hubbard, S. & Young, R. C. (1975) Advanced diffuse histiocytic lymphoma, a potentially curable disease. *Lancet*, 1, 248–250.

Freeman, C., Berg, J. W. & Cutler, S. J. (1972) Occurrence and prognosis of extranodal lymphomas. *Cancer*, 29, 252–260.

Fuks, Z. & Kaplan, H. S. (1973) Recurrence rates following radiation therapy of nodular and diffuse malignant lymphomas. *Radiology,* **108,** 675–684.

Griffin, J. W., Thompson, R. W., Mitchinson, J. M., Kiewief, J. C. & Welland, F. H. (1971) Lymphomatous leptomeningitis. *American Journal of Medicine,* **51,** 200–208.

Hanks, G. E., Terry, L. N., Bryan, J. A. & Newsome, J. F. (1972) Contribution of diagnostic laparotomy to staging non-Hodgkin's lymphomas. *Cancer,* **29,** 41–43.

Hass, A. C., Brunk, S. F., Gulesserian, H. P. & Guiler, R. L. (1971) The value of exploratory laparotomy in malignant lymphomas. *Radiology,* **101,** 157–165.

Hellman, S., Rosenthal, D. S., Moloney, W. C. & Chaffey, J. T. (1975) The treatment of non-Hodgkin's lymphoma. *Cancer,* **36,** 804–808.

Johnson, R. E., O'Connor, G. T. & Levin, D. (1970) Primary management of advanced lymphosarcoma with radiotherapy. *Cancer,* **25,** 787–791.

Johnson, R. E., De Vita, V. T., Kun, L. E., Chabner, B. R., Chretien, P. B., Berard, C. W. & Johnson, S. K. (1975) Patterns of involvement with malignant lymphoma and implications of treatment decision making. *British Journal of Cancer,* **31,** 237–241.

Jones, S. E., Fuks, Z., Bull, M., Kadin, M. E., Dorfman, R. F., Kaplan, H. S., Rosenberg, S. A. & Kim, H. (1973) Non-Hodgkin's lymphoma IV. Clinicopathological correlation in 405 cases. *Cancer,* **31,** 806–823.

Jones, S. E., Fuks, Z., Kaplan, H. S. & Rosenberg, S. A. (1973) Non-Hodgkin's lymphoma. V. Results of radiotherapy. *Cancer,* **32,** 682–691.

Jones, S. E. (1974) Clinical features and course of the non-Hodgkin's lymphomas. *Clinics in Haematology,* **3,** 131–160.

Law, I. P., Dick, F. R., Blom, J. & Bergevin, P. R. (1975) Involvement of the central nervous system in non-Hodgkin's lymphoma. *Cancer,* **36,** 225–231.

Lister, A. et al (1977) *British Journal of Cancer,* in press.

Lukes, R. J. & Collins, R. D. (1975) New approaches to the classification of the lymphomata. *British Journal of Cancer,* **31,** 1–28.

Muriel, F. S., Pavlovsky, S., Penalver, J. A., Hidalgo, G., Bonesana, A. C., Eppinger-Helft, M., Demacchi, G. H. & Pavlovsky, A. (1974) Evaluation of induction of remission intensification and central nervous system prophylactic treatment in acute lymphoblastic leukaemia. *Cancer,* **34,** 418–426.

Pinkel, C., Johnson, W. & Aur, R. J. A. (1975) Non-Hodgkin's lymphoma in children. *British Journal of Cancer,* **31,** 298–323.

Rappaport, M., Winter, W. J. & Hicks, S. B. (1956) Follicular lymphoma. A re-evaluation of its position in the scheme of malignant lymphoma based on a survey of 253 cases. *Cancer,* **9,** 792–821.

Rosenberg, S. A., Dorfman, R. F. & Kaplan, H. S. (1975) The value of sequential bone marrow biopsy and laparotomy and splenectomy in a series of 127 consecutive untreated patients with non-Hodgkin's lymphoma. *British Journal of Cancer,* **31,** 221–227.

Rosenberg, S. A., Diamond, H. D., Jaslowitz, B. & Craver, L. F. (1961) Lymphosarcoma — a review of 1269 cases. *Medicine,* **40,** 31–84.

Schein, P., De Vita, V. T., Canellos, G. P., Chabner, B. & Young, R. C. (1975) A new combination chemotherapy program for diffuse histiocytic and mixed non-Hodgkin's lymphomas: BACOP. *Abstract 1108.* American Society of Clinical Oncology.

Veronsei, U., Musumeci, R., Pizzetti, F., Gennari, L. & Bonadonna, G. (1974) The value of staging laparotomy in non-Hodgkin's lymphomas. *Cancer,* **33,** 446–459.

Williams, H. M., Diamond, H. D., Craver, L. F. & Parsons, H. (1959) *Neurological Complications of Lymphomas and Leukaemias.* Springfield, Ill.: Charles C. Thomas.

4
THE TREATMENT OF ACUTE LEUKAEMIA

J. S. Malpas

Less than 25 years ago acute leukaemia was a short devastating illness frequently painful and usually terminated by haemorrhage or infection. Occasionally the disease ran a less acute course and very rarely long-term survival was seen. A reversal of the natural history of this disease occurred with the introduction of folic acid antagonists (Farber et al, 1948). Few therapeutic results are as dramatic. A pallid, feverish, bleeding child, unable to walk because of painful bony deposits is treated, and within a few days returns to health, and at the end of a few weeks may be fit to return to school. It is not surprising therefore that a tremendous effort has been made to understand what happens during such recovery and to find out, having once achieved remission, how it may be sustained. Only within the last decade has it appeared that a therapeutic cure, rather than the very rare fortuitous natural recovery, is possible. Progress has been greatest in acute lymphoblastic leukaemia (ALL) of childhood. Nevertheless, considerable progress has also been made in acute myelogenous leukaemia (AML). It is the purpose of this review to consider the major factors that have resulted in the improvement in outlook.

CLASSIFICATION OF ACUTE LEUKAEMIA

A detailed account of the morphological classification of the leukaemias is outside the scope of this chapter, but since it considerably influences many aspects of management it must be considered. Using Romanowsky stains and cytochemical techniques it is possible to define four main groups of the disorder (Hayhoe, Quaglino and Doll, 1964; Clein, 1974).

Acute lymphoblastic leukaemia

The first is ALL in which the marrow contains more than 30 per cent of blast cells. These are cells with a high nuclear cytoplasmic ratio, the nuclei are not indented or twisted, Auer rods are absent and blast cells show coarse granules or blocks when stained by periodic-acid-Schiff (PAS) but are negative to Sudan black or peroxidase.

Acute myeloblastic leukaemia

The other major group is AML. This has been variously subclassified. Clein (1974) has defined the features of AML as cells having a regular cell outline, a lower nuclear cytoplasmic ratio, often Auer rods and a negative PAS reaction.

Because of possible dangers to technicians from the carcinogenic effects of peroxidase, Sudan black is to be preferred and is positive in AML. Acute myelomonocytic leukaemia (AMML) has these features but the nuclei are characteristically indented and twisted. Acute erythroleukaemia again has many features of AML but erythroblasts are present and predominate in the marrow. Because anaemia is such a feature of the latter condition and megaloblastic changes may be seen with gross red cell abnormalities, it may be mistaken for a megaloblastic anaemia.

The further subvariant of promyelocytic leukaemia (APML) should be described because of its association with fulminating haemorrhage (Rosenthal, 1963) and the fact that if it is correctly managed, prognosis may be relatively good (Bernard et al, 1973). In this form promyelocytes predominate in the marrow and the blood, numerous granules or Auer rods may be seen and occasionally these granules may be very large. Acute monocytic leukaemia is a rare variant of AML.

A useful working classification (Table 4.1) has been given by Beard and Hamilton Fairley (1974).

Table 4.1   A classification of acute leukaemia

1. Myelogenous leukaemia
     Myeloblastic
     Promyelocytic
     Myelomonocytic (and monocytic)
     Di Guglielmo syndrome
       Erythroleukaemia
       Erythremic myelosis
2. Lymphoblastic leukaemia
3. Undifferentiated leukaemia

After Beard and Hamilton Fairley (1974)

There is an important group of AML which is identified as much on clinical as on cytological grounds. In this group the marrow contains less than 30 per cent of blast cells, there is good preservation of normal marrow elements for a long time, and even when untreated deterioration is slow. Clinically it is essential to recognise these 'smouldering acute leukaemias'.

Finally there is undoubtedly a group of acute leukaemias whose morphology defies classification. The absence of characteristic features in the nucleus, the lack of granulation in the cytoplasm, failure to show Auer rods or react with cytochemical stains make it impossible to assign these leukaemias to any group. The Medical Research Council Working Party on Acute Leukaemia in Adults (1975), reviewing the classification of 272 cases of AML based on May–Grünwald–Giemsa staining alone, was unable to classify 42 (15.4 per cent). Fraumeni, Manning and Mitus (1971) found that 24.6 per cent of a series of 1263 children with ALL were unclassifiable on morphology alone. If cytochemistry is added to the criteria for classification, fewer cases remain as undifferentiated. Beard and Hamilton Fairley (1974), analysing 212 cases of acute leukaemia on both morphological and cytochemical grounds, found only 2.8 per cent which were unclassifiable (Table 4.2).

There has been relatively little practical impact yet of electron microscopy on the classification of acute leukaemia, but a comment on membrane cell markers

Table 4.2 Analysis of 212 cases of acute leukaemia[a]

Myelogenous		
1. Myeloblastic	99 (10^b)	46.7% (4.7)
2. Promyelocytic	3	1.4%
3. Myelomonocytic	38	17.9%
4. Di Guglielmo syndrome	4	1.9%
Lymphoid		
1. PAS positive (definitely lymphoid)	39	18.4%
2. PAS negative (probably lymphoid)	13	6.1%
Undifferentiated	6	2.8%

[a] This is a selected series
[b] In these 10 patients Romanowsky staining was insufficient to determine the nature of the cells. Correct diagnosis was made after staining by Sudan black
   After Beard and Hamilton Fairley (1974)

is necessary, for in the lymphoid leukaemias they would appear to have a relation to prognosis.

Surface markers in acute lymphoblastic leukaemia

Surface markers for human thymus-derived (T) or bone-marrow derived (B) cells have been found on the surface membranes of leukaemic cells and these antigens have recently provided another method of classifying ALL which is likely to increase in importance. Membrane-bound immunoglobulin (Ig) detectable by immunofluorescence is the most reliable method of detecting B cells whilst the formation of rosettes with sheep red cells indicates the presence of thymus-derived lymphocytes. Seligman (1975) has reviewed the limitations of these methods. In studies of lymphoblastic leukaemias the proportion bearing the various surface markers have been shown to be non-B or T 75 per cent, T only 23 per cent, B only 2 per cent. The presence of T cells is associated with a high initial white count, a high tumour cell mass (mediastinal tumours for example), a characteristic morphology of the malignant nucleus which shows numerous folds and clefts, and a bad prognosis.

Recently a specific antiserum to acute leukaemia cells has been produced, Greaves et al (1975) having raised a specific antibody to human ALL in rabbits. A conjugated fluorescent antiserum which reacts only with 'malignant' lymphoblasts has considerable potential not only in helping to elucidate so-called undifferentiated leukaemia, but also in following the response of the leukaemic cell population in the marrow to therapy.

Exact classification of acute leukaemia is not always possible even after applying all available diagnostic tests. This poses a difficult therapeutic problem for the treatment of ALL uses less toxic regimes and is less hazardous. It is reasonable in any patient under the age of 20 with an unclassifiable leukaemia in relatively good clinical condition to attempt to induce remission with the less toxic ALL regimes. Similarly, patients in the older age groups would probably best be treated with the AML protocols. The most difficult problem is with the patient in very poor clinical state in whom only one essay at remission is likely to be possible. In these patients it is better to use a regime suitable for inducing remission in AML as these are also nearly always effective in ALL.

REMISSION IN ACUTE LEUKAEMIA

The effectiveness of management is measured by the frequency and duration of remission and the survival time.

Definition of remission

It is important to discuss the criteria by which remission is measured.

In acute leukaemia the bone marrow is infiltrated with blast cells which impair the production of red cells, granulocytes and platelets. Many other organs are also involved; a comprehensive study of 604 autopsies of leukaemic patients has been reported by Anromin (1968). In particular the central nervous system, kidneys and genital organs are infiltrated. Eventually there is such a burden of tumour tissue that the patient dies. This occurs when there are approximately 10^{12} leukaemic cells which would weigh between 1 and 2 kg. In studies on the mouse L1210 leukaemia, Skipper, Schabel and Wilcox (1964) showed that there is a progressive increase in tumour cells and if the increase is recorded on a log scale the disease only becomes detectable when a tumour of some 10^9 to 10^{10} cells is present. Only a further '2 logs' increase is required to cause death. An ill child with ALL with, say, 1 kg of malignant cells could be restored to health and have less than 1 per cent of blast cells with a 2-log reduction of cells after treatment, at which time only 10 g of leukaemic cells would be present. The term complete remission is therefore only relative; leukaemic cells remain in considerable numbers. Mathé et al (1966) in a study in which numerous biopsies were performed in leukaemic subjects in remission judged by blood and bone marrow examination, were able to demonstrate leukaemic cells in the liver, kidneys, testes, cerebrospinal fluid and other sites. A practical working definition of complete remission has been given by Hewlett, Battle and Bishop (1964). They stated that the patient should have no signs or symptoms attributable to acute leukaemia, the haemoglobin should be more than 10 g/dl, the neutrophil granulocytes more than 1.5×10^9/litre, and platelets more than 100×10^9/litre. The bone marrow smear should show less than 5 per cent blast cells. A number of centres have produced modifications of this definition.

The Southwest Oncology Group (1964) have produced a category rating for the state of the bone marrow in terms of the degree of infiltration with lymphoblasts and other lymphocytic cells. The marrows are rated M1, M2 and M3. An M1 marrow contains zero to 5 per cent lymphoblasts, zero to 40 per cent in total of lymphocytes and lymphoblasts. An M2 marrow contains 6 to 25 per cent of lymphoblasts and 41 to 69 per cent of lymphocytes and lymphoblasts. An M3 marrow contains more than 25 per cent lymphoblasts and more than 69 per cent of lymphocytes and lymphoblasts together.

Beard and Hamilton Fairley (1974) consider that in AML a complete remission is not obtained until all the blast cells and mature granulocyte precursors in the remission marrow no longer resemble the pretreatment leukaemic cells. This appears to be a very stringent criterion, but it would seem illogical to consider a marrow to be in complete remission when it contains undoubted leukaemic cells.

Duration of remission

The duration of complete remission has been defined by the St Jude group for ALL and is generally accepted (Pinkel, 1972). It is the time from which the patient is well, with the peripheral blood showing no abnormal cells, more than 0.5×10^9/litre neutrophils, more than 75×10^9/litre platelets and an M1 marrow, to the onset of persistent M2 or M3 marrow changes described above. Meningeal relapse, testicular infiltration or signs or symptoms definitely attributable to acute leukaemia also indicate the end of remission.

Frequency of complete remission

The frequency with which a regime induces complete remission in patients with acute leukaemia has for some time been used as a measure of the efficacy of the regime. In considering therapeutic data of this kind it is important to know whether there has been any selection of patients. Special centres may have referred to them a higher proportion of very ill patients or the data may exclude patients who, for example, die in the first six weeks after the start of therapy.

With increasing success in inducing remission another factor has become important. This is what Mathé has called the 'toxic cost' of a regime (Mathé and Weiner, 1973). It is evident with drugs which are myelosuppressive, immuno-suppressive, cardiotoxic and neurotoxic or have some other toxicity, that they will cause their own morbidity or mortality. A potentially effective regime for inducing remission may have an unacceptable mortality. The early risk must be considered in relation to the ultimate prognosis.

THE TREATMENT OF ACUTE LYMPHOBLASTIC LEUKAEMIA

The last five years has seen a dramatic improvement in the prognosis of children with ALL. The best modern management now aims at a 50 per cent five-year survival rate at which time the hope of cure may be entertained (Aur, 1974). Inappropriate or inadequate treatment at the beginning of the illness may preclude the child's chances of achieving long-term survival; the occasional therapy of childhood acute leukaemia, particularly if it does not include prophylactic central nervous system treatment, is to be deprecated.

The principles of therapy are first, the induction of complete remission with combinations of drugs that are as effective as possible but have minimal toxicity, then the eradication of leukaemia from the central nervous system, and finally, maintenance therapy or what is more properly continuation therapy in which the minimal leukaemic state is treated for a period of at least two years with effective combinations of chemotherapeutic agents.

A great deal of success has been obtained in each of these stages but it is important to recognise that each one is the subject of intensive investigation and therapeutic trial. Consequently, textbooks are usually out of date, and even current journals report only the results of a previous trial. To give the child every advantage it should be referred to a centre with experience and special facilities.

The induction of remission

It is not possible to detail the pharmacology of the drugs which may be used to induce remission in acute lymphoblastic leukaemia. The chief features of the eight drugs that have been used to treat ALL (Lascari, 1973) are given in Table 4.3 together with an assessment of their effectiveness as judged by the complete remission rate in large series.

The specific drug therapy for inducing remission in ALL has undergone a number of changes. The induction of remission in ALL should not be difficult and the risk attached is usually low. Following a period in which intensive cyclical combinations of such drugs as vincristine, prednisolone, methotrexate, and mercaptopurine were given to maximum tolerance, there has been a return in most centres to milder induction regimes. This is because a steadily increasing initial mortality was being seen with combinations of four or more drugs, and

Table 4.3 Effectiveness of single drugs in acute leukaemia

Drug	Route	Dose	Complete rem. ALL (%)	AML (%)	Median dur. compl. rem. ALL	AML	Year intro.
Methotrexate	Oral	1.25–5.0 mg/day	22	11	17 wk	21 wk	1947
	i.m. or Oral	30 mg/m^2×2 wk	—	—	10 mth	—	
	i.v.	3–6 mg/kg every 2 wk	—	—	7.7 mth	—	
Prednisone	Oral	2 mg/(kg·day)	60–76	14	1.5 mth	—	1950
6-Mercaptopurine	Oral	3 mg/(kg·day)	27	9	21 wk	26 wk	1952
Cyclophosphamide	Oral	3 mg/(kg·day)	28	Rare	16 wk	—	1957
Vincristine	i.v.	1.5–2.0 mg/m^2 weekly	57–85	36	9–18 wk	—	1960
Daunomycin	i.v.	45–60 mg/m^2 daily×5	40	25–50	9 wk	—	1964
L-Asparaginase	i.m. or i.v.	Variable	62	Uncommon	9 wk	—	1967
Cytosine arabinoside	i.v.	25 mg/kg×2 a week	32	33	10 wk	—	1968
	i.v.	3–5 mg/kg daily for 10 days	26				

i.v., intravenous; i.m., intramuscular; ALL, acute lymphoblastic leukaemia; AML, acute myeloblastic leukaemia; rem., remission; dur., duration; compl., complete; intro., introduced
After Lascari (1973)

there was no evidence that the remissions produced were lasting any longer than those induced just as effectively but less dangerously by vincristine and prednisolone (Henderson, 1970). Vincristine and prednisolone have become the drugs most commonly used for the induction of remission. Remission rates vary between 80 and 95 per cent for previously untreated children in most centres. Complete remission rates are given in Table 4.4. Vincristine is usually given in a dose of 1.5 mg/m^2 once a week while prednisolone is given daily. In children there is no advantage in giving more than 2 mg of vincristine. The dose of prednisolone is similarly curtailed to 40 mg daily.

The success rate for remission induction falls with increasing age. In patients with ALL over the age of 25 remission rates are far lower, three out of four achieving remission (Clarkson et al, 1975). Similarly a less satisfactory rate of remission can be seen in children who are in the so-called poor risk group. There is general agreement that the presence of an initial high total white cell count (above 30×10^9/litre), a mediastinal mass or leukaemia presenting in Negro children carries a definitely worse prognosis. There is debate on whether lymph node masses, a large liver or spleen, and the presence of macrolymphoblasts affect prognosis. It has been shown that more intensive treatment than vincristine and prednisolone is required to produce remission in the poor prognosis group. Cyclophosphamide and ara-C may be added to vincristine (Oncovin) and prednisolone to produce the COAP regime which has been well tolerated and achieved a good remission rate.

A regime which has produced an improvement in the remission induction rate of adults at St Bartholomew's Hospital has been a combination of vincristine, prednisolone, asparaginase, and adriamycin. This has produced a complete remission rate of 68 per cent in adult patients (Lister, personal communication).

Table 4.4 Combinations of two drugs in childhood acute lymphatic leukaemia

Drugs and dosages Prednisone	Vincristine	No. of patients	Bone marrow remissions (%)
40 mg/(m^2·day)	1.5 mg/(m^2·wk)	31	87
40 mg/(m^2·day)	2.0 mg/(m^2·wk)	63	84
		30	83
40 mg/(m^2·day)	2.0 mg/(m^2·wk)	121	86
120 mg/(m^2·day)	2.0 mg/(m^2·wk)	166	84

After Henderson (1970)

Improvement in remission duration

So great is the number of satisfactory induction regimes for both average and poor risk children with ALL that it would be impossible to review them all. It is important to consider some principles and some evidence brought forward recently by Simone (personal communication) that although the prednisolone and vincristine regime is simple and well tolerated, it is not the optimum treatment. Simone points out that the main obstacle to cure in ALL since the introduction of successful central nervous system prophylaxis is haematological relapse. He has reviewed all the patients admitted to Studies I to VIII reported from St Jude Children's Research Hospital since 1962 and has prepared curves of the number of children in continuous complete remission against time for all previously untreated patients who attained an M1 marrow. The number remaining in remission at 6, 12, 18, and 24 months have been determined. Curves were constructed for each study (Fig. 4.1). Study VII showed inferior results and in analysing the reason for this, it became apparent that the patients in this study received only vincristine and prednisolone for remission induction and no further intensification of therapy. Simone concludes that if therapy in the first eight weeks does not contain three drugs than the opportunity for cure may be gone for ever; aggressive therapy later may not compensate for the initial deficiency. He advocates the use of a third drug during remission induction and suggests the use of either daunorubicin or asparaginase. An alternative is to give an intensive period of therapy early in remission. The numbers in the St Jude studies give a statistically satisfactory basis for this argument and it must be concluded that vincristine and prednisolone alone for the child in the good risk group are inadequate. It is unlikely that the addition of a third drug such as asparaginase to vincristine and prednisolone would produce significant increase in morbidity or mortality, especially when it is given immediately after achieving complete remission. It is reasonable to give children who have all the prognostic features in their favour for long survival and possible cure the optimal treatment available at the beginning.

In summary, it is recommended that children with good prognosis ALL are treated initially with vincristine and prednisolone, but that a third drug such as asparaginase, adriamycin, or daunorubicin is used early in remission. Children in the poor prognosis group need a regime with four drugs from the start of their treatment. Should these measures fail, the likeliest cause is an incorrect

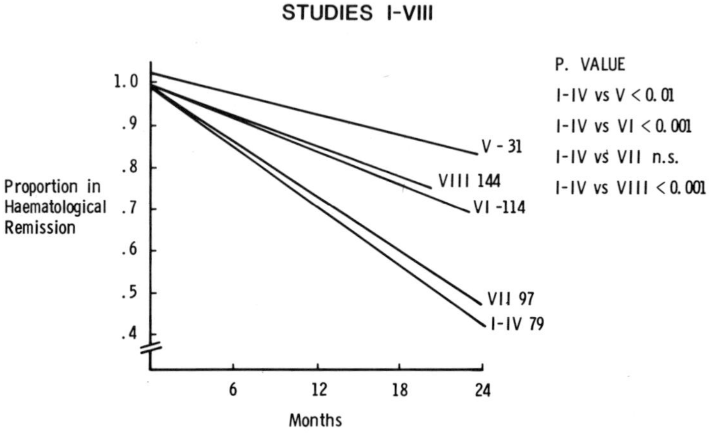

STUDIES I-VIII

P. VALUE

I-IV vs V < 0.01
I-IV vs VI < 0.001
I-IV vs VII n.s.
I-IV vs VIII < 0.001

Figure 4.1 Children in continuous haematological remission during the first two years of the various St Jude Children's Research Hospital studies (Simone, personal communication)

diagnosis. The child may have an acute undifferentiated malignancy or may have an acute or chronic myeloid leukaemia. If the diagnosis is revised then more appropriate treatment will need to be instituted. It is inadvisable simply to intensify the regime already used.

Central Nervous System in Acute Leukaemia

With increasing duration of both remission and survival in ALL the frequency of relapse in the central nervous system increased. Hardisty and Norman (1967) reviewed the symptomatology and incidence of meningeal leukaemia and found that some 50 to 70 per cent of children developed this complication. About half were in haematological remission when they relapsed in the central nervous system. It was evident also that relapse in the central nervous system was followed soon afterwards by systemic relapse and this of course had a deleterious effect on survival. A clear distinction must be made between the treatment of established meningeal leukaemia and so-called prophylactic therapy.

Meningeal leukaemia begins with the appearance of leukaemic cells in the superficial arachnoid, in trabeculae, and in the walls of veins (Price and Johnson, 1973). Later the deep perivascular arachnoid is involved down to the precapillary arterioles and postcapillary venules. The cells are still separated from the brain by the pia-glial membrane at this stage, but with further progression this membrane is split and the leukaemic cells enter the substance of the brain. Cells that have penetrated the brain deeply are inaccessible to drugs injected into the subarachnoid space. Aur (1974) describes how early minimal disease present in the central nervous system may be eradicated by so-called 'prophylactic therapy'.

Radiotherapy of the central nervous system

Early attempts using craniospinal irradiation at from 500 to 1200 rad were ineffective and the results were similar to those in children who were given no prophylactic therapy. In Study V when the dose was increased to 2400 rad (24 Gy) cranial irradiation with intrathecal methotrexate, only 3 out of 31 children developed meningeal leukaemia. The results of the various trials are summarised in Table 4.5.

Table 4.5 'Prophylactic' CNS therapy in ALL

		No. of patients	Prophylactic CNS therapy	Frequency of initial relapse in CNS
I–II	1962–64	13	DXT low	3 (23%)
III	1964–65	24	DXT low	12 (50%)
IV	1965–67	42	None	25 (59%)
V	1967–68	31	DXT 2400 rad +i.t. MTX	3 (10%)
VI	1968–70	45	DXT 2400 rad	2 (4.4%)
		49	None	33 (67%)
VIII	1970–72	45	DXT 2400 rad +i.t. MTX	6 (13%)
		49	DXT 2400 rad	3 (6%)

DXT, irradiation; i.t., intrathecal; MTX, methotrexate
After Aur (1974)

Irradiation is begun within one month of obtaining remission. The cerebrospinal fluid must be examined, preferably using a cytocentrifuge, to establish that overt disease is not present. Great care must be taken to give the appropriate dose to the correct cranial portal. Failure to irradiate the retro-orbital extension of the arachnoid for example, may negate the whole manoeuvre. Doses of 1500 rad (15 Gy) are used for children under one year old, 2000 rad (20 Gy) for children one to two years old, and 2400 rad (24 Gy) for older children. Adults require up to 3500 rad (35 Gy). Cranial irradiation together with five injections of intrathecal methotrexate 12 mg/m^2 with a maximum of 12 mg administered evenly throughout the radiation is as effective as irradiation of the cranium and the spine (Aur et al, 1971; Simone, 1974; Aur, 1974). The methotrexate is administered at a concentration of 1 mg/ml. It is inadvisable to use greater concentrations of methotrexate as this may lead to headaches, convulsions and other toxic side effects.

Using prophylactic therapy in a randomised trial (Study VI) a four-year continuous complete remission in excess of 55 per cent was achieved in the children treated with craniospinal irradiation (Aur et al, 1972) (Fig. 4.2). Similar good results are obtained with less side effects from marrow suppression by cranial irradiation and intrathecal methotrexate. Of 35 children with acute leukaemia treated in this way, 18 remain in continuous complete remission for at least six years (Aur et al, 1973).

It might be expected that such intensive prophylactic therapy would have either short- or long-term complications. Drugs given intrathecally may act systemically and therefore prejudice the bone marrow which may already be depressed from continuation therapy. This needs to be kept in mind when intrathecal therapy is being given to children with pancytopenia. If intrathecal methotrexate is used, systemic protection by parenteral folinic acid may be advisable in such patients. There appears to be no immediate effect of irradiation on the central nervous system clinically. Freeman, Johnston and Voke (1973)

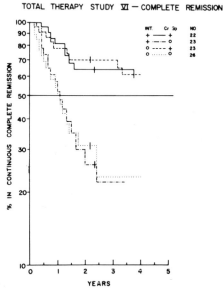

Figure 4.2 Children in continuous remission in Study VI showing the improved rate in children given prophylactic cranial irradiation (Aur, 1974)

described the occurrence of somnolence, anorexia, lethargy and irritability in 22 out of 28 children in the United Kingdom Acute Leukaemia Trial occurring some six to eight weeks after radiotherapy. This 'somnolence syndrome' may be severe with a child sleeping most of the day or falling asleep at inappropriate times. The syndrome usually improves spontaneously in about a week and recovery is the rule. Since it occurs in children having either prophylactic therapy with craniospinal irradiation or cranial irradiation and intrathecal methotrexate, it is attributed to irradiation and on indirect evidence appears to be a delayed radiation induced encephalopathy. Versoza et al (1974) and Soni et al (1975) in a prolonged follow-up of these children have discovered no significant neurological or psychological sequelae. Malpas, Freeman and Sheaff (1975) have found that the characteristic slow wave abnormality of the EEG observed in these children gradually returns to normal and at two years there is no evidence of any abnormality. The only long-term abnormality noted has been some stunting of growth due to a shortened crown–rump length in children receiving the spinal component of irradiation (Versoza et al, 1974). The likelihood of other long-term sequelae of which the secondary radiation-induced tumours are probably the most sinister is not known.

Central nervous system prophylaxis by chemotherapy alone

If the prevention of CNS relapse by intrathecal methotrexate alone were possible it would have much to recommend it, and a number of groups have investigated this point. Komp et al (1975) treated 192 children with intrathecal methotrexate, cytosine arabinoside and hydrocortisone for one year following an M1 marrow remission. Eighty-eight children were randomised to receive 2400 rad (24 Gy) cranial irradiation. Two out of the 104 children receiving intrathecal drugs only, and 1 of the 88 children receiving intrathecal drugs and cranial irradiation, developed meningeal leukaemia during the first bone marrow remission. The duration of haematological remission and survival is no different so far in the two groups. At three years their results are identical, and they conclude that the addition of radiotherapy has conveyed no advantage when added to an effective intrathecal regime. These results are interesting, but the total time that has elapsed is probably still too short to allow judgement, for it is possible that the long initial course of chemotherapy has suppressed but not eliminated central nervous system infiltration. In an attempt to improve chemoprophylaxis, Freeman, Wang and Sinks (1975a) have suggested the use of high-dose methotrexate followed by folinic acid to inhibit the folic acid antagonistic action. Three courses of methotrexate 500 mg/m^2 are given; a third of the dose is given as a single intravenous injection and the remaining two-thirds as a 24 h infusion. These courses are given at three-weekly intervals, combined with intrathecal methotrexate in a dose of 12 mg/m^2 given $\frac{1}{2}$ to 2 h before the i.v. methotrexate. A single dose of i.m. leucovorin in a dose of 15 mg/m^2 is given to counter the effects of the high-dose methotrexate 24 h later. So far 16 patients have been treated in this way and 15 are in continuous complete remission at 4 to 27 months with a median of 10 months. Insufficient time has elapsed to know if this approach is justifiable, but the early results are promising. It must be emphasised, however, that the combination of radiotherapy and intrathecal methotrexate is a well-proven method of preventing meningeal relapse; the occurrence of short-term complications such as the somnolence syndrome do not contraindicate the use of irradiation.

Established meningeal leukaemia

The treatment of leukaemic infiltration of the meninges is usually by combined craniospinal irradiation and intrathecal drugs. Ten injections of either methotrexate or cytosine arabinoside are usually necessary. The course may consist half of methotrexate and half of cytosine arabinoside. In some centres an Ommaya subcutaneous cerebrospinal fluid reservoir is used. In this a reservoir is connected by a fine tube to the anterior horn of the lateral ventricle. In this way chemotherapy can be given easily and painlessly, and if the cannula is correctly placed a good distribution of the drug occurs. Problems of infection and blockage have prevented wide acceptance.

Continuation Therapy

It has been mentioned above that a patient in clinical and haematological remission in ALL still has a number of leukaemic cells present, but they are not detectable using the usual diagnostic methods. This minimal leukaemic state soon reverses and the patient relapses if no further treatment is given. In a study of patients given no further therapy, Freireich et al (1963) showed a median haematological remission of only two months.

A situation similar to the minimal leukaemic state can be produced in mice. Goldin et al (1956) showed that it was possible to cure mice inoculated with L1210 leukaemic cells by the use of intermittent methotrexate when the tumour burden was low. It is therefore logical when discussing the strategy of this part of the leukaemia programme to talk of continuation therapy rather than maintenance therapy, as continuous therapy of the minimal leukaemic state implies an active attempt to eliminate residual disease. If this strategy is accepted, there are a number of tactical possibilities. The first is to use drugs which are known to be effective singly in sequence. The theoretical advantages are that the regime would minimise the production of resistance to all agents. A second method would be to use combinations of drugs sequentially. This would be more effective in eliminating leukaemic cells, but the number of combinations of drugs available is limited. The periodic or cyclical use of combinations of drugs might delay or prevent the emergence of resistant cell lines. A compromise is one in which single or multiple drugs such as vincristine and prednisolone, which are known to be effective in producing remission, are given at intervals. This is the principle of pseudo-reinduction.

Comparison of these regimes is difficult unless groups have had the same remission induction, cranial prophylaxis and supportive therapy.

The Australian Cancer Society (1968), in a controlled trial, found that the median duration of survival of children treated with cyclical agent combinations was no better than the use of single sequential agents. Bernard, Jacquillat and Weil (1972), reviewing their treatment schedules for acute lymphoblastic leukaemia, showed that in sequential studies the introduction of vincristine and prednisolone improved the median duration of survival to over three years in their children, and some cooperative studies in the United States have confirmed this. The use of intensive periods of treatment shortly after remission has been induced, so-called consolidation therapy, has met with varying success. In the VIth total study at St Jude Children's Research Hospital (Aur et al, 1972; Simone, 1974) no benefit was obtained when consolidation therapy was used.

These findings are disturbing for they raise the possibility that in some children there is a small fraction of the leukaemic cell population which is resistant from the beginning to all drugs presently available, and a completely different mode of therapy may be necessary to eliminate these cells. This view is confirmed by the results of an extension of the cyclical drug regime, the L2 schedule of treatment reported by Haghbin et al (1974) and reviewed by Clarkson et al (1975). Following remission induction intensive cycles of drugs comprising thioguanine, cyclophosphamide, hydroxyurea, daunorubicin, methotrexate, nitrosourea, cytosine arabinoside, and vincristine have been used. Seventy-four out of 75 children (99 per cent) achieved complete remission. Fifty-four out of these 74 children have been in continuous complete remission for 1 to 58 months. The projected median duration of remission is about four and a half years. The regime has been well tolerated, the main toxic side effect being marrow suppression. These results are certainly an improvement, but relapse still occurs and the answer would not appear to be in the administration of even more drugs. The solution may lie in recognising the resistant subfractions of the leukaemic population of cells and 'tailoring' a regime to treat that particular leukaemia.

Until such time as more specific therapy becomes available the problem that remains is the optimum number of drugs that can be used in combination. This problem is being considered in Study VIII of St Jude Children's Research Hospital (Simone, 1974). In this study children are randomised to four different continuation regimes — methotrexate alone, methotrexate and 6-mercaptopurine, methotrexate, 6-mercaptopurine and cyclophosphamide, and finally all three drugs and cytosine arabinoside. All drugs are given weekly except 6-mercaptopurine which is given daily. Treatment with methotrexate alone has been discontinued because of severe toxic side effects on the nervous system. The relapse rate has been approximately equal in the other three groups; 6 of the 44 patients receiving two drugs having relapsed and the rates for the other two groups are 10 out of 45 and 3 out of 41 respectively. In the four-drug group, however, two deaths have occurred in remission. The morbidity in the three groups as judged by admission to hospital for infections, etc., is markedly different and the two-drug regime is outstandingly the best in this respect (Simone et al, 1975). The 'toxic cost' as a result of destruction of defence mechanisms has not been emphasised in this chapter but is of great importance as it is the most important factor in limiting the duration of continuation therapy.

The duration of continuation therapy

There would be no need to discuss the length of continuation therapy if it was so innocuous that it could be continued for many years with no evidence of morbidity or mortality. Unfortunately this is not the case, deaths from infection have reached 15 per cent (Simone, 1974), and these children die with no evidence of leukaemia. Temporary growth retardation occurs and in the long term there is evidence of liver damage, sterility, and secondary neoplasia. There would also be no need to discuss the problem if continuation therapy produced only a very short-lived remission. However, most centres now achieve remission rates of 90 per cent and half the children are still in continuous remission at three years (Aur, 1974).

Burchenal (1968) showed in a study of long-term survivors that therapy could be stopped without subsequent relapse. In children surviving seven years from the time of diagnosis and who had had no evidence of leukaemia for four years, it was possible to stop continuation therapy with little risk of relapse. This implies that either the leukaemic cells had been eliminated or they had lost their malignant properties. Since many of these children had minimal treatment by modern standards, it could be argued that they represent a special subpopulation and it would be unwise to apply these results generally. Nevertheless it remains the only guide there is to a perplexing problem.

In the St Jude studies (Aur et al, 1974) therapy is stopped after two or three years. These children relapse most frequently in the first year after stopping treatment, especially those who were in earlier treatment protocols and received no CNS prophylaxis. They were unable to find any other feature that predicted which children would relapse. It is of considerable interest that many of their long-term survivors, having stopped therapy, were those who initially had had poor prognostic features.

Since it has not been possible to identify children who are likely to relapse early it was reasonable to try to answer the question with a randomised trial. This was done by Children's Cancer Study Group A (Krivit, Gilchrist and Beatty, 1970). Fifteen patients were randomised after long-term chemotherapy for continuation or cessation of therapy. After five years, four out of eight who stopped therapy have relapsed compared with four out of seven who continued therapy.

There is, therefore, no answer as to when therapy should be stopped, but between two and three years after remission induction seems reasonable. If treatment has not eliminated or modified the leukaemic cell population by then, it is unlikely to do so.

When therapy is stopped there is usually a rapid rebound in the lymphocytic population and this has to be carefully distinguished from relapse. The bone marrow should be examined serially when the lymphocyte population is seen to fall if the patient remains in remission.

THE TREATMENT OF ACUTE MYELOGENOUS LEUKAEMIA

There are differences between AML (or what is more accurately but less euphoniously described as acute non-lymphoblastic leukaemia) and ALL both in natural history and specific therapy. Whereas ALL commonly occurs in children, AML occurs mostly in adults. Since AML may occur in the elderly it may be associated with degenerative disease such as myocardial ischaemia or even with other malignancies such as Hodgkin's disease or myeloma. Instead of a previously fit and healthy person the physician treating AML may be presented with a patient in poor general health, and this must influence him in the choice of the rigorous and toxic treatment required to induce remission. The child with ALL will almost always require prompt treatment. This is not the case in AML where smouldering forms of acute leukaemia may be best managed by general measures with treatment of infection or anaemia by antibiotics and blood transfusion.

In general, however, the classic form of AML is much more aggressive than childhood ALL, many patients presenting with haemorrhage, anaemia, infection and a variety of metabolic disturbances which, if not treated promptly, are rapidly fatal. Tivey (1954) has shown that the median survival time was longer in children with ALL than adult patients with AML even when both groups received only supportive therapy (Table 4.6).

Table 4.6 Survival of untreated leukaemic patients

	Median survival (months)
Childhood ALL	
1937–53	3–5
Childhood AML	
1937–53	1–2
Adult ALL	
1937–53	1–4
Adult AML	
1937–53	2

After Tivey (1954)

The induction of remission

The incidence of complete remission has risen considerably in the last decade except in patients over 70 years of age. It is justifiable to consider using supportive therapy alone in the elderly, especially if there are pre-existent complications such as heart disease or diabetes. In patients with a low blast count in the marrow (25–35 per cent) and who have a relatively well-preserved bone marrow function, it is reasonable to observe progress before starting specific therapy. Many of these patients undoubtedly do badly with intensive therapy, whereas some of those untreated survive considerably longer than the median survival times of 7 to 13 months reported (Clarkson, 1972; Crowther et al, 1973) in treated patients.

Combination therapy in AML

In younger patients a number of effective drugs are available, which when given in combinations may achieve complete remission rates of over 50 per cent (Table 4.7).

There are so many induction regimes that their very number indicates the unsatisfactory position at the moment. The major difficulty is that the amount of drug necessary to eliminate the leukaemic cells will destroy all normal marrow elements. The marrow becomes aplastic and infection and haemorrhage result. This happens so frequently that some workers (Bernard et al, 1972; Beard and Hamilton Fairley, 1974) consider it to be almost inevitable if remission is to be obtained, and that these complications must be accepted.

Examples of effective regimes are those described by Gee, Yu and Clarkson (1969), Clarkson (1972), Crowther et al (1971, 1973), Dowling et al (1973) and Spiers (1974) and the regime of the Southwest Oncology Group reported by McCredie et al (1975). Clarkson (1972) described the 'L6' protocol and reviewed the results three years later. In the 'L6' protocol 10-day courses of cytosine arabinoside 3 mg/kg given 12-hourly i.v. are accompanied by thioguanine 2.5 mg/kg given 12-hourly orally. A 20-day interval to allow bone marrow recovery is followed by a further course of the same drugs. This programme is repeated until remission is obtained. Following this, vincristine, methotrexate, BCNU, hydroxyurea, daunorubicin, and asparaginase are given in succession. The principle is to eliminate the cells that are dividing by first using drugs such as cytosine arabinoside and thioguanine which act specifically on cells synthesising DNA, and to follow these with alkylating agents which affect cells which are

Table 4.7 Combination therapy for induction of remission in acute myelogenous leukaemia

Drug combination	Dose and administration	CR rate (%)	Med. dur remission (mth)	Patient numbers	Author
'L6' protocol					
Cytosine arabinoside	3.0 mg/(kg·q 12h) } i.v. for 10 days	56	10	88	Clarkson (1975)
Thioguanine	2.5 mg/(kg·q 12h) }				
	Six courses at 10-day intervals				
St Bartholomew's Hospital regime					
Cytosine arabinoside	2.0 mg/(kg·q 24h) i.v. for 5 days	54	7	72	Crowther et al (1973)
Daunorubicin	1.5 mg/kg i.v. on day 1 only given at 10-day intervals until CR				
MRC Leukaemia Unit (TRAP)					
Thioguanine	100 mg/(m²·day) p.o. for 5 days	40	9	17	Spiers (1974)
Rubidomycin (daunorubicin)	40 mg/(m²·day) i.v. on day 1 only				
Ara-C (cytosine arabinoside)	100 mg/(m²·day) i.v. for 5 days				
Prednisolone	30 mg/(m²·day) p.o. for 5 days				
Southwest Oncology Group					
Vincristine	1.5 mg/m² i.v. on day 1, 19 and subsequently	68	Not available	77	McCredie et al (1975)
Adriamycin	40 mg/m² i.v. on day 1, 19 and subsequently				
Cytosine arabinoside	100 mg/m² i.v. cont. infusion day 5 to 9				
Prednisolone	25 mg/q 6h p.o. day 1 to 5				
BCG	3 mg in 0.6 ml intradermally days 1, 12, 17				

CR, complete remission; Med. dur, median duration: mth, months; i.v., intravenous; p.o., orally in a non-synthetic phase. Cyclophosphamide and BCNU will do this. In 88 previously untreated patients, 49 achieved complete remission (56 per cent). The median duration of remission was 10 months. The median survival of those responding was about two years, whereas survival of non-responders was slightly less than two months.

The regime described by Crowther et al (1973) consists of repeated 5-day courses of daunorubicin and cytosine arabinoside. Daunorubicin is given in a dose of 1.5 mg/kg body weight (55 mg/m^2 of body area) by fast i.v. infusion on day 1, and cytosine arabinoside 2 mg/kg body weight (70 mg/m^2) is given on days 1 to 5 by intravenous injection every 24 h. Courses are repeated at 10-day intervals until remission is achieved. A further single 'consolidation' course is given. Complete remission was achieved in 39 out of 72 patients (54 per cent). Some three to seven courses were required. In the patients treated by these methods in the St Bartholomew's Hospital trial who were maintained with chemotherapy alone, the medial survival of all patients was just over seven months. For the patients who went into complete remission it was $11\frac{1}{2}$ months. This regime is relatively non-toxic and is feasible when reversed isolation facilities are not available. The cumulative dose of daunorubicin given in this induction protocol does not give rise to cardiotoxicity as the upper limit of about 600 mg/m^2 is rarely reached. Because of the synergism which is known to occur between cytosine arabinoside and thioguanine, and cytosine arabinoside and daunorubicin, these three drugs have been used together with prednisolone as the basis for a four-drug induction regime referred to as TRAP. The literature on chemotherapy is now beset with acronyms such as TRAP, COAP, COPP, TRAMCOL, etc., which are produced by using the first letter of the approved or proprietary name. COPP for example, consists of Cyclophosphamide, Oncovin (proprietary name for vincristine) Procarbazine and Prednisolone. TRAP consists of Thioguanine, Rubidomycin (daunorubicin), Ara C (cytosine arabinoside) and Prednisolone. This shorthand may give rise to confusion, VAC for example, contains vincristine and cyclophosphamide but A may represent either actinomycin D or adriamycin. Although these acronyms are sometimes misleading, they are widely used and regrettably must be accepted. COAP introduced by Whitecar et al (1972) is similar to TRAP but cyclophosphamide and vincristine (Oncovin) are used instead of thioguanine and rubidomycin. These drug combinations have been used by themselves or on occasion alternated with the aim of eliminating drug resistant cell lines. Given intermittently and in a cyclical manner drug toxicity is reduced. Using TRAP to produce remission and then alternating TRAP and COAP, Paolin et al (1973) reported one year's experience in which 13 out of 27 patients (48 per cent) with AML remained in remission. Spiers (1974) reviewing his experience with a similar programme of TRAP and COAP records an overall remission rate of 10 out of 26 patients (40 per cent).

The search continues for effective combinations. Glucksberg et al (1975), using a 5-drug combination of daunorubicin, cytosine arabinoside, thioguanine, prednisolone and vincristine, claim a complete remission rate of 18 patients out of 23 (78 per cent). The possibility that drugs hitherto regarded as more useful in the lymphomas may be effective is emphasised in the report by Jacobs et al

(1975b) that the epipodophyllotoxin VP 16213 when combined with cytosine and adriamycin produces rapid complete remission. Six out of eight of these patients responded and passed into remission after only one or two courses; this is exceptional in AML. The latest results show a complete remission rate of 80 per cent in previously untreated patients (Jacobs and Dubovsky, personal communication).

The Southwest Oncology Group in the United States, who have not separated the adult forms of acute leukaemia but treated all by the same protocol, including drugs which have been of proven value in ALL rather than AML, have recorded a remarkable success with the use of vincristine, prednisolone, cytosine, and adriamycin. The regime also includes the use of BCG, an agent which will be discussed later. They report remissions in 52 out of 77 adult patients (68 per cent) (McCredie et al, 1975). Their regime consists of vincristine 1.5 mg/m^2 i.v. and adriamycin 40 mg/m^2 i.v. on day 1, cytosine arabinoside 100 mg/m^2 daily by continuous infusion on days 5 to 9 together with BCG 3 mg diluted in 0.6 ml of saline intradermally on days 1, 12 and 17, and prednisolone 25 mg four times a day on days 1 to 5. On day 19 the marrow is examined, if it still contains blast cells the whole cycle is repeated except that BCG is omitted. Using this regime at St Bartholomew's Hospital in 26 patients, the remission rate was 50 per cent (Whitehouse, personal communication). The regime causes marked marrow suppression and support with antibiotics, blood and platelet transfusions is necessary.

The results of remission induction are in general still unsatisfactory in AML. It remains to be seen whether remission rates reported with recent regimes will be maintained.

Continuation therapy

Unless the patient is treated with some immuno- or chemotherapeutic programme following the induction of remission, relapse occurs in a few weeks. Chemotherapy has been as disappointing in maintaining long-term remission in AML as it has been in inducing remission. Acute promyelocytic leukaemia which, because of its association with life-threatening haemorrhagic complications, is one of the most lethal of all the leukaemias, is an exception. With the recognition of disseminated intravenous coagulation as the cause of the haemorrhagic tendency, many patients who have been supported through the initial severe illness experience prolonged survival. Bernard et al (1973) report a median duration of remission of 26 months in this condition.

Agents used for continuation therapy in ALL are unsatisfactory in AML. Methotrexate and 6-mercaptopurine have been found to be of little value. It is necessary, therefore, to continue to use drugs given in obtaining remission (Crowther et al, 1973) or to use a variety of uncommon agents as in the L6 protocol. Chemotherapy (see Table 4.7) has produced median survival times of from six months to under a year in the groups as a whole.

One successful chemotherapeutic maintenance programme reported is that of Manaster et al (1975). They record that 13 patients out of 29 who achieved remission with cyclophosphamide, cytosine arabinoside and vincristine reported by Abu-Zahra et al (1972) and then were maintained with 1,3-bis(2-chloroethyl)-

1-nitrosourea (BCNU) and cyclophosphamide at 8-weekly intervals had a projected median duration of complete remission of 65 weeks and of survival from diagnosis of 144 weeks. These good results were achieved with considerably less time in hospital than in most regimes.

The use of androgens for induction and continuation of remission has been reported by Sotto et al (1975) and represents an entirely new approach to the management of AML. Thirty-six patients were treated with vincristine, daunorubicin, and prednisolone, and 16 (44 per cent) achieved complete remission. The remission was continued with 6-mercaptopurine and methotrexate. In addition during induction and remission they received stanozolol, an androgen, in a dose of 0.15 mg/kg per day. Using this therapy, only four patients have relapsed during a period of four and a half years. If the study is confirmed, hormone therapy may prove to be an important adjunct to continuation therapy. Survival of patients in their study are compared to other standard regimes in Figure 4.3.

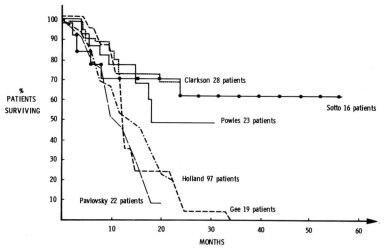

Figure 4.3 Survival of adult patients on various maintenance regimes (After Sotto, 1975)

An alternative approach to chemotherapy, either with cytostatic agents or hormones, has been the use of immunotherapy. Mathé et al (1969) showed that BCG and irradiated leukaemic cells from other children or adults with ALL could, when given to patients in remission with leukaemia, prolong its duration. The present status of immunotherapy has been reviewed by Hamilton Fairley (1975). In man, BCG alone was not found to be effective in ALL in trials by the Medical Research Council (MRC Report, 1971) and Heyn et al (1975). A cooperative study by the European Organisation for the Research in and Treatment of Cancer (EORTC, 1975) in ALL, in which BCG and allogeneic non-irradiated cells were given, has not so far shown any difference between the group receiving immunotherapy and the group receiving chemotherapy. It is important not to judge too quickly the results of this trial, but there would appear to be no extra benefit from immunotherapy. Heyn et al (1975) in a trial comparing a group without maintenance therapy. with groups treated by chemotherapy (methotrexate, vincristine and prednisolone), and BCG, showed that BCG produced a median duration of remission of 4.3 months compared with four months for the no maintenance group, while the chemotherapy group had most of the children still in remission at eight months. These results demonstrate that BCG had no effect. The excellent results now being achieved in several centres using induction, cranial prophylaxis, and chemotherapy maintenance in ALL renders it difficult to devise an acceptable trial. How and when immunotherapy might be fitted into a 'total' care programme for ALL awaits further study.

The position is clearer in AML where the duration of remission is so short. In patients who have been treated with BCG alone and with chemotherapy, a number of groups have now reported increased duration of remission (Vogler and Chan, 1974; Gutterman et al, 1974; Whiteside et al, 1974; Weiss, Stupp and Izak, 1974). Approximate doubling of the median duration of remission occurs (Gutterman et al, 1974; Vogler and Chan, 1974), and duration of survival is improved to 89 weeks with chemotherapy and BCG, compared with 53 weeks with chemotherapy alone (Whiteside et al, 1974). At St Bartholomew's Hospital and the Royal Marsden Hospital BCG and allogeneic cells have been used together in one arm of a randomised trial in which both groups of patients received chemotherapy. Median duration of remission in the group treated with immunotherapy and chemotherapy was 313 days compared to 191 days with chemotherapy alone. The median survival time was 520 days compared with 295 days (Powles et al, 1973; Hamilton Fairley, 1975). Powles (1974) has treated patients with BCG and allogeneic irradiated cells alone and has found that such treatment produces remission and survival times similar to those of patients who receive chemotherapy as well. In a larger study, Freeman et al (1975b) have 10 patients out of 20 alive after treatment with immunotherapy alone with a median survival of 65 weeks compared with four alive out of nine patients treated with immunotherapy and chemotherapy who have a very similar median duration of survival at 64 weeks. They have confirmed their earlier results (Freeman, C. B. et al, 1973) which showed that remission durations were shorter with immunotherapy alone, but survival was just as good because second and third remissions are so much easier to induce than when chemotherapy has been used. It is surprising that out of the 20 patients who relapsed in the immunotherapy group, 14 (70 per cent) gained a second remission, compared with only four out of eight (50 per cent) in the group treated with chemotherapy. Whether this is due to the lessened chance of drug resistance if immunotherapy only is used or whether immunotherapy supports the normal marrow and enables it to tolerate more intensive induction therapy is not yet known. Some evidence that the latter may be true comes from the work by Mathé, Halle-Pannerko and Bourot (1974) who have shown that BCG protects the bone marrow in animals treated with cyclophosphamide.

SUPPORTIVE THERAPY

It is no exaggeration to say that the success of various regimes employed in the treatment of acute leukaemia depends as much on the general supportive care as on the composition of the regime. The rapid and effective treatment of infections, the replacement of erythrocytes, granulocytes, and platelets, the use of allopurinol to prevent hyperuricaemia, and the recognition and avoidance when possible of the side effect of specific drugs, contribute to success or failure. This is particularly notable in AML, and it has been shown that in a joint cooperative trial in which many centres participated in using the same induction protocol, those centres that had readily available platelet and white cell transfusions had remission rates of 45.5 per cent compared to an overall remission rate of 29 per cent (EORTC, 1974).

In children with ALL prolonged aplasia of the bone marrow is unusual with the regimes now commonly employed to induce remission. Protected environments are not usually required except in those units using experimental intensive treatment. The value of protected environments as compared with prophylactic antibiotics is still debatable, although the final verdict must await studies which are in progress. A detailed account of antibiotic therapy for infections complicating leukaemia is beyond the scope of this review, but in general the prompt use of effective antibiotics such as gentamycin, tobramycin, and flucloxacillin, covering both the Gram-positive and Gram-negative organisms that are commonly found — that is, resistant staphylococci, coliform and pyocyaneous organisms, is probably as effective as elaborate isolation methods. The regular use of white cell transfusion is now possible, but there is as yet no conclusive evidence for its efficacy. The management of infections in patients with leukaemia has been reviewed by Levine, Graw and Young (1972).

A number of factors may result in a haemorrhagic tendency in acute leukaemia (Rosner et al, 1972), the commonest cause being thrombocytopenia. The haemorrhagic tendency may be increased in the presence of anaemia or infection. The thrombocytopenia is best treated with ABO compatible platelets. Suitable prepared platelet concentrates will successfully, but only temporarily, stop haemorrhage. Disseminated intravascular coagulation (DIC) is another cause of bleeding in leukaemia. It may occur in all forms of leukaemia, but it is characteristic of APML when it may be the cause of death (Bernard et al, 1973). APML has an incidence of 7 per cent in large series (Medical Research Council, 1975). The abnormality is probably related to the granular contents; certainly when the cells undergo destruction the DIC is exacerbated, and measures to combat bleeding should be started before the specific therapy if possible. Heparin, aminocaproic acid, and transylol have been reported as effective. Heparin, although requiring great care in its use, is probably most effective (Gralnick, Bagley and Abrell, 1972). DIC is recognised by an increased prothrombin and partial thromboplastin time, and a low-serum fibrinogen with an increase of fibrin degradation products. It is essential to give platelets for the accompanying thrombocytopenia. Heparin should be infused continuously at the low dosage of 1000 units hourly and adjusted to give a thrombin time of about 30 s. Within a few hours of starting heparin, specific chemotherapy can be instituted.

Hypokalaemia occurs particularly in AMML and monocytic leukaemia (Pickering and Catowsky, 1973). Potassium replacement may be necessary as hypokalaemia may result from the administration of gentamycin and cephalenin — antibiotics frequently used to combat infection in these patients (Young, Sullivan and Hurley, 1973).

CONCLUSION

The present position in the treatment of acute leukaemia in adults has been reviewed by Clarkson et al (1975). The results are clearly less satisfactory in adults than in children. The effectiveness of drugs against adult leukaemic cells is less and their toxicity greater than in children. There is a lack of effective drugs to continue remission in adults, and although other methods such as immunotherapy have been proved useful in some centres, they have to be developed for general use. The same is true for marrow transplantation. However, many adult patients are now living as long as a year, and just a few are well for as long as four years.

This review has concentrated on the specific methods of treating acute leukaemia now available. These are increasingly complex and there is no doubt that if progress is to be made, patients will need to be treated in centres where special facilities are available. This is particularly so in ALL in children where there is increasing optimism that this disease in potentially curable. AML remains an intractable problem but progress is being made with methods of treatment which are as yet in their infancy.

REFERENCES

Abu-Zahra, H., Clarysse, A., Cowan, D. H., Hasselback, R. & Bergsagel, D. E. (1972) Treatment of acute myeloblastic leukaemia in adults. *Canadian Medical Association Journal,* **107**, 1073.

Anromin, G. D. (1968) *Pathology of Leukaemia.* New York and London: Hoeber.

Aur, R. J. A., Simone, J., Hustu, H. O., Walters, T., Borella, L., Pratt, C. & Pinkel, D. (1971) Central nervous system therapy and combination chemotherapy of childhood lymphocytic leukaemia. *Blood,* **37**, 272.

Aur, R. J. A., Simone, J. V., Hustu, H. O. & Versoza, M. S. (1972) A comparative study of central nervous system irradiation and intensive chemotherapy early in remission of childhood acute lymphocytyc leukaemia. *Cancer,* **30**, 334.

Aur, R. J. A., Hustu, H. O., Versoza, M. S., Wood, A. & Simone, J. V. (1973) Comparison of two methods of preventing central nervous system leukaemia. *Blood,* **42**, 349.

Aur, R. J. A. (1974) Management of acute lymphocytic leukaemia in children. In *Advances in Acute Leukaemia,* ed. Cleton, F. J., Crowther, D. & Malpas, J. S., Vol. 1, Ch. 4. Amsterdam, Oxford, New York: North-Holland.

Aur, R. J. A., Simone, J. V., Hustu, H. O., Versoza, M. S. & Pinkel, D. (1974) Cessation of therapy in childhood acute lymphocytic leukaemia. *New England Journal of Medicine,* **291**, 1230.

Australian Cancer Society (1968) Cyclic drug regimen for acute childhood leukaemia. *Lancet,* **1**, 313.

Beard, M. E. J. & Hamilton Fairley, G. (1974) Acute leukaemia in adults. *Seminars in Haematology,* **11**, 5.

Bernard, J., Jacquillat, C. & Weil, M. (1972) Treatment of the acute leukaemias. *Seminars in Haematology,* **9**, 181.

Bernard, J., Weil, M., Boiron, M., Jacquillat, C., Flandrin, G. & Gemon, M. F. (1973) Acute promyelocytic leukaemia. *Blood,* **41**, 489.

Burchenal, J. H. (1968) Long-term survivors in acute leukaemia and Burkitt's lymphomas. *Cancer,* **21**, 595.

Clarkson, B. D. (1972) Acute myelocytic leukaemia in adults. *Cancer,* **30**, 1572.

Clarkson, B. D., Dowling, M. D., Gee, T. S., Cunningham, B. & Burchenal, J. H. (1975) Treatment of acute leukaemia in adults. *Cancer,* **36**, 775.

Clein, G. P. (1974) The classification of acute leukaemia. In *Advances in Acute Leukaemia,* ed. Cleton, F. J., Crowther, D. & Malpas, J. S., Ch. 2. Amsterdam, Oxford, New York: North-Holland.

Crowther, D., Bateman, C. J. T., Vartan, C. P., Whitehouse, J. M. A., Malpas, J. S., Hamilton Fairley, G. & Bodley Scott, R. (1970) Combination chemotherapy using L-asparaginase, daunorubicin and cytosine arabinoside in adults with acute myelogenous leukaemia. *British Medical Journal,* **4**, 513.

Crowther, D., Powles, R. L., Bateman, C. J. T., Beard, M. E. J., Gauci, C. L., Wrigley, P. F. M., Malpas, J. S., Hamilton Fairley, G. & Bodley Scott, R. (1973) Management of adult acute myelogenous leukaemia. *British Medical Journal*, **1**, 131.

Dowling, M. D., Haghbin, M., Gee, T. S., Cunningham, B., Tan, C. T. C., Clarkson, B. D. & Burchenal, J. H. (1973) Comparative results obtained in the treatment of acute leukaemia. *Recent Results in Cancer Research*, **43**, 133.

European Organisation for Research on the Treatment of Cancer. Leukaemia and Haematosarcoma Cooperative Group (1974) A second comparative trial of remission induction in acute myeloid leukaemia. *European Journal of Cancer*, **10**, 413.

European Organisation for Research on the Treatment of Cancer. Hemopathies Working Party (1975). Immuno- versus chemotherapy during complete remission of acute lymphoblastic leukaemia. *International Society of Hematology Abstract*, 21: 06.

Farber, S., Diamond, L. K., Mercer, R. D., Sylvester, R. F. & Wolff, J. A. (1948) Temporary remission in acute leukaemia in children. *New England Journal of Medicine*, **238**, 787.

Fraumeni, J. F., Manning, M. D. & Mitus, W. J. (1971) Acute childhood leukaemia. *Journal of National Cancer Institute*, **46**, 461.

Freeman, A. I., Wang, J. J. & Sinks, L. F. (1975a) High dose methotrexate in acute lymphocyte leukaemia. *American Society of Clinical Oncology Abstracts*, **16**, 232.

Freeman, C. B., Taylor, G. M., Harris, R., Geary, C. G., MacIver, J. E. & Delamore, I. W. (1975b) Maintenance of acute myeloid leukaemia patients with irradiated allogeneic leukaemia cells and BCG. *International Society of Haematology Abstract*, 21: 10.

Freeman, C. B., Harris, R., Geary, C. G., Leyland, M. J., MacIver, J. E. & Delamore, I. W. (1973) Active immunotherapy used alone for maintenance of patients with acute myeloid leukaemia. *British Medical Journal*, **4**, 565.

Freeman, J. E., Johnston, P. G. B. & Voke, J. M. (1973) Somnolence after prophylactic cranial irradiation in children with acute lymphoblastic leukaemia. *British Medical Journal*, **4**, 523.

Freireich, E. J., Gehan, E., Frei, E., Schroeder, L. R., Wolman, I. J., Anbari, R., Bugert, E. D., Mills, S. D., Pinkel, D., Selawry, O. S., Moon, J. H., Gendel, B. R., Spurr, C. L., Storrs, R., Haurani, F., Hoogstraten, B. & Lee, S. (1963) The effect of 6-mercaptopurine on the duration of steroid induced remission in acute leukaemia. *Blood*, **21**, 699.

Gee, T. S., Yu, K. P. & Clarkson, B. D. (1969) Treatment of adult acute leukaemia with arabinocyclocytosine and thioguanine. *Cancer*, **23**, 1019.

Glucksberg, H., Coleman, D., Rudolph, R., Fass, L., Fefer, A. & Thomas, E. D. (1975) Combination chemotherapy in adult non-lymphoblastic acute leukaemia. *American Association for Cancer Research Abstract*, **16**, 120.

Goldin, A., Venditti, J. M., Humphreys, S. R. & Mantel, N. (1956) Modification of treatment schedules in the management of advanced mouse leukaemia with amethopterin. *Journal of the National Cancer Institute*, **17**, 203.

Gralnick, H. R., Bagley, J. & Abrell, E. (1972) Heparin treatment for the haemorrhagic diathesis of acute promyelocytic leukaemia. *American Journal of Medicine*, **52**, 167.

Greaves, M. F., Brown, G., Capellaro, D., Reves, Z. T., Lister, A. & Rapson, N. (1975) Cell surface markers of leukaemic cells. *International Society of Haematology Abstract*, 21: 13.

Gutterman, J. U., Hersh, E. M., Rodriguez, V., McCredie, K. B., Mavligit, G., Reed, R., Burgess, M. A., Smith, T., Gehan, E., Bodey, G. P. & Freireich, E. J. (1974) Chemoimmunotherapy of adult acute leukaemia. *Lancet*, **4**, 1405.

Haghbin, M., Tan, C. C., Clarkson, B. D., Mike, V., Burchenal, J. H. & Murphy, M. L. (1975) Treatment of acute lymphoblastic leukaemia in children with prophylactic intrathecal chemotherapy and intensive systemic chemotherapy. *Cancer Research*, **35**, 807.

Hamilton Fairley, G. (1975) Immunotherapy in the management of leukaemia. *British Journal of Haematology*, **31**, 181, Suppl.

Hardisty, R. M. & Norman, P. M. (1967) Meningeal leukaemia. *Archives of Disease in Children*, **42**, 441.

Hayhoe, F. G. J., Quaglino, D. and Doll, R. (1964) The cytology and cytochemistry of acute leukaemias. *MRC Special Report Series No. 304*, London: HMSO.

Henderson, E. S. (1970) Treatment of acute leukaemia. In *Leukaemia and Lymphoma*, ed. Holland, J. F., Miescher, P. A. & Jaffe, E. R. New York and London: Grune & Stratton.

Hewlett, J. S., Battle, J. D., & Bishop, R. C. (1964) Criteria for complete remission. *Cancer Chemotherapy Reports*, **42**, 25.

Heyn, R. M., Joo, P., Karon, M., Nesbit, M., Shore, N., Breslow, N., Weiner, J., Reed, A. & Hammond, D. (1975) BCG in the treatment of acute lymphoblastic leukaemia. *Blood*, **46**, 431.

Jacobs, P., King, H. S. & Sealy, G. R. H. (1975a) Epipodophyllotoxin (VP 16–213) in the treatment of diffuse histiocytic lymphoma. *South African Medical Journal*, **49**, 483.

Jacobs, P., Dubovsky, D., Hougaard, M. & Comay, S. (1975b) Epipodophyllotoxin in acute non-lymphoblastic leukaemia. *British Medical Journal*, 1, 396.

Komp, D., Falletta, J., Ragab, A. & Humphrey, G. B. (1975) Is cranial irradiation necessary for CNS prophylaxis in ALL of childhood? *American Society for Clinical Oncology Abstracts*, 16, 232.

Krivit, W., Gilchrist, G. & Beatty, E. C. (1970) The need for chemotherapy after prolonged complete remission in acute leukaemia of childhood. *Journal of Pediatrics*, 76, 138.

Lascari, A. D. (1973) In *Leukaemia in Childhood*. Springfield, Illinois: C. C. Thomas.

Levine, A. S., Graw, R. G. & Young, R. C. (1972) Management of infections in patients with leukaemia and lymphoma. *Seminars in Haematology*, 9, 141.

Malpas, J. S., Freeman, J. E. & Sheaff, P. C. (1975) EEG changes following cranial irradiation in childhood leukaemia and lymphoma. *International Society of Haematology Abstract*, 46: 09.

McCredie, K. B., Hester, J. P., Gutterman, J. U., Gehan, E. A. & Freireich, E. J. (1975) Survival of adults with acute leukaemia. *American Association for Cancer Research Abstracts*, 16, 141.

Manaster, J., Cowan, D. H., Curtis, J. E., Hasselback, R. & Bergsagel, D. (1975) Maintenance of acute non-lymphoblastic remission with 1,3-bis(2-chloroethyl)-1-nitrosourea and cyclophosphamide. *Cancer Chemotherapy Reports*, 59, 537.

Mathé, G., Schwarzenberg, L., Mery, A. M., Cattan, A., Schneider, M., Amiel, J. L., Schlumberger, J. R., Poisson, J. & Wajcner, G. (1966) Extensive histological and cytological survey of patients with acute leukaemia in 'complete remission'. *British Medical Journal*, 1, 640.

Mathé, G., Amiel, J. L., Schwarzenberg, L., Schneider, M., Cattan, A., Schlumberger, J. R., Hayat, M. & de Vassal, F. (1969) Active immunotherapy for acute lymphoblastic leukaemia. *Lancet*, 1, 697.

Mathé, G. & Weiner, R. (1973) Criteris for short-term results in the treatment of acute leukaemia. *Recent Results in Cancer Research*, 43, 110.

Mathé, G., Halle-Pannerko, O. & Bourot, C. (1974) Immune manipulation by BCG administered before or after cyclophosphamide for chemoimmunotherapy of L1210 leukaemia. *European Journal of Cancer*, 10, 661.

Medical Research Council (1971) Treatment of acute lymphoblastic leukaemia (Concord Trial). *British Medical Journal*, 4, 189.

Medical Research Council's Working Party on Leukaemia in Adults (1975). The relation between morphology and other features of acute myeloid leukaemia. *British Journal of Haematology*, 31, suppl., 165.

Paolino, W., Resegotti, L., Rossi, M. & Infelise, V. (1973) Treatment of acute myeloid leukaemia according to the Hammersmith protocol: preliminary report. *British Medical Journal*, 3, 567.

Pickering, T. G. & Catowsky, D. (1973) Hypokalaemia and raised lysozome levels in acute myeloid leukaemia. *Quarterly Journal of Medicine*, 42, 677.

Pinkel, D. (1972) Treatment of acute lymphocytic leukaemia. In *Leukaemia Research Fund Publication*. London: Queen Anne Press, 1973.

Powles, R. L., Crowther, D., Bateman, C. J. T., Beard, M. E. J., McElwain, T. J., Russell, J., Lister, T. A., Whitehouse, J. M. A., Wrigley, P. F. M., Pike, M., Alexander, P & Hamilton Fairley, G. (1973) Immunotherapy for acute myelogenous leukaemia. *British Journal of Cancer*, 28, 365.

Powles, R. L. (1974) Immunotherapy for acute myelogenous leukaemia. *Cancer*, 34, 1558.

Price, R. A. & Johnson, W. W. (1973) The central nervous system in childhood lymphocytic leukaemia. *Cancer*, 31, 520.

Rosenthal, R. L. (1963) Acute promyelocytic leukaemia associated with hypofibrinogenemia. *Blood*, 21, 495.

Rosenthal, D. S. & Maloney, W. C. (1972) The treatment of acute granulocytic leukaemia in adults. *New England Journal of Medicine*, 286, 1176.

Rosner, F., Dobbs, J. V., Ritz, N. D. & Lee, S. L. (1970) Disturbances of haemostasis in acute myeloblastic leukaemia. *Acta haematologica*, 43, 65.

Seligman, M. (1975) Membrane call markers in human leukaemia and lymphomas. *British Journal of Haematology*, 1, 31, suppl.

Simone, J. V. (1974) Acute lymphocytic leukaemia in childhood. *Seminars in Haematology*, 1, 25.

Simone, J. V., Aur, R. J. A., Hustu, H. O. & Versoza, M. (1975) Acute lymphocytic leukaemia in children. *Cancer*, 36, 775.

Skipper, H. E., Schabel, F. M. & Wilcox, W. S. (1964) Experimental evaluation of potential anticancer agents. *Cancer Chemotherapy Reports*, 35, 1.

Soni, S. S., Marten, G. W., Pitner, S. E., Duenas, D. A. & Powazek, M. (1975) Neuropsychologic functioning of children after CNS irradiation. *New England Journal of Medicine*, 293, 113.

Sotto, J. J., Hollard, D., Schaerer, R., Bensa, J. C. & Seigneurin, D. (1975) Androgens and prolonged complete remissions in acute non-lymphoblastic leukaemias. *Nouvelle Revue Francaise d'Hematologie*, 15, 57.

Southwest Oncology Group (1964) Criteria for evaluating chemotherapy in acute leukaemia. *Cancer Chemotherapy Reports*, **42**, 27.

Spiers, A. S. D. (1974) Management of the different forms of leukaemia. In *Leukaemia*, ed. Gunz, F. & Backie, A. G., Ch. 18. New York, San Francisco, London: Grune & Stratton.

Tivey, H. (1954) The natural history of untreated acute leukaemia. *Annals of the New York Academy of Sciences*, **60**, 322.

Versoza, M., Aur, R. J. A., Hustu, H. O., Simone, J. V. & Pinkel, D. (1974) CNS status 5 years after preventive CNS therapy for childhood acute lymphocytic leukaemia. *American Association for Cancer Research Abstracts*, **15**, 98.

Vogler, W. R. & Chan, Y. K. (1974) Prolonging remission in myeloblastic leukaemia by Tice-strain BCG. *Lancet*, **2**, 128.

Weiss, D. W., Stupp, Y. & Izak, G. (1974) Treatment of acute myelocytic leukaemia patients with the MER tubercle bacillus fraction. *Proceedings of the 5th Congress of the Transplantation Society*, Jerusalem, August 1974, p. 74.

Whitecar, J. P., Bodey, G. P., Freireich, E. J., McCredie, K. B. & Hart, J. S. (1972) Cyclophosphamide, vincristine, cytosine arabinoside and prednisolone combination chemotherapy for acute leukaemia in adults. *Cancer Chemotherapy Reports*, **56**, 543.

Whiteside, M. G., Cauchi, M. N., Paton, C. M., Foy, A. & Stone, J. M. (1974) Immunotherapy in the maintenance period acute non-lymphatic leukaemia. *Proceedings of the XV Congress of the International Society of Haematology*, Jerusalem, 1974, Abstract Part II, p. 295.

Young, G. P., Sullivan, J. & Hurley, T. (1973) Hypokalaemia due to gentamycin and cephalenin in leukaemia. *Lancet*, **2**, 855.

5
SLOW VIRUS DISEASES OF THE CENTRAL NERVOUS SYSTEM

H. E. Webb

As yet no generally acceptable definition of 'slow virus disease' has been found, and, indeed, the viral aetiology of some of the diseases to be discussed in this chapter has yet to be proved. However, their causative agents are of ultramicroscopic size, filterable, able to replicate and transmit the disease to another host.

There is no agreement as to exactly what viral diseases should come under this heading. Reviews of the subject are plentiful (Gajdusek, Gibbs and Alpers, 1965; Dick, 1972; Fucillo, Kurent and Sever, 1974; Kimberlin, 1976). In 1954, Sigurdsson suggested the following criteria for slow diseases of viral, bacterial or other microbiological origin.

1. A long initial period of latency of several months or years.
2. A protracted illness usually ending in death.
3. Limitation of the infection to one host species and lesions in one organ or tissue system.

He gave the following examples of slow virus disease:

Rida (Icelandic form of scrapie)
Visna (encephalitis in sheep) ⎱
Maedi (progressive pneumonia in sheep ⎰ Same agent
Jaagsiekete (infectious adenomatosis in sheep)
'Bittner' mammary carcinoma in mice
'Gross' leukaemia in mice.

He suggested that Rous sarcoma, Leuke's renal carcinoma of the leopard frog and Shope's rabbit papilloma should also be included. Many of these are diseases caused by oncogenic viruses and further comments will be made about this aspect in the section on 'Future Research'. This concept has had to be modified as knowledge has increased and it is no longer a criteria of slow virus diseases that infections are limited to a single host or a single organ.

A modern list of naturally occurring slow virus diseases would omit the oncogenic virus diseases and include:

Scrapie in sheep ⎫
Mink encephalopathy ⎬ The spongiform encephalopathies
Kuru in man ⎪
Creutzfeldt–Jacob disease ⎭

Subacute sclerosing panencephalitis in man
Progressive multifocal leucoencephalopathy
Adenovirus 32 encephalitis in man
Cytomegalovirus (herpes virus group)
Rubella (congenital)
Arboviruses in man and animals, e.g. epilepsia partialis continua — Kozhevnikov's epilepsy
Visna ⎫
Maedi ⎭ In sheep
Aleutian disease of mink
Hepatitis viruses in animals and man
Lymphocytic choriomeningitis virus infections in mice where tolerance has been produced.

This second list contains nine human diseases compared to none in the first list. It emphasises how the concept of slow virus diseases in animals led to the recognition of similar disorders in man. Animals provide the experimental models for the human diseases, and the investigation of slow virus diseases of the CNS in man and animals should naturally proceed together where possible.

It is important to realise that the pathogenic mechanisms involved in damage to the CNS by slow viruses are also observed in slow virus diseases affecting other organs, such as the lungs in maedi of sheep. This is a particularly relevant example because what appears to be the same virus can cause a CNS demyelinating disease in the same animal.

VIRUS/HOST RELATIONSHIP

Later in this chapter it will be necessary to refer to slow virus diseases which affect organs other than the CNS in man or animals, to illustrate the part the host state at the time of infection plays in the genesis of a slow rather than acute process.

The Nature of the Virus

The result of infection will obviously depend upon the particular type and strain of virus, but is also dependent upon the *state* of the virus, i.e. does it consist mostly of higly virulent, non-virulent or even defective infectious particles. An example is the wide variation of infectivity of the arbovirus Semliki Forest (Bradish, Allner and Maber, 1972). The virus may be highly virulent or almost totally avirulent when it will not kill animals such as mice even when inoculated intracerebrally (i.c.); nevertheless, both strains multiply in the brain to produce a very high level of infectivity. However, there is evidence that avirulent strains can produce chronic disease months after the acute infection (Zlotnik, Grant and Batter-Hatton, 1972).

The Immune State of the Host

When an animal becomes infected it may be in a 'fit' state to deal with the virus but occasionally its immune mechanisms may be suppressed. Immune suppression may be caused by other infections, particularly viral, immunosuppressive drugs and irradiation as used in the treatment of cancer, or the animal may not develop either a cell mediated and/or soluble antibody response to an infection. This is seen in the immunological deficiency states, the hypogammaglobulinaemias and cell-mediated deficiency diseases in humans.

An example of these problems can be seen in one of the human slow virus diseases — progressive multifocal leucoencephalopathy (PML). This occurs in patients with various malignant diseases in which the tumour itself may have caused immune deficiency (e.g. Hodgkin's disease). It is even more common in patients who have been further immunosuppressed by cytotoxic drugs or irradiation. The age of the host may also be an important factor in determining the response to infection, as for example, when lymphocytic choriomeningitis (LCM) virus is inoculated into baby mice either in utero or immediately postnatally. If virus is given at these times the mice may become 'tolerant' and regard the virus as 'self'. Large quantities of virus are produced in the blood, brain and other organs but acute meningoencephalitis does not develop as it does when the virus is inoculated into mice with a competent immune response. However, over a length of time a chronic glomerulonephritis develops because of deposition of immune complex in the kidney and the animals eventually die many months later. Similar tolerance can be induced in adult mice by cytotoxic drugs such as cyclophosphamide. However, an acute meningoencephalitis can be produced by reconstituting the cell mediated side of the immune response by the intraperitoneal (i.p.) administration of lymphocytes sensitised to LCM virus (Cole et al, 1971).

It is perhaps instructive to mention here the differing types of disease which can be produced by canine hepatitis virus depending on the state of the host. Gocke et al (1967) showed that canine hepatitis virus, inoculated into non-immune dogs, caused an acute fulminating hepatitis, with death on the fourth to the ninth day. However, if by chance some of the dogs infected had a low level of antibody at the time of inoculation, some of them developed an illness which ran a subacute course and died between 8 and 21 days after infection; others developed a chronic hepatitis with little or no sign of illness. In the non-immune group the liver histology was one of acute necrosis. Virus could be labelled by fluorescent antibody techniques and isolated. In the subacute and chronic forms, the histology in the early stages was similar and the virus could be labelled but not isolated. At 27 days the dogs with chronic disease showed histological changes in the liver consisting of dense accumulations of lymphoid and plasma cells. This subsequently progressed to extensive hepatic fibrosis. The authors were able to reproduce these results exactly, by infecting dogs which had been passively immunised. All fully immune dogs had no illness or pathological changes when infected with the virus. Hepatitis viruses are interesting in that certain of them, such as mouse hepatitis virus, can be used to produce experimental demyelination in the CNS (Herndon et al, 1975).

Genetic Factors in the Host

The genetic constitution of the host is an important factor in its susceptibility and response to infection, e.g. in scrapie and Aleutian disease of mink and to a lesser extent visna/maedi in sheep. There also appears to be some genetic influence in kuru and in multiple sclerosis (MS) which some research workers feel shows some of the features of slow virus disease.

In view of the above considerations, the criteria for slow virus disease may be restated as follows:

Slow virus diseases are prolonged illnesses presenting months or years after infection by a wide range of viruses some of which are known to cause acute diseases and by virus-like agents as yet unidentified but which are known to be transmissable. The length of the interval between infection and the clinical manifestations of disease depends upon the infectivity of the virus, its route of entry and the immune competence of the host at the time of infection.

SPONGIFORM VIRUS ENCEPHALOPATHIES

The spongiform encephalopathies compose scrapie of sheep and goats, mink encephalopathy, kuru of the Fore tribe of New Guinea and Creutzfeldt–Jacob disease (C–J).

Scrapie

Historical

It is proper to consider scrapie of sheep first, as historically it has provided the impetus for the search for slow virus diseases in man. It is so called because in the early stages the animals rub and scrape themselves against objects. They go on to develop a progressive ataxia especially of the hind legs, and finally collapse.

As early as 1755 Lincolnshire farmers petitioned Parliament to make it illegal to mix sheep ill in this way with healthy animals, but only in this century has the transmissibility of the scrapie agent been established. Vertical transmission through the mother is a factor in some breeds. Much is now known about genetic factors which influence the incubation period in sheep (and to a much larger extent in scrapie-infected mice). Known experimental hosts for scrapie are sheep, goats, mice, rats, hamsters, voles, two species of Old World monkeys (cynomologous and rhesus) and three species of New World Monkeys (capuchin, spider and squirrel). The incubation period for this disease varies widely not only in each animal but in different genetic strains of each animal. The incubation period may extend from months to five or more years.

Pathology

Although the scrapie agent infects the reticuloendothelial system early in the incubation period and is also found in other organs, abnormal pathology is only found in the brain and spinal cord where there is hypertrophy and proliferation of astrocytes and vacuolisation within the cytoplasm of neurones — the spongiform changes. The change seen in monkeys is indistinguishable to that caused by experimental infection with kuru and C–J disease. There is no evidence of an inflammatory reaction or a primary demyelinating process. In sheep the cerebellum, medulla and hypothalamic nuclei are particularly affected. In mice the distribution and extent of the neurological lesions depend on the strain of the scrapie agent used and the genetic strain of the mouse (Frazer and Dickinson, in Kimberlin, 1976).

The agent

This is very fully described by Hunter and Millson (1977) who quote many references to past work. The agent has many properties common to the agents of the other spongiform encephalopathies. It is remarkable in that it can survive treatment by boiling, proteolytic enzymes, β-propriolactone, acetylethylene-amine, formaldehyde, RNase, DNase, and high doses of ultraviolet light. Superficially it appears that the agent of scrapie is at least 1000 times more resistant to ultraviolet inactivation and has at most only a tenth of the nucleic acid content than that of any other known viral agent. It is possible to pass the agent through 50 nm filters with reasonable success. Its size is thought to be about 25 to 35 nm.

Millson, Hunter and Kimberlin (1971) established the fact that the scrapie agent had a very close relationship with membrane and certainly membrane-disrupting substances cause inactivation. The biological activity of the scrapie agent is destroyed by extremes of pH, detergents, chaotropic agents, organic solvents and by inorganic salts. Great interest was aroused by Diener (1973) when he showed that the plant viroids shared some of these extreme physicochemical properties with the scrapie agent and in particular its extraordinary resistance to ultraviolet light. These plant viroids, such as potato spindle virus, citrus exocortic virus and chrysanthemum stunt virus, have very small RNA components of less than 50 000 daltons. It is not fully understood how such small RNA membrane-bound agents react to various inactivations. Hunter and Millson (1977) suggest that the biological activity of the scrapie agent is mediated by a two-component system and even if one component is a small viroid-like nucleic acid, the component donated by the plasma membrane, probably a hydrophobic protein or glycoprotein, almost certainly plays an important role in the pathogenesis of this disease.

Mink Encephalopathy

Historical

Several mink encephalopathies occur but the important one in this context is that which is characterised by spongy degeneration. It was first observed in 1947 in the USA and the disease was characterised by Hartsough and Burger (1965) and Burger and Hartsough (1965). It is a disease of animals over one year old. Epidemics of the disease are infrequent but if they occur they may affect 100 per cent of the stock.

Pathology

Gross examination of the CNS reveals no abnormality. On microscopical examination there is intense astroglial proliferation, neuronal degeneration and vacuolation associated with a status spongiosis of the grey matter. An inflammatory response in the CNS is rarely observed.

The agent

The agent has been studied by Burger and Hartsough (1965) and Marsh and Hanson (1969). It appears to have a particle size of 50 nm. It is resistant to boiling for 15 min and to ultraviolet light at 253.7 nm. It is sensitive to ether, formalin and to cell membrane-disrupting substances such as hot phenol and pronase. It has been shown to persist and to replicate in cell cultures of brain from infected animals. The agent may be passed by intracerebral and intramuscular routes when the incubation period shortens to four to five and six and a half to eight months respectively. Although lesions are only found in the brain, virus can be isolated from liver, spleen, lung, kidney, bladder muscle and faeces, but not from the urine or blood. An immunological or interferon response has not been reported as yet in this disease.

Clinical features

Field observations suggest that the incubation period is 6 to 12 months. The disease lasts two to six weeks and is usually fatal. The baby mink do not develop this disease even when housed with and suckling from affected mothers. The onset is insidious with the animal developing symptoms of excitability and loss of control of the limbs. This continues to a frank ataxia associated with stiff and jerky movement. Periods of pathological somnolence occur and the animal becomes anaemic.

Host susceptibility

The disease has been passed successfully to other mink, goats, mice, golden hamsters, albino ferrets, skunk, racoon, rhesus and squirrel monkeys and considerable discussion continues as to whether mink encephalopathy and scrapie are the same diseases in different hosts. The problem is well reviewed by Barlow (in Dick, 1972).

Kuru of the Fore Tribe of New Guinea

Historical

Kuru is the first slow transmissible infection recorded in man. It was discovered in 1957 by Gajdusek and Zigas in a mesolithic cannibal tribe of the Fore linguistic group who live in a very isolated area of the Eastern Highlands of New Guinea. The disease when discovered was the commonest cause of death and had reached frightening endemic proportions. It affected predominantly adult females and to a lesser extent children of both sexes over the age of five years. If adult manhood was reached the incidence was significantly less in this group. There were scattered cases amongst neighbouring groups of natives which may have been due to intermarriage with a member of the Fore tribe. Since that time the incidence of kuru has decreased greatly probably due to the suppression of ritual cannibalism (Hornabrook and Moir, 1970). This was practised chiefly by the females of the tribe who handled highly infectious brain tissue during ritual ceremonies carried out during mourning for the dead. This tissue was distributed to the children present and not only was it eaten but it almost certainly contaminated open abrasions on the body. It is this route rather than ingestion which is probably the most important method of infection.

A genetic factor also appears to play a role in susceptibility. It was Hadlow (1959) who first compared this disease to scrapie of sheep because of its very similar epidemiology and suggested that it might be passed to subhuman primates.

Pathology

The basic pathology consists of clearing of neuronal cytoplasm, formation of vacuoles in pre- and postsynaptic terminals and eventually neuronal destruction creating the picture of what is now called 'a status spongiosus of grey matter'. There is also astroglial hypertrophy and hyperplasia and the formation of amyloid plaques which resemble those seen in the ageing nervous system (Gajdusek, in Dick, 1972). This latter finding will be commented on more fully in the section on 'Future Research'.

The agent

This has many of the physicochemical characteristics of the scrapie agent but it has not as yet been passed through membranes of 100 nm minimal pore size, in sharp contrast to the easy passage of the scrapie and mink encephalopathy agents through this size of filter. It has been passed from over 10 human patients to many chimpanzees with incubation periods of 14 to 39 months. With passage through further chimpanzees the average incubation period has fallen from 22 to 11 months.

The clinical features

The disease starts insiduously with a mild tremor of the trunk (kuru means tremor in the Fore language). Severe cerebellar ataxia develops until walking becomes impossible and any attempt at movement of any limb is associated with gross ataxic jerks. In the terminal stages of the disease abnormalities of eye movements develop and alterations in personality and behaviour occur. Finally, total immobilisation occurs with incontinence, impaired swallowing and hence starvation. Convulsions and disturbance of sensory modalities are not seen. Death usually occurs three to six months after the onset of symptoms. During the disease process the patients are afebrile unless intercurrent infections occur, and the CSF and blood show no abnormality or immunological reaction which can be related to the disease.

Creutzfeldt–Jacob Disease

Historical

Jacob (1921, 1923) described five patients aged between 30 and 50 years who presented with comparable symptoms including mental changes and jerky movements and who at necropsy showed changes of a fairly specific disease process in the CNS. An earlier case described by Creutzfeldt appeared to be similar and the disease came to be known as Creutzfeldt–Jacob (C–J) disease. Daniel (in Dick, 1972) using the distribution of lesions as a basis for classification refers to the Jacob, the Heidenhain, the diffuse, and the ataxic forms of the disease. Jacob (1923) described these cases as having spastic pseudosclerosis and likened it to what is seen in amyotrophic lateral sclerosis. Heidenhain emphasised marked changes in the visual cortex and early symptoms were visual disturbances. The diffuse type describes what it suggests and forms a large group in which the emphasis is a widespread nerve cell degeneration with proliferation of astrocytes throughout the cortex. The ataxic form described by Brownwell and Oppenheimer (1965) emphasises the clinical features and pathological changes relating to the cerebellum. However, it must be made quite clear that there is a wide overlap between each group. The most important histological feature as regards the transmissibility of an agent from these brains is the presence of the spongiform change described in more detail below.

Pathology

Pathological changes are limited to the CNS which shows diffuse neuronal degeneration with cytoplasmic vacuolisation, astrocytic proliferation and hypertrophy. Satellitosis and neuronaphagia are often seen. The microcystic spaces, i.e. the spongiform changes, are scattered in the grey matter and according to Beck et al (1969) may be very difficult to see in advanced cases because the spaces collapse. The proliferation and hypertrophy of astrocytes and microglial proliferation was most marked where the status spongiosus was most severe. By electron microscope studies Lampert, Gajdusek and Gibbs (1971) showed that the spongiform changes occur mainly in the nerve cells. There is no evidence of inflammation or demyelination as seen in multiple sclerosis (Roos, Gajdusek and Gibbs, 1973).

The agent

This has not been identified or seen under the electron microscope. It produces no cytolytic pathology in cell cultures and no immune response has been found in humans or experimentally infected animals. Like kuru the agent of C–J disease passes through a millipore filter of 220 nm but has not been detected after filtration through smaller pores. The agent has not been isolated as yet from visceral tissues, blood, CSF or urine from humans or animals infected with the disease. This agent like the kuru agent can persist in explanted animal and human tissues (Gajdusek et al, 1972). The kuru agent persisted in vitro for at least 70 days in chimpanzee brain cells kept at 37°C and the C–J agent for over 255 days in human brain cells at the same temperature. Further inoculation of these cultures with 14 different viruses showed no evidence of interference. There was no production of interferon detectable in any of the infected cells and incidentally the treatment of kuru affected chimpanzees with interferon inducers had no effect on the clinical course of the disease (Gibbs and Gajdusek, in Dick, 1972).

The agent is thought to have many physicochemical properties similar to the kuru agent but investigations have not been in progress long enough for definitive conclusions to be reached.

At the time of writing the animals to which this disease has been passed are the following: chimpanzee, four types of New World monkey (spider, squirrel, woolly, and marmoset), seven types of Old World monkey (bushbaby, mangabey, African green, rhesus, stump-tailed, cynomologus, and pig-tailed) and the domestic cat (Gibbs and Gajdusek, 1973). The incubation period varies greatly from 11 to 26 months in chimpanzees and up to 47 months or more in other monkeys; in the cat it was 30 months and a recent publication suggests the possibility of transmission to random bred albino laboratory mice after 18 to 24 months (Brownwell et al, 1975).

Of considerable concern is a case report of possible human transmission of C–J disease by transplantation of a cornea from a 55-year-old male who died of pneumonia and was known to have a two-month history of progressive loss of memory. The diagnosis of C–J disease was not made until the brain had been examined histologically. A 55-year-old female who received the cornea developed neurological symptoms and signs 18 months later and died eight months after that. The autopsy showed the characteristic histology of C–J disease (Duffy et al, 1974).

The clinical features

The disease has a world-wide incidence and there are a few recorded familial cases (Roos et al, 1973). It is a presenile dementia starting between 31 and 70 or more years of age but the maximum incidence occurs between 40 and 70. The mental deterioration is often rapid and may be evident from day to day. The dementia is followed by a progressive spastic quadraparesis, pseudobulbar palsy and myoclonus. In approximately 50 per cent of cases psychiatric abnormalities, ataxia, basal ganglia signs and disturbances of vision are seen. Disorders of higher cortical function also occur such as aphasia, dysgraphia, dyslexia, agnosia, and spatial and visual disorientation. Lower motor neurone involvement is uncommon but when it does occur it is accompanied by fasciculation. The myoclonus which occurs is often produced by sensory stimuli. The patient is frequently dead within two years of the start of the illness.

Laboratory studies

Investigations of blood and CSF show no constant or significant abnormality. The EEG in the early stages shows generalised slow activity replacing the normal rhythms. As the disease progresses the degree of EEG abnormality increases progressively and polyphasic complexes soon appear. These tend to be of high voltage, are frequently bilaterally synchronous although not necessarily symmetrical and alternate with periods of lower voltage slow activity. In some patients the complexes are periodic while in others they are irregular. Sometimes myoclonic jerks accompany the complexes but they are not related to either their form or amplitude. In the final stages of the disease the amplitude of the EEG diminishes and becomes flat for long periods in between the bursts of slow or sharp waves.

SUBACUTE SCLEROSING PANENCEPHALITIS

Historical

This rare disease was first associated with the measles virus by Connolly et al (1967). It is difficult to trace cases before this time but it is unlikely that this was a new disease. The clinical syndrome itself is very variable (Freeman, 1969; Lowenthal et al, 1972) and the pathological picture of diffuse perivascular cuffing, gliosis, neuronal degeneration and slight to severe demyelination is seen with other virus diseases. The Cowdrey type A (eosinophilic) nuclear inclusions in brain cells seen in this disease were first described by Dawson (1933).

Pathology

The brain appears grossly normal but on section there is a multifocal abnormality of tissue necrosis, perivascular cuffing, primary and secondary demyelination and astrocytosis. the perivascular cuffs consist mostly of lymphocytes and plasma cells. As mentioned before eosinophilic nuclear and cytoplasmic inclusions are present in neurones and glial cells.

The agent

Measles virus was successfully isolated from a case of subacute sclerosing panencephalitis (SSPE) by using the important new technique of cocultivation by cell culturing the SSPE brain biopsy with HeLa cells, the latter being cells in which measles virus replicates very efficiently (Horta-Barbosa et al, 1969). Horta-Barbosa et al (1971) used a similar technique successfully to isolate measles virus from a lymph gland of an additional two patients with SSPE indicating that the virus is not confined to the brain alone. Fluorescent antibody techniques have played an important part in identifying the measles virus in the brain (Connolly et al, 1967). Electron microscopic studies of brain tissue by Bouteille et al (1965) also suggested a viral aetiology. These workers found intranuclear tubular filaments in brain which resembled those seen in dog kidney cells infected with measles virus (Tawara, 1965). The eosinophilic nuclear inclusions may show a massive collection of tubular measles nucleocapsids under the electron microscope (Herndon and Rubinstein, 1968).

Clinical features

The disease was first described in three boys aged 12, 15 and 17 at an interval of 11 to 13 years after their experiencing childhood measles (Connolly et al, 1967). It affects predominantly children of school age and the incubation period varies from months to many years. The diagnosis is made by the combination of the clinical features, the periodic complexes in the EEG and serological studies.

The disease usually begins with an alteration in personality and performance. Visual disturbances may develop which can frequently be related to a progressive chorioretinitis (Font, Jenis and Tuck, 1973). These are followed by focal myoclonic jerking and focal or generalised convulsions which may be severe enough to throw the patient off a bed or seat. Finally, there is severe dementia, increasing stupor, marked rigidity with upper motor neurone signs and alterations in autonomic function. As stated earlier the clinical course is very variable and may last up to three to four years. During this time there may be phases of improvement, and remissions of months to several years have been noted (Donner et al, 1972). It is causing some concern that a few cases of SSPE continue to be reported after the administration of live attenuated measles vaccine (Schneck, 1968).

Laboratory investigations

The EEG has already been mentioned. Initially the basic rhythms of the EEG become slower and irregular, very high voltage paroxysms (1400 μV) soon appear consisting of a single diphasic slow wave with brief runs of delta activity occasionally associated with sharp waves. The form of these complexes differs from patient to patient. As the disease progresses the complexes become established and they recur at frequent intervals between 6 and 16 times a minute. They tend to become more frequent as the illness evolves. The paroxysms are bilateral and synchronous and as a rule generalised and symmetrical. These are seldom affected by afferent stimulation and tend to become reduced during sleep. Later in the course of the illness the background activity between the paroxysms becomes lower in voltage and in some patients sporadic sharp waves are seen. Frequently myoclonic phenomena are seen to occur in synchrony with the complexes.

The CSF shows a raised protein and the percentage of gamma-globulin is elevated. The globulins in the CSF have been shown to be specific antibodies directed against various antigenic components of measles virus (Vandick and Norrby, 1973). All patients have unusually high titres of measles antibody in both serum and CSF, in fact a higher titre than that usually seen after the acute disease. IgM antibody persists at high levels suggesting the persistence of measles antigen whereas following ordinary measles it has disappeared by the forty-sixth day. The amount of antibody seen in the CSF as compared to the serum suggests that antibody is being released within the CNS (Connolly, 1968). The antibody titre may rise very significantly during the course of the disease.

PROGRESSIVE MUTLIFOCAL LEUCOENCEPHALOPATHY

Historical

Progressive multifocal leucoencephalopathy (PML) is an unusual demyelinating disease of man first described by Astrom, Mancall and Richardson in 1958. It is a disease of the CNS particularly associated with lymphomas but has been seen in other malignant disorders. It was not until 1965 that ZuRhein and Chou demonstrated under the electron microscope particles within the inclusions in the oligodendrocytes which had the appearance characteristic of the papova viruses. Further work by Howatson, Nagai and ZuRhein (1965) indicated that the PML virus was smaller than the only known human papova virus — the wart virus — but was of similar size and morphology to the Simian virus 40 (SV40) — polyoma subgroup of papova viruses. In 1971 Padgett et al isolated a virus which they named JC virus (which must not be confused with Creutzfeldt–Jacob and the C–J agent) from one of their patients; this turned out to be a papova virus. In 1972 Weiner et al (1972a) isolated agents from two more PML patients and these viruses appeared antigenically similar to SV40. The JC virus and SV40 (PML) virus are distinguishable from one another but have antigens in common with SV40 (Penney et al, 1972).

Pathology

There is focal myelin loss but sparing of axis cylinders. No inflammation is seen but the astrocytes have unusual chromatin patterns and the oligodendrocytes around the areas of demyelination frequently contain eosinophilic intranuclear inclusions. The oligodendrocytes contain the majority of virus which can frequently be seen in the inclusions (Narayan et al, 1973).

The agents

The JC virus was originally isolated from a case of Hodgkin's disease complicated by PML (Padgett et al, 1971). It has been isolated from a further five cases of PML (Weiner et al, 1973; Walker, 1974). It only grows well in human fetal glial cells and can agglutinate human type O red cells which has not yet been achieved with SV40 or the SV40-PML strain. Its properties in other animals and in tissue culture will be discussed further in the section on 'Future Research'. Padgett and Walker (1973) have shown in an antibody survey carried out in Wisconsin that antibody to JC virus was present to significant levels in 69 per cent of adults and that the highest rate of sero-conversion occurred during the first 14 years of life. This indicates that infection with this virus throughout the world may be common though to date the occurrence of PML is rare. This rarity may only represent our difficulties to date of making a positive diagnosis.

The SV40-PML virus has only been isolated in two cases and they appear to be perfectly valid isolations (Weiner et al, 1972b). Antibodies to this virus do occur in man (Shah et al, 1971) but the normal hosts are monkeys. There did not appear to be a relationship in either of the two cases to the use of killed polio vaccine used between 1955 and 1961 which was contaminated with the SV40 virus.

Clinical features

Any abnormal focal neurological signs appearing in patients in the terminal stages of malignant disease and particularly in those suffering from lymphoma who have been treated by immunosuppression, is suggestive of PML. There may be mental disturbances, disturbances of vision with blindness, dysphasia leading to aphasia, upper motor neurone and cerebellar signs. Secondary deposits, other space occupying lesions and meningitis due to more common viruses, fungi or coccidiosis need to be excluded. The patient is often afebrile. The CSF is usually normal but the EEG may show a generalised dysrhythmia. Other specialised investigations such as air encephalography show no abnormalities. A precise diagnosis can be made by brain biopsy before death with examination of the material under the electron microscope and in tissue culture, but this is infrequently done. Patients may survive over two years but death usually occurs earlier and may be from pre-existing malignant disease.

HUMAN CYTOMEGALOVIRUS INFECTIONS

Approximately 1 per cent of infants born in the USA excrete cytomegalovirus (herpes group) in their urine at birth and may continue to do so for the first four years of life. Observable CNS damage occurs in approximately 17 per cent of those 1 per cent (Hanshaw, 1971) and it has been suggested that about 3200 children are born each year in the USA with brain damage because of congenital infection with this virus. The CNS problem is characterised by microcephaly, mental retardation, epilepsy and progressive cerebral calcification. The virus reaches the fetus from the mother via the placenta. Reynolds et al (1974) observed that some infants who appear normal at birth but excrete virus in their urine may develop sequelae of mental retardation and neural deafness three to five years later.

Pathology

In the fetus cells can be found in the parenchymatous organs which are enlarged, contain inclusions and are surrounded by a mixed population of inflammatory cells. These changes are also seen in the CNS where areas of focal necrosis develop which may become calcified.

HERPES SIMPLEX INFECTIONS OF THE CNS

Herpes simplex virus may produce an acute, chronic or recurrent encephalitis in human beings; this is well reviewed by Illis and Gostling (1972). It is also responsible for the repeated attacks of nasal, lip and genital herpes. For a long time the mechanisms involved in this recurrence were not at all clear. Recently herpes virus has been isolated from both trigeminal and sacral ganglia and this has confirmed that virus can lie latent in the nervous system (Barringer, 1974; Lehrer, Wilton and Shillitoe, 1975). Very recently it has been shown, using an antibody-mediated cell-dependent immune lysis system, that people with recurrent 'cold sores' have both CSF and serum antibodies to herpes simplex virus. It is suggested that these antibodies may be responsible for maintaining the latency of the virus. This virus affects many animals including mice; experimental models are therefore available.

VARICELLA–ZOSTER INFECTIONS OF THE CNS

As this virus produces CNS damage both in relation to chickenpox (varicella) and to shingles (zoster) it should be included in a discussion of slow viruses affecting the CNS. The latency of this virus is reviewed by McArthy (in Dick, 1972). It is accepted now that all those who develop zoster have had varicella in the past. Recurrent attacks of zoster are frequent. It is thought that after varicella the virus may be dormant like herpes simplex in the sensory ganglia in a form which enables it to multiply at a later date. Then when some repressor mechanism on virus replication is removed the virus multiplies and zoster develops. The path to and from the sensory ganglia is probably the continuum of the Schwann cells surrounding sensory nerves. There may be a relationship between the breakdown of immunological protection and the development of zoster. Certainly the wise clinician looks for occult malignant disease when zoster appears in the elderly. The nervous tissue involvement with varicella–zoster is very difficult to investigate because of the lack of a suitable experimental animal and human autopsy specimens.

The herpes virus group are of great interest in the field of slow virus diseases as they frequently damage the CNS, have a considerable capacity for persistence and latency and are also associated with many and varied malignancies in animals. The oncogenicity of the herpes virus group is well reviewed in a

Symposium in *Cancer Research*(1973). The virus has been associated with sheep and pulmonary adenomatosis (Jaagsiekte), monkey and rabbit lymphomas, American leopard frog and Leuke's renal carcinoma, domestic chicken lympho-proliferative (Marek's) disease and guinea-pig lymphoblastic leukaemia. In man a herpes type virus, EB virus, is not only associated with infectious mononuc-leosis but may be of aetiological importance in Burkitt's lymphoma and nasopharyngeal carcinoma. A herpes virus has also been associated with carcinoma of the cervix. The relevance of herpes virus to malignant disease and the overall significance of proliferation of cells associated with slow virus disease of the CNS is discussed further in the section on 'Future Research'.

RUBELLA

Rubella virus is teratogenic in man and causes well-known and widespread problems. Perhaps not so well known is the damage the virus may produce in the CNS, causing focal neurological lesions, microcephaly, mental retardation, hemiparesis, quadriparesis, convulsions and CSF abnormalities. It has been possible to isolate virus from the CSF for at least 18 months after birth (Desmond et al, 1967). There is usually a mild meningitis and recurrent pleocytosis occurs. Perivascular cuffing is present, and of considerable interest is the calcification seen in the walls of vessels within the brain substance. Myelination is defective or incomplete and suggests abnormal metabolism or functioning of the oligodendrocytes (Rorke and Spiro, 1967). Recently two important publications have appeared showing that rubella can produce a chronic progressive panen-cephalitis in the second decade of life and this has been likened to subacute sclerosing panencephalitis because of the high antibody titre to rubella in serum and CSF. The features of this disease are progressive dementia, ataxia and seizures. In one case perimacular pigmentation occurred (Townsend et al, 1975; Weil et al, 1975).

MAEDI-VISNA COMPLEX

Historical

Visna is the neurological disease caused by a virus which also causes maedi, a pulmonary disease of sheep. The neurological component of the maedi-visna complex was first observed in Iceland in 1935 but had been eradicated from the natural sheep population by 1951. Maedi was recognised from about 1939 and persisted in certain flocks in circumscribed areas until 1965. The maedi-visna diseases are well reviewed by Thormar (in Gajdusek et al, 1965) and Palsson (in Dick, 1972). They deserve extensive discussion as these diseases are an excellent example of what experimentally appears to be virtually the same virus producing two different conditions. If the virus is taken from the lung disease, extensive pulmonary pathology and little CNS damage is caused in recipient sheep but if it is taken from animals with damage to the CNS the virus will produce further damage in the CNS on passage to other sheep. However, it is important to appreciate that intracerebral inoculation of the maedi (lung) strain can produce the neurological symptoms associated with visna (brain) strain and that the visna strain can produce maedi.

The nature of the viruses of maedi-visna

These viruses contain RNA and an RNA-dependent DNA polymerase. This enzyme has previously only been found in RNA tumour viruses (Stone et al, 1971) and this point will be discussed later. They can be seen under the electron microscope and have a myxovirus-like structure (Pautrat et al, 1971). Replication takes place in the cytoplasm and the virus reaccumulates later at the cell surface (Thormar, 1969). The physicochemical properties of these viruses which are not particularly unusual have been reviewed by Palsson (in Dick, 1972). The two viruses are almost identical but at pH 4.2 maedi virus was inactivated three times more rapidly than visna virus (Thormar, 1966).

Neutralising antibodies usually appear three to six months after infection but complement-fixing antibodies frequently appear after a few weeks and in some cases are found when neutralising antibodies are not detectable. Antibodies persist in high titre for many years, and the sheep with high levels of antibody often show pronounced pathological lesions when killed (Gudnadottir and Kristinsdottir, 1967). Both viruses grow well in tissue culture and the cytopathic effect with maedi is characterised by the formation of multinucleated synctia. This leads eventually to the complete disintegration of the cell culture (Sigurdardottir and Thormar, 1964). Of particular interest is the effect of visna on tissue cultures of human glia in which virus persistence for long periods of time may be demonstrated (MacIntyre, Wintergill and Vatter, 1974).

In transmission experiments a prolonged leucocytosis in the blood occurs in both diseases. In visna 50 to 200×10^6 cells/litre may be found in the CSF within a few weeks of inoculation, but sometimes these do not appear for several months. There is also an increase in the gamma-globulin levels in the CSF.

Visna

Pathology

In sheep dying of uncomplicated visna no specific macroscopic postmortem changes are seen. There is evidence of proliferation of the cells of the reticuloendothelial system. The major feature on microscopical examination of the CNS is a subependymal and meningeal infiltration of cells. Lesions can be found in every part of the white matter of the brain and cord. The lesions start as foci of microglial infiltration which may become invasive and associated with cystic degeneration. Myelin degeneration is thought to be secondary; it is usually mild and the axis cylinders are well preserved. In the affected areas there is extensive perivascular cuffing with lymphocytes, plasma cells and histiocytes. The peripheral nerves are also involved and show diffuse lymphocytic infiltration, but changes in the myelin sheaths are mild.

Clinical features

Visna, which means 'wasting' in old Norse, was never observed in animals under two years of age in natural conditions. Weakness of the hind limbs appear first, associated with general loss of condition. The paralysis of the limbs progresses slowly and usually takes from several months to several years before it is complete. Sometimes trembling of the lips and eye lids is seen and the head is often turned a little to one side.

Maedi

Pathology

The postmortem changes are usually confined to the lungs and associated lymph nodes. The weight of the lungs may be four times that of the normal. They are voluminous and collapse only slightly when the thoracic cavity is opened.

The main microscopical lesion is a chronic interstitial inflammation with a diffuse thickening of the alveolar septa, sometimes causing total obliteration of the alveoli. The thickening of the alveolar septa is mostly due to an excess number of large mononuclear cells and to a lesser extent lymphocytes. Hyperplasia of smooth muscle in the interalveolar wall is often seen and peribronchial and perivascular proliferation of lymphoid tissue is always marked. Hyperplasia of the epithelium in small bronchioles is often found sometimes in association with disorganisation and epithelialisation of neighbouring alveoli (Georgsson and Palsson, 1971).

Clinical features

The word maedi means 'short of breath'. Leucocytosis is often seen before any clinical abnormality is noticed. Loss of general condition is followed by increasing dyspnoea requiring the increased use of the accessory muscles of respiration. This is often accompanied by rhythmic jerks of the head and flanks. The sheep frequently die of a secondary pneumonia.

ALEUTIAN MINK DISEASE

Aleutian disease is a chronic virus infection of mink which has caused serious financial problems in the mink industry. There is a genetic determinant involving the blue mink originally derived from Aleutian mink but other mink may become infected. Proliferation of plasma cells and marked hypergammaglobulinaemia, glomerulonephritis, degenerative arterial lesions and proliferation of intrahepatic bile ducts are commonly seen. Virus can persist for indefinite periods and can be found in the cytoplasm of macrophages, spleen, lymph glands and the Küpffer cells of the liver. High levels of antibody are detectable and deposits of immune complexes can be identified in the glomeruli. The animals eventually develop renal failure and die. The renal lesions can be prevented by immunosuppression with drugs such as cyclophosphamide. The whole problem is well reviewed by Kimberlin (1976).

NEUROLOGICAL DISEASE IN MAN OF POSSIBLE VIRAL AETIOLOGY

Certain common and less common diseases of the CNS in man have features sharing some of the characteristics of slow virus disease, e.g. multiple sclerosis,

Parkinson's disease, motor neurone disease, Vilyuisk encephalitis, and other meningoencephalitides. Although a viral aetiology remains purely speculative the evidence that exists will be discussed.

Multiple Sclerosis

Multiple sclerosis (MS) is a disease which usually starts in early adult life. It is almost unknown at the Equator but may reach a prevalence up to 150 per 100 000 of the population in the more northern latitudes. A similar situation exists moving towards the southern latitudes but these areas have not as yet been extensively studied. Epidemiological surveys (Dean, 1970; Brody, 1972) suggest an infective aetiology. People moving from high- to low-risk areas appear to retain their high risk. There is evidence for a higher incidence in families. The possibility of MS being related in some way to scrapie even though this disease bears little resemblance clinically or pathologically to MS has been considered. However, certain studies still need to be explained. Palsson, Pattison and Field (in Gajdusek et al, 1965) produced scrapie in Icelandic sheep 16 to 21 months after intracerebral inoculation of brain from a patient dying of acute MS (Field, Miller and Russell, 1962). Inoculum from this patient's brain failed to produce scrapie-like lesions in mice (Field, 1966) but some scrapie-like lesions were produced in a second passage in mice from the brain of another MS patient. This work has not been confirmed (Dick et al, 1965; Palsson et al, in Gajdusek et al, 1965) and no condition like MS has been observed in monkeys and chimpanzees (Gibbs, Gajdusek and Alpers, 1969). Carp et al (1972) indicated that intraperitoneal or intracerebral inoculation of mice with MS tissue produced a granulocytopenia but no other detectable change. Serum from mice with granulocytopenia was able to cause a fall in the cell levels in other mice and this suggested the possibility of a filterable agent with a possible filtration size of 25 to 50 nm.

More recently Carp, Merz and Licursi (1974) inoculated a transformed line of mouse fibroblasts with MS material. No abnormality was detected at the first subculture but subsequent subcultures, at weekly intervals, showed a reduction in cell yield by two to four-fold or more in the MS infected cultures. The cell-free lysate from the eighteenth passage produced a granulocytopenia when inoculated into mice. Success was claimed with materials from MS patients' brain, spleen, serum, CSF, kidney and lymph node and from every stage of the disease. No positives were found from other materials. Henle et al (1975) and Kodovsky et al (1975) have also managed to produce the granulocytopenia using MS material in mice and have shown that sera from MS patients and a few of their close relatives neutralise this activity whereas sera from patients with other diseases so far tested do not do this. For some reason, as yet unexplained, sera from people indigenous to East Africa have high titres of neutralising antibody although MS is virtually unknown in this area. Licursi et al (1972) found a similar granulocytopenia using scrapie-infected tissue but no such neutralisation has yet been detected from scrapie-infected animals. All this evidence strongly suggests a viral aetiology but a lot needs to be done to identify the agent or agents which may produce these findings.

Electron microscopic studies

Three types of 'virus-like' particles have been seen from either autopsy or biopsy material from MS patients (Perier and Gregaire, 1965; Rinne, 1968; Perier, 1969; Suzuki et al, 1969; Andrews, 1972; Field et al, 1972; Prineas, 1972). The most important, perhaps, are the tubular structures resembling myxovirus nucleocapsids and particularly their relationship to serological studies implicating measles virus, itself a myxovirus.

Serological studies

In 1962 Adams and Imagawa reported that the titre of measles antibody was higher in MS patients than in controls. Twenty out of 22 subsequent studies in the US and Europe have confirmed this finding in serum and/or cerebrospinal fluid.

However, measles has not been the only virus to which higher antibody titres appear to occur in MS. Rises in antibody titre to herpes simplex, varicella, mumps, influenza C or parainfluenza 3 viruses, have also been reported (Brody, 1972).

Cell culture studies

Ter Meulen et al (1972) established brain cell cultures from two patients dying of MS and one of these cultures showed tubules resembling paramyxovirus nucleocapsids under the electron microscope. After using cell fusion techniques in the presence of lysolecithin with CV-1 and human diploid cells, the cells appeared to become transformed, haemadsorbed red cells and showed abundant cytoplasmic nucleocapsid-like structures. Haemadsorption and infectivity for CV-1 cells could be neutralised by antisera against parainfluenza type 1 but neither the particles nor parainfluenza 1 antigen could be found in the brains of the patients. Field et al (1972) also showed an agent suggestive of measles virus in cell cultures from the brain of an MS patient but laboratory contamination could not be ruled out for certain.

These findings are all inconclusive but provide a strong stimulus for further studies particularly of the relationship of measles to MS. The whole problem is made much more difficult by the probability that all animal brains contain viruses which are not necessarily pathogenic as shown by the isolation of a variety of viruses from chimpanzee brains (Rogers et al, 1967).

Parkinson's Disease

Following von Economo's disease (encephalitis lethargica) which was presumed to have a viral aetiology, approximately one-third of the surviving cases developed a syndrome like classical Parkinson's disease but with abnormal eye movements (oculogyric crises) 6 months to 20 years later. Parkinsonism also occurs as a complication of other virus CNS infections but usually appears with the acute illness.

Motor Neurone Disease

Textbooks and teachers use all the following titles, motor neurone disease, progressive muscular atrophy, amyotrophic lateral sclerosis (ALS), to refer to the same disease and a standardisation of nomenclature is long overdue. Similarly, because of the preference of the disease for damaging the motor neurone it has been related to poliomyelitis and in some of the older textbooks it has even been named chronic poliomyelitis. It is a disease limited to the lower and upper motor neurones (corticospinal tract) although at autopsy it is not uncommon to find histological lesions in the other spinal tracts especially the posterior column, even though sensory symptoms may not arise during life. Amyotrophic lateral sclerosis does not appear to have any geographical localisation except on the island of Guam which lies in a chain of islands — the Marianas — in the Western Pacific and on the Kii peninsula of Japan (Yase, 1970; Brody, Hirano and Scott, 1971). It is of considerable interest that another syndrome, Parkinsonian dementia (PD), is also prevalent in this area. This disease which also shows Alzheimer's neurofibrillary changes and intracytoplasmic inclusion bodies may be related to the Guam ALS disease. Twelve per cent of the people in the terminal stages of ALS showed evidence of the PD syndrome whereas about a third of those who started with the PD syndrome developed ALS before they died (Kurland, in Gajdusek et al, 1965). It is interesting that the neurofibrillary changes can be seen in patients as young as 28 years of age (Hirano, in Gajdusek et al, 1965). Neurofibrillary changes were not observed in the classic cases of ALS seen at Montefiore Hospital, New York (Hirano and Zimmerman, 1962) and this may differentiate the condition from the Guam ALS which on clinical grounds would otherwise be very difficult.

Viruses are able to produce both upper and lower motor neurone lesions particularly those of the tick-born encephalitis group (TBE) and Russian scientists have postulated that a chronic TBE infection might be one virus that could cause ALS disease. Zilber et al (1963) reported transmission of ALS to monkeys after one to three years latency and Gardashian et al (1970) have reported further transmissions. However, Gibbs and Gajdusek (in Dick, 1972) using these and other inocula from patients in the USA and from Guam have not been able to confirm these findings. In Northern Siberia ALS has been reported as a sequelae of Vilyuisk encephalitis (Petrov, 1970). A virus resembling encephalomyocarditis virus has been isolated from CSF, blood and brain of patients with this disease but the causative relationship of the virus to the disease has not been proven.

Vilyuisk Encephalitis

Historical

This disease occurs in Yakutia (Siberia), USSR, a region inhabited by the Yakut tribe. Visitors to this area at the end of the last century described an unpleasant neurological condition which affected those people who lived alongside the Vilyui river. It has been investigated since but the majority of the literature is in Russian. A description can be found in Gajdusek et al (1965) with references to the Russian literature.

Pathology

There is frequently a panencephalitis with inflammation and loss of neurones occurring throughout the CNS. Hydrocephalus is common. Petrov (1973) describes microgranulomatous foci in the grey matter of the brain with some areas of status spongiosus, inflammatory reactions, gliofibrosis and neuronal loss. It must be of considerable interest that this is a chronic neurological disease which combines status spongiosus with an inflammatory reaction; inflammation is conspicuously absent in the four spongiform encephalopathies described previously.

The agent

Eleven strains of virus have been isolated in this disease after infected material had been inoculated into mouse brain. Unfortunately, the viruses so far identified are related to known mouse viruses (Mengo and EMC) and may have no relation to the disease at all. At the present time a viral aetiology to this disease is not proven. However, the illness and its pathology are very strongly suggestive of a virus infection.

Clinical features

The disease apparently occurs between the ages of 8 and 45 years and is more common in females. It occurs in an acute, subacute or chronic form. Sometimes the illness starts with a depressive state and may be suddenly complicated by multiple cranial nerve abnormalities, extrapyramidal rigidity and tremor accompanied by a mild pyrexia. Intense somnolence may develop and death ensue. The chronic condition is characterised by increasing spasticity and abnormalities of the cranial nerves and extrapyramidal tracts. Dementia becomes an important feature with the patient in some cases surviving up to 20 years. There are reports that a small number of cases have the symptoms and signs of classical amyotrophic lateral sclerosis. In the acute disease there may be headache, vomiting, meningeal irritation and acute psychosis.

Other Meningoencephalitides

Behçet's disease, characterised by recurrent oral and genital ulcers and CNS involvement (Wolf, Schotland and Phillips, 1965), has some CNS pathological features suggesting a chronic viral disease (Sugihara, Mutch and Tuchiyama, 1969). Alm and Oberg (1945) produced similar lesions in a rabbit from the CSF of one patient and the sputum from another. Sezer (1953, 1956) isolated a possible virus on chorioallantoic membranes from vitreous and subretinal exudates of three patients and claimed further isolation of the agent from the blood of 20 more patients. Others have also reported isolations from patients with this disease (Alm and Oberg, 1945; Evans, Pallis and Spillane, 1957; Nakagawa and Shingu, 1958). However, these agents have not as yet been identified and therefore a viral aetiology of this disease must remain in doubt.

Vogt–Koyanagi–Harada encephalitis syndrome is in the same category as Behçet's disease in that ophthalmic lesions have been induced in rabbits. This disease is reviewed by Reed et al (1958). Further virological studies have been carried out and have been discussed by Mortada (1969).

FUTURE RESEARCH

In the introduction to this chapter reference was made to Sigurdsson (1954) and his original examples of slow virus disease. Included were several diseases caused by oncogenic viruses, e.g. infectious adenomatosis (Jaagsiekte) in sheep, 'Bittner' mammary carcinoma and 'Gross' leukaemia in mice. He also suggested that other oncogenic viral diseases might be included, i.e. Rous sarcoma, Leuke's renal carcinoma of the leopard frog and Shope's rabbit papilloma. In more modern lists these diseases are omitted because they are caused by oncogenic viruses, but as cell proliferation may be a feature of accepted slow virus disease, oncogenic virus diseases ought possibly to be included.

Cell proliferation in slow virus disease

Abnormal proliferation of cells is seen in many of the slow virus diseases, particularly of elements of the neuroglial cells, the epithelium and smooth muscle of the bronchioles in maedi, and the reticuloendothelial cells both in visna and maedi. It has been shown that human glia, cultured in vitro, can maintain a visna infection for a long time, multiplying abnormally with loss of contact inhibition (MacIntyre et al, 1974). It has already been stated that this virus contains an RNA-dependent DNA polymerase, an enzyme which has only been found previously in RNA tumour viruses (Stone et al, 1971). Research is needed to determine whether proliferation of cells is caused by a destructive effect of the virus-damaging neurones followed by a reactive glial response, or if viruses primarily stimulate the cells to multiply more rapidly? If this last case applies these viruses may be considered to have some oncogenic properties and factors related to this possibility are discussed below.

The glia proliferates in response to many differing insults including inflammation, trauma, toxins, anoxia. They are cells which are easily stimulated to multiply. There is considerable evidence in many of the neurological diseases discussed in this chapter that the glial abnormality commences before the human or animal subject is ill or shows any evidence of weakness or sensory changes suggestive of neuronal fall-out. In scrapie in mice and other animals, in C–J disease and kuru in monkeys, histopathological examination shows that there is hypertrophy and proliferation of the astrocyte some time before the disease can be detected clinically.

Studies of cultures of mouse and sheep brain cells have shown that infection with scrapie increases growth potential (Field and Windsor, 1965; Gustafson and Kanitz, in Gajdusek et al, 1965; Haig and Pattison, 1967). Caspary and Bell (1971) suggested that the increased activity of the cells resembled those of tumour cells. Glia from the brains of animals infected with the agent from kuru, C–J disease and milk encephalopathy also appears to be stimulated in cell culture (Marsh and Hanson, 1969; Haig and Clarke, 1971; Gajdusek et al, 1972). Zlotnik (1968) has shown that a number of peripherally inoculated arboviruses cause both hypertrophy and proliferation of astrocytes as one of the earliest pathological changes. Transformed areas (i.e. areas showing abnormal growth patterns suggestive of tumour-like growth) have recently been seen in subcultures of cells derived from the brain of two patients with SSPE (Katz, Koprowski and

Moorhead, 1969) and from the brain of a patient with C–J disease (Hooks et al, 1972). In the latter case particles morphologically resembling the oncogenic RNA viruses was detected. Ter Meulen et al (1972) observed abnormal growth in fused cell cultures containing MS brain tissue from which was isolated a parainfluenza type virus. Webb, Illavia and Laurence (1971) using measles virus vaccine in human fetal brain culture showed that loss of contact inhibition occurred and virus continued to be produced in significant quantities for over 10 weeks. Similar results were obtained by using several mosquito and tick-borne arboviruses. (Illavia and Webb, 1972; Precious, Webb and Bowen, 1974) and in all cultures virus continued to be produced for long periods of time. This evidence adds, incidentally, some support to the possibility that chronic tick-borne encephalitis may be a reality. The appearance of the cultures were similar to that seen with SV40, an oncogenic DNA virus (papova group), when inoculated into primary mouse kidney cells (Black, 1968). This is of considerable interest in relation to PML in which papova-type viruses, JC and SV40, are seen particularly in the oligodendrocytes and have been isolated from brain cultures. Recently it has been reported that 83 per cent of new-born hamsters inoculated with JC virus developed malignant gliomas within six months. Virus could only be recovered after using cocultivation techniques (Walker et al, 1973).

In order to emphasise the difficulties which may be encountered in diagnosing the cause of CNS signs which may occur in association with malignant disease it is of note that Roos et al (1972) isolated an adenovirus 32 strain from a patient dying of subacute encephalitis and a lymphosarcoma treated by x-irradiation. The diagnosis made during life was PML. The histopathology indicated a subacute focal encephalitis with neuronal intranuclear inclusion bodies containing adenovirus-like particles. Adenovirus infections of man may cause CNS disturbances (Sohier, Chardonnet and Prunieras, 1965) but adenovirus isolation from brain is rare. Again this virus is of interest because it is known to produce malignant disease in animals.

The CNS of animals and insects is a site where a wide range of viruses have been isolated from brains previously thought to be sterile (Rogers et al, 1967). Some of the factors in the host–virus relationship which may affect the course of CNS infection are discussed by Webb (1968).

To consider now the cells of the lung in maedi, there is undoubtedly similar proliferation of the mesenchymal tissue of the lung so that the lung sometimes weighs four times that of the normal. The increased weight is not due to fluid. These findings suggest the real possibility that primary excessive stimulation of cell multiplication by the infecting agent plays an important part in the pathogenesis of these diseases. If research finds that this is due to an oncogenic-like effect, concepts of treatment will be altered considerably. The role of the glia in the CNS would also be altered because abnormalities in these cells might be the cause of the degeneration of both neurones and myelin. Cathala et al (1974) have shown that in a chimpanzee infected with the C–J agent, EEG abnormalities preceded the clinical signs by a very significant period. The EEG abnormality might well be arising from abnormalities of the glia, the first cells which appear abnormal in the histopathology of this disease. It is also relevant to note that EEG changes occur after infections with measles virus vaccine in which overt CNS abnormalities were minimal (Pampiglione, Griffiths and Bramwell, 1971). These may perhaps arise from vaccine virus affecting the glia. This is an example of a live vaccine reaching the brain and causing changes that may not at the time cause concern. SSPE has been reported (Schneck, 1968) and continues to be reported in relation to measles vaccine. This is particularly relevant in view of the length of time measles virus vaccine appears to be able to survive and the changes it produces in human fetal brain cultures (Webb et al, 1971).

Genetic factors

Considerable interest has arisen in the relationship between histocompatibility leucocyte antigens (HLA) and disease processes. Recognition of these antigens came from tissue typing work associated with transplant compatibility. Patients with various diseases including MS, lupus erythematosis, ankylosing spondylitis and chronic active hepatitis seem to have an unusually high incidence of certain of the HLA antigens. It has been determined that people suffering from MS are much more likely to possess the HLA antigens A3, B7 and DW2 than people who do not have the disease. It may be that tissue typing would be very helpful in assessing prognosis and types of treatment potentially available, including immunotherapy (Lance et al, 1975).

Some interesting results concerning genetic influence are available from experiments with scrapie. It has been shown that a bi-allelic gene (termed *sinc*, short for scrapie incubation) controls the length of the incubation period of the disease in mice. It was also shown that the agents of scrapie caused diseases which differed not only in their incubation period but also in the extent and site of the histopathological lesions they produced. It was found that one agent produced a short incubation period in one strain of mice and a long incubation period in another, causing an apparent reversal of gene roles (Frazer and Dickinson, in Kimberlin, 1976). This stresses once again the importance of the host–agent relationship. It is this sort of work which has been done in scrapie that would provide much useful information if it could be applied to the agent of C–J disease.

The Agents

Work will continue on defining the remarkable physicochemical properties of the agents of the spongiform encephalopathies, particularly as to their relationship to cell membranes. Recently under the electron microscope particles have been seen which may be related to the scrapie agent (Cho and Greig, 1975). Substantiation of this would be an important advance.

The Creutzfeldt–Jacob agent

The whole spectrum of disease pathology which the C–J agent can produce is not at all clear as yet. For example it has been isolated from the brain of a patient with the familial type of Alzheimer's disease and from another with papulosis atrophicans maligna of Kohlmerer–Degos (Gajdusek et al, 1973). The significance of this latter isolation is not at all clear and it may be that the patient was also suffering from C–J disease which was in fact suggested by the histopathological lesions in the CNS. If so it was certainly not clinically obvious and emphasises how these agents may be occurring more frequently and in a much wider range of patients than expected. The brains of more patients dying of malignant disease should be examined for evidence of virus infection. In addition to the ethical problems of biopsying brain, the problem of expense has greatly curtailed investigations in this field. Monkeys are very expensive and to wait several years for the result of an experiment involves a large capital outlay. However, as indicated previously, smaller animals which are cheaper and easier to breed and house are being shown to be susceptible to many of these agents but the number of laboratories in the world where it would be considered really safe to work with them are few. Meanwhile for the more simple and less well-equipped laboratories and for investigators studying the effect of viruses on the CNS there are many simple and relatively safe models with which to work, e.g. mouse hepatitis virus and Semliki forest virus.

Herndon et al (1975) have been able to produce a recurring demyelination in the CNS of mice by using mouse hepatitis virus, emphasising again the ubiquity of certain viruses and the need to search for viruses naturally infecting other organs as potential CNS pathogens.

Semliki forest virus can produce a chronic neurological disease affecting chiefly the glia as described by Zlotnik (1968). It has also been shown to cause temporary demyelination when the avirulent strain is used for repeated infections (Chew-Lim, Suckling and Webb, 1977).

Embryonic and neonatal infections

The damage caused by cytomegalovirus and rubella virus, and their persistence in cells, has already been discussed (pp. 94, 96). It seems likely that research will show that other viruses may have the capacity to do this also, even if persistence of the virus is only confined to embryonic life. For example, remarkable hydrocephalic states can be produced in rodents particularly with mumps, influenza or parainfluenza viruses. This topic is fully discussed by Johnson (in Thompson and Green, 1974). It has particular relevance because it has been shown that children may develop aqueduct stenosis and hydrocephalus following mumps (Timmons and Johnson, 1970). Hypoplasia of the cerebellum can be produced in hamsters by infecting them with rat virus. This virus has a remarkable research potential. The virus was originally isolated from a rat tumour and has several similarities to polyoma virus. By using different doses of virus in animals of varying ages three responses can result in hamsters, an acute fulminating disorder, stunting of growth and tooth dysplasia, and a latent infection from which infective virus can be recovered. It can also produce a remarkable cerebellar hypoplasia by damaging the granular layer of the cerebellum during development, as well as hepatitis and cerebellar hypoplasia in rats, and cerebellar disease in cats (Margolis and Kilham, 1968). Other viruses can also produce cerebellar hypoplasia such as the feline panleukopenic virus in cats and ferrets (Kilham, Margolis and Colby, 1967, 1971). This again is a virus thought previously to produce only a pancytopenia, but which has been found, depending upon dose of virus and age of host, to produce an entirely different but highly significant disease.

Finally, to emphasise one of the major themes of this chapter that a single virus may produce more than one disease, depending upon virulence, dosage and the host's immune status, the example of blue tongue virus disease in sheep is given. If infection occurs in the embryo before immunological competence develops (75 days) cerebral atrophy results, between 75 and 100 days cystic areas appear in the brain, and after the hundredth day an insignificant meningoencephalitis without sequelae is observed.

In this chapter it has been suggested that in special circumstances many viruses can produce unusual and as yet unexplained disease. It is therefore very important to approach with an entirely open mind any clinical disease possibly associated with a slow virus infection.

REFERENCES

Adams, J. M. & Imagwa, D. T. (1962) Measles antibodies in multiple sclerosis. *Proceedings of the Society for Experimental Biology and Medicine*, **111**, 562–566.

Alm, L. & Oberg, L (1945) Animal experiments in connection with so-called Behçet syndrome; preliminary report. *Nordisk Medicin*, **25**, 603–604.

Andrews, J. M. (1972) The ultrastructural neuropathology of multiple sclerosis. In *Multiple Sclerosis: Immunology, Virology and Ultrastructure*, ed. Wolfgram, Ellison, Stevens & Andrews, pp. 23–52. New York: Academic Press.

Astrom, K. E., Mancall, E. L. & Richardson, E. P., Jr (1958) Progressive multifocal leuko-encephalopathy: a hitherto unrecognised complication of chronic lymphatic leukaemia and Hodgkin's disease. *Brain*, **81**, 93–111.

Barringer, J. R. (1974) Recovery of herpes simplex virus from human sacral ganglions. *New England Journal of Medicine*, **291**, 828–830.

Beck, E., Daniel, P. M., Matthews, W. B., Stevens, D. L., Alpers, M. P., Asker, D. M., Gajdusek, D. C. & Gibbs, C. J., Jr (1969) Creutzfeldt–Jacob disease: the neuropathology of a transmission experiment. *Brain*, **92**, 699–716.

Black, P. H. (1968) Malignant transformation in vitro by oncogenic viruses. *Journal of the American Medical Association*, **206**, 1258–1262.

Bouteille, M., Fontaine, C., Verdrenne, C. & Delarue, J. (1965) Sur un cas d'encephalite subaigüe à inclusion; etude anatoma-clinique et ultrastructurale. *Revue Neurologique (Paris)*, **113**, 454–458.

Bradish, C. J., Allner, K. & Maber, H. B. (1972) The virulence of original and derived strains of Semliki forest virus for mice, guinea-pigs and rabbits. *Journal of General Virology*, **12**, 141–160.

Brody, J. A. (1972) Epidemiology of multiple sclerosis and a possible virus aetiology. *Lancet*, **ii**, 173–176.

Brody, J. A., Hirano, A. & Scott, R. M. (1971) Recent neuropathologic observation in amyotrophic lateral sclerosis and Parkinsonism dementia of Guam. *Neurology (Minneapolis)*, **21**, 528–536.

Brownwell, B. & Oppenheimer, D. R. (1965) An ataxic form of subacute presenile polio-encephalopathy (Creutzfeldt–Jacob disease). *Journal of Neurology, Neurosurgery and Psychiatry*, **28**, 350–361.

Brownwell, B., Campbell, M. J., Greenham, L. W. & Peacock, D. B. (1975) Experimental transmission of Creutzfeldt–Jacob disease. *Lancet*, **ii**, 186–187.

Burger, D. & Hartsough, G. R. (1965) Encephalopathy of mink. II. Experimental and natural transmission. *Journal of Infectious Diseases*, **115**, 393–399.

Carp, R. I., Licursi, P. C., Merz, P. A. & Merz, G. S. (1972) Decreased percentage of polymorphonuclear neutrophils in mouse peripheral blood after inoculation with material from multiple sclerosis patients. *Journal of Experimental Medicine*, **136**, 618–629.

Carp, R. I., Merz, G. S. & Licursi, P. C. (1974) Reduced cell yields of mouse cell line cultures after exposure to homogenates of multiple sclerosis tissues. *Infection and Immunity*, **9**, 1011–1056.

Caspary, E. A. & Bell, T. M. (1971) Growth potential of scrapie mouse brain in vitro. *Nature (London)*, **229**, 269–270.

Cathala, F., Court, L., Rohmer, F., Gajdusek, D. C., Gibbs, C. J., Jr & Castaigne, P. (1974) Experimental transmission of Creutzfeldt–Jacob disease to a chimpanzee, with an electroencephalographic study using indwelling electrodes. *Proceedings of the 10th International Congress of Neurology,* 9th–14th September 1973, pp. 381–389.

Chew-Lim, M., Suckling, A. J. & Webb, H. E. (1977) Demyelination in mice after two or three infections with avirulent Semliki forest virus. *Veterinary Pathology,* 14, 67–72.

Cho, H. J. & Greig, A. S. (1975) Isolation of 14 nm virus-like particles from mouse brain infected with scrapie agent. *Nature (London),* 257, 685–686.

Cole, G. A., Gilden, D. H., Monjan, A. A. & Nathanson, N. (1971) Lymphocytic choriomeningitis virus. Pathogenesis of acute central nervous system disease. *Federation Proceedings. Federation of American Societies for Experimental Biology,* 30 (6), 1831–1841.

Connolly, J. M. (1968) Additional data on measles virus antibody and antigen in subacute sclerosing panencephalitis. *Neurology (Minneapolis),* 18, 87–89.

Connolly, J. M., Allen, I. V., Murwitz, L. J. & Millar, J. M. D. (1967) Measles virus antibody and antigen in subacute sclerosing panencephalitis. *Lancet,* i, 542–544.

Dawson, J. R., Jr (1933) Cellular inclusions in cerebral lesions of lethargic encephalitis. *American Journal of Pathology,* 9, 7–15.

Dean, G. (1970) The multiple sclerosis problem. *Scientific American,* 233, 40–46.

Desmond, M. M., Wilson, G. S., Melnick, J. L., Singer, D. B., Zion, T. E., Rudolph, A. J., Peneda, R. G., Ziai, M. & Blattner, R. (1967) Congenital rubella encephalitis. *Journal of Pediatrics,* 71, 311–331.

Dick, G. (1972) Host–virus reactions with special reference to persistent agents. *Journal of Clinical Pathology,* 25; Suppl. Royal College of Pathologists, 6, 1–158.

Dick, G., McAlister, J. J., McKeown, F. & Campbell, A. M. G. (1965) Multiple sclerosis and scrapie. *Journal of Neurology, Neurosurgery and Psychiatry,* 28, 560–562.

Diener, T. O. (1973) Similarities between the scrapie agent and the agent of potato spindle tuber diseases. *Annals of Clinical Research,* 5, 268–278.

Donner, M., Waltimo, O., Porras, J., Forsius, H. & Saukkonen, A. L. (1972) Subacute sclerosing panencephalitis as a cause of chronic dementia and relapsing brain disorder. *Journal of Neurology, Neurosurgery and Psychiatry,* 35, 180–185.

Duffy, P., Wolf, J., Collins, G., Devoe, A. G., Streeten, D. & Cowen, D. (1974) Possible person-to-person transmission of Creutzfeldt–Jacob disease. *New England Journal of Medicine,* 290, 692.

Evans, A. D., Pallis, C. A. & Spillane, J. D. (1957) Involvement of the nervous system in Behçet's syndrome. Report of three cases and isolation of virus. *Lancet,* ii, 349–353.

Field, E. J. (1966) Transmission experiments with multiple sclerosis. An interim report. *British Medical Journal,* ii, 564–565.

Field, E. J. & Windsor, G. D. (1965) Cultural characters of scrapie mouse brain. *Research in Veterinary Science,* 6, 130–132.

Field, E. J., Miller, H. & Russell, D. S. (1962) Observations on glial inclusion bodies in a case of acute disseminated sclerosis. *Journal of Clinical Pathology,* 15, 278–284.

Field, E. J., Cowshall, S., Naring, H. K. & Bell, T. M. (1972) Viruses in multiple sclerosis. *Lancet,* ii, 280–281.

Font, R. L., Jenis, E. H. & Tuck, K. D. (1973) Measles maculopathy associated with subacute sclerosing panencephalitis. *Archives of Pathology,* 96, 168–174.

Freeman, J. M. (1969) The clinical spectrum and early diagnosis of Dawson's encephalitis. *Journal of Pediatrics,* 75, 590–603.

Fuccillo, D. A., Kurent, J. E. & Sever, J. L. (1974) Slow virus diseases. *Annual Review of Microbiology,* 28, 231–264.

Gajdusek, D. C., Gibbs, C. J. & Alpers, M. (1965) *Slow, Latent and Temperature Virus Infections,* NINDB Monograph No. 2, Public Health Service Publication No. 1378. Washington, DC: US Government Printing Office.

Gajdusek, D. C., Gibbs, C. J., Jr, Earle, K., Dammin, G. J., Schoene, W. C. & Tyler, H. R. (1973) Transmission of subacute spongiform encephalopathy to the chimpanzee and squirrel monkey from a patient with papulosis atrophicans maligna of Kohlmeier–Degos. *Proceedings of the 10th International Congress of Neurology,* 9th–14th September 1973, pp. 390–392.

Gajdusek, D. C., Gibbs, C. J., Jr, Rogers, N. G., Basnight, M. & Hooks, J. (1972) Persistance of viruses of kuru and Creutzfeldt–Jacob disease in tissue cultures of brain cells. *Nature (London),* 235, 104–105.

Gajdusek, D. C. & Zigas, V. (1957) Degenerative disease of the central nervous system in New Guinea: the endemic occurrence of 'kuru' in the native population. *New England Journal of Medicine,* 257, 974–978.

Gardashiyan, A. M., Khondkarian, O. A., Bunina, T. L., Popova, J. M. & Katkin, S. G. (1970)

Experimental data on the study of the aetiology of amyotrophic lateral sclerosis. *Vestnik Akademii Medical Science*, **25** (10), 80–83.

Georggson, G. & Palsson, P. A. (1971) The histopathology of maedi, a slow viral pneumonia of sheep. *Veterinary Pathology*, **8**, 63–80.

Gibbs, C. J., Jr & Gajdusek, D. C. (1973) Experimental subacute spongiform virus encephalopathies in primates and other laboratory animals. *Science (New York)*, **182**, 67–68.

Gibbs, C. J., Jr, Gajdusek, D. C. & Alpers, M. P. (1969) Attempts to transmit subacute and chronic neurological diseases to animals, pathogenesis and aetiology of demyelinating diseases. *International Archives of Allergy*, **36**, 519–552.

Gocke, D. J., Preisig, R., Morris, T. Q., McKay, D. G. & Bradley, S. E. (1967) Experimental viral hepatitis in the dog: production of persistent disease in partially immune animals. *Journal of Clinical Investigation*, **46**, 1506.

Gudnadottir, M. & Kristinsdottir, K. (1967) Complement-fixing antibodies in sera of sheep affected with visna and maedi. *Journal of Immunology*, **94**, 663–667.

Hadlow, W. J. (1959) Scrapie and kuru. *Lancet*, **ii**, 289.

Haig, D. A. & Clarke, M. C. (1971) Multiplication of the scrapie agent. *Nature (London)*, **234**, 106–107.

Haig, D. A. & Pattison, I. H. (1967) In-vitro growth of pieces of brain from scrapie-affected mice. *Journal of Pathology and Bacteriology*, **93**, 724–727.

Hanshaw, J. B. (1971) Congenital cytomegalovirus infection: a fifteen year perspective. *Journal of Infectious Diseases*, **123**, 555–561.

Hartsough, G. R. & Burger, D. (1965) Encephalopathy of mink. Epizootiologic and clinical observations. *Journal of Infectious Diseases*, **115**, 387–392.

Henle, G., Koldowsky, U., Koldowsky, P., Henle, W., Ackerman, R. & Haase, G. (1975) Multiple sclerosis associated agent: neutralisation of the agent by human sera. *Infection and Immunity*, **12**, 1367–1404.

Herndon, R. M., Griffin, D. E., McCormick, V. & Weiner, L. P. (1975) Mouse hepatitis virus induced recurrent demyelination. *Archives of Neurology (Chicago)*, **32**, 32–35.

Hirano, A. & Zimmerman, H. M. (1962) Alzheimer's neurofibrillary changes: a topographic study. *Archives of Neurology (Chicago)*, **7**, 227–242.

Hooks, J., Gibbs, C. J., Jr, Chopra, H., Lewis, M. & Gajdusek, D. C. (1972) Spontaneous transformation of human brain cells grown in vitro and description of associated virus particles. *Science (New York)*, **176**, 1420–1422.

Hornabrook, R. W. & Moir, D. J. (1970) Kuru epidemiological trends. *Lancet*, **ii**, 1175–1179.

Horta-Barbosa, L., Fuccillo, D. A., Sever, J. L. & Zeman, W. (1969) Subacute sclerosing panencephalitis isolation of measles virus from a brain biopsy. *Nature (London)*, **221**, 974.

Horta-Barbosa, L., Hamilton, R., Wittig, B., Fuccillo, D. A., Sever, J. L. & Vernon, M. L. (1971) Subacute sclerosing panencephalitis: isolation of suppressed measles virus from lymph node biopsies. *Science (New York)*, **173**, 840–841.

Howatson, A. F., Nagai, M. & ZuRhein, G. M. (1965) Polyoma-like virions in a human demyelination brain disease. *Canadian Medical Association Journal*, **93**, 379–386.

Hunter, G. D. & Millson, G. C. (1977) The scrapie agent: the present position about its nature. *Recent Advances in Clinical Virology*, 61–78. Edinburgh: Churchill-Livingstone.

Illavia, S. J. & Webb, H. E. (1972) The effect of encephalitogenic viruses on tissue cultures of non-neuronal cells of mouse and human brain. *Neurology (Minneapolis)*, **22**, 619–627.

Illis, L. S. & Gostling, J. V. T. (1972) *Herpes Simplex Encephalitis*. Bristol, England: Scientechnica Ltd.

Jacob, A. (1921) Uber eigenartige erkrankungen des zentral nerven systems mit bemerkenswerten anatomischen befunde (spastiche pseudosclerose encephalomyelopathie mit disseminierten degenerationsherden). *Zeitschrift für die gesamte Neurologie und Psychiatrie*, **64**, 147–228.

Jacob, A. (1923) *Die extrapyramidalen erkrankungen*, pp. 215–245. Berlin: Springer.

Katz, M., Koprowski, H. & Moorhead, P. (1969) Transformation of cells cultured from human brain tissue. *Experimental Cell Research*, **57**, 149–153.

Kilham, L., Margolis, G. & Colby, E. D. (1967) Congenital infections of cats and ferrets by feline panleukopenic virus manifested by cerebellar hypoplasia. *Laboratory Investigation*, **17**, 465–480.

Kilham, L., Margolis, G. & Colby, E. D. (1971) Cerebellar ataxia and its congenital transmission in cats by feline panleukopenia virus. *Journal of the American Veterinary Medical Association*, **158**, Suppl., **2**, 888.

Kimberlin, R. H. (1976) *Slow virus diseases of animals and man*. Amsterdam: Elsevier.

Koldowsky, U., Koldowsky, P., Henle, W., Ackerman, R. & Haase, G. (1975) Multiple sclerosis associated agent: transmission to animals and some properties of the agent. *Infection and Immunity*, **12**, 1355–1366.

Lampert, P. W., Gajdusek, D. C. & Gibbs, C. J., Jr (1971) Experimental spongiform encephalopathy (Creutzfeldt–Jacob disease) in chimpanzees: electron microscopic studies. *Journal of Neuropathology and Experimental Neurology*, **30**, 20–32.

Lampert, P. W., Hooks, J., Gibbs, C. J., Jr & Gajdusek, D. C. (1971) Altered plasma membranes in experimental scrapie. *Acta Neuropathology (Berlin)*, **19**, 81–93.

Lance, E. M., Kremer, M., Abbosa, J., Jones, V. E., Knight, S. & Medawar, P. B. (1975) Intensive immunosuppression in patients with disseminated sclerosis. *Clinical Experimental Immunology*, **21**, 1–12.

Lehrer, T., Wilton, J. M. A. & Shillitoe, E. J. (1975) Immunological basis for latency, recurrences and putative oncogenicity of herpes simplex virus. *Lancet*, **ii**, 60–62.

Licursi, P. C., Merz, P. A., Merz, G. S. & Carpi, R. I. (1972) Scrapie-induced changes in the percentage of polymorphonuclear neutrophils in mouse peripheral blood. *Infection and Immunity*, **6**, 370–376.

Lowenthal, A., Moya, G., Poire, R., Macken, J. & De Smedt, R. (1972) Subacute sclerosing panencephalitis. A clinical and biological reappraisal. *Journal of Neurological Sciences*, **15**, 267–270.

MacIntyre, E. H., Wintersgill, C. J. & Vatter, A. E. (1974) Prolonged culture of visna virus in human astrocytes. *Beiträge zur Pathologie (Budapest)*, **152**, 163–178.

Margolis, G. & Kilham, L. (1968) Virus-induced cerebellar hypoplasia. In *Infections of the Nervous System*, Research Publication ARNMD, Vol. XLIV, pp. 113–146. Association for Research in Nervous and Mental Disease.

Marsh, R. F. K. & Hanson, R. P. (1969) Transmissible mink encephalopathy neurological response. *Americal Journal of Veterinary Research*, **30**, 1643–1653.

Marsh, R. F. & Hanson, R. P. (1969) Physical and chemical properties of the transmissible mink encephalopathy agent. *Journal of Virology*, **3**, 176–180.

Meulen, V., ter, Koprowski, H., Iwasaki, Y., Kackell, Y. M. & Muller, D. (1972) Fusion of cultured multiple sclerosis brain cells with indicator cells: presence of nucleocapsids and virions and isolation of parainfluenza-type virus. *Lancet*, **ii**, 1–5.

Millson, G. C., Hunter, G. D. & Kimberlin, R. H. (1971) An experimental examination of the scrapie agent in cell membrane mixtures. II. The association of scrapie activity with membrane fractions. *Journal of Comparative Pathology*, **81**, 255–265.

Mortada, A. (1969) Virus aetiology of Harada's disease. *Bulletin of the Ophthalmic Society (Egypt)*, **62**, 119–124.

Nakagawa, Y. & Shingu, M. (1958) Studies of the pathogenic agent of Behçet's disease. I. The isolation of the Behçet's disease virus on the choria-allantois of developing chick embryo. *Journal of the Japanese Association of Infectious Diseases*, **32**, 270–278.

Narayan, O., Penney, J. B., Jr, Johnson, R. T., Herndon, R. M. & Weiner, L. P. (1973) The etiology of progressive multifocal leukoencephalopathy. Identification of virus in brains of 13 patients. *New England Journal of Medicine*, **289**, 1278–1282.

Padgett, B. L., Walker, D. L., ZuRhein, G. M. & Echroade, R. J. (1971) Cultivation of papova-like virus from human brain with progressive multifocal leukoencephalopathy. *Lancet*, **i**, 1257–1260.

Padgett, B. L. & Walker, D. L. (1973) Prevalence of antibodies in human sera against JC virus, an isolate from a case of progressive multifocal leucoencephalopathy. *Journal of Infectious Diseases*, **127**, 467–470.

Pampiglione, G., Griffith, A. H. & Bramwell, E. C. (1971) Transient cerebral changes after vaccination against measles. *Lancet*, **ii**, 5.

Pautrat, G., Tamalet, J., Chippaux-Hippolite, C. & Brahic, M. (1971) Etude de la structure du virus visna en microscopie electronique. *Comptes rendus hebdomadaire des séances de l'Academie des sciences (Paris)*, **273**, 653–655.

Penney, J. B., Jr, Weiner, L. P., Herndon, R. M., Narayan, O. & Johnson, R. T. (1972) Virions from progressive multifocal leukoencephalopathy. Rapid serological identification by electron microscopy. *Science (New York)*, **178**, 60–62.

Perier, O. (1969) Electron microscopic observations on human demyelinating diseases. *International Archives of Allergy*, **36**, Suppl., 452–462.

Perier, O. & Gregaire, A. (1965) Electron microscopic features of multiple sclerosis lesions. *Brain*, **88**, 937–952.

Petrov, P. A. (1970) Vilyuisk encephalitis in the Yakut Republic (U.S.S.R.). *American Journal of Tropical Medicine and Hygiene*, **19**, 146–150.

Petrov, P. A. (1973) Vilyuisk encephalitis in Yakutia (Siberia), U.S.S.R. Abstracts of invited papers. *IXth International Congress on Tropical Medicine and Malaria*, Athens, **1**, 219.

Precious, S. W., Webb, H. E. & Bowen, E. T. W. (1974) Isolation and persistance of Chikungunya virus in cultures of mouse brain cells. *Journal of General Virology*, **23**, 271–279.

Prineas, J. (1972) Paramyxovirus-like particles associated with acute demyelination in chronic relapsing multiple sclerosis. *Science (New York)*, **178**, 760–763.

Reed, H., Lindsay, A., Silversides, J. L., Speakman, J., Monckton, G. & Rees, D. L. (1958) The uveo-encephalitis syndrome or Vogt–Koyanagi–Harada disease. *Canadian Medical Association Journal*, **79**, 451–459.

Reynolds, D. W., Stagno, S., Stubbs, K. G., Dahle, A. J., Livingstone, M. M., Saxon, S. S. & Alford, C. A. (1974) Inapparent congenital cytomegalovirus infection with elevated cord IgM levels. Causal relation with auditory and mental deficiency. *New England Journal of Medicine*, **290**, 291–296.

Rinne, U. K. (1968) Electron microscopy of a multiple sclerosis brain biopsy. *Annales de Médecine Interne (Fenn)*, **58**, 179–183.

Rogers, N. G., Basnight, M., Gibbs, C. J., Jr & Gajdusek, D. C. (1967) Latent viruses in chimpanzees with experimental kuru. *Nature (London)*, **216**, 446–449.

Roos, R., Chou, S. M., Rogers, N. G., Basnight, M. & Gajdusek, D. C. (1972) Isolation of adenovirus 32 strain from human brain in a case of subacute encephalitis (36204). *Proceedings of the Society for Experimental Biology and Medicine*, **139**, 636.

Roos, R., Gajdusek, D. C. & Gibbs, C. J., Jr (1973) The animal characteristics of transmissible Creutzfeldt–Jacob disease. *Brain*, **96**, 1–20.

Rorke, L. B. & Spiro, A. J. (1967) Cerebral lesions in congenital rubella syndrome. *Journal of Pediatrics*, **70**, 243–255.

Russell, A. S. & Saertre, M. T. A. (1976) Antibodies to herpes-simplex virus in 'normal' cerebrospinal fluid. *Lancet*, **i**, 65–65.

Schneck, S. A. (1968) Vaccination with measles and central nervous system disease. *Neurology (Minneapolis)*, **18**, 29–82.

Sezer, F. N. (1953) Isolation of virus as cause of Behçet's disease. *American Journal of Ophthalmology*, **36**, 301–315.

Sezer, F. N. (1956) Further investigations on virus of Behçet's disease. *American Journal of Ophthalmology*, **41**, 41–55.

Shah, K. V., Ozer, H. L., Pond, H. S., Palma, L. D. & Murphy, G. P. (1971) Appearance of SV40 neutralising antibodies in sera of U.S. residents without history of polio immunisation. *Nature (London)*, **231**, 448–449.

Sigurdardottir, B. & Thormar, H. (1964) Isolation of a viral agent from the lungs of sheep affected with maedi. *Journal of Infectious Diseases*, **114**, 55–60.

Sigurdsson, B. (1954) Rida, a chronic encephalitis of sheep with general remarks on infections which develop slowly and some of their special characteristics. *British Veterinary Journal*, **110**, 341–354.

Sohier, R., Chardonnet, Y. & Prunieras, M. (1965) Adenoviruses. Status of current knowledge. *Progress in Medical Virology*, **7**, 253–325.

Stone, L. B., Scolnick, E., Takemoto, K. K. & Aardnson, S. A. (1971) Visna virus: a slow virus with an RNA-dependent DNA polymerase. *Nature (London)*, **229**, 257–258.

Sugihara, H., Mutoh, Y. & Tsuchiyama, H. (1969) Neuro-Behçet's syndrome. Report of two autopsy cases. *Acta pathologica japonica*, **19**, 95–101.

Suzuki, K., Andrews, J. M., Waltz, J. M. & Terry, R. D. (1969) Ultrastructural studies of multiple sclerosis. *Laboratory Investigation*, **20**, 444–454.

Symposium (1973) Herpes virus and cervical cancer. *Cancer Research*, **33**, 1351–1563.

Tawara, J. (1965) Fine structure of filaments in dog kidney cell cultures infected with measles virus. *Virology*, **25**, 322.

Thormar, H. (1966) A study of maedi virus in lung tumours in animals. *Proceedings of the 3rd Quadrennial Conference on Cancer*, University of Perugia, 1965, ed. Severi, L., pp. 393–402. *A Study of Visna- and Maedi-viruses and Their Relationship to Other Viruses of Animals*, pp. 1–29. Copenhagen: Dansk Videnskabs Forlag.

Thormar, H. (1969) Visna- and maedi-virus antigen in infected cell cultures studied by the fluorescent antibody technique. *Acta pathologica et microbiologica scandinavica*, **75**, 296–302.

Timmons, G. D. & Johnson, K. P. (1970) Aqueductal stenoses and hydrocephalus after mumps encephalitis. *New England Journal of Medicine*, **283**, 1505–1507.

Townsend, J. J., Baringer, J. R., Wolinsky, J. S., Malamud, N., Mednick, J. P., Panitch, H. S., Scott, R. A. T., Lyndon, S. O. & Cremer, N. E. (1975) Progressive rubella panencephalitis. *New England Journal of Medicine*, **292**, 990–993.

Vandvik, B. & Norrby, E. (1973) Oligoclonal IgG antibody response in the central nervous system to different measles virus antigens in subacute sclerosing panencephalitis. *Proceedings of the National Academy of Science (New York)*, **70**, 1060–1063.

Walker, D. L. (1974) Current study of an opportunistic papovavirus. In *Slow Virus Diseases*, ed. Zeman, W. & Lennette, E. Baltimore: Williams & Wilkins.

Walker, D. L., Padgett, B. L., ZuRhein, G. M., Albert, A. E. & Marsh, R. F. (1973) Human papovavirus (JC): induction of brain tumours in hamsters. *Science (New York)*, **181**, 674–676.

Webb, H. E. (1968) Factors in the host–virus relationship which may affect the course of an infection. *British Medical Journal*, **iv**, 684–686.

Webb, H. E., Illavia, S. J. & Laurence, G. D. (1971) Measles-vaccine viruses in tissue culture of non-neuronal cells of human fetal brain. *Lancet*, **ii**, 4–5.

Weil, M. L., Hideo, H. I., Cremer, N. E., Oshiro, L. S., Lenette, E. H. & Carnay, L. (1975) Chronic progressive panencephalitis due to rubella virus. *New England Journal of Medicine*, **292**, 994–998.

Weiner, L. P., Herndon, R. M., Narayan, O. & Johnson, R. T. (1972a) Further studies of a simian virus 40-like virus isolated from human brain. *Journal of Virology*, **10**, 147–149.

Weiner, L. P., Herndon, R. M., Narayan, O., Johnson, R. T., Shah, K., Rubinstein, L. P., Preziosi, T. J. & Conley, F. K. (1972b) Isolation of virus related SV40 from patients with progressive multifocal leukoencephalopathy. *New England Journal of Medicine*, **286**, 385–390.

Weiner, L. P., Narayan, O., Penney, J. B., Jr, Herndon, R. M., Tourtellotte, W. W. & Johnson, R. T. (1973) Progressive multifocal leukoencephalopathy. Rapid identification and subsequent isolation of a papovavirus, JV type. *Archives of Neurology (Chicago)*, **39**, 1–3.

Wolf, S. M., Schotland, D. L. & Phillips, L. L. (1965) Involvement of nervous system in Behçet's syndrome. *Archives of Neurology (Chicago)*, **12**, 315–325.

Yale, Y. (1970) Neurologic disease in the western Pacific islands, with a report on the focus of amyotrophic lateral sclerosis found in the Kii Peninsula, Japan. *Journal of Tropical Medicine and Hygiene*, **19**, 155–166.

Zilber, L. A., Bajdakoua, Z. L., Gardas'Jan, A. N., Konavalov, N. V., Bunina, T. L. & Barabadze, E. M. (1963) Study of the etiology of amyotrophic lateral sclerosis. *Bulletin of the World Health Organisation*, **29**, 449–456.

Zlotnik, I. (1968) Reaction of astrocytes to acute virus infections of the central nervous system. *British Journal of Experimental Pathology*, **49**, 555–564.

Zlotnik, I., Grant, D. P. & Batter-Hatton, D. (1972) Encephalopathy in mice following inapparent Semliki forest virus (SFV) infection. *British Journal of Experimental Pathology*, **53**, 125–129.

ZuRhein, G. M. & Chou, S. M. (1965) Particles resembling papovaviruses in human cerebral demyelination disease. *Science (New York)*, **148**, 1477–1479.

6
HEPATITIS
Jenny Heathcote

The discovery of the Australia antigen (Blumberg, Alter and Visnich, 1965) as a serum marker of infection with the hepatitis B virus (Prince, 1968a; Giles et al, 1969) and the recent recognition of the probable virus thought to be responsible for type A hepatitis (Feinstone, Kapikian and Purcell, 1973) have greatly enhanced our understanding of hepatitis. The greater part of this chapter will be concerned with types A and B hepatitis with particular reference to their epidemiological, clinical and immunological manifestations. The long-term sequelae of hepatitis will also be discussed and mention of some other agents, e.g. drugs responsible for hepatitis, will be made.

ACUTE VIRAL HEPATITIS

There are two common forms of acute, viral hepatitis; short incubation, type A hepatitis and long incubation, type B hepatitis (Krugman, Giles and Hammond, 1967). More recently, it has been suggested that there may be a non-B, long incubation hepatitis, but as yet there is no evidence that this is related to a virus infection (Prince, Brotman and Grady, 1974).

Less commonly an acute hepatitis may be the result of infection with any one of the following viruses: cytomegalovirus, Epstein–Barr, rubella, herpes simplex, varicella, or yellow fever virus.

Acute Type A Hepatitis

Aetiology

Human transmission experiments in the 1940s demonstrated that there was an infectious, filterable agent in the stools and blood of cases of short incubation hepatitis (Havens, Ward and Drill, 1944; MacCallum and Bradley, 1944; Paul, Havens and Sabin, 1945). Deinhardt et al (1967) have shown that serum taken from cases of acute, short incubation hepatitis can transmit hepatitis to marmoset monkeys. This work has been confirmed by others (Mascoli et al, 1973) who have now developed techniques using infected marmoset liver extracts for assaying antibody in the sera taken from convalescent cases of type A hepatitis (Miller et al, 1975; Provost et al, 1975). The tests appear to be specific for type A hepatitis (Krugman, Friedman and Lattimer, 1975) but the exact nature of the infectious agent remains unclear. Feinstone et al (1973) have reported finding 27 nm particles in stool filtrates taken from cases of type A hepatitis, during the acute phase of the disease and they have been able to demonstrate a serological response to these particles in convalescent sera. Similar reports have been made, showing aggregation of particles obtained from stool extracts, with human immunoglobulin (Zuckerman et al, 1974). However, Almeida, Gray and Wreghitt (1974) have pointed out that seroconversion to a variety of virus-like particles may take place during the course of acute hepatitis, so that the above reports should be interpreted with caution.

Epidemiology

Typically type A hepatitis occurs in epidemics. Volunteer experiments have shown that blood, faeces, duodenal juice and urine from acute cases are infective when given either parenterally or orally (Havens et al, 1944; MacCallum and Bradley, 1944; Paul et al, 1945; Krugman et al, 1967). Faeces and blood have been found to be infective three to four weeks after exposure and remain so for about three weeks, the period of infectivity generally terminating a few days after the appearance of jaundice. Airborne transmission has also been proposed (Aach, Evans and Losee, 1968) but it is likely that this route plays only a minor role in the spread of the disease. Spread is probably most commonly a result of faeco-oral transmission. In the past, outbreaks have occurred predominantly in rural areas (Pickles, 1939), thought to be a consequence of poor hygienic conditions. Outbreaks have also followed contamination of drinking supplies (Raska et al, 1966; Morse et al, 1972) and food sources (Joseph, Millar and Henderson, 1965; Koff and Sear, 1967). The increase in type A hepatitis now seen in some urban areas (Lobel and McCollum, 1965) is attributed in part to the influx of non-immune persons and to the poor living conditions found particularly amongst the drug addict community in cities. Children are most commonly affected in epidemics and the sex distribution is equal. But now that living standards have improved, certainly in the Western world, a population of non-immune, hence susceptible adults is emerging. Infection amongst adults occurs more frequently in men.

In temperate climates a seasonal variation in the incidence of hepatitis is reported (Kurylowicz, 1972) epidemics tending to occur in winter. But in the warmer climates the disease is endemic.

Acute Type B Hepatitis

Aetiology

In 1964, Blumberg described a new serum antigen which formed a precipitin line with sera from multiply tranfused haemophiliacs. This antigen was noted to be more common in the blood of Asians and Australian Aborigines than in persons coming from the West, hence it became known as the Australia antigen. Later, reports described the presence of this antigen in the sera of subjects with leukaemia, Down's syndrome, and hepatitis (Blumberg et al, 1967). An independent study in Japan detected this same antigen in some blood donor sera and in patients with acute and chronic liver disease (Okochi and Murakami, 1968). Meanwhile, Prince (1968a) was describing an antigen which he could detect during the incubation period and development of acute, serum transmitted hepatitis. He later demonstrated that his SH antigen was identical to Blumberg's Australia antigen (Prince, 1968b). Gradually it became clear that the Australia antigen was in some way associated with long-incubation hepatitis.

Electron microscope studies of serum containing this antigen revealed three different particles (Fig. 6.1): small spheres approximately 20 nm in diameter, tubules of varying length, up to 300 nm, and occasional larger, spherical particles, 42 nm in diameter. The latter contains a central core particle about 27 nm in diameter (Bayer, Blumberg and Werner, 1968; Almeida et al, 1969; Dane, Cameron and Briggs, 1970). Almeida, Rubenstein and Stott (1971)

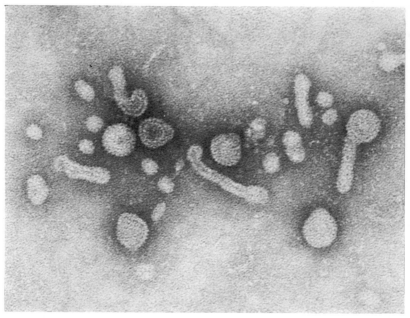

Figure 6.1   Hepatitis B antigen. The three morphological forms. There are pleomorphic spheres and tubules approximately 20 nm diameter and the more regular double-shelled 'Dane' particles, considered the most likely candidate for the HBV. (Electronmicrograph kindly given by Dr J. D. Almeida). ×225 000

showed that this central core was immunologically distinct from its coat and the small spheres and tubules. They demonstrated that there was one antibody system which agglutinated only with core particles (once they had been released from their coat covering by detergent) and another which agglutinated the small spheres, tubules, and coat fraction of the large spherical particles. Particles similar in size to the core of these 42 nm serum particles have been seen in the liver cell nuclei of persons with Australia antigen in their serum (Almeida et al, 1970; Nowoslawski et al, 1970; Huang, 1971). It seems likely that these intranuclear particles, and the central core of the 42 nm serum particles, represent the hepatitis B virus (HBV). Following intranuclear viral replication it is probable that the free core particles become enveloped, once they are in the liver cell cytoplasm, by the coat material. The small spheres and tubules are comprised of the excess coat material. The terminology now adopted to denote these various components are:

Hepatitis B surface (i.e. coat) antigen	HB_sAg
Hepatitis B core antigen	HB_cAg
Antibody to HB_sAg	anti-HB_s
Antibody to HB_cAg	anti-HB_c

Free HB_cAg particles probably exist mainly within the liver cell nuclei; recently HB_cAg has been detected in serum at a time when hepatic damage is at a maximum (Hollinger et al, 1975).

Absolute proof that HB_cAg is the hepatitis B virus is still lacking. All attempts to propagate the virus in tissue culture have failed. Nucleic acid studies have been hampered by the instability of the core fraction of the 42 nm serum particle once it has been separated from its coat. Kaplan et al (1973) however have presented evidence that the core particle contains a DNA template as well as a DNA polymerase. Further indirect evidence that HB_sAg positive serum contains the hepatitis B virus has been obtained from transmission studies in rhesus monkeys and chimpanzees (London et al, 1972; Barker et al, 1973a) and until an in vitro system is developed, such animal models are the only method we have to study further the hepatitis B virus.

There are different HB_sAg subtypes, the best worked out being the 'd'/'y' (Le Bouvier, 1971) and the 'w'/'r' (Bancroft, Mundon and Russell, 1972) systems. All HB_sAg positive sera seem to have a common antigenic determinant called 'a', whereas 'd' and 'y' and 'w' and 'r' are virtually always mutually exclusive. These antigenic determinants are present on the surface of all three types of serum particle. There is a marked difference in the geographical distribution of the different subtypes: 'y' is common in the East and Mediterranean (Saidi et al, 1972) and 'd' everywhere else; 'r' is predominant in Asia and 'w' in the USA (Bancroft et al, 1972). No pathological significance can be attached to any one subtype (Pons-Romero, Heathcote and Sherlock, 1974). Recently a further antigenic specificity 'e' has been described (Magnius et al, 1975). But this antigenic determinant does not always appear to be physically related to the HB_sAg particles. Now 'e' is most commonly detected in carriers of HB_sAg who have chronic liver disease, whereas antibody to 'e' is found in asymptomatic HB_sAg carriers (Eleftheriou et al, 1975a). It is possible that the 'e' antigen is a marker of infectivity and is related to the presence of the large, 42 nm particles and long tubules in the serum (Neurath et al, 1975).

Epidemiology

The Willowbrook studies (Giles et al, 1969) showed conclusively that serum HB_sAg is associated only with long incubation (formerly called serum) hepatitis.

It has long been recognised that any procedure involving parenteral exposure to serum may be complicated by the development of a long incubation hepatitis. Blood transfusions have been incriminated the most (Gocke and Kavey, 1969) but today the problem of type B hepatitis amongst drug addicts (Nordenfelt, Kaij and Ursing, 1970), tattooed persons (Mowat et al, 1973), dental patients (Levin et al, 1974), and hospital employees (Garibaldi et al, 1973) is being increasingly recognised. So, too, are the possibilities of non-parenteral transmission. In the 1950s it was noted that some uninoculated contacts of soldiers, who developed jaundice following influenza vaccination, also became jaundiced (Mirick and Shank, 1959). With the advent of a serum marker for infection with the hepatitis B virus, it became obvious that cases of HB$_s$Ag positive hepatitis often had no history of parenteral exposure (Cossart and Vahrman, 1970). The Willowbrook experiments demonstrated that HB$_s$Ag positive serum was infective when given orally as well as parenterally (Krugman et al, 1967). HB$_s$Ag has been sought in virtually all body secretions and has been found in the urine (Tripatzis and Horst, 1971), saliva (Ward et al, 1972), semen (Heathcote, Cameron and Dane, 1974a), bile (Akdamar et al, 1971), breast milk (Boxall et al, 1974), nasal washings (Villarejos et al, 1974), vaginal secretions (Durani and Gerber, 1974), sweat (Telatar et al, 1974), and cerebrospinal fluid (Dankert et al, 1975) of subjects with HB$_s$Ag in their serum. It remains unknown whether HB$_s$Ag in body fluids other than blood is infective. It is also possible that very often these secretions are contaminated with blood in microscopic amounts. But, undoubtedly, transmission of HB$_s$Ag in the absence of overt parenteral exposure takes place. Such transmission has been noted to be particularly common between sexual, especially male homosexual, partners.

Within the community the type B hepatitis virus does not seem to be as infectious as the type A hepatitis virus. Epidemics of type B hepatitis rarely occur except in particular circumstances, most notably in units caring for immuno-suppressed patients who have become HB$_s$Ag carriers, e.g. renal (Garibaldi et al, 1973) and oncology units (Wands et al, 1974). In general, person to person contact must be close for transmission to take place. Type B hepatitis also differs from type A in that transmission of the presumed virus takes place not only from cases of acute, type B hepatitis but also from HB$_s$Ag carriers (Heathcote et al, 1973). Such a carrier state would not appear to exist for the type A hepatitis virus. Evidence suggests that not all HB$_s$Ag carriers are equally infectious. It appears that it is those HB$_s$Ag carriers with underlying liver disease and those who are immunosuppressed who are most likely to transmit the virus (Reinicke et al, 1972; Heathcote, Gateau and Sherlock, 1974b).

The HB$_s$Ag carrier rate varies enormously from country to country. In the United Kingdom and the USA, the carrier rate among the volunteer blood donor population is less than 1 per cent (Blumberg, Sutnick and London, 1968), whereas in Greece it may be as high as 3 per cent (Hadziyannis et al, 1972a). In Asia a carrier rate amongst military personnel of 14 per cent has been recorded (Blumberg et al, 1969). No adequate explanation has been put forward to explain this geographical variation. It has been suggested that there may be an inherited susceptibility to becoming an HB$_s$Ag carrier (Blumberg et al, 1969). It has also been proposed that the mosquito may harbour the hepatitis B virus and act as a vector for transmission, accounting for the high HB$_s$Ag carrier rate in tropical areas (Prince et al, 1972). However, there is more recent evidence which suggests that replication of the hepatitis B virus is more likely to occur in bed bugs than in mosquitoes (Newkirk, Downe and Simon, 1975). Tribal scarification has also been incriminated as a method of transmission of the hepatitis B virus and maintenance of the HB$_s$Ag carrier rate in certain areas (Kew et al, 1973). In many countries a large proportion of HB_sAg carriers are drug addicts (Singleton et al, 1971). The liver pathology in asymptomatic HB_sAg carriers varies enormously: inactive cirrhosis, chronic active liver disease with or without cirrhosis, chronic persistent hepatitis, mild focal necrosis, or even an entirely normal liver may be found, regardless of whether the liver function tests are normal or not.

Acute, type B hepatitis tends to affect a slightly older age group than does type A, the peak being the 20 to 30 year age group. Population screening for HB_sAg suggests that in high carrier rate areas there may be two age groups particularly affected, young children and young adults.

The early childhood cases could be a result of transmission from an HB_sAg carrier parent to child (Steven et al, 1975). Epidemiological studies have shown that such transmission tends to take place between the mother and the offspring and not between father and child. There is much argument as to whether this is a result of vertical transmission or whether infection occurs only at the time of delivery or in the puerperium. It is likely that both routes are possible. The chances of the child being infected are much higher if the mother has acute, HB_sAg positive hepatitis during the last trimester of pregnancy than if she is an asymptomatic carrier of HB_sAg at the time of delivery (Skinhøj et al, 1972; Schweitzer et al, 1973). It is probably this mother to child transmission which maintains the HB_sAg carrier rate in any community.

The second HB_sAg peak seen in population screening is in the age group commonly affected by acute, HB_sAg positive hepatitis. As with type A hepatitis, in the adult population males are more commonly affected than females.

Clinical course of acute type A and type B hepatitis (Table 6.1)

As many of the clinical features of acute, type A and type B hepatitis are the same, they will be considered together.

It is hard to define the exact incubation period of type A hepatitis from natural epidemics as the disease is of such an infectious nature that numerous contacts are possible. However, 'point' source epidemics and experimental studies have suggested that the interval between exposure and the first sign of hepatic involvement ranges between 31 and 42 days (Krugman et al, 1967). The mode of transmission does not apparently alter the incubation time.

The incubation period for type B hepatitis is much longer and can range between 39 and 160 days. The length of the incubation period probably depends on a number of factors. Volunteer experiments have shown that the more dilute the icterogenic serum, the longer the incubation period (Barker and Murray, 1972). Other studies have demonstrated that orally administered infective serum leads to a longer incubation period than when the same serum is given parenterally (Krugman et al, 1967).

Large-scale population screening of biochemical liver function tests during outbreaks of acute, type A hepatitis have shown that the majority of cases in any outbreak are subclinical, particularly amongst children (Havens, 1962). The same probably applies to acute, type B hepatitis. The prodromal symptoms of type A and type B hepatitis are similar, vague abdominal upsets and malaise predominating. The symptoms of those who develop clinically overt disease are variable. Fever is more common with type B hepatitis as are the manifestations of the serum sickness syndrome (Hawley et al, 1944). These symptoms, seen in the early phase of the illness, may include rashes, arthralgia, headache, urticaria and even angioneurotic oedema. Henoch–Schönlein purpura has been described (Gitlin, 1973) and so has acute glomerulonephritis (Combes et al, 1971), although these latter two complications tend to be seen in those who progress to a more chronic hepatitis, following an acute infection.

The clinical course of both types of infection is generally short, complete recovery taking place within a few weeks in the majority. Rare complications, such as cardiac arrhythmias (Bell, 1971), autoimmune haemolytic anaemia (Raffensberger, 1958), and occasionally aplastic anaemia (Rubin, Gottlieb and Vogel, 1968) may occur.

Prolonged jaundice accompanied by severe pruritus may be seen in those who have the cholestatic form of the disease. This course tends to be peculiar to

Table 6.1   Course of acute viral hepatitis

C.P.H. = chronic persistent hepatitis

C.A.H. = chronic active hepatitis

P.L.C.C. = primary liver cell cancer

-------- = uncertain

specific epidemics (Dubin et al, 1960) and occurs probably more often in type A. The eventual outcome of cholestatic hepatitis is as good as for the non-cholestatic form.

Recurrences or more likely relapses of acute, viral hepatitis are seen more frequently amongst those who have been given corticosteroids during their initial illness (Blum, Stutz and Haemmerli, 1969; Dudley, Scheuer and Sherlock, 1972b) and amongst subjects who are immunosuppressed when they become infected (Blumberg, Sutnick and London, 1970). Probably because of the immature status of the immune system in neonates, they too tend to develop a chronic hepatitis following infection with the hepatitis B virus (Schweitzer et al, 1972). Persistent hepatitis with progression to chronic liver disease of varying severity is rare, but probably occurs more frequently following type B infections (Chiaramonte et al, 1974). Progression of acute, HB_sAg positive hepatitis to chronic hepatitis has been reported to be as high as 11 per cent in one follow-up series (Nielsen et al, 1971) but the majority of patients in this series were drug addicts and so are probably not representative of the general population. Although there is some evidence that acute type A hepatitis may become chronic (Galbraith et al, 1975) there is little epidemiological evidence to suggest that a chronic carrier state exists for the type A virus as it does for the type B.

Since the introduction of highly sensitive techniques for HB_sAg testing, it has become clear that the majority of cases of fulminant viral hepatitis are due to type B infections (Trepo et al, 1976). Particularly virulent outbreaks have been seen amongst the patients and staff of renal dialysis units (Bone et al, 1971). Fulminant hepatitis rarely affects children. The most severe cases are seen in postmenopausal women. Hepatitis in pregnancy is usually a mild illness, although a particularly high fatality rate in some parts of Asia has been reported (Borhanmanesh et al, 1973). The survival rate for fulminant hepatitis of any aetiology is extremely poor, (about 11 per cent). The survival rate for fulminant type B hepatitis is less than for type A (Trepo et al, 1976). However, if recovery occurs, virtually normal resolution of liver function takes place (Karvountzis, Redeker and Peters, 1974).

Laboratory features

The serum aspartate transaminase reaches its peak early in the course of the illness. In type B infections there tends to be a more gradual and prolonged rise of this enzyme. However, the total duration of aspartate transaminase abnormality rarely exceeds a month (Krugman et al, 1967). However, alanine transaminase levels may remain abnormal for very much longer (Wacker et al, 1972). The majority of cases of acute hepatitis remain anicteric. However, cholestatic forms of the disease are associated not only with a prolonged elevation of serum conjugated bilirubin concentrations but also with a marked rise in serum alkaline phosphatase levels. There may be a rise in total serum cholesterol levels during the early phases of the disease, which may become marked in those with obvious cholestasis. A fall in total serum cholesterol may be seen in particularly severe hepatitis and heralds a poor prognosis. Fasting triglycerides may be elevated and abnormalities in plasma lipoproteins are seen, lipoprotein X occurring in those with cholestasis (Ritland, 1975).

The serum sickness syndrome seen commonly in the early phase of acute type B hepatitis is associated with a fall in the total serum haemolytic complement (CH_{50}) and C_4 levels. This fall is thought to be a result of consumption by immune complexes of HB_sAg and anti–HB_s rather than of decreased hepatic synthesis (Alpert, Isselbacher and Schur, 1971). Such complexes have been demonstrated in various extrahepatic sites including the kidney (Combes et al, 1971) and synovial fluid (Onion, Crumpacker and Gilliland, 1971).

As the majority of cases of acute, viral hepatitis are mild and short-lived, little disturbance of the serum proteins takes place. Because the half-lives of the clotting factors manufactured in the liver are short, they are the first proteins to be affected. In cholestatic forms of the disease marked prolongation of the prothrombin time may be seen in the absence of severe hepatocellular dysfunction; this is reversed by parenteral vitamin K administration. It has been reported that in fulminant hepatitis increased consumption of the coagulation factors may take place as well as decreased synthesis (Rake et al, 1970). As the half-life of albumin is much longer than for the clotting factors, serum albumin levels rarely become abnormal in uncomplicated cases of acute, viral hepatitis. A rise in total serum gamma-globulin concentration is commonly seen over a two to three week period. In patients with acute, type A hepatitis this has been shown to be in part due to a rise in IgM levels (Wollheim, 1968). But in acute, type B hepatitis a rise in IgG levels is more common. This may be related to the fact that the viral antigen in type B infections has generally been present for a considerable time before the onset of overt disease, and thus the primary immune response may be missed. Persistent hypergammaglobulinaemia may suggest the development of chronic liver disease. The transient appearance of smooth muscle antibodies, to a maximum titre of 1 : 80 in the acute phase, contributes to the rise in total serum globulins (Ajdukiewicz et al, 1972). Antinuclear factor, antimitochondrial antibodies, and rheumatoid factor have all been reported in low titre, in some cases, as has the appearance of some organ specific antibodies (Berg, 1974).

The appearance of elevated levels of serum alpha-fetoprotein occurring a week or so after the peak of the serum aspartate transaminase activity has been reported during the course of acute hepatitis. The production of alpha-fetoprotein is thought to result from rapid hepatic regeneration and as such may be used as a prognostic marker in those with particularly severe attacks (Karvountzis and Redeker, 1974). The appearance of alpha-fetoprotein has been said to be more common following type B infections (Smith, 1971). This is probably because severe, acute viral hepatitis is more commonly type B.

Acute type A hepatitis — immunity

It has long been recognised that an attack of acute, type A hepatitis confers long-lasting immunity to further type A infections but affords no protection against type B infections (Pickles, 1939; McFarlen and Chesney, 1944). Only now, since the development of tests for hepatitis A antibody can the immunological pattern of the disease be mapped out. Antibody can be detected, in high titre, within one to four weeks after the onset of hepatitis and in a group of 20 patients tested, antibody was detectable in all of them for a follow-up period of 5 to 10 years (Krugman et al, 1975). Antibody determinations performed on batches of human immune globulin have shown titres of 1 : 8000 or more (Miller et al, 1975). The administration of immune globulin appears to afford partial protection inasmuch as it appears to reduce the incidence of icteric hepatitis if given before exposure or during the incubation period (Krugman, 1963). It has been suggested that subsequent exposure to the type A virus, following immune globulin administration, may lead to active immunisation, thus explaining the apparent prolonged effectiveness of passive immunisation (Stokes et al, 1951). Until the hepatitis A virus can be purified no active immunisation is possible.

Acute, type B hepatitis — immunity

It must be realised that unless sensitive techniques are used, many of the serological findings in acute, type B hepatitis may be missed. This fact in part explains why there have been many varying reports on the serological findings during the course of the disease.

Following exposure to the hepatitis B virus there is a delay in the appearance of HB_sAg in the serum, presumably whilst viral replication is initiated within the liver cell nuclei. Serum HB_sAg may be detected at any time between 14 and 120 days following exposure (Hirshman et al, 1969). A gradual rise in the HB_sAg titre occurs, reaching a peak, following which there is a rise in the serum aspartate transaminase activity. The onset of symptoms may follow the appearance of serum HB_sAg some two weeks to two months later, by which time the serum HB_sAg titre and the transaminase levels are decreasing (Krugman and Giles, 1970). By the time the patient presents with jaundice, the HB_sAg titre may have fallen to such a degree that it can only be detected by sensitive techniques. Hence, if insensitive methods of HB_sAg detection are being employed, the period of antigenaemia may be missed altogether and the case wrongly diagnosed as a non-type B infection. The duration of HB_s antigenaemia once clinical symptoms are manifest is extremely variable. In cases of fulminant hepatitis the titre of HB_sAg may fall so rapidly that it is commonly missed, unless radioimmunoassay techniques are used (Trepo et al, 1976). It is usual in uncomplicated cases for serum HB_sAg to be cleared within one month of the start of symptoms. If HB_sAg persists in the serum for longer than three months after the acute episode, the likelihood of a chronic hepatitis developing is high (Nielsen et al, 1971). However, the reverse is not true, in that a chronic hepatitis may develop even if the patient has apparently cleared serum HB_sAg, although this is unusual.

The results of searching for anti-HB_s following acute, type B hepatitis have been confusing. Again, this is partly due to the differing sensitivities of the techniques used. In general, anti-HB_s is not detected until some weeks or even months after the onset of the illness, and delays of up to six years have been reported (Krugman et al, 1974). The titre of anti-HB_s is usually low and probably as a result may or may not remain detectable in the serum thereafter. It is for this reason, that, to look for serum anti-HB_s following an attack of acute hepatitis is not a particularly reliable method of diagnosing the particular type of viral hepatitis. In some instances, anti-HB_s may be detected early on in the illness, when HB_sAg is still present in the serum, suggesting that immune complexes may be present. It is possible that the development of anti-HB_s does not offer complete immunity to further infection with the hepatitis B virus, particularly if the re-exposure dose is massive (Holland et al, 1969; Barker et al, 1972). Experimental studies have shown that sometimes an early anti-HB_s response occurs following exposure to the hepatitis B virus, anti-HB_s appearing prior to HB_sAg in the serum, yet, hepatitis may occur (Barker et al, 1973b). However the administration of high titre anti-HB_s, shortly after exposure to the hepatitis B virus, would seem to offer protection in the majority (Seeff et al, 1975; Prince et al, 1975), and has not been followed by any complications suggestive of an immune complex disease.

The role of immune complexes in the pathogenesis of the liver injury in acute, type B hepatitis has been debated. Although they can be detected in the serum on occasions during the hepatitic phase of the illness, it seems unlikely that such complexes are responsible for the liver injury although they may well be responsible for the extrahepatic manifestations (Combes et al, 1971; Onion et al, 1971). It is also unlikely that the liver damage is a direct result of invasion with the hepatitis B virus, but rather a delayed hypersensitivity response to the virus infection within the liver. It is probable that both the humoral and cellular immune processes are involved in the pathogenesis of the disease.

The presence of anti-HB_c rather than anti-HB_s may be a more reliable marker of recent hepatitis B virus infection. It is found in the serum after the appearance of HB_sAg but before the onset of clinical hepatitis and the appearance of anti-HB_s. Testing for serum anti-HB_c is still in its infancy but early results have shown anti-HB_c to be present only transiently although sometimes it appears to persist in the serum for some years after infection with the hepatitis B virus. DNA polymerase activity is only detected transiently before the onset of hepatitis and is therefore of little diagnostic value in the clinical context (Krugman et al, 1974).

Active immunisation against hepatitis B virus infection is not yet available. Experimental studies have shown that HB_sAg positive serum, heated to 98°C for 1 min, is still antigenic but not infective (Krugman and Giles, 1973). At present, further trials with formalin inactivated HB_sAg given to chimpanzees are proceeding and it is hoped that a hepatitis B vaccine will be available in the not too distant future.

DRUG-INDUCED HEPATITIS

Alcoholic Hepatitis

Aetiology

Alcoholic hepatitis may result from excessive consumption of any alcoholic beverage. Those heavy drinkers who develop only fatty infiltration of the liver are more fortunate than those who develop alcoholic hepatitis, as the former is a relatively benign condition. Total abstinence is followed by complete resolution to normal (Seife, Kessler and Lisa, 1950).

Consumption of more than 160 g ethanol daily for 10 years or more is an average history obtained from subjects with alcoholic hepatitis. It has been reported that heavy drinking for as little as three months may be all that is necessary (Lischner, Alexander and Galambos, 1971); conversely others may drink heavily for 20 years or more and sustain little or no liver injury (Lelbach, 1966). There are probably many factors which contribute towards this discrepancy. It has been claimed that there is an association between colour blindness and cirrhosis due to alcohol (Cruz-Coke and Varela, 1966). Although most would discredit this, it is likely that some genetic factors play a role. For instance, alcoholic cirrhosis is relatively rare amongst American Jews compared with American Indians (Lieber, 1973) but of course this may be largely due to differences in consumption. It is suggested that women are more susceptible to liver damage from alcohol than men and they need to drink less ethanol for liver damage to ensue. One American survey has shown a marked predominance of alcoholic hepatitis amongst Negro females (Lischner et al, 1971). It may be that these racial and sex differences are due to differences in rates of ethanol metabolism (Fenna et al, 1971) as well as sensitivity to alcohol. Experimental studies have shown that liver damage due to alcohol occurs independently of nutritional factors (Rubin and Lieber, 1968). Whether this hepatotoxic effect of alcohol is direct or is lymphocyte-mediated is not clear. Studies in subjects with alcoholic liver disease have shown that their lymphocytes are sensitised to ethanol. However, this could also be found in some patients with non-ethanolic chronic active liver disease (Sorrell and Leevy, 1972). One group of workers have demonstrated lymphocyte sensitisation to HB$_s$Ag in alcoholics with liver disease not found in alcoholics without liver disease (Pettigrew et al, 1972). However this work has not been substantiated.

All patterns of excessive drinking behaviour may lead to the development of alcoholic hepatitis. Some may be 'binge' drinkers' but the majority affected are those who drink continuously, either the 'skid-row' type or, as is often seen in the United Kingdom, persons from social classes I and II who manage to continue to work regularly and who are only found to have liver dysfunction when attending for medical check-ups (Brunt et al, 1974).

Morphology

The typical histological findings in alcoholic hepatitis include focal areas of liver cell necrosis, surrounded by an infiltrate of neutrophils and swollen liver cells, some of which may contain Mallory's hyalin (Lischner et al, 1971). The lesions tend to be centrilobular in distribution. Collagen fibres are commonly seen surrounding the central veins, so much so that the veins may be hard to visualise. This lesion has been termed 'central hyaline sclerosis' (Edmondson et al, 1963). This collagen may spread from the central veins, through the liver parenchyma to the portal tracts. It is probably the overall degree of scarring which is the most important factor in the development of cirrhosis in the alcoholic. The histological picture of alcoholic hepatitis may be superimposed on a normal, fatty or cirrhotic liver. Even following abstinence, the lesions of alcoholic hepatitis may take months or years to resolve. It has been reported that progression of alcoholic hepatitis to cirrhosis may take place in the absence of continued drinking (Galambos, 1972; Brunt et al, 1974).

Clinical features

The clinical findings in a subject with biopsy-proven alcoholic hepatitis may range from the completely asymptomatic to the moribund. Perhaps the most common complaints are anorexia often accompanied by weight loss, nausea and vomiting, particularly in the morning, and abdominal pain (Green, Mistilis and Schiff, 1963). The latter symptom is often only mild. However, it is sometimes sufficiently severe to suggest an intra-abdominal emergency (Edmondson et al, 1963). Other features of this illness include diarrhoea and occasionally gastrointestinal haemorrhage.

Jaundice is not a universal finding although in some instances a particularly cholestatic picture is found. Prominent vascular spiders are often seen. Other skin lesions include pellagra, palmar erythema, and ecchymoses. Hepatomegaly is practically universal, whereas splenomegaly is not so often found. Gross ascites may be present in the more severe cases. Although fever and a leucocytosis in the absence of infection is a recognised feature of alcoholic hepatitis, the presence of an underlying infection should always be ruled out, not forgetting that tuberculosis in such subjects is not at all uncommon.

Gastrointestinal haemorrhage may be due to alcoholic gastritis, tears, peptic ulceration, or portal hypertension. The latter may be a transient phenomenon in the absence of cirrhosis. Neurological abnormalities include various degrees of mental impairment due to hepatic precoma and/or delirium tremens. Peripheral neuropathy is common. Cardiomyopathy due to vitamin B_1 deficiency or as a direct toxic effect of alcohol may be present. A myopathy affecting predominantly the proximal limb muscles, sometimes giving rise to tender swollen limbs, occurs (Hed et al, 1962). Associated alcoholic pancreatitis may be present and can confuse the clinical picture since then one is not sure whether any cholestasis present is intra- or extrahepatic in origin.

The clinical course will depend on the severity of the hepatic lesion. Despite withdrawal from alcohol, further deterioration may occur following hospital admission. Inappropriate surgical intervention carries a serious prognosis. It is important to remember that deterioration resulting in terminal liver failure may take place in the absence of jaundice.

Laboratory findings

The haematological picture in alcoholic hepatitis may be extremely confusing. Anaemia is common, and may be due to iron deficiency, folate deficiency, or the direct toxic effect of alcohol upon the bone marrow (Beard and Knott, 1966). Rarely, haemolysis is seen. The term Zieve's syndrome has been used to describe the complex of haemolysis, leucocytosis, and hyperlipidaemia (Zieve, 1966). Leucocytosis alone is frequent and the total white cell count may exceed 20×10^9 cells per litre even in the absence of infection. Clotting abnormalities are common and the degree of prolongation of the prothrombin time is a sensitive indicator of the severity of the liver disease.

Elevation of the serum bilirubin, when present, is mainly in the conjugated fraction. Elevation of the serum alkaline phosphatase and the transaminase is usual. The rise in transaminase activity is much less than that seen in acute viral hepatitis. Total serum albumin levels are depressed in about 60 per cent depending on the severity and duration of the liver disease. Total gammaglobulin levels may be mildly elevated, more particularly if the hepatitis is superimposed on a cirrhosis. Hypokalaemia is common; hypoglycaemia, generally transitory, may occur. A rise in the blood urea may be seen, particularly if poorly regulated diuretic therapy has been given. One survey has suggested that the height of the serum bilirubin, the white cell count, and the blood urea are the most valid markers of the severity of the illness (Hardison and Lee, 1966).

Management

There is no satisfactorily proven specific treatment for alcoholic hepatitis, but attention to general supportive measures and early recognition of developing complications and their treatment are vital (Resnick and Iber, 1972). In subjects without hepatic precoma or ascites a high energy, high protein diet is recommended, and vitamin supplementation, particularly the B and C group, should be given even though overt vitamin deficiency is absent. However, this dietary regimen may not be feasible either because of profound anorexia and vomiting or from the severity of the liver disease. The presence of hepatic precoma will necessitate the removal of protein from the diet as well as the introduction of other measures. The value of intravenous feeding in the alcoholic has not been assessed. It may well be that parenteral lipid preparations, as well as intravenous amino acid feeding, are poorly tolerated by the damaged liver. Resort to nasogastric tube feeding may be necessary. The presence of fluid retention will necessitate a marked reduction in sodium intake. Potassium supplementation is frequently required. Cessation of alcohol intake is mandatory; however, it is probably wise to be prepared for the development of withdrawal symptoms. Many would advise sedation for the first few days following alcohol withdrawal. This picture may be complicated by the presence of hepatic precoma; however, if delirium tremens is present, carefully monitored sedation is necessary to avoid a grossly agitated state.

Gastrointestinal bleeding may be troublesome. Gastroscopy is valuable to diagnose the source of the bleeding. Apart from replacing the blood lost, parenteral vitamin K and fresh frozen plasma should be given in an attempt to improve the clotting status. Surgical intervention should be avoided.

The results of biochemical tests are of little value in determining the aetiology of the sometimes marked cholestasis seen in patients with alcoholic hepatitis, which may be due to gallstones, pancreatitis, tumour, or intrahepatic cholestasis. The introduction of endoscopic retrograde cholangiopancreatography has done much to alleviate this diagnostic problem.

Bacteraemia, due to both anaerobes and aerobes, is common and so repeated blood cultures should be carried out.

A rise in blood urea with or without other evidence of deteriorating renal function may be due to a number of factors, each requiring different management. Excessive amounts of blood in the gastrointestinal tract from a gastrointestinal haemorrhage may lead to a rise in blood urea. However, such a bleed may lead to prerenal uraemia and/or acute tubular necrosis. Urinary osmolality measurements are helpful in distinguishing the two. The so-called hepatorenal syndrome is probably a combination of a number of functional disorders (Lieberman, 1970).

The value of corticosteroids in the treatment of alcoholic hepatitis is uncertain. Some trials have shown an improved survival rate in those with the more severe disease, given steroids; although it has been argued that the improvement was secondary only to the increased calorie intake in the treated patients (Helman et al, 1971). Other reports have suggested that prednisolone therapy is of no value at all in the treatment of ethanolic hepatitis (Porter et al, 1971) and may even precipitate further deterioration due to infection.

Prognosis

The mortality rate from acute alcoholic hepatitis, amongst patients requiring hospital admission, may be as high as 50 per cent. However, this figure depends on the method of patient selection. The presence of a background cirrhosis worsens the prognosis.

The course of alcoholic hepatitis in the absence of cirrhosis appears to be variable. Despite continued abstinence it would seem that progression to cirrhosis is inevitable in some individuals. It has been suggested that there may be two forms of the disease, a benign, non-progressive variety and a more severe form (Galambos, 1972).

Halothane Hepatitis

Aetiology

Halothane was first introduced as an anaesthetic agent in 1956; in 1958 the first report was made of hepatic necrosis following the use of this agent (Virtue and Payne, 1958). There have been several further reports concerning the possibility of halothane-induced acute hepatitis (Klion, Schaffner and Popper, 1969; Peters et al, 1969; Moult and Sherlock, 1975). There has been one report suggesting that in a sensitised subject, repeated exposure to halothane may lead to the development of chronic liver disease (Klatskin and Kimberg, 1969). It is still the belief of some that the development of an acute hepatitis following halothane administration is fortuitous. (Simpson, Strunin and Walton, 1971). Although there is at present no simple way that this argument can be completely resolved, there are features of hepatitis following exposure to halothane which differ from those of acute, viral hepatitis, or any other cause of postoperative jaundice. The report of the National Halothane Study, states that the number of deaths attributable to massive hepatic necrosis following halothane anaesthesia is about 1 in 10 000. The overall mortality following halothane anaesthesia is still less than with other anaesthetics (Summary of the National Halothane Study, 1966). The morbidity of halothane hepatitis remains an unknown quantity as it is highly likely that in many instances it is undiagnosed.

The mechanism of injury remains unknown but the pattern of the illness, and some of the immunological and histological findings, suggest a hypersensitivity phenomenon. There is no evidence to suggest that subjects with prior hepatic or biliary tract disease are more susceptible. The majority of cases are seen when more than one halothane anaesthetic has been given (Belfrage, Ahlgren and Axelson, 1966). Nearly all reports on halothane hepatitis following multiple exposures to this anaesthetic agent have been of patients in whom the repeat exposure occurred within a period of a month. It would seem that this is in part the reason why so often the underlying surgical condition requires eye surgery, radium insertions, skin grafts, i.e. procedures requiring repeated short-term anaesthesia. However, intervals of some years have been noted between the two anaesthetics.

There has been one report demonstrating in vitro lymphocyte sensitisation to halothane, using lymphocytes from affected subjects (Paronetto and Popper, 1970). However, this has not been confirmed (Walton et al, 1973).

Several studies have stressed that obesity is a common feature amongst subjects with halothane hepatitis (Klion et al, 1969; Moult and Sherlock, 1975). As halothane is found in particularly high concentrations in adipose tissue, obesity may well be relevant.

But there still remains no hard and fast proof that halothane is responsible for a hepatitis. However, there are many factors which make it hard to incriminate any virus infection. No association with HB_sAg has been shown. The age group affected by halothane hepatitis is much older than that commonly affected by type

A hepatitis. One recent survey attempted to rule out all other possible causes of postoperative jaundice, bacterial infection, other drugs, 'shock', pulmonary embolism, and background chronic liver disease (Moult and Sherlock, 1975).

Morphology

The histological appearances depend very much on the timing of the hepatic biopsy with regard to the development of the hepatitis. However, if the clotting mechanisms are sufficiently unimpaired to allow the biopsy to be taken early in the course of the illness, then the features of a typical hepatitis, often indistinguishable from acute, viral hepatitis will be seen. Coagulative necrosis tends to be overwhelmingly confined to the central zones in halothane hepatitis. There may be differences, including the presence of clusters of eosinophils, occasional granulomata, and sometimes fatty change in surviving parenchymal cells. Electron microscope studies have shown more specific changes, quite different from those seen in acute, viral hepatitis. They include the segmental loss of the outer membrane and infolding of the inner membrane of the mitochondria (Klion et al, 1969). If the hepatic biopsy is taken somewhat later during the course of the illness, a noteworthy feature is the presence of significant amounts of collagen, more than would be expected following severe viral hepatitis (Peters et al, 1969).

Clinical features

The prodromal symptoms of malaise, anorexia, and upper abdominal pain are similar to those preceding any form of acute hepatitis, although they may often be overlooked in the light of recent surgery. Postoperative pyrexia, although not a universal finding, is a predominant feature of halothane hepatitis (Hughes and Powell, 1970). Retrospective analysis of temperature charts generally shows them to be of little diagnostic value following the first exposure to halothane, unless on the rare occasion hepatitis ensues after only one exposure. When hepatitis follows repeated administration of halothane, a delayed pyrexia, some four to seven days after the second exposure occurs and if still overlooked and the same anaesthetic is again administered, fever occurring some few hours after the third anaesthetic may be noted. The peak temperature is generally around 38 to 40°C.

Jaundice generally develops 1 to 12 days after the final operation. Hepato-megaly is found in about 50 per cent, splenomegaly is unusual. Most published series of cases have come from specialist centres and therefore there is probably a bias towards describing the more severe cases. A marked deterioration of hepatic function with the development of encephalopathy and ascites is reported to occur in more than 50 per cent of the published cases. All the usual complications of acute hepatic failure, coma, renal failure, hypoglycaemia, and bleeding diatheses may ensue.

Laboratory findings

Elevation of the total serum bilirubin may be marked. Concentrations greater than 700 μmol/l (40 mg/dl) have been recorded; the majority is conjugated. Similarly, there is often a massive rise in serum aspartate transaminase activity in the early stages of the illness. The levels are often seen to decline both in those with gradually improving liver function and in those who progress to fulminant hepatic failure. Elevation of the serum alkaline phosphatase is not usually more than two-fold. An alteration in the serum proteins may be seen. A fall in serum albumin may be found in those with the more protracted illness. Elevation of serum IgG and IgM has been reported. At one time, the detection of serum mitochondrial antibodies was thought to be a feature which would distinguish halothane hepatitis from viral hepatitis (Doniach et al, 1966), but recent studies have not shown these antibodies in cases of halothane hepatitis. Low titre, smooth muscle antibody and antinuclear factor may be detected. Very recently, it has been reported that a microsomal antibody can be detected in 25 per cent of cases of halothane hepatitis, this being absent in acute, viral hepatitis (Walton et al, 1976).

A rise, sometimes marked, of the total white cell count along with a peripheral eosinophilia may be found. A rigorous search for bacterial infection should be sought, although the fever and leucocytosis may occur in the absence of infection. The degree of abnormality of the coagulation tests is dependent on the severity of the hepatic disturbance. Similarly a rise in blood urea in association with other evidence of poor renal function indicates a poor prognosis.

Management

There is no specific treatment for halothane hepatitis. The usual measures taken with cases of fulminant hepatitis should be instituted when indicated, i.e. dextrose infusions, parenteral vitamin K_1, oral neomycin, enemas, protein restriction, and clotting factor replacements when necessary.

Prognosis

The mortality rate of halothane hepatitis in reported series ranges between 40 and 50 per cent. However, it must be stressed that these figures are probably not representative as undoubtedly many cases are never diagnosed as the patients often return home only a day or so after a minor operation. Once fulminant hepatic failure has developed, death is usual. Death is most common within the first week of jaundice. The earlier jaundice appears postoperatively, the worse the prognosis. Two other features, the degree of the clotting abnormality and obesity, were seen in one series to indicate a poor prognosis (Moult and Sherlock, 1975). However, in those who do survive, recovery would seem to be complete. Although not histologically proven, chronic liver disease does not apparently follow. Repeated non-halothane anaesthesia has been given to survivors, with no complications. Although unintentioned challenge with halothane has been seen to give rise to a further episode of hepatitis, this would not always appear to be the case (Dykes et al, 1965).

Other Drug-induced Hepatitis

The number of drugs declared responsible for inducing a hepatitis is rapidly increasing. Elevation of serum transaminases, if looked for, may often be noted following the administration of a vast number of drugs, but commonly the enzyme levels return to normal, despite the drug being continued. Persistent elevation of serum transaminase activity however should alert one to suspect a definite hepatitis.

Predictable drug injury

Some drugs, if given in sufficient dosage, will always induce liver damage, i.e. the drug reaction is 'predictable'. Such reactions may be seen following the use of a wide variety of drugs; for example, following exposure to carbon tetrachloride fumes or its ingestion in a suicide attempt, following an overdose of acetominophen, and with cytotoxic agents when given in sufficient dosage for long periods of time. Often, as in the case of acetominophen (paracetamol) poisoning, there may be a delay between the taking of the drug and the development of overt liver damage. The onset of hepatic coma heralds a poor

Table 6.2   Drug-induced hepatocellular damage

Predictable	Unpredictable	Controversial
Carbon tetrachloride	Alcohol	Antituberculous agents
Acetominophen	α-Methyldopa	
(paracetamol)		
Methotrexate	Monoamine oxidase	Oxyphenisatin
	inhibitors	

prognosis (Clark et al, 1973). But direct toxicity to other organs, particularly the kidneys, may often play a greater role in the eventual outcome. Apart from withdrawing the noxious agent, and general supportive measures, there is rarely any specific therapy. However, it has recently been suggested that the liver damage which follows acetominophen poisoning may be prevented if large doses of glutathione, given as its precursor, cysteamine, are administered within a few hours of ingestion (Prescott et al, 1974). The principle behind this is that the highly reactive, toxic intermediate metabolite of acetominophen is preferentially bound to the glutathione, rather than to the liver cell macromolecule. Unfortunately, a more recent series suggests that cysteamine is ineffective (Douglas, Hamlyn and James, 1976).

Unpredictable drug injury

No list of drugs which fall into this category will ever be complete. But the drugs in this group which are most commonly used in clinical practice, and which therefore are most frequently incriminated, are several of the anti-tuberculous drugs and the antihypertensive, agent α-methyldopa; halothane-induced hepatitis having been previously discussed. It has recently been suggested that the hepatic damage seen to follow isoniazid or methyldopa ingestion is not a sensitivity phenomenon; that, in fact, the damage is 'predictable' to a degree. One large survey of isoniazid-induced hepatitis has suggested that hepatotoxicity depends on the rate of acetylation occurring within the liver. Eighty-six per cent of subjects with isoniazid-induced hepatitis were found to be fast acetylators (Black et al, 1975). It is felt that the metabolite acetylhydrazine is responsible for the hepatic damage secondary to isoniazid ingestion. Similarly it has been reported that the toxic effect of methyldopa may be dependent on the rate of production of a toxic metabolite (Mitchell, Dybing and Nelson, 1975). If indeed drug-induced hepatic injury is dependent on the efficiency of the various hepatic enzyme systems, this would in part explain why such drug reactions are rarely seen in the young, presupposing that a certain degree of immaturity of such enzyme systems is present in childhood.

Nearly all the first line drugs used in the treatment of tuberculosis have been reported to cause a hepatitis. But, as sometimes occurs in the case of isoniazid toxicity, the damage may be mild and transient, this being particularly so with rifampicin (Lal et al, 1972). Nevertheless, if elevation of serum transaminases is persistent, it is wise to withdraw the incriminating drug. It may be difficult to assess which drug is responsible for the liver damage, if combination therapy is being employed (Scheuer et al, 1974).

Chronic use of oxyphenisatin, a constituent of aperients, now not available in the United Kingdom, may lead to the development of either an acute (Pearson et al, 1971) or chronic hepatitis (Reynolds, Peters and Yamanda, 1971). The liver injury is reversible after withdrawal of the drug, as is so with all the other hepatotoxic agents.

CHRONIC HEPATITIS

A chronic hepatitis may be defined as an inflammatory lesion of the liver, which has persisted for more than six months. Some would argue for extending this to one year as, occasionally, cases of acute hepatitis lasting longer than six months resolve, others, however, restrict the period to 10 weeks. Chronic hepatitis may be classified as chronic persistent or chronic active in type, the diagnostically distinguishing features being morphological (De Groote et al, 1968) although there are usually marked clinical differences between the two.

Chronic Persistent Hepatitis

Morphology

The characteristic histological feature of chronic persistent hepatitis is chronic inflammatory cell infiltration which is confined to the portal tracts. There may be some portal fibrosis but there is no disturbance of the lobular architecture. In HB$_s$Ag positive cases, immunofluorescence techniques and orcein staining (Deodhar, Tapp and Scheuer, 1975) have demonstrated the presence of HB$_s$Ag and possibly HB$_c$Ag within the liver cells.

Aetiology

It is likely that chronic persistent hepatitis is most commonly the result of infection with the type A or type B hepatitis viruses. Now that we have a serum marker for the type B infection, this group can be identified and would seem to represent approximately 40 per cent of the cases, depending on the country of origin of the subjects. In a series of 20 cases of HB$_s$Ag negative chronic persistent hepatitis, more than half gave a history suggestive of an acute hepatitis a year or more previously, at a time when other family members were affected similarly (Becker et al, 1970). This would suggest that type A virus was responsible.

The histological appearances of chronic persistent hepatitis can also occur as a result of drug hypersensitivity, e.g. oxyphenisatin (Dietrichson, 1975), and in polyarteritis nodosa associated with the presence of serum HB_sAg. Immunological studies have shown that whereas circulating HB_sAg and anti-HB_s immune complexes may be involved in the pathogenesis of the vasculitis, they do not appear to be responsible for the liver damage (Trepo et al, 1974). Portal 'triaditis' which is subsumed under chronic persistent hepatitis may be found in association with various non-hepatic diseases, predominantly chronic inflammatory disease of the gastrointestinal tract.

Epidemiology

As with acute hepatitis, chronic persistent hepatitis seems to affect males more than females (Dietrichson, 1975), particularly in the HB_sAg positive cases, and the same age group, i.e. 20 to 30 years. However, it may well be that it is this age group who are more likely to be detected, as asymptomatic HN_sAg positive blood donors or drug addicts. As chronic persistent hepatitis is often an asymptomatic disease, it may be more widespread than is at present realised.

Clinical course

Fifty to eighty per cent of patients with biopsy-proven chronic persistent hepatitis give a history of a preceding illness suggestive of acute hepatitis. There are two main presentations. First, with vague complaints of abdominal pain, malaise and perhaps some weight loss and secondly, through HB_sAg screening of blood donors. A history of jaundice is rarely obtained from the HB_sAg positive blood donors, which supports the observation that it is more often cases of anicteric hepatitis who progress to chronic liver disease. A number of follow-up studies have been reported (Becker et al, 1970; Van Waes et al, 1974; Dietrichson, 1975). In general, there is little progression of the disease, tender hepatomegaly may persist, but signs of liver failure do not develop. However, most studies have been limited to a two to three year follow-up period. Some cases resolve completely, most remain static but progression to a more active lesion with the development of cirrhosis has been noted, but rarely (Tapp, Hollanders and Dymock, 1975). It could be argued that those who appear to develop a more severe disease may have been misdiagnosed originally, because of the sampling error of needle liver biopsies.

Laboratory findings

The biochemical liver function tests are not always abnormal in cases of chronic persistent hepatitis, as they tend to fluctuate. Jaundice is uncommon, but may occur transiently, although the total serum bilirubin is unlikely to rise above 85 μmol/l (5 mg/dl). If the serum aspartate transaminase level is raised, it is rarely more than four-fold. If the disease is due to drug sensitivity, then challenge with the drug generally leads to a sudden rise in the serum transaminase concentrations. The serum alkaline phosphatase is usually normal. The IgG level is raised in about 50 per cent of cases, but IgM and IgA levels remain within normal limits

(Dietrichson, 1975). In a few instances, non-organ-specific antibodies have been detected, including smooth muscle antibody, antinuclear factor and rheumatoid factor, but the presence of antimitochondrial antibodies has not been recorded.

The percentage of cases of chronic persistent hepatitis found to be HB$_s$Ag positive varies in accordance with the carrier rate of the community. Results suggest that acute, type B hepatitis is more likely to become chronic, than type A (Chiaramonte et al, 1974). The persistence of serum HB$_s$Ag beyond three months, following an episode of acute, type B hepatitis, suggests that some form of chronic liver disease is developing. Cases of HB$_s$Ag positive, chronic persistent hepatitis tend to maintain a high titre antigenaemia (Chiaramonte et al, 1977), although this finding has been disputed (Gentilini et al, 1972). Clearance of HB$_s$Ag has been noted with resolution of the disease, which may occur spontaneously or following immunosuppressive therapy.

Management

As chronic persistent hepatitis rarely progresses to a more severe form of chronic liver disease, no treatment is thought necessary. Follow-up studies have so far been few but they do suggest that cases should be repeatedly reviewed. As the serum biochemical findings do not necessarily indicate the severity of the underlying liver damage, repeat histology is necessary (Tapp et al, 1975). Should drug sensitivity be suspected, then removal of that drug will result in resolution of the disease. If thought justifiable, challenge with the drug often leads to a rapid biochemical response.

Chronic Active Hepatitis

Morphology

Chronic active hepatitis differs from chronic persistent hepatitis in that the inflammatory cell infiltration is not confined to the portal tracts, but invades the liver parenchyma. Liver cell necrosis is frequently seen and its severity along with the degree of inflammatory cell infiltration indicates the activity of the disease. Intralobular fibrous septa are commonly seen, leading to a disturbance of the architecture of the liver. Nodular regeneration, although not one of the diagnostic criteria, is often present by the time the affected subject is first biopsied. The lesion of chronic active hepatitis is often very patchy and thus sampling errors sometimes lead to confusion. As in HB$_s$Ag positive chronic persistent hepatitis, various methods can be used to demonstrate the presence of both HB$_s$Ag and HB$_c$Ag within the liver cells of HB$_s$Ag carriers with chronic active liver disease.

Aetiology

The term chronic active hepatitis is purely a morphological description, and this pathology is not pathognomonic of one particular aetiology. A number of diseases may be associated with the histological picture of chronic active hepatitis. Perhaps the two most common associations are either as the 'lupoid' hepatitis syndrome or as a chronic hepatitis associated with the presence of serum HB$_s$Ag. It has been argued that these two types of chronic active hepatitis may have the same aetiology (Popper and Mackay, 1972; Eddleston and Williams, 1974). However, there are a number of distinguishing features, hence they will be dealt with separately.

It is now becoming apparent that there is a group of subjects, predominantly male, who have chronic active hepatitis which is neither of the classical 'lupoid' variety or associated with the HB$_s$Ag, but in whom a serum microsomal antibody can be detected (Rizzetto, Swana and Doniach, 1973). At the present time, the precipitating factor has not been recognised.

The morphological picture of chronic active hepatitis may also be found in subjects with Wilson's disease (Sternlieb and Scheinberg, 1972) or as a result of drug hypersensitivity, e.g. oxyphenisatin (Reynolds et al, 1971), methyldopa (Rehman, Thomas and Gall, 1973) and isoniazid (Black et al, 1975). Whether chronic active hepatitis resulting from drug hypersensitivity ever progresses to cirrhosis is uncertain. This same morphological picture is being increasingly recognised as part of the spectrum of liver disease resulting from alcohol abuse (Galambos, 1975), and may also be seen following neonatal infection with the rubella or cytomegalovirus. It has been reported that many children with neonatal hepatitis have α_1-antitrypsin deficiency, and some do progress to a more chronic form of liver disease (Berg and Eriksson, 1972).

'Lupoid' Hepatitis

Epidemiology

'Lupoid' hepatitis may affect any age group and either sex, but it is most commonly seen in females aged between 20 and 30 years (Mackay, Taft and Cowling, 1956). It is not associated with the presence of serum HB$_s$Ag but rather with the presence of various non-organ specific auto-antibodies. Family studies have shown an increased incidence of these same antibodies amongst unaffected relatives (Galbraith et al, 1974) and HL-A typing has shown an increased incidence of HL-A types 1 and 8 in affected subjects (Mackay and Morris, 1972). These findings suggest that there may be a genetic factor which predisposes to the development of this disease. The role of the type A virus is uncertain as yet. Some cases of 'lupoid' hepatitis seem to follow a typical attack of acute hepatitis; however, this is rarely biopsy-proven and may represent the first clinical manifestation of an already established chronic disease. Nevertheless, acute, HB$_s$Ag negative hepatitis may progress to chronic liver disease (Galbraith et al, 1975), and may well be an aetiological factor in some cases of 'lupoid' hepatitis.

Clinical features

If 'lupoid' hepatitis presents as an apparent attack of acute, viral hepatitis, certain features are often atypical. The illness may be particularly prolonged or there may be recurrent episodes of jaundice. About a third of cases seem to present in this way, whilst the majority have a more insidious onset of jaundice associated with generalised malaise, frequent amenorrhoea in females and easy bruising. Occasionally, one of the manifestations of liver cell failure or an extrahepatic complication of the disease may be the presenting feature.

Physical examination generally reveals hepatomegaly unless the disease has reached a late stage, by which time the liver may have become small due to heavy fibrosis. Spider naevi are common. Skin striae and a wide variety of skin lesions including vasculitis, urticaria, acne, purpura, vitiligo, and nodular lesions resembling erythema nodosum, may be present. Other extrahepatic manifestations of the disease include polyarthritis, glomerulonephritis, renal tubular acidosis, thyroiditis, diabetes, a Cushing-like syndrome, ulcerative colitis, myocarditis, pericarditis, and various neurological abnormalities (Mistilis and Blackburn, 1970). A number of pulmonary changes may be found. Cyanosis may be due to the development of pulmonary arteriovenous anastomoses, or to fibrosing alveolitis. Primary pulmonary hypertension has been described.

Various haematological abnormalities may be present, including a Coombs' positive haemolytic anaemia, and autoimmune neutropenia, as well as the clotting defects which may be seen with any form of liver disease.

It is generally felt that the disease is gradually progressive. Death is inevitable once cirrhosis has developed but the clinical course is generally one of intermittent episodes of liver cell failure, which may respond well to therapy for a number of years. It is well recognised that the disease may become inactive for considerable periods of time, and survival for as long as 20 years from the time of diagnosis has been observed.

Laboratory findings

The term 'lupoid' hepatitis was coined because 15 per cent of patients are found to have LE cells (Joske and King, 1955). The biochemical criteria for entry to the most recent trial of therapy for chronic active hepatitis was a 5 to 10-fold rise in serum transaminase activity (Soloway et al, 1972). However, in the later stages when the disease has often become inactive the serum aspartate transaminase may not be raised but a low serum albumin and total cholesterol will reflect the severity of the underlying liver disease. Sometimes, the serum alkaline phosphatase and bilirubin are raised, on occasions to the extent that there appears to be considerable overlap with primary biliary cirrhosis. The other common feature is a marked elevation of the total serum gammaglobulin. This is predominantly due to a rise in IgG although other immunoglobulin levels may be elevated. A variety of serum antibodies are in part responsible for this elevation. Smooth muscle antibody is found in 67 per cent, antinuclear factor is somewhat less commonly seen (Doniach et al, 1966) and more recently anti-DNA antibodies have been described (Davis and Read, 1975). Anti-mitochondrial antibodies are rarely present. Organ-specific antibodies found include those against thyroid, adrenal and gastric mucosa. High titre antibodies to various gut bacteria have been described (Triger, Alp and Wright, 1972a). This response has been attributed to the failure of the damaged hepatic phagocytes to sequester gut bacterial antigens efficiently, so that continual antigenic stimulation takes place (Triger and Wright, 1973). However, high titre antibody to the rubella and particularly to the measles viruses, have also been described in chronic liver disease, the latter being virtually limited to cases of 'lupoid' hepatitis, and so there must be an alternative explanation for these findings, which remains unknown (Triger et al, 1972b).

With relevance to the involvement of the humoral immune system, a fall in serum complement concentrations may be seen, particularly when liver cell failure is evident. Although it is likely that this reduction is due to decreased synthesis, complement consumption by immune complex formation cannot be excluded (Potter, Trueman and Jones, 1973).

There is much experimental evidence to suggest that the cellular immune system is also disturbed in cases of 'lupoid' hepatitis. A depressed response to cutaneous testing for delayed hypersensitivity has been noted as well as impaired in vitro lymphocyte transformation to non-specific mitogens (Toh et al, 1973). Whether these findings are primary defects or secondary to the development of chronic liver disease is unclear. More recent studies have shown that subjects with both 'lupoid' and HB_sAg associated chronic active hepatitis have a functional abnormality of circulating T cells (De Horatius, Strickland and Williams, 1974). The presence of serum antibodies and the often massive lymphocyte infiltration of the liver and the impaired T-cell function has led to much speculation about 'autodestruction' of the liver being responsible for the disease. There is now good evidence to suggest that sensitisation to a liver-specific lipoprotein does exist (Miller et al, 1972). Experimental studies have shown that injection of liver-specific lipoprotein into rabbits is followed by the development of an hepatic lesion very similar to human 'lupoid' hepatitis (Meyer zum Buschenfelde and Hopf, 1974). What triggers off part of the liver cell to become antigenic is unknown, although it has been suggested that it is a viral infection, the virus acting as a 'neoantigen'.

Finally, transient elevation of serum α_1-fetoprotein has been reported in subjects with chronic active hepatitis (Silver et al, 1974). Increased production of this foetal protein is probably due to rapid liver cell regeneration.

Management

It is now well recognised that steroid therapy prolongs the survival of subjects with 'lupoid' hepatitis (Cook, Mulligan and Sherlock, 1971; Soloway et al, 1972). However, the results of different controlled trials have varied. The controlled trial carried out by Cook et al (1971) employed 15 mg prednisolone in the treated group, initially, the dose being reduced once the biochemical tests became normal. A significant improvement in serum bilirubin and albumin levels was seen in those given steroids. The difference in the mortality rate between the untreated and the treated was significant ($P<0\cdot01$) and it was concluded that corticosteroid therapy used during the early active phase of chronic active hepatitis improved life expectancy. More recently, the results of a further trial (Soloway et al, 1972) suggest that corticosteroids, (20 mg prednisone daily was used as the initial dose) may in fact induce a complete remission. Patients without histological evidence of cirrhosis did better than those with cirrhosis, although the difference was not significant. Similar results were seen by the same group, when they used half this dose of prednisone in combination with 50 mg azathioprine daily. Not surprisingly, fewer serious steroid side effects were seen with this latter regime. By contrast, deterioration was seen in the majority of those given a placebo or azathioprine 100 mg daily, although remission was noted in 20 per cent. It may well be argued that as the requirement for the minimum duration of liver disease was only 10 weeks in this trial, some of the cases included may well have had acute rather than chronic liver disease. As prednisone needs to be converted to prednisolone by the liver before it becomes active, it is possible that a smaller dose of prednisolone may be used to obtain remission (Powell and Axelsen, 1972). To explain the ineffectiveness of azathioprine when given alone, it may well be that prednisolone is required to improve liver function sufficiently so that azathioprine can be converted to its active metabolite 6-mercaptopurine. The introduction of azathioprine may be valuable in subjects who develop marked side effects to the steroids, enabling the dose of the latter to be reduced. Other trials have confirmed that used alone, azathioprine is ineffective (Mackay, 1968; Murray-Lyon, Stern and Williams, 1973) and its metabolite, 6-mercaptopurine may even be hepatotoxic on occasions (Krawitt et al, 1967). All trials have shown that even amongst corticosteroid treated subjects, relapse is common and experience would suggest that steroid therapy should be continued for some six months or more after the biochemical tests have returned to normal. The value of repeated liver biopsies is questionable in view of the problems of sampling error, and the difficulty of assessing the degree of activity, whilst the patient is taking steroids.

The complications of liver cell failure and portal hypertension should be treated by the standard methods. Unfortunately, shunt surgery is on the whole not well tolerated by subjects with 'lupoid' hepatitis (Hourigan et al, 1971). It is possible that the mesocaval 'jump' graft operation may give better results as there is less diminution of hepatic blood flow.

Prognosis

If left untreated 'lupoid' chronic active hepatitis is generally a progressive disease, terminating in liver cell failure, the mortality being 50 per cent or more within the first five years after diagnosis (Joske and Kings, 1955; Cook et al, 1971), death within the first two years being most common. Treatment with corticosteroids markedly improves survival. Recent reports suggest that if treatment is instituted early, during the precirrhotic phase, permanent remission may occasionally take place (Soloway et al, 1972).

HB$_s$Ag Positive Chronic Active Hepatitis

Epidemiology

Chronic active liver disease associated with the presence of a serum HB$_s$Ag predominantly affects men over the age of 30 years (Dudley et al, 1972b). This form of chronic liver disease is much more commonly seen in Mediterranean and tropical countries (Bianchi et al, 1972) than in the United Kingdom (Fox, Niazi and Sherlock, 1969) or Australia (Matthews and Mackay, 1970), the incidence in the USA being about midway between these two extremes. It is probably equally prevalent in all social classes, but in one reported series, 20 per cent of affected subjects were doctors (Dudley et al, 1972b). This finding may be partly explained by the supposition that certain sections of society, who by virtue of their employment are more likely than others to become exposed to HB$_s$Ag, are therefore more likely to become infected. In areas where there is a high HB$_s$Ag carrier rate, familial cases have been reported (Ohbayashi, Okochi and Mayumi,

1972). In such households, the HB$_s$Ag subtype tends to be the same, although no one particular subtype is associated with the HB$_s$Ag positive chronic active liver disease (Pons-Romero et al, 1974). Although studies have not been extensive, there seems to be no association between HL-A type and this disease (Galbraith et al, 1974).

Aetiology
There seems little doubt that the hepatitis B virus is involved in the pathogenesis of HB$_s$Ag positive chronic active hepatitis. Progression from acute HB$_s$Ag positive hepatitis to chronic active hepatitis has been noted (Nielsen et al, 1971; Chiaramonte et al, 1974). However, it seems unlikely that the liver cell damage is due to the direct action of the virus. Immunofluorescence studies on the livers of asymptomatic, HB$_s$Ag carriers, with relatively little liver damage, have shown massive quantities of HB$_s$Ag within the liver (Hadziyannis et al, 1972b). Serum HB$_s$Ag may be found very occasionally in subjects with chronic liver disease due to alcohol but it is felt that, in this situation, the hepatitis B virus is not involved in the pathogenesis of the disease, but rather the association is a fortuitous one (Reed et al, 1973a; Chiaramonte et al, 1977). It is felt that infection with the hepatitis B virus leads to 'autosensitisation' to the host's liver cells. It has been suggested that HB$_s$Ag in some way alters the liver cell membrane so that it becomes antigenic and hence sensitises both the host's humoral and cellular immune system (Eddleston et al, 1974). It is possible that such sensitisation occurs in any subject infected with the hepatitis B virus and that it is the response of an individual's immune system which determines the type of ensuing liver damage (Dudley, Fox and Sherlock, 1972a). In vitro lymphocyte studies have shown that subjects with HB$_s$Ag positive chronic active liver disease have partial impairment of their cellular immune system (Giustino, Dudley and Sherlock, 1972) and it is suggested that this may be in part responsible for the continuing liver cell necrosis. Subjects who have recovered completely from acute, type B hepatitis and cleared HB$_s$Ag seem to have fully competent delayed hypersensitivity mechanisms.

Other have suggested that immune complexes of HB$_s$Ag and anti-HB$_s$, which have been found in the serum of subjects with HB$_s$Ag positive chronic active liver disease may be responsible for the liver damage (Almeida and Waterson, 1969). However, Trepo et al (1974) could find no correlation between the presence of such immune complexes present in the serum and the activity of liver disease present. Dudley, Fox and Sherlock (1971) found normal serum levels of the third component of complement in the majority of patients with chronic hepatitis. It would therefore seem unlikely that the formation of immune complexes of HB$_s$Ag and anti-HB$_s$ is directly responsible for liver damage.

Clinical features
The presenting features of this disease vary very much according to the method of selection. Biochemical and histological studies on asymptomatic HB$_s$Ag carriers, detected in blood donor surveys, may reveal a small number of completely symptom-free cases of chronic active hepatitis. Even the symptomatic subjects referred to liver disease clinics tend to have only mild symptoms,

compared to their HB$_s$Ag negative counterparts. Fatigue, anorexia and vague abdominal discomfort generally predominate. Extrahepatic complications are rare and even the usual stigmata of chronic liver disease are often absent. Although no extensive studies have been made, a two-year follow-up carried out by Dudley et al (1972b) showed deterioration to be minimal. Surveys carried out in Greece by Hadziyannis (1974) confirm this finding, However, as with all forms of chronic liver disease, once cirrhosis is established the disease becomes irreversible leading to liver cell failure and portal hypertension. There is one complication peculiar to long-term HB$_s$Ag positive chronic active liver disease, that is the development of primary liver cell carcinoma (Dudley et al, 1972b). Thus any subject with HB$_s$Ag positive chronic active hepatitis who shows signs of rapid deterioration should be suspected of this.

Laboratory findings

In subjects with HB$_s$Ag positive chronic active hepatitis, the titre of HB$_s$Ag is often less than 1:256, which means that unless highly sensitive methods of HB$_s$Ag detection are used, it may not be detected (Chiaramonte et al, 1977). Generally, serum HB$_s$Ag persists but its disappearance has been noted (Reed, Eddleston and Stern, 1973b) and may be associated with resolution of the disease (Gentilini et al, 1972). Anti-HB$_s$ as well as HB$_s$Ag may sometimes be detected in the serum and electron microscopic examination of sera from cases of HB$_s$Ag positive chronic active hepatitis often reveals the presence of immune complexes, although there is little evidence to suggest that such complexes play a role in the pathogenesis of the liver disease. Recently, the 'e' antigenic determinant has been described in high frequency in HB$_s$Ag carriers with evidence of chronic liver disease, contrasting with those HB$_s$Ag carriers with minimal evidence of liver damage (Nielsen, Dietrichson and Juhl, 1974; Eleftheriou et al, 1975b). Anti-HB$_c$ can be detected in the majority of HB$_s$Ag carriers (Hoofnagle et al, 1974), but the finding of DNA polymerase activity is variable (Krugman et al, 1974).

The biochemical tests in subjects with HB$_s$Ag positive chronic active hepatitis are often only minimally deranged. Jaundice is uncommon and only moderate rises in serum transaminase activity are found. Serum albumin levels are well maintained and the total serum globulin levels are generally not markedly elevated. The presence of serum autoantibodies is reported and some would argue that their presence is no less frequent than in 'lupoid' hepatitis (Reed et al, 1973b). However, when smooth muscle antibody and antinuclear factor are present, they tend to be in low titre and often transient. The finding of LE cells is not reported.

Transient elevations of serum α-fetoprotein may be found as with 'lupoid' hepatitis. Persistent elevations, particularly when in increasing concentrations, would seem to indicate the presence of a developing primary liver cell carcinoma (Eleftheriou et al, 1975b). Unfortunately, the growth rate of such tumours is so rapid that such measurements tend to be of academic interest only.

Management

No formal trial of therapy for HB$_s$Ag positive chronic active hepatitis has been reported. Fourteen per cent of the patients included in the trial carried out by

Soloway et al (1972) were HB_sAg positive. Their response to therapy with either corticosteroids alone or in combination with azathioprine was poorer than that seen in cases of 'lupoid' hepatitis (Summerskill et al, 1975).

It is sometimes hard to justify long-term immunosuppressive therapy in subjects, who, despite the presence of considerable 'activity' in their liver biopsy, feel very well. Attempts have been made to eradicate the hepatitis B virus, thereby hoping to discontinue lymphocyte sensitisation to the virus and subsequent liver cell destruction. Both infusion of anti-HB_s (Reed et al, 1973b) and transfer factor have been tried (Kohler et al, 1974).

Unfortunately, there is still no effective therapy for primary liver cell carcinoma. Hepatic resection in the majority of cases is not feasible, either due to the size of the tumour or the severity of the background liver disease.

Prognosis

The long-term survival of cases of HB_sAG positive chronic active liver disease is very much better than for 'lupoid' hepatitis. We await the results of prospective controlled drug trials being carried out, to see whether life expectancy can be improved. It could well be that the development of primary liver cell carcinoma is in part related to the continued presence of the hepatitis B virus, which may have oncogenic properties. It would therefore seem desirable to attempt to eradicate the virus, in any therapeutic regimen.

REFERENCES

Aach, R. D., Evans, J. & Losee, J. (1968) An epidemic of infectious hepatitis possibly due to airborne transmission. *American Journal of Epidemiology*, **87**, 99–109.

Ajdukiewicz, A. B., Dudley, F. J., Fox, R. A., Doniach, D. & Sherlock, S. (1972) Immunological studies in an epidemic of infective short incubation hepatitis. *Lancet*, **i**, 803–806.

Akadamar, K. A., Maumus, L., Epps, A. C., Leach, R. & Warren, S. (1971) S. H. antigen in bile. *Lancet*, **i**, 909.

Almeida, J. D. & Waterson, A. P. (1969) Immune complexes in hepatitis. *Lancet*, **ii**, 983–986.

Almeida, J. D., Zuckerman, A. J., Taylor, P. E. & Waterson, A. P. (1969) Immune-electron microscopy of the Australia-SH (serum hepatitis) antigen. *Microbios*, **2**, 117–123.

Almeida, J. D., Waterson, A. P., Trowell, J. M. & Neale, G. (1970) The finding of virus-like particles in two Australia antigen-positive human livers. *Microbios*, **6**, 145–153.

Almeida, J. D., Rubenstein, D. & Stott, E. J. (1971) New antigen–antibody system in Australia-antigen-positive hepatitis. *Lancet*, **ii**, 1225–1227.

Almeida, J. D., Gay, F. W. & Wreghitt, T. G. (1974) Pitfalls in the study of hepatitis A. *Lancet*, **ii**, 748–750.

Alpert, E., Isselbacher, K. J. & Schur, P. H. (1971) The pathogenesis of arthritis associated with viral hepatitis: complement component studies. *New England Journal of Medicine*, **285**, 185–189.

Bancroft, W. H., Mundon, F. K. & Russell, P. K. (1972) Detection of additional antigenic determinants of hepatitis B antigen. *Journal of Immunology*, **109**, 842–848.

Barker, L. F. & Murray, R. (1972) Relationship of virus dose to incubation time of clinical hepatitis and time of appearance of hepatitis-associated antigen. *American Journal of Medical Sciences*, **263**, 27–33.

Barker, L. F., Chisari, F. V., McGrath, P. P., Dalgard, D. W., Kirschstein, R. L., Almeida, J. D., Edington, T. S., Sharp, D. G. & Peterson, M. R. (1973a) Transmission of type B viral hepatitis to chimpanzees. *Journal of Infectious Diseases*, **127**, 648–662.

Barker, L. F., Peterson, M. R., Shulman, N. R. & Murray, R. (1973b) Antibody responses in viral hepatitis, type B. *Journal of the American Medical Association*, **223**, 1005–1008.

Bayer, M. E., Blumberg, B. S. & Werner, B. (1968) Particles associated with Australia antigen in the sera of patients with leukaemia, Down's syndrome and hepatitis. *Nature*, **218**, 1057–1059.

Beard, J. D. & Knott, D. H. (1966) Hematopoietic response to experimental chronic alcoholism. *American Journal Medical Sciences*, **252**, 518–525.

Becker, M. D., Scheuer, P. J., Baptista, A. & Sherlock, S. (1970) Prognosis of chronic persistent hepatitis. *Lancet*, **i**, 53–56.

Belfrage, S., Ahlgren, I. & Axelson, S. (1966) Halothane hepatitis in an anaesthetist. *Lancet*, **ii**, 1466–1467.

Bell, H. (1971) Cardiac manifestations of viral hepatitis. *Journal of the American Medical Association*, **218**, 387–391.

Berg, N. O. & Eriksson, S. (1972) Liver disease in adults with alpha$_1$ antitrypsin deficiency. *New England Journal of Medicine*, **287**, 1264–1267.

Berg, P. A. (1974) Immune response in acute viral hepatitis. In *Clinics in Gastroenterology*, ed. Tygstrup, N., Vol. 3, Ch. 2. London: W. B. Saunders Company Ltd.

Bianchi, P., Bianchi Porro, C., Coltorti, M., Dardanoni, L., Del Vecchio Blanco, C., Faglolo, U., Farini, R., Manozzi, I., Naccarato, R., Pagliaro, L., Spano, G. & Verme, G. (1972) Occurrence of Australia antigen in chronic hepatitis in Italy. *Gastroenterology*, **63**, 482–485.

Black, M., Mitchell, J. R., Zimmerman, H. J., Ishak, K. G. & Epler, G. R. (1975) Isoniazid-associated hepatitis in 114 patients. *Gastroenterology*, **69**, 289–302.

Blum, A. L., Stutz, R. & Haemmerli, U. P. (1969) A fortuitously controlled study of steroid therapy in acute viral hepatitis. *American Journal of Medicine*, **47**, 82–92.

Blumberg, B. S. (1964) Polymorphisms of the serum proteins and the development of iso-precipitins in transfused patients. *Bulletin of the New York Academy of Medicine*, **40**, 377–386.

Blumberg, B. S., Alter, H. J. & Visnich, S. (1965) A 'new' antigen in leukaemia sera. *Journal of the American Medical Association*, **191**, 541–546.

Blumberg, B. S., Gerstley, B. J. S., Hungerford, D. A., London, W. T. & Sutnick, A. I. (1967) A serum antigen (Australia antigen) in Down's syndrome, leukaemia and hepatitis. *Annals of Internal Medicine*, **66**, 924–931.

Blumberg, B. S., Sutnick, A. I. & London, W. T. (1968) Hepatitis and leukaemia: their relation to Australia antigen. *Bulletin of the New York Academy of Medicine*, **44**, 1566–1586.

Blumberg, B. S., Friedlaender, J. S., Woodside, A., Sutnick, A. I. & London, W. T. (1969) Hepatitis and Australia antigen: autosomal recessive inheritance of susceptibility of infection in humans. *Genetics*, **62**, 1108–1115.

Blumberg, B. S., Sutnick, A. I. & London, W. T. (1970) Australia antigen as a hepatitis virus. Variation in host response. *American Journal of Medicine*, **48**, 1–8.

Bone, J. M., Tonkin, R. W., Davison, A. M., Marmion, B. P. & Robson, J. S. (1971) Outbreak of dialysis-associated hepatitis in Edinburgh 1969–1970. *Proceedings of the European Dialysis and Transplant Association*, **8**, 189–193.

Borhanmanesh, F., Haghighi, P., Hekmat, K., Rezaizadeh, K. & Ghavami, A. G. (1973) Viral hepatitis during pregnancy. *Gastroenterology*, **64**, 304–312.

Boxall, E. H., Flewett, T. H., Dane, D. S., Camerson, C. H., MacCallum, F. O. & Lee, T. W. (1974) Hepatitis B surface antigen in breast milk. *Lancet*, **ii**, 1007–1008.

Brunt, P. W., Kew, M. C., Scheuer, P. J. & Sherlock, S. (1974) Studies in alcoholic liver disease in Britain. *Gut*, **15**, 52–58.

Chiaramonte, M., Dardoni, L., Farini, R., Filipozzo, G., Genova, G., Naccarato, R., Pagliaro, L. & Spano, G. (1974) Observations on acute phase and follow-up of similar series of cases of HBAg positive and HBAg negative hepatitis. *Rendiconti di Gastro-enterologia*, **6**, 1–5.

Chiaramonte, M., Heathcote, J., Crees, M. & Sherlock, S. (1977) The detection, by three techniques, of hepatitis B surface antigen (HB$_s$Ag) and the determination of HB$_s$Ag and anti-HB$_s$ titres in patients with chronic liver disease. *Gut*, **18**, 1–6.

Clark, R., Thompson, R. P. H., Borirakchanyavat, V., Widdop, B., Davidson, A. R., Goulding, R. & Williams, R. (1973) Hepatic damage and death from overdose of paracetamol. *Lancet*, **i**, 66–70.

Combes, B., Stastny, P., Shorey, J., Eigenbrodt, E. H., Barrera, A., Hull, A. R. & Carter, N. W. (1971) Glomerulonephritis with deposition of Australia antigen–antibody complexes in glomerular basement membrane. *Lancet*, **ii**, 234–237.

Cook, G. C., Mulligan, R. & Sherlock, S. (1971) Controlled prospective trial of corticosteroid therapy in active chronic hepatitis. *Quarterly Journal of Medicine*, **40**, 159–185.

Cossart, Y. E. & Vahrman, J. (1970) Studies of Australia-SH antigen in sporadic viral hepatitis in London. *British Medical Journal*, **i**, 403–405.

Cruz-Coke, R. & Varela, A. (1966) Inheritance of alcoholism. *Lancet*, **ii**, 1282–1284.

Dane, D. S., Cameron, C. H. & Briggs, M. (1970) Virus-like particles in serum of patients with Australia-antigen associated hepatitis. *Lancet*, **i**, 695–698.

Dankert, J., Postma, A., de Vries, J. A. & Zijlstra, J. B. (1975) HB$_s$Ag in spinal fluid from leukaemia children. *Lancet*, **i**, 690.

Davis, P. & Read, A. I. (1975) Antibodies to double-stranded (native) DNA in active chronic hepatitis. *Gut*, **16**, 413–415.

De Groote, J., Desmet, V. J., Gedigk, P., Korb, G., Popper, H., Poulsen, H., Scheuer, P. J., Schmid, M., Thaler, H., Uehlinger, E. & Wepler, W. (1968) A classification of chronic hepatitis. *Lancet*, **ii**, 626–628.

De Horatius, R. J., Strickland, R. G. & Williams, R. C., Jr (1974) T and B lymphocytes in acute and chronic hepatitis. *Clinical Immunology and Immunopathology*, **2**, 353–360.

Deinhardt, F., Holmes, A. W., Capps, R. B. & Popper, H. (1967) Studies on the transmission of human viral hepatitis to marmoset monkeys. *Journal of Experimental Medicine*, **125**, 673–687.

Deodhar, K. P., Tapp, E. & Scheuer, P. J. (1975) Orcein staining of hepatitis B antigen in paraffin sections of liver biopsies. *Journal of Clinical Pathology*, **28**, 66–70.

Dietrichson, O. (1975) Chronic persistent hepatitis. A clinical, serological and prognostic study. *Scandinavian Journal of Gastroenterology*, **10**, 249–255.

Doniach, D., Roitt, I. M., Walker, J. G. & Sherlock, S. (1966) Tissue antibodies in primary biliary cirrhosis, active chronic (lupoid) hepatitis, cryptogenic cirrhosis and other liver diseases and their clinical implications. *Clinical and Experimental Immunology*, **1**, 237–262.

Douglas, A. P., Hamlyn, A. N. & James, O. (1976) Controlled trial of cysteamine in treatment of acute paracetamol (acetominophen) poisoning. *Lancet*, **i**, 111–115.

Dubin, I. N., Sullivan, B. H., Jr, LeGorvan, P. C. & Murphy, L. C. (1960) The cholestatic form of viral hepatitis. *American Journal of Medicine*, **29**, 55–72.

Dudley, F. J., Fox, R. A. & Sherlock, S. (1971) Relation of hepatitis associated antigen (HAA) to acute and chronic liver injury. *Lancet*, **ii**, 1–3.

Dudley, F. J., Fox, R. A. & Sherlock, S. (1972a) Cellular immunity and hepatitis-associated Australia antigen liver disease. *Lancet*, **i**, 723–726.

Dudley, F. J., Scheuer, P. J. & Sherlock, S. (1972b). Natural history of hepatitis associated antigen positive chronic liver disease. *Lancet*, **ii**, 1388–1393.

Durani, M. & Gerber, M. (1974) Hepatitis B antigen in vaginal secretions. *Lancet*, **ii**, 1008.

Dykes, M. H. M., Walzer, S. G., Slater, E. M., Gibson, J. M. & Ellis, D. S. (1965) Acute parenchymatous hepatic disease following general anaesthesia. *Journal of the American Medical Association*, **193**, 339–344.

Eddleston, A. L. W. F. & Williams, R. (1974) Inadequate antibody response to HBAg or suppressor T-cell defect in development of active chronic hepatitis. *Lancet*, **ii**, 1543–1545.

Edmondson, H. A., Peters, R. L., Reynolds, T. B. & Kuzma, O. T. (1963) Sclerosing hyaline necrosis of the liver in the chronic alcoholic. *Annals of Internal Medicine*, **59**, 646–673.

Eleftheriou, N., Heathcote, J., Thomas, H. C. & Sherlock, S. (1975a) Serum alphafetoprotein levels in patients with acute and chronic liver disease: relation to hepatocellular regeneration and the development of primary liver cell carcinoma (in preparation).

Eleftheriou, N., Thomas, H. C., Heathcote, J. & Sherlock, S. (1975b) Incidence and clinical significance of 'e' antigen and antibody in acute and chronic liver disease. *Lancet*, **ii**, 1171–1173.

Feinstone, S. M., Kapikian, A. Z. & Purcell, R. H. (1973) Hepatitis A: detection by immune electron microscopy of a virus-like antigen associated with acute illness. *Science*, **182**, 1026–1028.

Fenna, D., Mix, L., Schaefer, O. & Gilbert, J. A. L. (1971) Ethanol metabolism in various racial groups. *Canadian Medical Journal*, **105**, 472–475.

Fox, R. A., Niazi, S. P. & Sherlock, S. (1969) Hepatitis-associated antigen in chronic liver disease. *Lancet*, **ii**, 609–612.

Fulford, K. W. M., Dane, D. S., Catteral, R. D., Woof, R. & Denning, J. V. (1973) Australia antigen and antibody among patients attending a clinic for sexually transmitted diseases. *Lancet*, **i**, 1470–1473.

Galambos, J. T. (1972) Natural history of alcoholic hepatitis. III. Histological changes. *Gastroenterology*, **63**, 1026–1035.

Galambos, J. T. (1975) Chronic active hepatitis and ethanol — a form of drug hepatitis? *Gastroenterology*, **68**, 1075 (Abstract).

Galbraith, R. M., Eddleston, A. L. W. F., Smith, M. G. M., Williams, R., McSween, R. N. M., Watkinson, G., Dick, H., Kennedy, L. A. & Batchelor, J. R. (1974) Histocompatibility antigens in active chronic hepatitis and primary biliary cirrhosis. *British Medical Journal*, **iii**, 604–605.

Galbraith, R. M., Portmann, B., Eddleston, A. L. W. F. & Williams, R. (1975) Chronic liver disease developing after outbreak of HBₛAg negative hepatitis in haemodialysis unit. *Lancet*, **ii**, 886–890.

Garibaldi, R. A., Forrest, J. N., Bryan, J. A., Hanson, B. F. & Dismukes, W. E. (1973) Hemodialysis-associated hepatitis. *Journal of the American Medical Association*, **225**, 384–389.

Gentilini, P., Surrenti, C., Chiarantini, E. & Lamanna, A. (1972) H.A.A. in chronic liver disease. *Lancet*, **ii**, 378.

Giles, J. P., McCollum, R. W., Berndtson, L. W. & Krugman, S. (1969) Viral hepatitis. Relation Australia/SH antigen to Willowbrook MS-2 strain. *New England Journal of Medicine*, 281, 119–122.

Gitlin, N. (1973) Extrahepatic manifestations of long incubation hepatitis (MS-2 hepatitis): an association with Henoch–Schönlein syndrome. *Liver. Proceedings of the International Liver Conference, Cape Town*, pp. 47–48. London: Pitman Medical.

Giustino, V., Dudley, F. J. & Sherlock, S. (1972) Thymus dependent lymphocyte function in patients with hepatitis-associated antigen. *Lancet*, ii, 850–853.

Gocke, D. J. & Kavey, N. B. (1969) Hepatitis antigen. Correlation with disease and infectivity of blood donors. *Lancet*, i, 1055–1059.

Green, J., Mistilis, S. & Schiff, L. (1963) Acute alcoholic hepatitis. *Archives of Internal Medicine*, 112, 67–78.

Hadziyannis, St., Vissoulis, Ch., Moussouros, A. & Afroudakis, A. (1972a) Cytoplasmic localisation of Australia antigen in the liver. *Lancet*, i, 976–979.

Hadziyannis, St., Merikas, G., Panetsos, S. & Kourepi, M. (1972b) Hepatitis associated antigen carriers among blood donors in Greece. *American Journal of Disease of Children*, 123, 381–383.

Hadziyannis, St. (1974) Chronic viral hepatitis. In *Clinics in Gastroenterology*, ed. Tygstrup, N., Vol. 3, Ch. 9. London: W. B. Saunders Company Ltd.

Hardison, W. G. & Lee, F. I. (1966) Prognosis in acute liver disease of the alcoholic patient. *New England Journal of Medicine*, 275, 61–66.

Havens, W. P., Jr, Ward, R. & Drill, V. A. (1944) Experimental production of hepatitis by feeding icterogenic materials. *Proceedings of the Society for Experimental Biology and Medicine*, 57, 206–208.

Havens, W. P. (1962) Viral hepatitis. Clinical pattern and diagnosis. *American Journal of Medicine*, 32, 665–678.

Hawley, W. L., McFarlen, A. M., Steigman, A. J., McMichael, J. & Dible, J. H. (1944) Hepatitis following infection of mumps convalescent plasma: clinical and laboratory study. *Lancet*, i, 818–821.

Heathcote, J., Cameron, C. H. & Dane, D. S. (1974a) Hepatitis B antigen in saliva and semen. *Lancet*, i, 71–73.

Heathcote, J., Gateau, Ph. & Sherlock, S. (1974b) Role of hepatitis B antigen carriers in non-parenteral transmission of the hepatitis B virus. *Lancet*, ii, 370–372.

Hed, R., Lundmark, C., Fahlgren, H. & Orell, S. (1962) Acute muscular syndrome in chronic alcoholism. *Acta medica scandinavica*, 171, 585–599.

Helman, R. A., Temko, M. H., Nye, S. W. & Fallon, H. J. (1971) Alcoholic hepatitis: natural history and evaluation of prednisolone therapy. *Annals of Internal Medicine*, 74, 311–321.

Hersch, T., Melnick, J. L., Gowal, R. K. & Hollinger, F. B. (1972) Non-parenteral transmission of viral hepatitis type B (Australia antigen-associated serum hepatitis). *New England Journal of Medicine*, 285, 1363–1364.

Hirschman, R. J., Shulman, N. R., Barker, L. F. & Smith, K. O. (1969) Virus-like particles in the sera of patients with infectious and serum hepatitis. *Journal of the American Medical Association*, 208, 1667–1670.

Holland, P. V., Walsh, J. H., Morrow, A. G. & Purcell, R. H. (1969) Failure of Australia antibody to prevent post-transfusion hepatitis. *Lancet*, ii, 553–555.

Hollinger, B. F., Dreesman, G. R., Fields, H. & Melnick, J. L. (1973) HB_cAg, anti-IIB_c and DNA polymerase activity in transfused recipients followed prospectively. *American Journal of the Medical Sciences*, 270, 343–348.

Hoofnagle, J. H., Gerety, R. J., Ni, L. Y. & Barker, L. F. (1974) Antibody to hepatitis B core antigen. *New England Journal of Medicine*, 290, 1336–1340.

Hourigan, K., Sherlock, S., George, P. & Mindel, S. (1971) Elective end-to-side portacaval shunt: results in 64 cases. *British Medical Journal*, iv, 473–477.

Huang, S. (1971). Hepatitis-associated antigen hepatitis. *American Journal of Pathology*, 64, 483–491.

Hughes, M. & Powell, L. W. (1970) Recurrent hepatitis in patients receiving multiple halothane anaesthetics for radium treatment of carcinoma of the cervix uteri. *Gastroenterology*, 58, 790–797.

Inman, W. H. W. & Mushin, W. W. (1974) Jaundice after repeated exposure to halothane: an analysis of reports to the Committee on Safety of Medicine. *British Medical Journal*, i, 5–10.

Joseph, P. R., Millar, J. D. & Henderson, D. A. (1965) An outbreak of hepatitis traced to food contamination. *New England Journal of Medicine*, 273, 188–194.

Joske, R. A. & King, W. E. (1955) The L.E. cell phenomenon in active chronic viral hepatitis. *Lancet*, ii, 477–479.

Kaplan, P. M., Greenman, R. L., Gerin, J. L., Purcell, R. A. & Robinson, W. S. (1973) DNA polymerase associated with human hepatitis B antigen. *Journal of Virology*, 12, 995–1005.

Karvountzis, G. G. & Redeker, A. G. (1974) Relation of alpha-fetoprotein in acute hepatitis to severity and prognosis. *Annals of Internal Medicine*, 80, 156–160.

Karvountzis, G. G., Redeker, A. G. & Peters, R. L. (1974) Long-term follow-up studies of patients surviving fulminant hepatitis. *Gastroenterology*, 67, 870–877.

Kew, M. C., Reis, P., Macnab, G. M., Seftel, H. C. & Bersohn, I. (1973) The witch-doctor and tribal scarification of the skin and the hepatitis B antigen. *South African Medical Journal*, 47, 2419–2420.

Klatskin, G. & Kimberg, D. V. (1969) Recurrent hepatitis attributable to halothane sensitisation in an anesthetist. *New England Journal of Medicine*, 280, 515–522.

Klion, F. M., Schaffner, F. & Popper, H. (1969) Hepatitis after exposure to halothane. *Annals of Internal Medicine*, 71, 467–477.

Koff, R. S. & Sear, H. S. (1967) Internal temperature of steamed clams. *New England Journal of Medicine*, 276, 737–739.

Kohler, P. F., Trembath, J., Merrill, D. A., Singleton, J. W. & Dubois, R. S. (1974) Immunotherapy with antibody lymphocytes and transfer factor in chronic hepatitis B. *Clinical Immunology and Immunopathology*, 2, 465–471.

Krawitt, E. L., Stein, J. H., Kirkendall, W. M. & Clifton, J. A. (1976) Mercaptopurine hepatotoxicity in a patient with chronic active hepatitis. *Archives of Internal Medicine*, 120, 729–734.

Krugman, S. (1963) The clinical use of gammaglobulin. *New England Journal of Medicine*, 269, 195–201.

Krugman, S., Giles, J. P. & Hammond, J. (1967) Infectious hepatitis: evidence for two distinctive, clinical, epidemiological and immunological types of infection. *Journal of the Americal Medical Association*, 200, 365–373.

Krugman, S. & Giles, J. P. (1973) Viral hepatitis, type B (MS-2 strain). Further observations on natural history and prevention. *New England Journal of Medicine*, 288, 755–760.

Krugman, S. & Giles, J. P. (1970) Viral hepatitis. New light on an old disease. *Journal of the American Medical Association*, 212, 1019–1029.

Krugman, S., Hoofnagle, J. H., Gerety, R. J., Kaplan, P. M. & Gerin, J. L. (1974) Viral hepatitis, type B. DNA polymerase activity and antibody to hepatitis B core antigen. *New England Journal of Medicine*, 290, 1331–1335.

Krugman, S., Friedman, H. & Lattimer, C. (1975) Viral hepatitis, type A. Identification by specific complement fixation and immune adherence tests. *New England Journal of Medicine*, 292, 1141–1143.

Kurylowicz, W. (1972) Epidemiology of viral hepatitis and its long-term sequelae in Poland. *American Journal of Diseases of Children*, 123, 335–340.

Lal, S., Singhal, S. N., Burley, D. M. & Crossley, G. (1972) Effect of Rifampicin and Isoniazid on liver function. *British Medical Journal*, i, 148–150.

Le Bouvier, G. L. (1971) The heterogeneity of Australia antigen. *Journal of Infectious Diseases*, 123, 671–675.

Lelback, W. K. (1966) Leberschäden bei chronischem Alkoholismus. *Acta hepato-splenologica*, 13, 321–349.

Levin, M. L., Maddrey, W. C., Wands, J. R. & Mendeloff, A. I. (1974) Hepatitis B transmission by dentists. *Journal of the American Medical Association*, 228, 1139–1140.

Lieber, C. S. (1973) Hepatic and metabolic effects of alcohol (1966 to 1973). *Gastroenterology*, 65, 821–846.

Lieberman, F. L. (1970) Functional renal failure in cirrhosis. *Gastroenterology*, 58, 108–109.

Lischner, M. W., Alexander, J. F. & Galambos, J. T. (1971) Natural history of alcoholic hepatitis. I. The acute disease. *American Journal of Digestive Diseases*, 16, 481–494.

Lobel, H. O. & McCollum, R. W. (1965) Some observations on the ecology of infectious hepatitis. *Bulletin of the World Health Organisation*, 32, 675–682.

London, W. T., Alter, H. J., Lander, J. & Purcell, R. H. (1972) Serial transmission in rhesus monkeys of an agent related to hepatitis-associated antigen. *Journal of Infectious Diseases*, 125, 382–389.

MacCallum, F. O. & Bradley, W. H. (1944) Transmission of infective hepatitis to human volunteers: effect on rheumatoid arthritis. *Lancet*, ii, 228.

Mackay, I. R. (1968) Chronic hepatitis: effect of prolonged suppressive treatment and comparison of azathioprine with prednisolone. *Quarterly Journal of Medicine*, 37, 379–392.

Mackay, I. R. & Morris, P. J. (1972) Association of autoimmune active chronic hepatitis with HL-A 1, 8, *Lancet*, ii, 793–795.

Magnius, L. O., Lindholm, A., Lundin, P. & Iwarson, S. (1975) A new antigen–antibody system. *Journal of the American Medical Association*, 231, 356–359.

Matthews, J. D. & Mackay, I. R. (1970) Australia antigen in chronic liver disease. *British Medical Journal*, **i**, 259–261.

Mascoli, C. C., Ittensohn, O. L., Villarejos, V. M., Argnedas, J. A., Provost, P. J. & Hilleman, M. R. (1973) Recovery of hepatitis agents in the marmoset from human cases occurring in Costa Rica. *Proceedings of the Society for Experimental Biology and Medicine*, **142**, 276–282.

McFarlen, A. M. & Chesney, G. (1944). Epidemiology of hepatitis. *Lancet*, **i**, 816–816.

Meyer zum Büschenfelde, K. H. & Hopf, U. (1974) Studies on the pathogenesis of experimental chronic active hepatitis in rabbits. *British Journal of Experimental Pathology*, **55**, 498-508.

Miller, W. J., Provost, P. J., McAleer, W. J., Ittensohn, O. L., Villarejos, V. M. & Hilleman, M. R. (1975) Specific immune adherence assay for human hepatitis A antibody. Application to diagnostic and epidemiologic investigations. *Proceedings of the Society for Experimental Biology and Mecicine*, **149**, 254–261.

Miller, J., Smith, M. G. M., Mitchell, C. G., Reed, W. D., Eddleston, A. L. W. F. & Williams, R. (1972) Cell-mediated immunity to a human liver-specific antigen in patients with active chronic hepatitis and primary biliary cirrhosis. *Lancet*, **ii**, 296–297.

Mirick, G. S. & Shank, R. E. (1959) An epidemic of serum hepatitis studied under controlled conditions. *Transactions of the American Clinical and Climatological Association*, **71**, 176–190.

Mistilis, S. P. & Blackburn, C. R. B. (1970) Active chronic hepatitis. *American Journal of Medicine*, **48**, 484–495.

Mitchell, J. R., Dybing, E. & Nelson, S. D. (1975) Metabolic activation of Methyldopa by superoxide anion in human liver and erythrocytes. *Gastroenterology*, **69**, 847 (Abstract).

Morse, L. J., Bryan, J. A., Hurley, J. P., Murphy, J. F., O'Brien, T. F. & Wacker, W. E. C. (1972) The Holy Cross Football Team hepatitis outbreak. *Journal of the American Medical Association*, **219**, 706–708.

Moult, P. J. A. & Sherlock, S. (1975) Halothane-related hepatitis. *Quarterly Journal of Medicine*, **68**, 99–114.

Mowat, N. A. G., Albert-Recht, F., Brunt, P. & Walker, W. (1973) Outbreak of serum hepatitis associated with tattooing. *Lancet*, **i**, 33-34.

Murray-Lyon, I. M., Stern, R. B. & Williams, R. (1973) Controlled trials of prednisone and azathioprine in active chronic hepatitis. *Lancet*, **i**, 735–737.

Neurath, A. R., Trepo, C., Chen, M. & Prince, A. M. (1975) Identification of additional antigenic sites on Dane particles and the tubular forms of hepatitis B surface antigen. *American Journal of Medical Sciences*, **270**, 205–206.

Newkirk, M. M., Downe, A. E. R. & Simon, J. B. (1975) Fate of ingested hepatitis B antigen in blood-sucking insects. *Gastroenterology*, **69**, 982–987.

Nielsen, J. O., Dietrichson, O. Elling, P. & Christoffersen, P. (1971) Incidence and meaning of persistance of Australia antigen in patients with acute viral hepatitis. Development of chronic hepatitis. *New England Journal of Medicine*, **285**, 1157–1160.

Nielsen, J. O., Dietrichson, O. & Juhl, E. (1974) Incidence and meaning of the 'e' determinant among hepatitis B antigen positive patients with acute and chronic liver diseases. *Lancet*, **ii**, 913–915.

Nordenfelt, E., Kaij, K. & Ursing, B. (1970) Presence and persistance of Australia antigen among drug addicts. *Vox sanguinis*, **19**, 371–378.

Nowoslawski, A., Brzosko, W. J., Madalinski, K. & Krawczynski, K. (1970) Cellular localisation of Australia antigen in the liver of patients with lymphoproliferative disorders. *Lancet*, **i**, 494–497.

Ohbayashi, A., Okochi, K. & Mayumi, M. (1972) Familial clustering of asymptomatic carriers of Australia antigen and patients with chronic liver disease or primary liver cancer. *Gastroenterology*, **62**, 618–625.

Okochi, K. & Murakami, S. (1968) Observations on Australia antigen in Japanese. *Vox sanguinis*, **15**, 374–385.

Onion, D. K., Crumpacker, C. S. & Gilliland, B. C. (1971) Arthritis and hepatitis associated with Australia antigen. *Annals of Internal Medicine*, **75**, 29–33.

Paronetto, F. & Popper, H. (1970) Lymphocyte stimulation induced by halothane in patients with hepatitis following exposure to halothane. *New England Journal of Medicine*, **283**, 277–280.

Pattison, C. P., Maynard, J. E., Berquist, K. R. — Webster, H. M. (1973) Serological and epidemiological studies of hepatitis B in haemodialysis units. *Lancet*, **i**, 172–174.

Paul, J. R., Havens, W. P., Jr & Sabin, A. B. (1945) Transmission experiments in serum jaundice and infectious hepatitis. *Journal of the American Medical Association*, **128**, 911–915.

Pearson, A. J. G., Grainger, J. M., Scheuer, P. J. & McIntyre, N. (1971) Jaundice due to oxyphenisatin. *Lancet*, **1**, 994–996.

Peters, R. L., Edmondson, H. A., Reynolds, T. B., Meister, J. C. & Curphey, T. J. (1969) Hepatic necrosis associated with halothane anaesthesia. *American Journal of Medicine*, **47**, 748–764.

Pettigrew, N. M., Goudie, R. B., Russell, R. I. & Chaudhuri, A. K. R. (1972) Evidence for a role of hepatitis virus B in chronic alcoholic liver disease. *Lancet*, **ii**, 724–725.

Pickles, W. N. (1939) Epidemic catarrhal jaundice. In *Epidemiology in Country Practice*, Ch. 7. Bristol: Wright.

Pons-Romero, F., Heathcote, J. & Sherlock, S. (1974) The epidemiological importance of 'ay' and 'ad' subtypes of the HBAg. *Gut*, **15**, 733–736.

Popper, H. & Mackay, I. R. (1972) Relation between Australia antigen and autoimmune hepatitis. *Lancet*, **i**, 1161–1164.

Porter, H. P., Simon, F. R., Pope, C. E., Volwiler, W. & Fenster, L. F. (1971) Corticosteroid therapy in severe alcoholic hepatitis. *New England Journal of Medicine*, **284**, 1350–1355.

Potter, B. J., Trueman, A. M. & Jones, E. A. (1973) Serum complement in chronic liver disease. *Gut*, **14**, 451–456.

Powell, L. W. & Axelsen, E. (1972) Corticosteroids in liver disease: studies on the biological conversion of prednisone to prednisolone and plasma protein binding. *Gut*, **13**, 690–696.

Prescott, L. F., Newton, R. W., Swainson, C. P., Wright, N., Forrest, A. R. W. & Matthew, H. (1974) Successful treatment of severe paracetamol overdosage with cysteamine. *Lancet*, **i**, 588–592.

Prince, A. M. (1968a) An antigen detected in the blood during the incubation period of serum hepatitis. *Proceedings of the National Academy of Sciences of the United States of America*, **60**, 814–821.

Prince, A. M. (1968b) Relation of Australia to SH antigens, *Lancet*, **ii**, 462–463.

Prince, A. M., Hargrove, R. L., Szmuness, W., Cherubin, C. E., Fontana, V. J. & Jeffries, G. H. (1970) Immunologic distinction between infectious and serum hepatitis. *New England Journal of Medicine*, **282**, 987–991.

Prince, A. M., Metselaar, D., Kafuko, G. W., Mukwaya, L. G., Ling, C. M. & Overby, L. R. (1972) Hepatitis B antigen in wild-caught mosquitoes in Africa. *Lancet*, **ii**, 247–250.

Prince, A. M., Brotman, B. & Grady, G. F. (1974) Long-incubation post-transfusion hepatitis without serological evidence of exposure to hepatitis B virus. *Lancet*, **ii**, 241–246.

Prince, A. M., Szmuness, W., Mann, M. K., Vyas, G. N., Grady, G. F., Shapiro, F. L., Suki, W. N., Friedman, E. A. & Stenzel, K. H. (1975) Hepatitis B 'immune' globulin: effectiveness in prevention of dialysis-associated hepatitis. *New England Journal of Medicine*, **293**, 1063–1067.

Provost, P. J., Ittensohn, O. L., Villarejos, V. M. & Hilleman, M. R. (1975) A specific complement fixation text for human hepatitis A employing CR 326 virus antigen. Diagnosis and epidemiology. *Proceedings of the Society for Experimental Biology and Medicine*, **148**, 962–969.

Raftensberger, E. C. (1958) Acute acquired haemolytic anaemia in association with acute viral hepatitis. *Annals of Internal Medicine*, **48**, 1243–1253.

Rake, M. O., Flute, P. T., Pannell, G. & Williams, R. (1970) Intravascular coagulation in acute hepatic necrosis. *Lancet*, **i**, 533–537.

Raska, K., Helcl, J., Jezek, J., Kubelka, Z., Litov, M., Novak, K., Radkovsky, J., Sery, V., Zeidl, J. & Zikmund, V. (1966) A milk born infectious hepatitis epidemic. *Journal of Hygiene, Epidemiology, Microbiology and Immunology*, **10**, 413–428.

Reed, W. D., Eddleston, A. L. W. F., Cullins, H., Williams, R., Zuckerman, A. J., Peters, D. K., Williams, D. G. & Maycock, W. D. (1973a) Infusion of hepatitis B antibody in antigen-positive active chronic hepatitis. *Lancet*, **ii**, 1347–1351.

Reed, W. D., Eddleston, A. L. W. F. & Stern, R. B. (1973b) Detection of hepatitis B antigen by radioimmunoassay in chronic liver disease and hepatocellular carcinoma in Great Britain. *Lancet*, **ii**, 690–693.

Rehman, O. U., Thomas, A. K. & Gall, E. A. (1973) Methyldopa induced submassive hepatic necrosis. *Journal of the American Medical Association*, **224**, 1390–1392.

Reinicke, V., Dybkjaer, E., Poulsen, H., Banke, O., Lylloft, K. & Nordenfelt, E. (1972) A study of Australia-antigen-positive blood donors and their recipients with special reference to liver histology. *New England Journal of Medicine*, **286**, 867-870.

Resnick, R. H. & Iber, F. L. (1972) Treatment of acute, alcoholic hepatitis. *Gut*, **13**, 68–73.

Reynolds, T. B., Peters, R. L. & Yamanda, S. (1971) Chronic active and lupoid hepatitis caused by a laxative, oxyphenisatin. *New England Journal of Medicine*, **285**, 813–820.

Ritland, S. (1975) Quantitative determination of the abnormal lipoprotein of cholestasis LP-X in liver disease. *Scandinavian Journal of Gastroenterology*, **10**, 5–15.

Rizzetto, M., Swana, G. & Doniach, D. (1973) Microsomal antibodies in active chronic hepatitis and other disorders. *Clinical and Experimental Immunology*, **15**, 331–344.

Rubin, E., Gottlieb, C. & Vogel, P. (1968) Syndrome of hepatitis and aplastic anaemia. *American Journal of Medicine*, **45**, 88–97.

Rubin, E. & Lieber, C. S. (1968) Alcohol-induced hepatic injury in non-alcoholic volunteers. *New England Journal of Medicine*, **278**, 869-876.

Saidi, S., Farrohi, Kh., McCollum, R. W. & Le Bouvier, G. L. (1972) Hepatitis B antigen in Iran: frequency and subtype. *Lancet*, ii, 1377–1378.

Scheuer, P. J., Summerfield, J. A., Lal, S. & Sherlock, S. (1974) Rifampicin hepatitis. *Lancet*, i, 421–425.

Schweitzer, I. L., Wing, A., McPeak, C. & Spears, R. L. (1972) Hepatitis and hepatitis associated antigen in 56 mother–infant pairs. *Journal of the American Medical Association*, 220, 1092–1095.

Schweitzer, I. L., Mosley, J. W., Ashcavai, M., Edwards, M. & Overby, L. B. (1973) Factors influencing neonatal infection by hepatitis B virus. *Gastroenterology*, 65, 277–283.

Seeff, L. B., Zimmerman, H. J., Wright, E. C., Felsher, B. F. et al (1975) Efficacy of hepatitis B immune serum globulin after accidental exposure. *Lancet*, ii, 939–941.

Seife, M., Kessler, B. J. & Lisa, J. R. (1950) Clinical, functional and needle biopsy study on the liver in alcoholism. *Archives of Internal Medicine (Chicago)*, 86, 658–670.

Silver, H. K. B., Gold, P., Shuster, J., Javitt, N. B., Freedman, S. O. & Finlayson, N. D. C. (1974) Alpha₁-fetoprotein in chronic liver disease. *New England Journal of Medicine*, 291, 506–508.

Simpson, B. R., Strunin, L. & Walton, B. (1971) The halothane dilemma: a case for the defence. *British Medical Journal*, iv, 96–100.

Singleton, J. W., Fitch, R. A., Merrill, D. A., Kohler, P. F. & Rettberg, W. A. H. (1971) Liver disease in Australia-antigen-positive blood donors. *Lancet*, ii, 785–787.

Skinhøj, P. Olesen, H., Cohn, J. & Mikkelsen, M. (1972) Hepatitis-associated antigen in pregnant women. *Acta pathologica et microbiologica scandinavica*, 80, 362–366.

Smith, B. J. (1971) Occurrence of alpha fetoprotein in acute viral hepatitis. *International Journal of Cancer*, 8, 421–424.

Soloway, R. D., Summerskill, W. H. J., Baggenstoss, A. H., Geall, M. G., Gitnick, G. L., Elveback, L. R. & Schoenfield, L. J. (1972) Clinical, biochemical and histological remission of severe chronic active liver disease: a controlled study of treatments and early prognosis. *Gastroenterology*, 63, 820–833.

Sorrell, M. F. & Leevy, C. M. (1972) Lymphocyte transformation and alcoholic liver injury *Gastroenterology*, 63, 1020–1025.

Soulier, J. P., Blatix, C., Couronce, A. M., Benamon, D., Amouch, P. & Drouet, J. (1972) Prevention of virus B hepatitis (SH hepatitis). *American Journal of Diseases of Children*, 123, 429–434.

Sternlieb, I. & Scheinberg, I. H. (1972) Chronic hepatitis as a first manifestation of Wilson's disease. *Annals of Internal Medicine*, 76, 59–64.

Stevens, C. E., Beasley, R. P., Tsui, J. & Lee, W. C. (1975) Vertical transmission of hepatitis B antigen in Taiwan. *The New England Journal of Medicine*, 292, 771–774.

Stokes, J., Jr, Farquhar, J. A., Drake, M. E., Capps, R. B., Ward, C. S. & Kitts, A. W. (1951) Infectious hepatitis: length of protection by immune serum globulin (gamma globulin) during epidemics. *Journal of the American Medical Association*, 147, 714–719.

Summary of the National Halothane Study (1966) *Journal of the American Medical Association*, 197, 775-788.

Summerskill, W. H. J., Korman, M. G., Ammon, H. V. & Baggenstoss, A. H. (1975) Prednisone for chronic active liver disease: dose titration, standard dose, and combination with azathioprine compared. *Gut*, 16, 876–883.

Tapp. E., Hollanders, D. & Dymock, I. W. (1975) Progression of histological changes in hepatitis B antigen carriers. *Gut*, 16, 836 (Abstract).

Telatar, H., Kayhan, B., Kes, S. & Karacadag, S. (1974) HBAg in sweat. *Lancet*, ii, 461.

Toh, B. H., Roberts-Thomson, I. C., Matthews, J. D., Whittingham, S. & Mackay, I. R. (1973) Depression of cell mediated immunity in old age and the immunopathic diseases, lupus erythematosus, chronic active hepatitis and rheumatoid arthritis. *Clinical and Experimental Immunology*, 14, 193–202.

Tong, M. J., Sun, S. C., Schaeffer, B. T., Chang, N. K., Lo., K. J. & Peters, R. L. (1971) Hepatitis-associated antigen and hepatocellular carcinoma in Taiwan. *Annals of Internal Medicine*, 75, 687–691.

Trepo, C. G., Zuckerman, A. J., Bird, R. C. & Prince, A. M. (1974) The role of circulating hepatitis B antigen/antibody immune complexes in the pathogenesis of vascular and hepatic manifestations in polyarteritis nodosa. *Journal of Clinical Pathology*, 27, 863-868.

Trepo, C. G., Robert, D., Motin, J., Trepo, D., Sepetjian, M. & Prince, A. M. (1976) Hepatitis B antigen (HB$_s$Ag) and/or antibodies (anti-HB$_s$ and anti-HB$_c$) in fulfilment hepatitis: pathogenic and prognostic significance. *Gut*, 17, 10–13.

Triger, D. R., Alp, M. H. & Wright, R. (1972a) Bacterial and dietary antibodies in liver diseases *Lancet*, i, 60–63.

Triger, D. R., Kurtz, J. B., MacCollum, F. O. & Wright, R. (1972b). Raised antibody titres to measles and rubella viruses in chronic active hepatitis. *Lancet*, i, 665-667.

Triger, D. R. & Wright, R. (1973) Hyperglobulinaemia in liver disease *Lancet*, i, 1494–1496.

Tripatzis, I. & Horst, H. G. (1971) Detection of Australia–SH–antigen in urine. *Nature*, 231, 266–267.

Tygstrup, N. (1963) Halothane hepatitis. *Lancet*, ii, 466–467.

Van Waes, L., Segers, J., Van Egmond, J., Van Nimmen, L., Barbier, F., Wieme, R. & Demeulenaere, L. (1974) Chronic liver disease and hepatitis B antigen: a prospective study. *British Medical Journal*, iii, 444–446.

Villarejos, V. M., Visona, K. A., Alvaro Gutierrez, D. & Antonio Rodriguez, A. (1974) Role of saliva, urine and feces in the transmission of type B hepatitis. *New England Journal of Medicine*, 191, 1375–1378.

Virtue, R. W. & Payne, K. W. (1958) Postoperative death after fluothane. *Anesthesiology*, 19, 562–563.

Wacker, W. E. C., Riordan, J. F., Snodgrass, P. J., Chang, L. W., Morse, L. J., O'Brien, T. F. & Reddy, W. J. (1972) The Holy Cross hepatitis outbreak: clinical and chemical abnormalities. *Archives of Internal Medicine*, 130, 357–360.

Walton, B., Dumonde, D. C., Williams, C., Jones, D., Strunin, J. M., Layton, J. M., Strunin, L. & Simpson, R. (1973) Lymphocyte transformation. Absence of increased responses in alleged halothane jaundice. *Journal of the American Medical Association*, 225, 494–498.

Walton, B., Perrin, J., Doniach, D., Strunin, L. & Simpson, G. B. R., Appleyard, A. J. (1976) London Hospital survey of postoperative jaundice. *British Medical Journal*, i, 1171–1176.

Wands, J. R., Walker, J. A., Davis, T. T., Waterbury, L. A., Owens, A. H. & Carpenter, C. C. J. (1974) Hepatitis B in an oncology unit. *New England Journal of Medicine*, 291, 1371–1375.

Ward, R., Borchert, P., Wright, A. & Kline, E. (1972) Hepatitis B antigen in saliva and mouth washings. *Lancet*, ii, 726–727.

Wollheim, F. A. (1968) Immunoglobulins in the course of viral hepatitis and in cholestatic and obstructive jaundice. *Acta medica scandinavica*, 183, 473–479.

Zieve, L. (1966) Hemolytic anaemia in liver disease *Medicine* (Baltimore), 45, 497–505.

Zuckerman, A. J., Bird, R. G., Darnell, R., Farrow, L. J., Stewart, J. S. & Lamb, S. G. (1974) Hepatitis A virus-like particles. *British Medical Journal*, i, 453.

7
SEXUALLY TRANSMITTED DISEASE

J. K. Oates   J. R. W. Harris

The last decade has seen considerable advances in our understanding of sexually transmitted disease. We have endeavoured to discuss certain aspects which we feel are both of interest to general physicians practising in the United Kingdom and of increasing importance in a world with changing patterns of sexual behaviour and an international epidemic of venereal disease.

Approximately 2000 cases of gonococcal septicaemia, with its varying clinical spectrum, present to physicians in the United Kingdom each year. As many as 40 per cent of the patients with hepatitis B may have contracted the infection as a sexually transmitted disease. Herpes (subgroup B) neonatal infection, which has serious and occasionally fatal consequences, can be attributed to a sexually transmitted infection. Infectious syphilis is still with us and ocular, renal, and hepatic involvement during the infectious phase may be more common than we at present realise. Recent tissue typing studies have shown that there is a hereditary predisposition to Reiter's syndrome, although medical microbiologists are still confused about the aetiology of non-specific urethritis.

HERPES GENITALIS

Genital herpes is due to infection with herpes simplex virus type II (HSV II) whilst the common oral lesions are caused by type I strains. The two strains can be separated and in most cases clearly identified in the laboratory (Dowdle et al, 1967). Both grow readily on the chorio-allantoic membrane of fertile hens eggs, HSV II strains producing large necrotic lesions or large plaques of growth which are not seen with type I strains. Other differences between them are apparent in the cytopathogenic effect obtained when they are grown in cell culture. Distinction between the two types is also possible serologically and immuno-fluorescent antibody testing has beem reported upon favourably (Gardner and McQuillan, 1968; Geder and Skinner, 1971). Neutralising antibodies (Hatfield, Wasley and Gray, 1967) can also be detected and a microneutralisation test clearly differentiates the circulating antibodies of the two strains (Nahmias et al, 1970). In spite of these apparently clear-cut differences there are cases in practice where it is not easy to type individual strains by any of these methods.

In routine clinical work the virus is easily grown in culture from a swab taken from suspect lesions into either Hansen's virus transport medium or Stuart's transport medium (Rodin, Hare and Barwell, 1971). Stuart's medium is almost universally available and the results seem to be as good when it is used as those obtained from the more specialised virus medium.

Primary HSV I infections probably occur early in childhood though there is some evidence that in the upper socioeconomic groups these infections are now occurring at a later age than formerly. Nevertheless, about 85 per cent of children will have antibodies to HSV I by about the age of 15 (Smith, Peutherer and MacCallum, 1967).

The incidence of antibodies to HSV II in the general population is not yet as well documented, but figures of 22 per cent in Houston, Texas, are quoted (Rawls et al, 1968) and 33 per cent in Belgium (Sprecher-Goldberger et al, 1970). Type I antibodies do not prevent infections with type II strains (Nahmias et al, 1970) though there is suggestive evidence that the genital strain antibodies do protect against type I infections.

Epidemiology

Much evidence, clinical and serological, exists to show that type II strains are sexually transmitted in the majority of cases though the division between the sites the viruses attack is far from absolute. The increased frequency of orogenital contacts in both homosexual and heterosexual activity gives ample scope for viruses to be found in either site.

Figures as to the incidence of the disorder are not very reliable though there is little doubt in the minds of experienced venereologists that this has increased greatly over the past 15 years. Shelley (1967) found an incidence of 1 case per 500 cytology specimens using as his criteria for diagnosis the presence of intranuclear viral inclusions, a method which is likely to give a considerable underestimate of the true numbers infected. That a considerable genitourinary reservoir exists in the male is made clear by the work of Centifanto et al (1972) who found positive cultures for HSV II in 15 per cent of 190 randomly selected males between the ages of 15 to 85.

Clinical picture

The typical clinical picture of itchy, sometimes painful, grouped vesicles on the genitals is well known. Primary attacks may be very severe with fever, local adenopathy, and systemic symptoms. In women a particularly unpleasant feature is the development of a severe necrotic cervicitis (Willcox, 1968). In women involvement of the urethral region is especially common and may lead to urinary difficulty and retention. Retention may occur without urethral disease and Goldmeier, Bateman and Rodin (1975) have also reported intestinal obstruction occurring in association with HSV II infections. Occasionally meningitis and encephalitis are associated with a primary genital lesion (Skoldenburg, Jeansson and Wolontis, 1973).

Herpes in pregnancy and the neonate

It has now become clear that HSV II infection in late pregnancy can be a serious danger to the fetus — no clear evidence exists that the virus can cross the placental barrier though Nahmias et al (1971b) have recorded in patients with genital herpes an abortion rate which is three times the normal, whilst in primary attacks the rate is even higher. Goldman (1970) has detected herpetic viral inclusions in samples of endometrium. Primary attacks of genital herpes after the thirty-second week of pregnancy appear to carry a high risk of neonatal infection — estimated by Nahmias, Alford and Korones (1971a) as being at least as high as 42 per cent regardless of antibody status. These authors gave details of 142 cases of herpetic infection in the newborn, the great majority of which were type II infections. They found that when the infection was disseminated, the mortality rate was 95 per cent and the overall mortality rate was 71 per cent. With such a serious disorder any measures which might help in its prevention should be considered and several authors now recommend caesarean section in all cases of genital herpes occurring in the last months of pregnancy provided that the membranes have not ruptured (Hare, 1974). In spite of this, clinical observation shows that some infants can be delivered of women with genital herpes virus infections during late pregnancy and escape apparent neonatal infection (St Geme et al, 1975) whilst Ng, Regan and Yen (1970) found no evidence of increased fetal mortality in a large series of pregnant women with genital herpes. Altschuler (1974) has produced evidence that ascending transcervical infection with HSV II can occur and that therefore the fetus of a woman whose herpes has subsided before delivery could theoretically still be at risk.

Relation to carcinoma of the cervix

Strong evidence exists that cancer of the cervix is in some way associated with sexual activity, there being a close relationship between adolescent promiscuity, age at first marriage, age at first pregnancy, and number of pregnancies with the disease (Wynder, 1969). It is likely that some coitally transmitted agent capable of producing mutation in the cervical epithelium leads to the development of cancer. Suspicion fell on the genital strain of herpes virus and many authors have produced striking evidence of an association between infection with the virus and cervical cancer. Neutralising antibodies to HSV II have been found in a far higher percentage of cancer patients than matched controls. Royston and Aurelian (1970) for example found 98 per cent of patients with invasive carcinoma, carcinoma in situ, or atypical cells showed antibodies to HSV II compared with only 55 per cent in controls. Skinner, Thouless and Jordan (1971) examined the serum from patients with cervical carcinoma, genital carcinoma of other sites, and a control group for serological evidence of infection with HSV II. The group with cervical carcinoma showed a higher incidence of infection than all other groups and this was independent of age and socioeconomic class. This epidemiological evidence was supported by the fact that certain herpes viruses are known to be implicated in oncogenesis in both man and animals. The Epstein–Barr virus is most likely the chief factor causing Burkitt's lymphoma (Epstein and Achong, 1973) and is associated with cancer of the postnasal space. Other members of the herpes group cause the Lucke kidney cancer of North American frogs, malignant lymphoma in some monkeys and Marek's lymphoma in chickens. At the moment a definite answer to the question 'Does HSV II virus cause cervical cancer' cannot yet be given. An association between most cases of cervical cancer and HSV II infections seems clear but much further work is required to establish the precise nature and significance of this relationship. It should seem to be prudent practice to ensure cytological follow-up of all patients known to have had genital herpes, especially those where the cervix has been known to be involved clinically.

Treatment

5-Iodo-2'-deoxyuridine, which acts by blocking thymidine and preventing the formation of viral DNA, can be used in a 40 per cent solution in dimethyl sulphoxide (Juel-Jensen, 1973). If applied in the early stages of infection to the lesions four times daily for four to five days, it can be very effective. Unfortunately the site of many lesions in women, for example, makes this an unsuitable form of treatment and symptomatic therapy has to be relied on. Laird and Roy (1975), however, claim that cotrimoxazole is very effective in both relieving symptoms and aiding healing of herpetic ulcers if given in the dosage of two tablets twice daily for five to seven days.

SYPHILIS

Serological Diagnosis

The last decade has seen the introduction of more simple specific tests for treponemal disease. These are based on *Treponema pallidum* as antigen and use immunofluorescence or haemogluttination techniques for the detection of antibody. Unfortunately none of these tests will distinguish syphilis from infections with the other pathogenic treponemes. The advent of these new more specific tests has resulted in a reappraisal of the classical tests for antilipoidal antibody (reagin). The classical tests for reagin have been adapted for automated procedures and tests for reagin would now be regarded as screening procedures (Wilkinson, 1975).

Since a variety of antibodies both anti-treponemal and non-specific are produced during infection with *T. pallidum* and the other pathogenic treponemes the tests to detect these antibodies can be divided into specific and non-specific. The specific tests in common use in hospital laboratories today are the *Treponema pallidum* haemaglutination assay (TPHA) and the fluorescent treponemal antibody absorption test (FTA-ABS) while the simplest and most commonly used reagin (non-specific) tests are the VDRL rapid plasma reagin and automated reagin.

Since patients' sera are negative to all tests in early primary syphilis, no serological test can be relied upon as a sole diagnostic aid in clinical situations where early primary syphilis is a possibility. The FTA-ABS is the most valuable specific test in primary syphilis and one would expect 86 per cent reactivity to the test at this stage. Comparisons of the TPHA and FTA-ABS have shown that both tests have a high sensitivity at all stages of the disease except in primary syphilis when the FTA-ABS is superior. As occasional false positive results have been reported in many of the published series involving both tests verification by the TPI is desirable.

The VDRL slide test has general acceptance as a test of high sensitivity for antilipoidal antibody (Wilkinson, 1972). The rapid plasma reagin (circle) cord

(RPR) test is a further modification which because of its simplicity is a suitable screening test for use in field surveys. Serial quantitative reagin tests are of value in situations where the possibility of repeated infection has to be considered.

Serum immunoglobulin levels in syphilis have been extensively investigated (Wilkinson, 1975). While some syphilitic patients have levels within the normal range the mean IgG and IgM levels are elevated in primary, secondary and latent syphilis. An increase in IgM at an early stage of infection has been noted and it has been suggested that estimations of IgM levels might be of use in assessing activity in late syphilis. FTA-ABS tests with a conjugate specific for IgM antibody were developed and felt to have particular relevance to the mother/neonate situation since the presence of specific IgM antitreponemal antibody was thought to indicate active production of antibody due to infection of the baby. However, many have reservations on the value of IgM studies in this situation.

It is important to remember that the Wassermann complement fixation test (WR) is rarely used nowadays and that the *Treponema pallidum* immobilisation test (TPI) while still used in national reference centres need only be applied to the evaluation of problem sera. It is important to appreciate that the TPI is of no value in clinical situations where reinfection is a possibility.

In practical terms the most simple technical combination of serological investigation on serum would be the VDRL and the TPHA. However, if early primary syphilis is a possibility then the FTA-ABS should also be used. In cases of maternal/neonatal infection and reinfection a study of serum immunoglobulin may be beneficial, and in situations where reinfection is a possibility in an individual whose sera shows persistent reactivity, quantitative reagin tests will be helpful.

The problem of Infectious Syphilis

Only by early diagnosis and treatment of infectious syphilis can tertiary complications be avoided. Early diagnosis also facilitates contact tracing and prevents disease spread. Recent developments in immunological and electron microscopy have improved our understanding of the pathogenesis of infection. As a result there has been a greater appreciation of the nature and degree of renal and hepatic involvement in secondary syphilis.

Infectious syphilis in the United Kingdom is predominantly a disease of males. As the initial inoculation lesion in the male homosexual is frequently anorectal or oropharyngeal, the patient progresses to the secondary stage of the infection with neither patient nor physician suspecting the correct diagnosis (Samenius, 1968).

Infectious Syphilis and the Liver

In the past there has been controversy over the association between syphilis and liver disease. Sherlock (1971) felt that there was only limited evidence for an active hepatitis solely due to spirochaetal infection. Many felt that the hepatic damage was either the result of prior arsphenamine therapy or was due to viral hepatitis which was acquired by infection during intravenous therapy (Harris et al, 1973). A viral aetiology was proposed by Papaevangelou et al (1974a) who noted that hepatitis B virus might be sexually transmitted.

Syphilitic hepatitis which responded dramatically to penicillin therapy was described as a distinct entity by Zellerman and Norcross (1967). Albertazzi, Strani and Sartoris (1970) considered a similar case and discussed the difficulty of distinguishing this condition from viral hepatitis. They felt that there was great similarity between the clinical and histopathological pictures of the two forms of hepatitis. Lee, Thornton and Conn (1971) and Baker et al (1971) felt that syphilitic hepatitis during the infectious phase of syphilis was a distinct entity. They reported cases of patients presenting with hepatic tenderness, jaundice, and the rash of secondary syphilis. They found gross elevation of alkaline phosphatase levels to more than 10 times the normal value and noted that this was a disproportionate increase in relation to the transaminase rise. Histological pictures unlike those found in viral hepatitis were noted by Baker et al (1971) and Sobel and Wolf (1972). As Australia antigen was not present in these patients and there was a rapid response to antibiotic therapy it was felt that active syphilitic hepatitis was a distinct entity.

Feher, Somogyi and Timmer (1975) reported a number of patients with early untreated syphilis who were found to have abnormal hepatic function tests, indicating liver damage. Fifteen of these patients had liver biopsies prior to therapy. All 15 had hepatomegaly and four had splenomegaly. Nine of the liver biopsy specimens showed focal liver necrosis in the lobules and proliferation in the walls of branches of central veins, portal veins and arterioles. Treponemes were demonstrated by light and electron microscopy in the hepatic lesions. Penicillin therapy was continued for two months in these cases, and post-therapy biopsy showed healing of liver damage and no treponemes. Many workers would feel that there was no need to continue antibiotic therapy for as long as two months in these cases. Certainly the four patients with this syndrome whom we have treated have responded completely with a 21-day antibiotic course. However, despite controversy over the dosage there is no doubt that hepatitis is definitely a significant clinical component of the secondary stage of syphilis.

Infectious Syphilis of the Kidney

McCracken, Hall and Pierce (1969) reported the association of the nephrotic syndrome and acute hepatitis in a patient with secondary syphilis. Brophy et al (1964) and Falls et al (1965) had already presented the pre-treatment and post-treatment electron microscopic findings on renal biopsy. They observed swelling of the endothelial cells and electron-dense deposits adjacent to either side of the basement membrane and noted fusion of the epithelial foot processes. The abnormalities returned to normal after adequate antibiotic therapy. These findings resemble those observed by Kaplan et al (1972) in the glomerulopathy of congenital syphilis. Braunstein et al (1970), in describing a case of glomerulopathy during secondary syphilis, also noted perivascular mononuclear infiltration and mesangial cell proliferation. They demonstrated that the electron-dense deposits were IgG but were unable to detect complement deposition in the same site. Bhorade, Carag and Lee (1971) were able to demonstrate the presence of these complement deposits (β_{1c}-globulin) on electron microscopy.

Neurosyphilis

Widespread use of antibiotics and psychoactive drugs may be responsible for altering the psychiatric, neurological, and serological components of neuro-syphilis (Gowardman, 1970). Undue reliance on clinical and laboratory features which were established in the pre-antibiotic era is outmoded (Mahony et al, 1972). There is an increasing awareness that neurosyphilis today has a widely variable symptomatology and clinical presentation (Wetherill, Webb and Catterall, 1965).

An excellent prospective study of neurosyphilis, from the Medical College of Virginia, was published in 1972 by Hooshmand, Escobar and Kopf. From July 1965 until July 1970 they evaluated 251 patients who were diagnosed as having neurosyphilis. The value of this study is that it gives a clinical spectrum of neurosyphilis in the antibiotic era. The diagnostic criteria used by the authors were as follows:

(a) Positive blood and CSF FTA-ABS with abnormal white cells counts in CSF (more than 5 white cells/mm^3 (5×10^6/litre), with no evidence of bacterial or viral meningitis).
(b) Positive blood FTA-ABS and ophthalmic or neurological findings sugges-tive of neurosyphilis.
(c) Positive blood and CSF FTA-ABS in patients with progressive neurological symptoms in whom other aetiological factors had been ruled out.

While one might not agree with a figure as low as 5 white cells/mm^3 (5×10^6/litre), there is no doubt that the non-specific tests, such as the Wassermann, which were previously used in the CSF, are of little value. Indeed, Fulford et al (1972) reported six patients with a neurological disorder associated with chronic biological false-positive Wassermann serology which resembled multiple sclerosis. Gowardman (1970) and Dewhurst (1968) both remarked that a negative serological or CSF non-treponemal test did not exclude the diagnosis of neurosyphilis. Grahmann (1969) showed the limitations of the Lange curve, while Scalla and Fucci (1970) observed that CSF leucocyte count and protein levels were frequently normal in the presence of neurosyphilis. This reliance on non-specific serological and CSF tests, CSF total protein levels and CSF leucocyte levels is unjustified nowadays.

DISSEMINATED GONOCOCCAL DISEASE

During the past 10 years there has been a progressive increase in the incidence of gonorrhoea in the United Kingdom. A commensurate increase might therefore be expected in the number of patients presenting with systemic manifestations of gonococcal infection. An estimated 1.9 per cent of patients with gonorrhoea will develop a disseminated infection (Barr and Danielsson,

1971) so one might postulate that at least 2000 patients would present each year to physicians in the United Kingdom with disseminated gonococcal disease. Yet there is a relative absence of reports of such cases in the literature from the United Kingdom as compared with the literature from North America and Europe (Harris, McCann and Mahony, 1973). Indeed, the three largest British series published to date — Wolff, Goodman and Vahrman (1970), Harris et al (1973) and Seifert, Miller and Warin (1973) — together discuss a total of only 24 patients, while Barr and Danielsson (1971) reported a series of 23 patients from a population of 250 000 in a rural area of Sweden.

Clinical features

The condition, in both its symptomatic and asymptomatic forms, has a wide spectrum of clinical presentation, including arthritis or arthralgia, tenosynovitis, intermittent pyrexia, a haemorrhagic vesiculopustular rash, abdominal pain, hepatomegaly, hepatitis, chest pain relating to pericarditis, and neck stiffness with meningitis. With such a degree of multisystem involvement the various series will be slanted towards the specialities in which the authors practise. Hence rheumatologists will report series where the majority of the patients will have arthropathies as the dominant feature while studies from infectious diseases units will show a predominance of cases presented with pyrexia and associated skin lesions. Disseminated gonococcal infection is much more common in women than in men (Graber, Sanford and Ziff, 1960), which would appear to be the result of adequate early treatment of acute urethritis in many males.

Asymptomatic gonorrhoea is a frequent source of disseminated infection. The dissemination may result from asymptomatic anorectal (Holmes, Counts and Beaty, 1971) and pharyngeal (Metzger, 1970) sites as well as from asymptomatic genital sources. Patients who have symptomatic infection or local complications of gonorrhoea, however, may also develop the disseminated form of the disease. Therefore, in addition to the multisystem clinical presentation referred to above, one can also find associated urethritis, pharyngitis, proctitis, salpingitis, or epididymitis.

There would appear to be several phases in the septicaemic process. Initially transient gonococcal bacteraemia occurs. The patients develop petechial, papular and vesiculopustular skin lesions with transient arthralgia, myalgia and pyrexia (Bjornberg, 1970). Many of these patients, if untreated, will progress to the 'septic' phase, although in some recovery appears to occur even before antibiotics are given (Abu-Nasser, Hill and Fred, 1963). In the 'septic' phase polyarthropathy, tenosynovitis, rigors and cutaneous lesions predominate, and hepatic involvement, as indicated by abnormal liver function tests, may also occur. Myocarditis or pericarditis is an infrequent accompaniment, and a number of cases of gonococcal meningitis and endocarditis (Holmes et al, 1971) have been reported.

Diagnosis

Diagnosis of disseminated gonococcal infection is dependent upon clinical suspicion and the recognition of *Neisseria gonorrhoeae*. Routine cultures using selective Thayer–Martin type media (Thayer and Martin, 1966) should be set up with material taken from the urethra, rectum and oropharynx in the male and from the cervix, urethra, rectum and oropharynx in the female. The simplest method is to heavily inoculate the appropriate agar medium directly with the culture swab at the time of examination. The medium should be placed in a candle jar. Various alternative methods for providing CO_2 by prepacking Thayer–Martin medium in small sealed bottles containing increased CO_2 (Transgrow) are convenient but not essential (Martin and Lester, 1971). It is much more rewarding to attempt to culture the gonococcus from the sites listed than from blood samples. Lack of appreciation of this fact is a frequent reason for delay or failure in diagnosis. Bacteriological diagnosis is dependent upon the particular case and the sites from which the specimens are taken, the use of viable transport systems and selective culture media (Bro-Jørgensen and Jensen, 1973; Babb, 1974; Holmes, 1974). A provisional diagnosis may be made on recognition of intracellular diplococci in Gram-stained specimens from the urethra, cervix and rectum (Harris et al, 1973) but, although this facilitates rapid treatment, it cannot replace cultures as a reliable diagnostic method.

Treatment

The treatment of disseminated gonococcal infection has not been systematically studied. Until 1973 it was assumed that the gonococcal strains involved were those with a high antibiotic resistance. Hence most patients were treated with parenteral aqueous or procaine penicillin G given in doses ranging from 2.4 to 10 million units daily. It was felt that the minimum dosage used should also be effective in controlling potentially serious complications such as meningitis and endocarditis. Antibiotic therapy was continued for 14 days, or until there was a complete remission of symptoms and follow-up studies were negative. Instillation of penicillin into joint cavities had by this time been discontinued (Schmid and Parker, 1969).

However, in 1973 Weisner, Handsfield and Holmes observed that the strains of gonococci causing disseminated infection had all a high degree of sensitivity to penicillin. Thus doses of 10 million units of penicillin daily are probably unnecessary. Certainly, we have treated more than 20 cases since then and have never used more than 2.4 mega procaine penicillin daily. Alternative effective drugs are tetracycline and trimethoprinsulphomethoxole. The latter combination has in our experience been most successful when the patient gave a history of penicillin hypersensitivity.

NON-SPECIFIC URETHRITIS

Non-specific genital infection provides the venereologist with one of his biggest problems. It is diagnosed whenever signs and symptoms of genital infection are present and efficient microbiological tests fail to demonstrate a pathogen. Such a definition is likely to cover a number of different entities and King (1972) reviewing the problem considered non-specific genital infection to include urethritis, abacterial or haemorrhagic cystitis, prostatitis and epididymitis in men; and cervicitis, Bartholinitis, abacterial pyuria and pelvic inflammatory disease in women. By far the commonest presentation of the condition is non-specific urethritis (NSU) and most of the research effort over the last 15 years has been directed towards attempts to isolate and define the causative agent or agents.

NSU is only notifiable in the United Kingdom and in 1951 there were 10 794 cases. There has been a steady increase year by year with 85 015 cases being reported in 1973 and NSU is now commoner than gonococcal urethritis. Microbiological research has tended to concentrate on two main groups of organisms as potential causes of NSU. These groups are the genital myco-plasmas and the genus *Chlamydia*.

Genital mycoplasmas

The varieties which produce large colonies on artificial culture medium now seem unlikely to be connected in any significant way with urethritis, but those which form tiny colonies ('T' strains) are still the subject of controversy as to their possible aetiological role. For example, 'T' strains have been found more commonly in NSU than in controls by Shephard (1966), Csonka, Williams and Corse (1966), Shipley, Bowman and O'Connor (1968), Sueltmann et al (1971). On the other hand the organisms have been found in roughly similar frequencies in control subjects and NSU sufferers by Fowler and Leeming (1969), Haas, Dorfman and Sacks (1971) and Lassus et al (1971). In one study more were found in the control subjects than patients (Black and Rasmussen, 1968). 'T' mycoplasmas are sensitive to tetracyclines and to erythromycin whilst being insensitive to lincomycin. As the first two are effective in treating NSU and lincomycin is not (Csonka and Spitzer, 1969), this information is at least compatible with the organisms being a cause of NSU. On balance as in the large colony mycoplasmas, there is as yet no convincing evidence that 'T' strains are a significant cause of NSU. It is possible that they may cause other manifestations of non-specific genital infection such as salpingitis as well as being possibly related to abortion, puerperal fever and infertility. Reviews of the genital mycoplasmas and their disease potential are given by Ford (1970), and McCormack et al (1973).

The genus Chlamydia

The *Chlamydia* group of agents are now known to be responsible for much infectious eye disease in the form of trachoma and inclusion conjunctivitis. T'ang et al (1957) isolated the agent from patients with trachoma by using the yolk sacs of fertile hen's eggs. Subsequently the disease was reproduced by inoculation of the conjunctivae of volunteers (Collier, Duke-Elder and Jones, 1958). The same agent was isolated by Jones, Collier and Smith (1959) from patients with ophthalmia neonatorum and subsequently from other babies, from the genital tracts of their mothers, and from their fathers who had NSU (Dunlop, Jones and Al-Hussaini, 1964; Dunlop et al 1967. *Chlamydia* were then isolated from 21 per cent of men who presented with NSU and 35 per cent of their female contacts were also found to be infected (Dunlop et al, 1967). Isolates from genital material have subsequently been made in many countries and it seems clear that the condition has a world-wide distribution. Improvements in the tests for chlamydial infection have included the use of irradiated McCoy cells (Magruder et al, 1963) instead of the less efficient yolk sac method, the addition of serum to the transport medium with storage in liquid nitrogen and high-speed centrifugation (Darougar et al, 1972). With these methods isolates have been obtained from 44 of 99 men with NSU and 10 of their 34 female partners (Dunlop et al, 1972). Other workers have had similar success (Oriel et al, 1972; Richmond, Hilton and Clarke, 1972) and the use of the cell culture method has permitted the isolation of *Chlamydia* from the rectum whereas in the past tests from this site had always given negative results. *Chlamydia* were isolated from the cervix of 33 per cent of women who were consorts of men with NSU by Oriel et al (1974) and Hilton et al (1974) who also noted an even higher rate in those women who were also infected with gonorrhoea.

Further evidence about the scope and extent of chlamydial infections may be obtained by the use of the micro-immunofluorescence test (Wang, 1971) which allows the identification of individual serotypes of *Chlamydia* which should be of great assistance in epidemiological studies. However, much further work is required before the test is of use in clinical work.

It seems clear that *Chlamydia* is emerging as a significant cause of NSU in the male. Much evidence points to the importance of infection of the female partner — it has been shown for example that salpingitis occurs frequently in the mothers of babies with chlamydial opthalmia (Dunlop et al, 1967; op. cit. Mordhurst and Dawson, 1971). This female reservoir of infection must play a large part in the sustained increase year by year of cases of NSU in males. Female contacts of NSU frequently either are not examined or do not receive treatment as physical examination and current routine tests show little, if any, abnormality.

Treatment

With most cases lacking a defined cause, treatment remains very largely empirical. There is general agreement that penicillin is of little use in the treatment of NSU whilst sulphonamides, alone or in combination with injections of streptomycin, also produce very disappointing results. The tetracyclines appear to be reasonably effective and are currently the most widely prescribed drugs for this disorder. Erythromycin and spiramycin are similarly effective and will sometimes produce a 'cure' when a tetracycline has failed. Holmes et al (1967) showed in a double blind trial the effectiveness of tetracycline compared with a placebo and Johns (1971) produced evidence suggesting that better results were obtained by giving tetracyclines for a longer period of time. His patients who were treated for 21 days with 250 mg of oxytetracycline six-hourly achieved a cure rate of 87.5 per cent compared with 55 and 75 per cent for 5 and 10 day treatment schedules of different dosages of the same drug. Battacharaya and Morton (1973) using a triple tetracycline (Deteclo) 300 mg twice daily for 21 days claimed a recurrence rate of only 11.8 per cent three months after treatment and no recurrences in the first month following treatment. However, as Fowler (1970) in a double blind trial of tetracycline 250 mg four times daily for four days found that this regime was only a little better than a placebo in the form of lactose tablets, it is possible that these results can be attributed to the short duration of treatment with the antibiotic.

REITER'S DISEASE

The clinical pattern of this confusing disorder has now been well documented and good general reviews are given by Hancock (1964) and Csonka (1965).

Epidemiology

The fact that Reiter's disease commonly follows attacks of diarrhoea or dysentery in some parts of the world such as Africa, Asia, and Eastern Europe whilst in others, for example, the United Kingdom and North America, it is seen following urogenital infection usually acquired by sexual intercourse has not yet been explained. These differences, however, may be more apparent than real as both forms of the illness can coexist in the community (Davis, Haverty and Boatwright, 1969). Historically, some of the earliest accounts of Reiter's disease describe it amongst military populations where sexually transmitted and dysenteric disorders are very common.

The incidence of the disorder is difficult to assess accurately. If for example it is assumed that Reiter's disease 'complicates' non-specific urethritis (NSU) in the male, figures of between 1 and 2 per cent are usually quoted. In 1972 62 498 men with NSU attended clinics for sexually transmitted disease in Britain and 447 developed arthritis, an incidence less than 1 per cent. Harris (1975) pointed out that it would be unwise to assume figures such as these to be representative of the whole community, as inevitably a disease's incidence is bound to be underestimated if the statistics relating to only one of the specialities where it may be present, are considered.

Aetiology

All races appear to be equally susceptible and there are no limitations as to age and sex though it is recognised at least 10 times more frequently in males than in females. As might be expected the majority of cases in childhood are associated with an attack of dysentery and Moss (1964) in reviewing the literature emphasised that iritis and, to a less extent, keratitis were both commoner and tended to be more severe than in adults. Research directed towards determining whether a specific infecting agent or agents play any part in inducing the disorder has continued. Mycoplasmas in view of their ability to cause arthritis in animals (Decker and Ward, 1966) and their undoubted ability, on occasion, to cause genital infection in man has led to their association with Reiter's disease being carefully investigated and a few workers have isolated the organisms from joint fluid (Claus et al, 1964; Dunlop et al, 1969). Other workers however have failed to confirm these observations (Sharp, 1970) and some have concluded that a relationship between mycoplasma infection and Reiter's disease is unlikely (Taylor-Robinson et al, 1969; McCormack et al, 1973). Perhaps the only way that these organisms could be implicated in the disease would be the concept of a strain which cannot be cultured by current techniques and whose presence (at a site possibly remote from the joints) may induce immunological changes which are themselves responsible for the disorder. No direct evidence for this concept exists. Ford (1970) and Smith and Ward (1971) agree that the association for Reiter's disease and mycoplasma infection still merits further study.

The association of chlamydial infection with many cases of NSU has led to work which suggests that they may also play some part in Reiter's disease. Isolates have been obtained from synovial fluid, synovial membrane, conjunctiva and urethra (Schachter et al, 1966; Schachter, 1967; Dunlop et al, 1967; Ostler et al, 1971) though these findings have to be interpreted in the light of the fact that the culture method employed, namely isolation in the yolk sac, is one known to be prone to cross-infection in the laboratory (Harper et al, 1967). Using the cell culture method which does not have this drawback and is also more sensitive, no isolates have so far been obtained from synovial fluids though urethral isolates were obtained from 3 of 10 untreated patients (Vaughn-Jackson et al, 1972) and from both urethral and conjunctival material (Gordon et al, 1973).

Serological evidence suggesting an association between chlamydial infection and some cases of Reiter's disease exists in the many studies showing significant titres (usually 1 in 16 or more) with the lymphogranuloma complement fixation test (Barwell et al, 1967; Kinsella, Norton and Ziff, 1968; Schachter, 1971). By using the much more specific micro-immunofluorescent test a considerable percentage of patients with Reiter's disease show evidence suggesting chlamydial infection (Dwyer et al, 1972). Finally the experimental inoculation of *Chlamydia* into the knee joints of macaque monkey produces a self-limiting arthritis (Smith et al, 1973) and in rabbits, a chronic arthritis. Treatment of these rabbits with penicillin or tetracycline could reverse the process though the longer the delay in starting treatment the longer the arthritis persisted (Gilbert et al, 1973).

The occurrence of familial cases of Reiter's disease has suggested that genetic factors may be of importance and Lawrence (1974) produced the first survey of relatives of patients with the disorder. He examined clinically and radiologically 110 relatives of patients with Reiter's disease and compared them with the relatives of patients with ankylosing spondylitis, psoriatic arthropathy and Still's disease. He found that psoriasis occurred about nine times more frequently in the male relatives of patients with Reiter's disease than in the normal population. In these relatives, ankylosing spondylitis was found eight times, and radiological evidence of sacro-iliitis, three times more frequently than in the normal population. This figure closely approaches that found in Still's disease and spondylitic families.

Some further insight into this genetic linkage has come with the study of the association of human leucocyte antigens and disease. Brewerton et al (1973a) showed that 97 per cent of their patients with ankylosing spondylitis possessed the antigen HLA B27 compared with a frequency in the normal population of 4 per cent. Subsequent work (Brewerton et al, 1973b; Harris et al, 1974) has shown that about 76 per cent of patients with Reiter's disease have HLA B27 and about 55 per cent of those with acute anterior uveitis (Brewerton et al, 1973c). What precise part the antigen plays in the development of any of these disorders is not clear, but it may be that its importance lies in the fact that it is linked to a number of immune response genes which are believed to control specific immune responses including those to infections. To the clinician, the determination of HLA status is not often of much help — for example, it has been estimated that less than 5 per cent of patients who possess HLA B27 will develop ankylosing spondylitis, so such information has little predictive value. However, in individual cases of diagnostic difficulty knowledge of HLA status may be enough to help the clinician to come to a firm conclusion.

Clinical Features

Though these in the main are well established some aspects of them deserve emphasis as do some more recent clinical observations.

Lesions of mucous membranes

Lesions of the genital mucous membrane in men in the form of circinate or Reiter's balanitis occur in about one-quarter of all patients but there is little doubt that this particular manifestation still frequently goes unremarked. Similar lesions on the mucous membrane of lips, mouth, tongue and palate are almost certainly as common but as they tend to appear early in the disease and to cause few symptoms they are not noted unless the mouth is routinely inspected. From time to time symptomatic stomatitis, which can be severe, develops and diagnosis may be difficult if development of the lesions has not been observed. Gatter and Moskowitz (1962) record the development of pneumonitis in a young man with such a stomatitis and they suggest the pulmonary lesion could have been due to the extension of the inflammatory process to the trachobronchial tree.

Lesions of skin

Keratoderma blenorrhagica (KD) the characteristic skin lesion of Reiter's disease, is present in only one-quarter of patients and is seen much more frequently (but by no means exclusively) in the more severe attack. Clinical and pathological observations of the developed lesions do not permit differentiation from those of pustular or rupioid psoriasis (Wright and Reed, 1964; Perry and Mayne, 1965; Maxwell, 1965). A few patients with Reiter's disease (which is always severe and recurrent) eventually exhibit the typical clinical features of severe psoriatic arthropathy (Khan and Hall, 1965; Maxwell et al, 1966).

Involvement of the eye

Mild, sometimes recurrent, conjunctivitis in about 25 per cent of cases is an accepted feature of the disorder as is the much more serious anterior uveitis which develops in a similar percentage of patients especially those with severe forms of disease. Uveitis however may develop after the acute manifestations have subsided so that the diagnosis may not be immediately apparent. Catterall (1960) showed that Reiter's disease was present in 52 of 176 unselected cases of anterior uveitis attending the Institute of Ophthalmology, an incidence of nearly 30 per cent.

Involvement of cardiovascular system

Conduction defects (Nossen et al, 1975), pericarditis, myocarditis, and aortic valve disease are all known to occur: valve disease which appears to be identical in every way to that seen in ankylosing spondylitis has attracted especial attention and has been reviewed by Collins (1972). The valve lesion has been observed to develop from 4 to 31 years after the first attack of Reiter's disease, and Block (1972) produced evidence that on occasion aortic incompetence may develop rapidly and suggested the need for careful follow-up of patients in order to detect such abnormalities as soon as possible.

Miscellaneous

Thrombophlebitis in association with the disease has been recorded by Csonka (1966 and Lemke (1965). Spontaneous rupture of the synovial capsule of the knee joint which has been noted in Reiter's disease (Weese and McCarty, 1969; Garner and Mowat, 1972) can closely mimic thrombophlebitis and arthograms may be necessary to establish the precise diagnosis.

Radiological changes

These have been studied by many authors, and comprise erosions and periosteal new bone formation as seen in many forms of arthritis. In some chronic cases of Reiter's disease there is a striking almost pathognomonic tendency for the development of large rough calcaneal spurs with extensive fluffy periosteal new bone formation (Mason et al, 1959). The sacro-iliac joints show abnormalities in a high percentage of chronic cases estimated at 75 per cent after five years (Delbarre, Amor and Panahi, 1969).

Laboratory diagnosis

No specific tests for the diagnosis of Reiter's disease exist. Pekin, Malinim and Zuafler (1967) drew attention to the finding of high levels of haemolytic complement in the synovial fluid of patients with Reiter's disease (in excess of 140 units and often over 170 units). High levels were also found in the serum and they suggested this may be of help in differential diagnosis especially from rheumatoid arthritis which typically has low values. They also described the presence of large macrophages of a unique character which they found in a high percentage of synovial fluids from affected joints in Reiter's disease. The cells ('Pekin cells') are large spherical vacuolated cells about 40 μm in diameter which frequently contain many polymorphs along with deeper staining basophilic structures. They suggested these cells could be the result of the response to whatever the provocative factor in Reiter's disease is — for example, macro-phages could be expected early in the inflammatory response to either a local endotoxin produced by an infective agent in the joint or in the necessary 'processing' of any foreign antigen in the same site.

Prognosis

Accurate date about the long-term outcome of Reiter's disease is still very scanty and therefore the study by Sarainen, Paronen and Mähonen (1969) who reviewed 100 of the 350 cases of Reiter's disease which occurred in an epidemic of dysentery in Finland in the early 1940s is of particular interest. They compared them with a control group of 100 males matched for age and occupation and found that 42 per cent of the Reiter's disease patients had some permanent disability. These disabilities included 32 per cent with 'rheumatoid spondylitis', 18 per cent with chronic arthritis and 7 per cent with recurrent iritis. A somewhat surprising finding was that only 20 per cent had remained symptom-free after recovering from the first attack. Others have recorded the development of amyloidosis in chronic cases (Bleehen, Everall and Tighe, 1966).

Treatment

This for the great majority of patients still consists of a combination of bed rest, choice of a suitable analgesic, and skilled physiotherapy. The choice of analgesic depends very much on the clinician though in general phenylbutazone, oxyphenylbutazone, and indomethacin seem to be of especial help. It is perhaps salutory to recall that most of the deaths recorded in Reiter's disease appear to be due to a complication of treatment — haemoptysis following large doses of aspirin (Welper, 1942, Denko et al, 1964) — hepatic necrosis with phenyl-butazone (Catterall, 1968). A common feature in many patients is the presence of a large tense effusion in the knee joint. Aspiration of this fluid affords rapid relief of pain and possibly speeds the process of recovery (Nicol, 1970; Boyle and Buchan, 1971).

Oral preparations of steroid hormones have in general been disappointing though some patients will respond extremely well.

The use of folic acid antagonists in the treatment of rupioid psoriasis led to these agents being successfully used in cases of Reiter's disease with extensive keratoderma (Mullins et al, 1967; Farber, Forshner and O'Quinn, 1967). Other authors have reported that methotrexate has in addition given good results in patients who have persistent active disabling joint disease (Jetton and Duncan, 1969; Krebs, Kung and Honnat, 1971). The use of these dangerous drugs for such a disease as Reiter's disease should only be undertaken after very careful consideration.

SEXUAL TRANSMISSION OF VIRAL HEPATITIS B
(see also Chapter 6)

The discovery of Australian antigen (HBAg) (Blumberg, Alter and Visnich, 1965) and its association with viral hepatitis type B (Prince, 1968; Giles et al, 1969) led to the observation that cases of infection could occur where there was clearly no history of parenteral exposure. Alternative routes of transmission were explored. Krugman, Giles and Hammond (1967) indicated the importance of an oral route. Since there was a predominance of males among those affected by the type B virus Blumberg, Sutnick and London (1968) postulated that homosexual practice might be responsible.

Prince et al (1970) noted that 55 per cent of adult patients with hepatitis who were HBAg positive gave no history of parenteral exposure. Vahrman (1970) endorsed the hypothesis of Blumberg et al (1968) that homosexual practice was in some way responsible for the male/female infection ratio. Hersh et al (1971), while being unable to establish the mechanism of transmission, presented evidence that hepatitis type B might spread between sexual partners by non-parenteral routes. Poulsen (1972) reported three cases of such infection developing after sexual contact. At this stage opinion was growing that the non-parenteral spread of the infection, in Western communities at least, was related to sexual contact and in particular to male homosexual contact. Various authors speculated that transmission might occur through the minor skin and mucous membrane lesions caused by sexual contact. Such a view was not incompatible with the belief that oral spread of HBAg was facilitated by blood and serous exudates (Krugman and Giles, 1970).

In 1973 Heathcote and Sherlock published the results of a survey of 67 patients admitted to two London hospitals with acute type B hepatitis. The aim of this survey was to establish the source of infection with the hepatitis B antigen HBAg. Following diagnosis each patient was questioned regarding transfusions, injection with non-disposable or shared needles and tattoos during the previous six months. Social contact with a jaundiced person during the same time was also investigated. Discreet enquiries were then made into the patient's sexual activities. Of the whole group, sexual or domestic contact was the definite or most likely source of infection in 27 patients (40 per cent). Fifteen of the 43 males in the survey admitted homosexual or bisexual habits. Vahrman (1973) in a review of his series of patients with viral hepatitis noted that 20 of the 32 male patients with HBAg positive hepatitis (60 per cent) were homosexual.

Two studies from London investigated the relationship between sexual practice and infection with type B hepatitis. Fulford et al (1973) and Jefferies et al (1973) determined the prevalence of HBAg among patients attending venereology clinical departments and compared this with the incidence of the antigen among blood donor populations. Both studies showed a high frequency of the antigen among patients attending venereology clinics. The antibody (HBAb) and the antigen were commonly found among promiscuous homosexual patients of British origin while the antigen occurred among non-promiscuous men of Mediterranean origin who were thought to be chronic carriers. A highly significant correlation was found for the HBAg group with a history of both syphilis and gonorrhoea. Since the immunodiffusion test which was used by the Middlesex Hospital group is relatively insensitive when compared with the haemagglutination test (Vyas and Schulman, 1970), Fulford and his colleagues speculated that over 80 per cent of the patients who admitted homosexual contact would have been HBAg positive.

Jefferies et al (1973), from St Mary's Hospital, London, also found that the great majority of patients who were HBAg positive were either male homosexuals or non-European heterosexuals. Indeed of all male homosexuals studied 3.8 per cent had HBAg on testing by immunoelectrophoresis and gel diffusion.

Certain objections to the use of blood donor populations as a control group in studies of this nature were raised by Wallace (1973) since anyone with a previous history of jaundice will be excluded from such populations. While these comments are relevant they in no way invalidate the observations that in the clinic population studied a highly significant correlation was demonstrated between the possession of HBAg, HBAb, homosexual practice, and prior infection with syphilis and gonorrhoea.

Until this time the emphasis in sexual transmission had been on male homosexual practice. The male homosexual seen in an urban cosmopolitan community frequently has a high promiscuity index (Harris et al, 1972), and the work of Papaevangelou et al (1973) and Henigst (1973) related the sexual transmission of type B hepatitis to promiscuity. Since both studied female prostitutes the suggestion that transmission was something specific to male homosexual relationships was negated.

Papaevangelou and his colleagues in Athens published a preliminary communication in 1973, and followed this in 1974 with a report of their study of 293 prostitutes who were compared serologically with 379 pregnant women of similar age and socioeconomic group. The prevalence of HBAb was significantly higher ($P<0.001$) in prostitutes than in controls and evidence of hepatitis B virus infections increased with the number of years of prostitution. Henigst (1973), in his series of female prostitutes in Hamburg, found that 2.2 per cent of females with high promiscuity ratings were HBAg carriers.

There would appear to be considerable evidence that in an urban cosmopolitan community the most important factor in the spread of active type B hepatitis is contact with jaundiced or HBAg carriers. The transmission is more likely to occur among sexual partners. Promiscuity favours transmission, as indicated by the high incidence among prostitutes and male homosexuals who appear particularly prone to the disease. There is a related high incidence of syphilis and gonorrhoea. In certain contexts active type B hepatitis behaves as a sexually transmitted disease. The observations of Heathcote, Cameron and Dane (1974) that HBAg was detectable in small quantities in the saliva and semen of patients who were serum carriers may indicate potential modes of transmission.

The physician who cares for patients with active type B hepatitis, being aware of this mode of transmission, should also seek to exclude the possibility of other sexually transmitted infections.

REFERENCES

Abu-Nasser, H., Hill, N. & Fred, H. L. (1963) Cutaneous manifestations of gonococcaemia. *Archives in Internal Medicine (Chicago)*, **112**, 731–737.

Albertazzo, A., Strani, G. F. & Sartoris, S. (1970) L'epatite luetica secondaria. Considerazioni cliniche e pathogenetiche presentazione di un caso. *Giornale Italiano di Dermatologia*, **45**, 440–445.

Altschuler, C. (1974) Pathogenesis of congenital herpes virus infection. Case report including a description of the placenta. *American Journal of the Diseases of Children*, **127**, 427–429.

Babb, R. R. (1974) Acute gonorrhoeal proctitis. *American Journal of Gastroenterology*, **61**, 143–144.

Baker, A. L., Kaplan, M. M., Wolfe, H. J. & McGowan, J. A. (1971) Liver disease associated with early syphilis. *New England Journal of Medicine*, **282**, 1422–1423.

Barr, J. & Danielsson, D. (1971) Septic gonococcal dermatitis. *British Medical Journal*, **i**, 482–484.

Bhorade, M. S., Carag, H. B. & Lee, H. J. (1971) Nephropathy of secondary syphilis. A clinical and pathological spectrum. *Journal of the American Medical Association*, **216**, 1159–1166.

Bjornberg, A. (1970) Benign gonococcal sepsis. *Acta detmato-venereologica (Stockholm)*, **50**, 313–316.

Black, F. T. & Rasmussen, O. G. (1968) Occurrence of T-strains and other mycoplasmata in non-gonococcal urethritis. *British Journal of Venereal Diseases*, **44**, 324–330.

Bleehen, S. S., Everall, J. D. & Tighe, J. R. (1966) Amyloidosis complicating Reiter's syndrome. *British Journal of Venereal Diseases*, **42**, 88–92.

Block, S. R. (1972) Reiter's syndrome and acute aortic insufficiency. *Arthritis and Rheumatism*, **15**, 218–220.

Blumberg, B. S., Alter, H. J. & Visnich, S. (1965) A 'new' antigen in leukaemic sera. *Journal of the American Medical Association*, **191**, 541–546.

Blumberg, B. S., Sutnick, A. I. & London, W. T. (1968) Hepatitis and leukaemia — their relation to Australia antigen. *Bulletin of the New York Academy of Medicine*, **44**, 1566–1586.

Boyle, J. A. & Buchanan, W. W. (1971) *Clinical Rheumatology*, pp. 262–281. Oxford and Edinburgh: Blackwell.

Braunstein, G. D., Lewis, E. J., Galvawek, E. G., Hamilton, A. & Bell, W. R. (1970) The nephrotic syndrome associated with secondary syphilis. An immune deposit disease. *American Journal of Medicine*, **48**, 643–648.

Brewerton, D. A., Caffrey, M., Hart, F. D., James, D. C. O., Nicholls, A. & Sturrock, R. D. (1973a) Ankylosing spondylitis and HLA-27. *Lancet*, **i**, 904–907.

Brewerton, D. A., Caffrey, M., Nicholls, A., Walters, D. & James, D. C. O. (1973b) Acute anterior uveitis and HLA-27. *Lancet*, **ii**, 994–996.

Brewerton, D. A., Caffrey, M., Nicholls, A., Walters, D., Oates, J. K. & James, D. C. O. (1973c) Reiter's disease and HLA-27. *Lancet*, **ii**, 996–998.

Bro-Jørgensen, A. & Jensen, T. (1973) Pharangeal gonorrhoea. *British Journal of Venereal Diseases*, **49**, 491–494.

Brophy, E. M., Ashworth, C. T., Arias, M. & Reynolds, I. (1964) Acute syphilitic nephrosis in pregnancy. *Obstetrics and Gynaecology*, **24**, 930–937.

Catterall, R. D. (1968) Fatal reaction to phenylbutazone in a patient with Reiter's disease. *British Journal of Venereal Diseases*, **44**, 151–153.

Centifanto, Y. M., Drylie, D. M., Deardourf, S. L. & Kaufman, H. E. (1972) Herpes virus type II in the male genito-urinary tract. *Science*, **178**, 318–319.

Claus, G., McEwen, C., Brunner, T. & Tsamparlis, G. (1964) Microbiological studies of Reiter's disease. *British Journal of Venereal Disease*, **40**, 170–180.

Collier, L. H., Duke-Elder, S. & Jones, B. R. (1958) Experimental trachoma produced by cultured virus. *British Journal of Ophthalmology*, **42**, 705–720.

Csonka, G. (1965) Reiter's syndrome. *Ergebnisse der inneren Medizin und Kinderheilkunde*, **23**, 125–189.

Csonka, G. W., Williams, R. E. O. & Corse, J. (1966) T-strain mycoplasma in non-gonococcal urethritis. *Lancet*, **i**, 1292–1296.

Csonka, G. (1966) Thrombophlebitis in Reiter's syndrome. *British Journal of Venereal Diseases*, **42**, 93–95.

Csonka, G. W. & Spitzer, R. J. (1969) Lincomycin non-gonococcal urethritis and mycoplasmata. *British Journal of Venereal Diseases*, **45**, 52–54.

Darougar, S., Kinnison, J. R. & Jones, B. R. (1971) Simplified irradiated McCoy cell culture for isolation of *Chlamydia*. *Trachoma and Related Disorders*, ed. Nichols, R. L. pp. 63–70. Amsterdam: Excerpta Medica.

Darougar, S., Jones, B. R., Kinnison, J. R., Vaughan–Jackson, J. D. & Dunlop, E. M. C. (1972) Chlamydial infections: advances in the diagnostic isolation of *chlamydia*, including TRIC agent, from the eye, genital tract and rectum. *British Journal of Venereal Diseases*, **48**, 416–420.

Davies, N. E., Haverty, J. R. & Boatwright, M. (1969) Reiter's disease associated with shigellosis. *Southern Medical Journal*, **62**, 1011–1014.

Decker, J. L. & Ward, J. R. (1966) The relationship of mycoplasma (PPLO) to rheumatoid arthritis and related diseases. *Bulletin on Rheumatic Diseases*, **16**, 412–413.

Delbarre, F., Amor, B. & Panahi, F. (1969) L'atteinte pelvispondylarthritique dans le rhumatisme de Fiersinger–Leroy–Reiter. *Semaine des hôpitaux; therapeutique (Paris)*, **45**, 563–570.

Denko, C. W. and van Haam, E. (1963) Reiter's syndrome: clinicopathological study of a fatal case. *Journal of the American Medical Association*, **186**, 632–636.

Dewhurst, K. (1968) Atypical serology in neurosyphilis. *Journal of Neurology, Neurosurgeru and Psychiatry*, **31**, 496–500.

Dowdle, W. R., Nahmias, A. J., Harwell, R. W. & Pauls, F. P. (1967) Association of antigenic type of herpes virus hominus with site of viral recovery. *Journal of Immunology*, **99**, 974–980.

Dunlop, E. M. C., Jones, B. R. & Al-Hussain, M. K. (1964) Genital infection in association with TRIC virus infection of the eye. III. *British Journal of Venereal Diseases*, **40**, 33–42.

Dunlop, E. M. C., Freedman, A., Garland, J. A., Harper, I. A., Jones, B. R., Race, J. W., Du Toit, M. S. & Treharne, J. D. (1967) Infection by bedsoniae and the possibility of spurious isolation. 2. Genital infection, disease of the eye, Reiter's disease. *American Journal of Ophthalmology*, **63**, supplement 1073–1081.

Dunlop, E. M. C., Vaughan-Jackson, J. D., Darougar, S. & Jones, B. R. (1972) Chlamydial infection: Incidence in non-specific urethritis. *British Journal of Venereal Diseases*, **48**, 425–428.

Dwyer, R. St C., Treharne, J. D., Jones, B. R. & Herring, J. (1972) Chlamydial infection: results of micro-immunofluorescence tests for the detection of type-specific antibody in certain chlamydial infections. *British Journal of Venereal Diseases*, **48**, 452–459.

Epstein, M. A. & Achong, B. C. (1973) Various forms of Epstein–Barr virus infection in man: established facts and a general concept. *Lancet*, ii, 836–839.

Falls, W. F., Ford, K. L., Ashworth, C. J. & Carter, N. W. (1965) The nephrotic syndrome in secondary syphilis: report of a case with renal biopsy findings. *Annals of Internal Medicine*, 63, 1047–1058.

Farber, G. A., Forshner, J. C. & O'Quinn, S. E. (1967) Reiter's syndrome: treatment with methotrexate. *Journal of the American Medical Association*, 200, 171–173.

Feher, J., Somogyi, T. & Timmer, M. (1975) Early syphilitic hepatitis. *Lancet*, ii, 896–899.

Ford, D. K. (1970) The role of myocoplasmas in genital tract infections of man. In *The Role of Mycoplasmas and L Forms of Bacteria in Disease*, ed. Sharp, J. T., pp. 137–146. Springfield, Illinois: C. C. Thomas.

Ford, D. K., Rasmussen, G. & Minken, J. (1967) T-strain pleuropneumonia-like organisms as one cause of non-gonococcal urethritis. *British Journal of Venereal Diseases*, 38, 22–25.

Fowler, W. & Leeming, R. J. (1969) T-strain mycoplasma in non–gonococcal urethritis: pathogen or commensal? *British Journal of Venereal Diseases*, 45, 287–293.

Fulford, K. W. M., Catterall, R. D., Delhanty, J. J., Doniach, D. & Kromer, M. (1972) A collagen disorder of the nervous system presenting as multiple sclerosis. *Brain*, 95, 373–386.

Fulford, K. W. M., Dane, D. S., Catterall, R. D., Woof, R. & Denning, J. V. (1973) Australia antigen and antibody among patients attending a clinic for sexually transmitted diseases. *Lancet*, i, 1470–1473.

Gardner, P. S. & McQuillin, J. (1968) Rapid diagnosis of herpes virus hominis infections in superficial lesions by immunofluorescent antibody techniques. *British Medical Journal*, iv, 89–92.

Garner, R. W. & Mowat, A. W. (1972) Joint rupture in Reiter's disease. *British Journal of Surgery*, 59, 657–659.

Gatter, R. A. & Moskowitz, R. W. (1962) Pneumonitis associated with Reiter's disease. Report of a case. *Diseases of the Chest*, 42, 433–436.

Geder, L. & Skinner, C. R. B. (1971) Differentiation between type 1 and type 2 strains of herpes simplex virus by an indirect immunofluorescent technique. *Journal of General Virology*, 12, 179–182.

Gilbert, R. J., Schachter, J., Engleman, E. P. & Meyer, K. P. (1973) Antibiotic therapy in experimental bedsonial arthritis. *Arthritis and Rheumatism (New York)*, 16, 30–33.

Giles, J. P., McCollum, R. W., Berndtson, L. W. & Krugman, S. (1969) Relationship of Australia/SH antigen to the Willowbrook MS-2 strains. *New England Journal of Medicine*, 281, 119–121.

Goldman, R. L. (1970) Herpetic inclusions in the endometium. *Obstetrics and Gynaecology*, 36, 603–605.

Goldmeier, D., Bateman, J. R. M. & Rodin, P. (1975) Urinary retention and intestinal obstruction associated with ano-rectal herpes simplex virus infection. *British Medical Journal*, i, 425.

Gowardman, M. G. (1970) Problems of diagnosis and management of neurosyphilis in psychiatric hospitals. *New Zealand Medical Journal*, 71, 178–182.

Graber, W. J. III, Sanford, J. P. & Ziff, M. (1960) Sex incidence of gonococcal arthritis. *Arthritis and Rheumatism*, 3, 309–313.

Grahmann, H. (1969) Die Sogenannte Paralysekurve der Goldsobreaktum bei Nichtsyphili. *Nervenarzt*, 40, 92–95.

Haas, H., Dorfman, M. L. & Sacks, T. G. (1971) T-strains of mycoplasma and non-gonococcal urethritis. *British Journal of Venereal Diseases*, 47, 131–134.

Hancock, J. A. H. (1964) Reiter's disease. In *Recent Advances in Venereology*, ed. King, A., pp. 395–471. London: Churchill.

Hare, M. J. (1974) Neonatal encephalitis following maternal genital herpes virus infection. *Proceedings of the Royal Society of Medicine*, 67, 15–16.

Harper, I. A., Dwyer, R. St C., Garland, J. A., Jones, B. R., Treharne, J. D., Dunlop, E. M. C., Fredman, A. & Race, J. W. (1967) Infection by bedsoniae and the possibility of spurious isolation. 1. Cross infection of eggs during culture. *American Journal of Ophthalmology*, 63, suppl., 1064–1073.

Harris, J. R. W., Mahony, J. D. H., Holland, J. & McCann, J. S. (1972) Sexually transmitted disease in homosexual relationships. *Journal of the Irish Medical Association*, 65, 62–66.

Harris, J. R. W., McCann, J. S. & Mahony, J. D. H. (1973) Gonococcal arthritis, a common rarity. *British Journal of Venereal Diseases*, 49, 42–46.

Harris, J. R. W., McCann, J. S., Mahony, J. D. H., Kennedy, J. & Fulton, T. T. (1974) Syphilis and chronic liver disease. *British Journal of Venereal Diseases*, 50, 267–269.

Harris, J. R. W. (1975) Epidemiology of Reiter's disease. In *Recent Advances in Sexually Transmitted*

Diseases, 1st edn, ed. Morton, R. S. & Harris, J. R. W., p. 303. Edinburgh, London and New York: Churchill Livingstone.

Harris, J. R. W., Gelsthorpe, K., Doughty, R. W., Lee, D. & Morton, R. S. (1975) HL-A27 and W10 in Reiter's syndrome and non-specific urethritis. *Acta dermato-venereologica (Stockholm)*, **55**, 127–130.

Hautfield, D. C., Wasley, G. D. & Gray, E. (1967) Immunological and epidemiological investigations of genital strains of herpes simplex virus. *British Journal of Venereal Diseases*, **43**, 48.

Heathcote, J., Cameron, C. H. & Dane, D. S. (1974) Hepatitis B antigen in saliva and serum. *Lancet*, **i**, 71–72.

Heathcote, J. & Sherlock, S. (1973) Spread of acute type B hepatitis in London. *Lancet*, **i**, 1468–1470.

Henigst, W. (1973) Sexual transmission of infections associated with hepatitis B antigen. *Lancet*, **ii**, 1395.

Hersh, T., Milnick, J. L., Goyal, R. K. & Hollinger, F. B. (1971) Non-parenteral transmission of viral hepatitis type B (Australia antigen associated serum hepatitis). *New England Journal of Medicine*, **285**, 1363–1364.

Hilton, A. L., Richmond, S. J., Milne, J. D., Hindley, F. & Clarke, S. K. R. (1974) Chlamydia A in the female genital tract. *British Journal of Venereal Diseases*, **50**, 1–10.

Holmes, K. K., Counts, G. W. & Beaty, H. N. (1971) Disseminated gonococcal infection. *Annals of Internal Medicine*, **74**, 979–993.

Holmes, K. K. (1974) Gonococcal infection. Clinical, epidemiological and laboratory perspectives. *Advances in Internal Medicine*, **19**, 259–285.

Hooshmand, H., Escobar, M. R. & Kopf, S. W. (1972) Neurosyphilis. A study of 241 patients. *Journal of the American Medical Association*, **219**, 726–729.

Jefferies, D. J., James, W. H., Jefferiss, F. J. G., MacLeod, K. G. & Willcox, R. R. (1973) Australia (hepatitis associated) antigen in patients attending a venereal disease clinic. *British Medical Journal*, **2**, 455–456.

Jetton, R. L. & Duncan, W. C. (1969) Treatment of Reiter's syndrome with methotrexate. *Annals of Internal Medicine*, **70**, 349–351.

Jones, B. R., Collier, L. H. & Smith, C. H. (1959) Isolation of virus from inclusion blennorrhoea. *Lancet*, **i**, 902–905.

Juel-Jensen, B. E. (1973) Herpes simplex and zoster. *British Medical Journal*, **i**, 406–410.

Kaplan, B. S., Wigglesworth, R. W., Marks, M. I. & Drummond, K. N. (1972) The glomerulopathy of congenital syphilis, an immune deposit disease. *Journal of Paediatrics*, **81**, 1154–1156.

Kinsella, T. D., Norton, W. L. & Ziff, M. (1968) Complement-fixing antibodies to bedsonia organisms in Reiter's syndrome and ankylosing spondylitis. *Annals of the Rheumatic Diseases*, **27**, 241–244.

Krebs, A., Kung, D. & Honnat, A. (1971) Syndrome de Feissinger–Leroy–Reiter accompagne d'un exantheme generalise et caracterise par une guerison rapide au methotrexate. *Bulletin de la Societé française de dermatologie et de syphiligraphie*, **78**, 239.

Krugman, S., Giles, J. P. & Hammond, J. (1967) Infectious hepatitis. Evidence for two distinctive clinical, epidemiological and immunological types of infection. *Journal of the American Medical Association*, **200**, 365–373.

Laird, S. M. & Roy, B. R. (1975) Treatment of primary attacks of genital herpes with co-trimoxazole. *British Journal of Clinical Practice*, **29**, 37–42.

Lassus, A., Purko, R.-I., Stubb, S., Mattila, R. & Jansson, E. (1971) Doxycycline treatment of non-gonococcal urethritis with special reference to T-strain mycoplasmas. *British Journal of Venereal Diseases*, **47**, 126–134.

Lawrence, J. S. (1974) Family survey of Reiter's disease. *British Journal of Venereal Disease*, **50**, 140–145.

McCracken, J. D., Hall, W. H. & Pierce, H. I. (1969) Nephrotic syndrome and acute hepatitis in secondary syphilis. *Military Medicine*, **134**, 682–686.

Magruder, G. B., Gordon, F. B., Quan, A. L. & Dressler, H. R. (1963) Accidental human trachoma with rapid diagnosis by a cell culture technique. *Archives of Ophthalmology*, **69**, 300–303.

Mahony, J. D. H., Harris, J. R. W., McCann, J. S., Kennedy, J. & Dougan, H. J. (1972) Evaluation of the CSF FTA-ABS test in latent and tertiary treated syphilis. *Acta dermato-venereologica (Stockholm)*, **52**, 71–74.

Martin, J. E., Jr & Lester, A. (1971) Transgrow, a medium for transport and growth of *Neisseria gonorrhoeae* and *Neisseria meningitidis*. *H.S.M.H.A. Health Report*, **86**, 30–36.

Maxwell, J. D., Greig, W. R., Boyle, J. A., Pascieczny, T. & Schofield, C. B. S. (1966) Reiter's syndrome and psoriasis. *Scottish Medical Journal*, **11**, 14–18.

Metzger, A. L. (1970) Gonococcal arthritis complicating gonorrheal pharyngitis. *Annals of Internal Medicine*, **73**, 267–269.

Mordhorst, C. H. & Dawson, C. (1971) Sequelae of neonatal inclusion conjunctivitis and associated disease in parents. *American Journal of Ophthalmology*, 71, 861–867.

Mullins, J. F., Maberry, J. D. & Stone, O. J. (1966) Reiter's syndrome treated with folic acid antagonists. *Archives of Dermatology*, 94, 335–339.

Nahmias, A. J., Josey, W. E., Naib, Z. M., Luce, C. F. & Duffey, A. (1970) Antibodies to herpes virus hominus — types 1 and 2 in humans. *American Journal of Epidemiology*, 91, 539–546.

Nahmias, A. J., Alford, C. A. & Korones, S. B. (1971a) Infection of the newborn with herpes virus hominis. *American Journal of Obstetrics and Gynecology*, 110, 825–837.

Nahmias, A. J., Josey, W. E., Naib, Z. M. Freeman, M. G., Fernandez, R. J. & Wheeler, J. H. (1971b) Perinatal risk associated with maternal genital herpes simplex virus infection. *American Journal of Obstetrics and Gynecology*, 110, 825–837.

Ng, A. B. P., Reagan, J. W. & Yen, S. S. C. (1970) Herpes genitalis: clinical and cytopathologic experience with 256 patients. *Obstetrics and Gynaecology*, 36, 645–651.

Oriel, J. D., Reeve, P., Powis, P., Miller, A. & Nicol, C. S. (1972) Chlamydial infection: isolation of *Chlamydia* from patients with non-specific genital infection. *British Journal of Venereal Diseases*, 48, 429–436.

Oriel, J. D., Powis, P. A., Reeve, P., Miller, A. & Nicol, C. S. (1974) Chlamydial infections of the cervix. *British Journal of Venereal Diseases*, 50, 11–16.

Ostler, H. B., Dawson, C. H., Schachter, J. & Engleman, E. P. (1971) Reiter's syndrome. *American Journal of Ophthalmology*, 71, 986–991.

Papaevangelou, G. (1973) Hepatitis associated antigen in V.D. clinic patients. *British Medical Journal*, iii, 172.

Papaevangelou, G., Trichopoulos, D., Kremastinou, T. & Papoutsakis, G. (1974a) Hepatitis B antigen and antibody in prostitutes. *British Medical Journal*, ii, 256–258.

Papaevangelou, G., Trichopoulos, D., Papoutsakis, G., Kremastinou, T. & Pavlides, E. (1974b) Hepatitis B antigen in prostitutes. *British Journal of Venereal Diseases*, 50, 228–231.

Pekin, T. J., Jr, Malinin, T. I. & Zuaifler, N. J. (1967) Unusual synovial fluid findings in Reiter's syndrome. *Annals of Internal Medicine*, 66, 677–684.

Perry, H. O. & Mayne, J. G. (1965) Psoriasis and Reiter's syndrome. *Archives of Dermatology*, 92, 129–136.

Poulsen, K. (1972) Three cases of serum hepatitis developing after sexual contact. *Ugeskrift for Laeger*, 134, 1854–1855.

Prince, A. M. (1968) An antigen detected in the blood during the incubation period of serum hepatitis. *Proceedings of the National Academy of Sciences, U.S.A.*, 60, 814–821.

Prince, A. M., Hargrove, R. L., Szmuness, W., Cherubin, C. E., Fontana, V. J. & Jefferies, G. H. (1970) Immunological distinction between infectious and serum hepatitis. *New England Journal of Medicine*, 282, 987–991.

Rawls, W. E., Laurel, D., Melnick, J. L., Glicksman, J. M. & Kaufman, R. H. (1968) A search for viruses in smegma, pre-malignant and early malignant cervical tissues. The isolation of herpes virus with distinct antigenic properties. *American Journal of Epidemiology*, 87, 647–655.

Richmond, S. J., Hilton, A. L. & Clarke, S. K. R. (1972) Role of chlamydia subgroup A in non-gonococcal and post-gonococcal urethritis. *British Journal of Venereal Diseases*, 48, 437–444.

Rodin, P., Hare, M. J. & Barwell, C. F. (1971) Transport of herpes simplex virus in Stuart's medium. *British Journal of Venereal Diseases*, 47, 198–199.

Royston, I. & Aurelian, L. (1970) The association of genital herpes virus with cervical atypia and carcinoma in situ. *American Journal of Hygiene*, 91, 531–538.

Sairanen, E., Paronen, I. & Mähonen, H. (1969) Reiter's syndrome: a follow-up study. *Acta medica scandinavica*, 185, 57–63.

Samenium, B. (1968) Primary syphilis of the anorectal region. *Diseases of the Colon and Rectum*, 11, 462–466.

Schachter, J. (1967) Isolation of bedsoniae from human arthritis and abortion tissues. *American Journal of Ophthalmology*, 63, suppl., 1082–1086.

Schachter, J. (1971) Complement-fixing antibodies to bedsonia in Reiter's syndrome, TRIC agent infection and control groups. *American Journal of Ophthalmology*, 71, 857–860.

Schachter, J., Barnes, M. G., Jones, J. P., Engleman, E. P. & Meyer, K. F. (1966) Isolation of bedsoniae from the joints of patients with Reiter's disease. *Proceedings of the Society of Experimental Biology, New York*, 122, 283–285.

Schmid, F. R. & Parker, R. H. (1969) Ongoing assessment of therapy in septic arthritis. *Arthritis and Rheumatism*, 12, 529–534.

Seifert, M. H., Miller, A. C. & Warin, A. P. (1973) Benign gonococcal arthritis with cutaneous lesions. *Annals of the Rheumatic Diseases*, 32, 392–393.

Sharp, J. T. (1970) Mycoplasmas and arthritis. *Arthritis and Rheumatism*, **13**, 263–271.

Shelley, W. B. (1967) Herpes simplex virus as a cause of erythema multiforme. *Journal of the American Medical Association*, **201**, 153–156.

Shepard, M. C. (1966) Human mycoplasma infections. *Health Laboratory Science*, **3**, 163–169.

Sherlock, S. (1971) The liver in secondary (early) syphilis. *New England Journal of Medicine*, **284**, 1437–1438.

Shipley, A., Bowman, S. J. & O'Connor, J. J. (1968) T-strain mycoplasmas in non-specific urethritis. *Medical Journal of Australia*, **1**, 794–796.

Skinner, G. R. B., Thouless, M. E. & Jordan, J. A. (1971) Antibody to type 1 and type 2 herpes virus in women with abnormal cervical cytology. *Journal of Obstetrics and Gynaecology of the British Commonwealth*, **78**, 1031–1038.

Skoldenberg, B., Jeansson, S. & Wolontis, S. (1973) Herpes simplex virus type 2 in acute aseptic meningitis. *British Medical Journal*, **ii**, 611.

Smith, I. Q., Peutherer, J. F. & MacCallum, F. O. (1967) The incidence of herpes virus hominis antibody in the population. *Journal of Hygiene (Cambridge)*, **65**, 395–408.

Smith, D. E., James, P. G., Schachter, J., Engleman, E. P. & Meyer, K. F. (1973) Experimental bedsonial arthritis. *Arthritis and Rheumatism (New York)*, **16**, 21–29.

Smith, C. B. & Ward, J. R. (1971) 'Chronic infectious arthritis' role of mycoplasmas. *Journal of Infectious Disease*, **123**, 313–315.

Sobel, H. J. & Wolf, E. G. (1972) Liver involvement in early syphilis. *Archives of Pathology*, **93**, 65–68.

Sprecher-Goldberger, S., Thiry, L., Cattoor, J. P., Hooghe, R. & Pestiau, J. (1970) Herpes virus type II infection and carcinoma of the cervix. *Lancet*, **ii**, 266.

St Geme, J. W., Bailey, S. R., Koopman, J. S., Hobel, W., Oh, C. J. & Imagawa, D. T. (1975) Neonatal risk following late gestational herpes virus infection. *American Journal of Diseases of Children*, **129**, 342–343.

Sueltmann, S., Allen, V., Inhorn, S. L. & Benforado, J. M. (1971) Study of mycoplasma in university students with non-gonococcal urethritis. *Health Laboratory Science*, **8**, 62–66.

Tang, F.-F., Chang, H.-L., Huang, Y.-T. & Wang, K.-C. (1957) Studies on the aetiology of trachoma with special reference to isolation of the virus in chick embryo. *Chinese Medical Journal*, **75**, 429–447.

Taylor-Robinson, D., Addey, J. P., Hare, M. J. & Dunlop, E. M. C. (1969) Mycoplasmas and 'non-specific' genital infection. 1. Previous studies and laboratory aspects. *British Journal of Venereal Disease*, **45**, 265–273.

Thayer, J. D. & Martin, J. E., Jr (1966) Improved medium selective for cultivation of *N. gonorrhoeae* and *N. meningitidis*. *Public Health Reports*, **81**, 559–564.

Vahrman, J. (1973) Spread of acute type B hepatitis in London. *Lancet*, **ii**, 157.

Vahrman, J. (1970) Transmission of hepatitis. *Lancet*, **ii**, 774.

Vaughan-Jackson, J. D., Dunlop, E. M. C., Darougar, S., Dwyer, E. St C. & Jones, B. R. (1972) Chlamydial infection: results of tests for *Chlamydia* in patients suffering from acute Reiter's disease, compared with results of tests of the genital tract and rectum in patients with ocular infection due to TRIC agent. *British Journal of Venereal Disease*, **48**, 445–451.

Vyas, G. N. & Schulman, N. R. (1970) Haemagglutination assay for antigen and antibody associated with viral hepatitis. *Science*, **170**, 332–333.

Wallace, J. (1973) Hepatitis B antigen in V.D. clinic patients/homosexuals. *British Medical Journal*, **iii**, 347.

Wang, S. P. (1971) A micro-immunofluorescent method. Study of antibody response to TRIC organisms in mice. *Trachoma and Related Disorders*. Ed. Nichols, Roger L., pp. 273–288. Amsterdam: Excerpta Medica.

Weese, W. C. & McCarty, D. J. (1960) Spontaneous rupture of the knee joint in Reiter's syndrome. *Journal of the Americal Medical Association*, **202**, 825–827.

Weisner, P. J., Handsfield, H. H. & Holmes, K. K. (1973) Low antibiotic resistence of gonococci causing disseminated infection. *New England Journal of Medicine*, **288**, 1221–1223.

Wepler, W. (1942) Zur Morphologie und Pathogenese der Post-Dysenterischen Polyarthritis. *Beitrage zur pathologischen Anatomie*, **106**, 289.

Wetherill, J. H., Webb, H. E. & Catterall, R. D. (1965) Syphilis presenting as an acute neurological illness. *British Medical Journal*, **i**, 1157–1158.

Wilkinson, A. E. (1972) Laboratory diagnosis of venereal disease. *Public Health Laboratory Service Monograph Series*, **1**, 1–24.

Wilkinson, A. E. (1975) Syphilis serology. *Recent Advances in Sexually Transmitted Diseases*, pp. 127–147. Churchill Livingstone.

Willcox R. R. (1968) Primary infection of herpes simplex causing necrotic cervicitis. *British Journal of Clinical Practice*, **22**, 358–363.

Wolff, C. B. Goodman, H. V. & Vahrman, J. (1970) Gonorrhoea with skin and joint manifestations. *British Medical Journal*, **ii**, 271–274.

Wright, V. & Reed M. W. B. (1964) The link between Reiter's syndrome and psoriatic arthritis. *Annals of the Rheumatic Diseases*, **23**, 12–21.

Wynder, E. L. (1969) Epidemiology of cancer in situ of the cervix. *Obstetrical and Gynaecological Survey*, **24**, 697–700.

Zellerman, H. E. & Norcross, J. W. (1967) *Lahey Clinical Foundation Bulletin*, **16**, 255.

8
ANTIMICROBIAL CHEMOTHERAPY

W. Brumfitt   D. A. Leigh   J. M. T. Hamilton-Miller

Antimicrobial chemotherapy is a subject that involves all doctors concerned with the care of patients. The first semisynthetic penicillin appeared in 1959, and this was followed by large numbers of new compounds. At first some of these represented important advances, but although the introduction of new substances continued, less practical benefit resulted. This was for two reasons: first, because many had little advantage over existing compounds and second, because of the vast number of possibilities, it became impossible to be aware of the proper place of individual compounds in therapy. Because of this situation, it will be suggested that a thorough knowledge of a relatively few compounds, which represent 'in-use groups' of antimicrobial agents, will serve the physician better than attempting to acquire a superficial knowledge of all new compounds.

PHARMACOKINETICS

The fate of an antibiotic after it has entered the body is clearly of crucial importance to the outcome of therapy. In order that antimicrobials should be effective the drug has to gain access to the infecting organisms. This may be relatively easy in the case of a septicaemia, but is much more difficult for tuberculosis, subacute bacterial endocarditis, gallbladder or urinary infections. As different drugs are handled differently in the body, and it is impossible to predict from first principles the way in which any particular compound will be dealt with, a certain amount of basic knowledge is clearly necessary. Although many different factors are involved, the most important ones are: absorption, distribution, excretion, and metabolism. The interplay of these factors determines the frequency and route of dosage. Each of these factors will be discussed separately.

Absorption
Oral. Many antimicrobial agents are absorbed sufficiently well from the gastrointestinal tract to enable their use by this route for the treatment of systemic infections. In terms of the amount of antibiotic activity recoverable from the urine, the absorption of several 'oral' antibiotics is not in fact very good, ampicillin, phenoxymethylpenicillin, and tetracycline being examples. The non-absorbability of some antibiotics, such as high molecular weight sulphonamides, and aminoglycosides as a group, is taken advantage of to treat

infections confined to the gut. However, their effectiveness for many of the conditions for which they are prescribed is open to doubt. For example, in enteritis due to non-invasive salmonellae antibiotic treatment of any kind has no effect on the acute disease and merely serves to prolong the carrier state. Compounds not normally well absorbed from the gut may be rendered absorbable by a variety of artifices — for instance enteric coatings to counteract stomach acid, or chemical modification (carfecillin — see below). For the majority of antimicrobial agents absorption from the gastrointestinal tract has been repeatedly demonstrated to be more variable than that after parenteral administration. Thus, in very ill patients, in those suffering from malabsorptive conditions or from vomiting, treatment by the parenteral route is preferred. Fortunately, most antibiotics are available in both oral and parenteral preparations.

Parenteral. The most common route by which antibiotics are injected is the intramuscular one. Absorption from the injection site, usually a bulky muscle such as the gluteus maximus, is usually rapid, and peak blood levels are obtained within about 20 min. There are available, however, slow-release preparations, such as the procaine, benzathine, and benethamine salts of benzylpenicillin. Antibiotics tend to be given in rather large amounts (1 g), and many are painful by the intramuscular route. On the other hand, some antibiotics, notably cephaloridine and clindamycin, are virtually painless, although the reasons for this are not fully understood. Absorption after intramuscular administration is more predictable than by the oral route, but is still subject to rather wide variations.

The intravenous route is often favoured in acutely ill patients, as direct infusion into the circulation is a certain way to attain desired blood levels. Practitioners in Britain usually prefer bolus injections, but a few clinicians infuse over the course of an hour or two. Still others (mainly in USA) favour the use of a constant infusion pump, which, in theory at least, enables a certain predetermined blood level to be maintained at a steady state. Much comparative work needs to be done to determine which of these methods gives the best overall results. The most commonly encountered side-effect of intravenous therapy is thrombophlebitis; cephalothin is the most notorious commonly used antibiotic that causes this complication.

When intravenous antibiotics are being administered the possibilities of incompatibility must always be borne in mind. Because of this, whenever practicable, the antibiotic should not be added to an existing drip fluid.

Certain antibiotics, such as lincomycin, clindamycin, and amphotericin B, must be prescribed by a small intravenous infusion which is given in a definitive volume over 10 to 45 min, depending on the dosage.

There are several other routes available for the parenteral administration of antibiotics. The intrathecal route is favoured by some in meningitis (intraventricular injection may also be indicated in certain circumstances). However, there are obvious inherent dangers, and this route should be avoided whenever possible. Intravesicular administration, particularly of antiseptics, is commonly used in the management of patients with indwelling urinary catheters and some workers have found it to be curative provided that the infection has not

ANTIMICROBIAL CHEMOTHERAPY 175

ascended into the ureters. Certain antibiotics may conveniently be given in dialysis fluids, since they reliably cross the peritoneal membrane and thus enter the circulation.

Distribution

General considerations. Once an antibiotic has entered the body it is distributed according to its physical and chemical properties; in this respect the two most important are lipid solubility and ionisation characteristics (pK). In general, an unionised substance with high lipid solubility will be well distributed throughout the body. Certain compounds equilibrate into extracellular fluids only; these substances, which include aminoglycosides, have a volume of distribution (V_d) equivalent to no more than 30 per cent of the total body water. Antibiotics of this sort, which fail to penetrate into body cells, will clearly be less desirable for use in the treatment of infections characterised by the presence of intracellular organisms, such as brucellosis and listerosis. Other compounds, like trimethoprim, have a V_d similar in size to the volume of total body water; these are the substances which are well distributed throughout body tissues.

Special cases. There are certain body compartments which present special problems from the point of view of accessibility to antibiotics. The cerebrospinal fluid is one example. Most antibiotics fail to enter the CSF under normal circumstances; only sulphadimidine, sulphadiazine, and chloramphenicol penetrate into normal CSF. When the meninges are inflamed, however, most antimicrobial agents diffuse into the CSF. Prostatic fluid is another example of a 'difficult' body compartment; only antibiotics which are substantially uncharged at pH 6.4 have any chance of entering the prostate. Of the agents in common use for the treatment of urinary tract infections, only trimethoprim would be expected to gain access to the prostate. Other compounds which might do so are sulphadimidine, erythromycin, chloramphenicol, and clindamycin. The treatment of prostatitis is difficult for this reason and presents some interesting and unusual problems.

Excretion

Most antibiotics are removed from the blood by the kidney; the rate at which this occurs is proportional to the concentration of antibiotic in the plasma passing at any one time through the kidney tubules. Thus, blood level vs. time curves (pharmacokinetic profiles) are governed by first-order kinetics. From a practical point of view, this means that the concept of 'half-life' ($T_{\frac{1}{2}}$) is applicable; each drug has a characteristic, fixed time period in which its concentration will halve. Half-lives vary from 15 min (for benzylpenicillin) to 140 h (for sulfametopyrazine). It follows that after a period equivalent to $4 \times T_{\frac{1}{2}}$ the blood level of an antibiotic will be down to about 5 per cent of the peak value; whether or not this is still inhibitory will depend upon the size of the initial dose (which determines the peak level) and the intrinsic activity of the drug. This type of simple calculation can be very useful for working out the required frequency of dosing, especially when the usual schedules cannot be adhered to, for instance because of kidney failure. Another example of the usefulness of simple pharmacokinetics is the ability to predict that dosing co-trimoxazole every 12 h (approximately $1 \times T_{\frac{1}{2}}$ for each component) will result in accumulation, with increased blood levels after five days' continuous therapy.

Half-lives can be increased only by decreasing the activity of the kidney. This is observed in renal failure, and can be induced in effect in certain cases (most notably many penicillins and cephalosporins) by administering probenecid, which prevents tubular excretion of these antibiotics.

Most antibiotics are thus concentrated in the urine, and it is not unusual to find mean levels of about 10 mg/ml shortly after a well-absorbed drug like cephalexin has been taken. For all β-lactam drugs, however, at least 95 per cent of the compound will have been excreted within 4 h (approx. $4 \times T_{\frac{1}{2}}$), and by this time urine concentrations may be becoming marginal. Examples of antibiotics not primarily excreted in the urine are fusidic acid, erythromycin and lower dosages of rifampicin (for latter see below).

Several antibiotics are excreted in the bile, but detailed information is lacking for many compounds. Of the β-lactam group, ampicillin, cephalexin, and cefazolin are well established to be present in the bile in higher concentrations than found in the blood. Without doubt the antibiotic best excreted in the bile is rifampicin. Small doses (up to 150 mg) are totally excreted by this route, but a threshold is reached and the increasing amounts of rifampicin are excreted by the kidney. Tetracyclines and trimethoprim are also concentrated in the bile, as are fusidic acid, lincomycin, and clindamycin. On the other hand, aminoglycosides and chloramphenicol, together with most of the β-lactam group, are poorly excreted by this route, and sulphonamides and polymyxins never appear in the bile. Where there is obstruction to the free flow of bile, even rifampicin may be only poorly excreted.

Little information is available on adjustment of antibiotic doses in liver failure.

Metabolism

Many drugs are modified in the body by detoxifying mechanisms. The 'detoxified' product is usually of reduced biological activity. On the other hand, certain antibiotic preparations, such as talampicillin and carfecillin (see below) depend absolutely on metabolism in vivo for the full realisation of their microbiological activity. In general, however, when antibiotics are metabolised in vivo the products are of reduced activity; for example, N^4-acetyl derivatives and glucuronides of sulphonamides are totally inactive, while deacetyl-cephalothin has only about 25 per cent the activity of the parent compound.

The group of antimicrobial agents for which metabolism is the most important is the sulphonamides. With these compounds the speed at which they are inactivated in vivo is as important a factor as is their rate of excretion. The extent to which sulphonamides are metabolised is a function of their structure; for instance, about 85 per cent of sulphamethoxazole ($T_{\frac{1}{2}}$ c.9 h) recovered in the urine is in an inactive form, while the inactivation of the ultra-long-acting compound sulfametopyrazine ($T_{\frac{1}{2}}$ c.140 h) is much slower, only about 50 per cent of the excreted compound being inactivated.

Penicillins are also broken down to penicilloic acids, probably in the liver; phenoxymethylpenicillin (penicillin V) is the most labile, approximately half of the absorbed dose being recoverable as the penicilloate. Other types of penicillin modification result in compounds which retain their microbiological activities. Cephalosporins are largely metabolically stable, on the other hand, except for cephalothin, which, in common with other analogues bearing an acetoxy group at the C-3 position, undergoes deacetylation in vivo.

The only other group of compounds for which in vivo metabolism is of importance is those bearing a nitro group. Nitrofurans are metabolised to a lesser or greater degree, but the situation remains unclear, as there is no biological assay for these compounds. Of the nitroimidazoles, metronidazole is partially converted into metabolites of reduced activity, while metabolites of nimorazole retain a great deal of their activity. As a consequence, care must be taken in interpreting pharmacokinetic studies of these drugs when assay techniques unable to distinguish between active and inactive substances are being used.

MICROBIAL DRUG RESISTANCE

Emergence of resistance

Over the years it has been an apparently inevitable feature that, following the introduction of a new antibiotic, resistant strains have emerged. In some cases, as for *Neisseria gonorrhoeae* and sulphonamides or *Staphylococcus aureus* and benzylpenicillin, this process has been rapid. In others, such as for *N. gonorrhoeae* and benzylpenicillin, it has been insidious. Only in the case of the polyene antibiotics and yeast has resistance not yet appeared. We may presently be witnessing the start of two new eras — of ampicillin-resistant *Haemophilus influenzae* and of the rapid spread of resistance to gentamicin among Gram-negative bacilli. Usually the spread, once the process has started, is inexorable, either by cross-infection or by genetic transfer, in global terms. Usually, but not always, resistance rises in proportion to the usage of an antibiotic. In some cases, however, there is no apparent correlation, and indeed resistance to methicillin by *Staph. aureus*, and apparently to gentamicin among Gram-negative bacilli, occurs in strictly localised geographical areas only. An encouraging feature to note is that the process of the spread of drug-resistance may be halted, and indeed reversed, by the firm application on a local scale of an antibiotic policy. Specific resistance problems have been dealt with by means of a total ban in the use of certain antibiotics.

Trimethoprim is an example of a drug to which resistance is still rare. However this fact may be obscured in some hospitals by the curious practice of reporting bacteria which are resistant to sulphonamides but sensitive to trimethoprim as 'resistant to co-trimoxazole'.

The emergence of resistance can be controlled, but a detailed knowledge of the origins and mechanisms of the phenomenon is necessary for this to be achieved in the most efficient way.

Mutation to high-level resistance

This phenomenon, which may involve a decrease in sensitivity of more than 1000-fold, occurs with such compounds as streptomycin and rifampicin, and is now regularly and successfully combated by using combined therapy, as in tuberculosis. Streptomycin may still be used alone for short periods (one week) when non-tuberculous conditions are involved, as mutation rates are too low for resistant variants to appear within this space of time. Rifampicin at present seems to be reserved by tacit agreement for use in tuberculosis only, although the logic behind this decision appears questionable. The limited experience gained with rifampicin short-term in non-tuberculous conditions suggests that it should be used in combination with another broad-spectrum antibiotic. Trimethoprim and sisomicin (an antibiotic closely related to gentamicin) have been suggested as possible candidates for the latter role.

Resistance transfer

In the laboratory, drug resistance may be transmitted from bacteria to bacteria by various processes: transformation (via naked DNA), transduction (genes are transferred by bacteriophage), and conjugation (direct cell-to-cell transfer mediated by the presence in the donor cell of an episome which confers fertility). It seems possible that transduction may be a significant means for the spread of drug resistance in burns, but other than this specific example only conjugation is of clinical importance. In this case the fertility-conferring episome (R-factor) also carries genes specifying resistance to various antimicrobial drugs.

R-factors are undoubtedly responsible for much of the resistance to ampicillin, sulphonamides, tetracyclines, and kanamycin which is seen among Gram-negative bacilli today. In terms of life-threatening infections, however, R-factors do not have great impact, as the antibiotics mentioned above (except for kanamycin in some hospitals) would not be considered as first-line drugs in such infections. In UK, R-factors have considerable nuisance value in burns units, as Lowbury's experience over the years has shown, and are also capable of exacerbating explosive but strictly limited and localised outbreaks of gastro-enteritis. Experience thus far has shown that withdrawal of antibiotics determinants of resistance to which are present will usually cause such troublesome R-factors to disappear. Advantage can be taken of the fact that resistance to some antibiotics is very rarely, if ever, carried on R-factors — examples are nalidixic acid, nitrofurans, rifampicin, polymyxin, and trimethoprim. Patience and a rigidly followed antibiotic policy constitute the basic formula for relief of those troubled by R-factor-bearing bacteria.

In other parts of the world, however, strains carrying R-factors are capable of causing extreme concern. The most obvious of these is the recent emergence of chloramphenicol-resistant *Salmonella typhi* in Mexico and Vietnam. Fortunately, alternative drugs effective in acute typhoid fever now exist, in the form of amoxycillin, co-trimoxazole, and mecillinam.

New drugs and resistance

Another way by which the resistance problem may be alleviated from time to time is, of course, the introduction of new drugs. The most dramatic example of this was when methicillin came into use in 1960, specifically to combat the penicillinase-producing *Staph. aureus*. An equally impressive result, in terms of chemical manipulation of a molecule with a specific biochemical purpose in mind, seems to have been achieved more recently with amikacin. Minocycline and rifampicin were derived empirically, and trimethoprim was synthesised with a specific purpose (inhibition of bacterial dihydrofolate reductase) in mind. However, rational or irrational, all these compounds have offered alternative compounds for therapeutic use against multiple-resistant strains. However, as it may take 10 years and as much as £10 million to develop a new antibacterial agent, physicians cannot go on accepting this way out of the problem. A radical new approach to the use of antibiotics is necessary if resistance is to be contained.

GENERAL MANAGEMENT OF INFECTIONS

Diagnosis of Bacterial Infection

The successful use of antibiotics must be based on a series of general principles. Antibiotic therapy should only be given to patients with bacterial infections that are likely to be susceptible, and the dosage and length of treatment must depend on the accessibility and chronicity of the infection. The route of administration will be governed by the clinical condition of the patient and the particular antibiotic. Although undesirable in principle, it may be necessary in some cases to combine two or more antibiotics to achieve a successful therapeutic result. Chemoprophylaxis has a special place in the case of certain patients with underlying diseases that make the risks and development of bacterial infections potentially more serious than in the population at large (see section on 'Indications for Prophylaxis').

In general, antibiotic therapy should only be given to patients in whom the presence of infection has been confirmed, or where bacteriological specimens have been collected. Diagnosis of the infection, which involves the collection of appropriate specimens, isolation and identification of the infecting organism, and determination of the antibiotic sensitivity, is an essential prerequisite to successful chemotherapy. Knowledge of the pharmacokinetics of the particular antibiotic is of course essential.

In the past, collection of the specimen for bacteriological culture has not received the attention it deserved. For example it was many years after reports that bacteria were able to multiply in urine and cause apparent infections when one was not present that the importance of clean collection techniques and rapid transport to the laboratory for examination were appreciated. Some infecting organisms have their origin in the intestinal tract, and thus the possible role of anaerobic bacteria must always be considered. The chance of isolation from infected sites is directly proportional to the care taken over the collection and transport of the specimen. The use of prereduced anaerobic containers or special media which maintain anaerobic conditions can result in a great increase in the isolation rate of anaerobic bacteria. It can be argued that bedside culture is the best way of isolating the bacteria that may be the cause of an infection, although unfortunately this method is not used in most hospitals. Collection of the best specimen depends on an understanding of the underlying pathological processes. Sampling of pus lying on the surface of a wound infection originating deep in the abdominal wall is unlikely to provide a true reflection of the bacteria present. In a large leg ulcer the bacteria present in the edge of the ulcer may be different from those in the centre and may be responsible for progression of the lesion. In patients with urethritis examination of a mid-stream specimen of urine will understandably fail to isolate bacteria present in the urethra, since the organisms causing the infection are washed out by the first part of the urine stream and will not be found in a mid-stream specimen. The carriage of bacteria through the genital tract of women may vary considerably, and a swab from the vaginal vault will not necessarily isolate the bacteria responsible for inflammation of the vulva or vestibule. In bacteraemia resulting from endocarditis the bacteriological culture of arterial blood specimens or bone marrow may be successful in isolating the infecting organism when a venous sample has failed to do so. The methods of laboratory culture of the specimen are equally important, since failure to use the correct procedures can lead to an inaccurate report. It is always necessary to use selective media for the isolation of anaerobic bacteria because these are usually slow-growing and can be hidden in a heavy growth of other bacteria which may not be the only pathogens. The use of standard culture media alone for the isolation of urinary pathogens will frequently fail to show the infecting organisms in urethritis, as many of these are anaerobic or microaerophilic and require blood for successful isolation. Because many of these bacteria are slow-growing, incubation should be continued for at least 48 h. Other possible causal organisms such as gonococci, chlamydia, and herpes must not be forgotten.

The methods used for the determination of antibiotic susceptibility are less important, although it is essential that each laboratory performs its own controls. In general hospitals the usual laboratory practice is to report the range of antibiotic sensitivities on the basis of the results of impregnated disc testing. The sensitivity of the infecting organism should be compared to that of a control organism, although a 'built-in' control on every culture plate is unnecessary and is not as reliable as is claimed by some workers. More accurate methods of sensitivity testing such as tube dilution or titration in agar may be needed in certain circumstances.

Control of Antibiotic Therapy

Although control of antibiotic therapy is impractical in most mild infections it is important in severe infections and in particular in those patients at special risk. Control can be exercised in two ways.

First, the route of administration should be chosen so that adequate blood and tissue levels of antibiotics are achieved. Absorption of orally administered antibiotics may be unpredictable in some patients, especially if there is vomiting or ileus, and under these circumstances it is essential to give the antibiotic systemically. The same applies to patients with circulatory failure. If absorption from an intramuscular site is thought to be unreliable because of circulatory failure, and therefore poor perfusion of blood through the muscles, intravenous injection or infusion is preferable. In a few cases where the infection is limited to a specific area such as a heart valve it may be possible by the use of an intravenous catheter to infuse the antibiotic in high concentrations in the locality of the infection. However it must be remembered that the use of the long intravenous line may itself be an important cause of infection. Where local therapy is possible, for example in abscess cavities. a high concentration of antibiotic can be achieved by local infusion (continuous if necessary), and in peritonitis complicating peritoneal dialysis an appropriate concentration of antibiotic can be added to the infusion fluid. With many antibiotics (but not cloxacillin) this is then absorbed into the circulation.

The second method of control is by the determination of the antibiotic concentration in various body fluids through the course of treatment. It is relatively simple to examine blood and urine samples, although in certain infections it is also desirable to estimate the antibiotic concentrations in bile, pus, prostatic secretions, cerebrospinal fluid, and sputum. Examination of expectorated sputum is the least satisfactory, owing to the difficulty in obtaining uncontaminated specimens in most patients. It is impossible in the very ill patient who cannot expectorate sputum. A routine method for collecting uncontaminated sputum specimens will enable an aetiological diagnosis to be made and greatly improve the prognosis.

It is necessary to collect specimens of blood at different times during therapy, and these are commonly arranged to provide a reflection of the 'peak' level, usually between 30 and 90 min after administration, and 'trough' level at the end of the dose interval. The 'trough' level is most important, since, where this is still high, lowering of the next dose avoids the danger of giving a dose capable of producing a potentially toxic blood level. The concentrations in urine are usually measured over time periods of 1 to 2 h or over the whole dose interval.

The correlation between the sensitivity of the infecting organism and the antibiotic level in the body fluid examined is not necessarily a direct one, since complicating factors such as protein binding, or the production of enzymes such as β-lactamases, may mean that the result does not reflect the true local conditions. For example, in certain infections such as subacute bacterial endocarditis the antibacterial activity of the blood (or serum) expressed as an inhibitory or bactericidal effect is a more accurate assessment, and provides important information in planning treatment. In this test the infecting organism (at various concentrations) is incubated in dilutions of the patient's serum, and the presence or absence of growth noted.

NEW ANTIMICROBIAL AGENTS
β-lactams

Penicillins
Since the introduction of carbenicillin in 1967 there have been no major advances in the penicillin field. Such advance as has been made is of a minor, technical nature. A significant event is that ampicillin came out of patent in September 1975, and we must now expect other brand names to join that of Penbritin (Beecham). Already Amfipen (Brocades), Pentrexyl (Bristol), and Vidopen (Berk) have appeared. It is important that the bioavailability of new brands should be carefully checked.

Talampicillin (Talpen, Beecham) has been introduced recently in order to solve the problem of the relatively poor absorption of ampicillin by the oral route. Talampicillin is a phthalyl ester of ampicillin, inactive per se, but hydrolysed in vivo to yield ampicillin. About 60 per cent of the ampicillin moiety of talampicillin is absorbed, making talampicillin, dose for dose, equivalent to approximately twice its weight of ampicillin. A consequence of the better absorption is said to be a lower incidence of gastrointestinal side-effects following talampicillin administration. Talampicillin is analogous to piv-ampicillin which, although not available in UK, is marketed on the Continent. Both compounds should prove useful substitutes, at reduced dosage schedules, for ampicillin, especially in paediatric patients, where ampicillin is absorbed very erratically. Also, for paediatric purposes, a syrup would be desirable but this has not yet been formulated.

Amoxycillin (Amoxil, Bencard) is a close chemical relative of ampicillin, and is also absorbed approximately twice as well as is ampicillin. Its antimicrobial spectrum is comparable to, but quantitatively slightly less than, that of ampicillin, and clinical experience so far suggests that it is a good substitute for ampicillin when given by mouth. Of particular interest is that amoxycillin has been reported to be as effective as chloramphenicol for the treatment of acute typhoid fever. A major problem with assessing the performance of antibiotics in typhoid fever, however, is that results from different geographical locations (i.e. South Africa, India, Mexico) are different. This strongly suggests that local factors, which may pertain to either host or parasite, have an important part to play.

Carfecillin (Uticillin, Beecham) is a form of carbenicillin (the phenyl ester at the sidechain carboxyl) which is absorbed by mouth. The ester is rapidly hydrolysed to free carbenicillin in vivo; however, the serum concentrations of the latter obtained after conventional doses (maximum of 3 g daily) are not sufficient to treat systemic infections even with sensitive organisms, and this compound should be reserved for treating urinary tract infections caused by *Pseudomonas aeruginosa* or indole-producing *Proteus* spp. Patients with this sort of infection should be thoroughly investigated because some underlying contributory factor (e.g. stone or ureteral stricture) is often present. *Escherichia coli* and *Pr. mirabilis* strains are also almost always sensitive to carbenicillin, but carfecillin is not indicated in urinary tract infections of this aetiology under normal cir-cumstances, owing to its high cost and its lack of advantage over ampicillin and amoxycillin.

Other derivatives. Indanyl carbenicillin is an analogous compound to carfecillin, but is not available in UK at the present time.

Ticarcillin is a close chemical analogue of carbenicillin, with the same antibacterial spectrum, but doubled intrinsic activity and superior phar-macokinetics. Although ticarcillin has not yet been marketed, several clinical trials have been carried out using it, and results have been satisfactory at a dose half that of carbenicillin.

Mecillinam, formerly called FL 1060 (Leo Laboratories), is a compound presently undergoing clinical evaluation. Its in vitro spectrum is remarkable in that it is more active against Gram-negative rods than against Gram-positive cocci. It is well absorbed by mouth in the form of its pivaloyl ester, FL 1039 (pivmecillinam). It therefore seems eminently suited for the treatment of urinary tract infections and salmonelloses. Preliminary reports have been encouraging, and it seems likely that mecillinam will soon be more generally available.

Cephalosporins

As with the penicillins, advances in cephalosporins have been gradual rather than dramatic. All bacteria are not equally sensitive to the various cephalosporins and for a particular species, one compound may be therapeutically superior.

Cephradine (Velosef, Squibb; Eskacef, Smith, Kline & French) is very similar chemically, pharmacokinetically and microbiologically to cephalexin. Its claim to novelty is that cephradine can be given orally, intramuscularly and intravenously, this being the only cephalosporin for which this can be said. Many clinicians prefer to initiate treatment with a cephalosporin, available by the parenteral route only, such as cephalothin, cephaloridine, or cefazolin, and substitute an oral compound later. Thus, the question arises as to whether the alternative compound is as effective against the pathogen concerned. Clearly, if the same compound is used this question cannot arise. It remains to be seen whether the existence of one cephalosporin for both roles is attractive.

Cephazolin (Kefzol, Lilly) is another new cephalosporin made generally available. This compound attains higher serum levels, gram for gram, than any related compound. It is administered by injection three times daily and is recommended for genitourinary and respiratory tract infections. Cephazolin has a considerable in vitro activity against anaerobic bacteria. Like all cephalosporins, it is expensive. Cephazolin is known to be excreted in the bile; for other cephalosporins biliary excretion is either poor, or badly documented. There are several new cephalosporins undergoing clinical evaluation, but none has obvious advantages over existing compounds. Cephoxitin, which is a cephamycin and closely related to the cephalosporins, on the other hand, has a very broad antibacterial spectrum (which includes species such as *Bacteriodes fragilis*), and preliminary trials appear to be very favourable.

Tetracyclines

Although several semisynthetic tetracyclines have been produced in the last 10 years, only two are worthy of serious consideration. Minocycline (7-dimethylamino-6-deoxy-6-demethyl-5-oxytetracycline) and doxycycline (6α-deoxy-5-oxytetracycline) both owe their peculiar properties to their increased lipophilicity compared with conventional tetracyclines. *Doxycycline* (Vibramycin, Pfizer) has a half-life of about 15 h, and the usual dosage is 100 mg every 24 h; *minocycline* (Minocin, Lederle) is given twice daily in 100 mg amounts. In addition to these improved pharmacokinetic properties, these two compounds also have enhanced intrinsic microbiological activities. These are more pronounced in the case of minocycline, which is active against many tetracycline-resistant strains, including Gram-negative anaerobic species and *Staph. aureus*. Minocycline has recently been reported to cause a worrying side-effect of light headedness, which is probably not vestibular in origin. Further detailed studies are needed to delineate fully the extent of this problem.

Unlike most tetracyclines, doxycycline may be used in the presence of impairment of renal function.

Aminoglycosides

Two new aminoglycosides have been introduced into clinical practice since gentamicin. One is *tobramycin* (Nebcin, Lilly), which is more intrinsically active against *Ps. aeruginosa* strains, and is regarded by some as drug of choice in infections caused by this species. There is a large measure of cross-resistance between gentamicin and tobramycin, and the compounds are of approximately equal toxicity.

Gentamicin resistance is beginning to take on serious proportions in certain geographical localities, and gentamicin-resistant strains are causing fatal infections more and more frequently. However, overall, gentamicin resistance is of low incidence, a fact for which we should be grateful, and the maintenance of which should exercise our minds constantly. Where this type of resistance is a problem, a new semisynthetic aminoglycoside, *amikacin* (Amikin, Mead Johnson), is proving very useful. Amikacin is a derivative of kanamycin, with which it shares pharmacokinetic and toxicological properties. It is stable towards many of the enzymes responsible for modifying aminoglycosides, and so remains active against the vast majority of bacteria which produce these type of enzyme. Resistance to amikacin is very unusual. As yet, amikacin is indicated only where gentamicin resistance is prevalent; otherwise, gentamicin remains the drug of choice.

Antifungal Agents

There have been some very welcome and much overdue developments in the field of antifungal agents in the past few years.

Griseofulvin (Fulcin, ICI; Grisovin, Glaxo) is the drug of choice for infections by dermatophytes (species of the genera *Trichophyton, Microsporum* and *Epidermophyton*) of hair, skin or nails. Griseofulvin is active only against dermatophytes, which have a chitinous cell wall. As the antibiotic is inactive against yeasts and filamentous fungi, the clinician must consider it mandatory to have laboratory confirmation of the precise microbial aetiology before prescribing a course of treatment with griseofulvin, which may have to be prolonged (6–12 months). Griseofulvin acts by altering keratin, upon which dermatophytes depend for nutrition. In order to do this, the antibiotic must be in the blood stream — topical application is useless.

Clotrimazole (Canesten, Bayer) is an oral, broad-spectrum non-polyene antifungal agent, which has proved especially useful for topical use. Parenterally, it gives rather low blood levels, and causes induction of liver enzymes, hastening its own metabolic inactivation. A closely related compound, *miconazole* (Daktarin, Jannsen) has very similar properties. A great advantage of these two compounds, both chlorimidazoles, is that laboratory diagnosis does not have to be made before their use, as they are, unlike griseofulvin, active against dermatophytes as well as yeasts and filamentous fungi.

Flucytosine (5-fluorocytosine; Alcobon, Roche) is a compound which, although not yet released for general use, is being more widely used for certain limited indications. It is active against *Candida, Cryptococcus* and *Aspergillus* spp., and can be given in large doses. It is excreted in the urine (unlike clotrimazole), and is therefore useful on the rare occasions when a urinary tract infection is caused by *C. albicans.* It has also been used for cryptococcal meningitis and candidal septicaemias. One disadvantage of this compound is that primary resistance occurs, and resistant mutants may be selected during therapy, so patients on flucytosine must be carefully monitored.

Some of the more important antimicrobial agents introduced into clinical practice over the past 10 years are shown in the Table 8.1.

Despite the introduction of these new drugs, amphotericin B remains the drug of choice for severe systemic fungal infections.

PROPHYLAXIS

In recent years more attention has focused upon antimicrobial prophylaxis. It is a commonplace that prevention is better than cure and experience over a century has shown that this is especially true of infection. However, the haphazard use of antibiotics for this purpose has been shown to be not only unjustified but positively dangerous.

Before recommending an antibiotic for prophylactic use it is vitally important to pay attention to the likely nature of the pathogen. A full history and examination of the patient is essential. For example, symptoms and clinical evidence of cholecystitis would not only allow the possible nature of the pathogen to be predicted, but also to select an appropriate antibiotic, which is excreted in the bile and effective against the likely pathogens.

Prophylactic antibiotics should not be given before collecting the appropriate specimens. It is also helpful to know the bacterial ecology of the hospital and the resistance pattern of the organisms.

As indicated in relation to the specific example of cholecystitis, knowledge of the pharmacokinetics of the antibiotic used is essential.

Planned prophylaxis such as that given before dental extraction in patients with rheumatic valvular disease must be given correctly since, if started too soon, selection of penicillin-resistant strains of streptococci may occur. Benzylpenicillin should be injected about 15 min before the extraction in order to reach its peak serum level at the time when bacteria are being shed into the blood.

Indications for Chemoprophylaxis

The indications for chemoprophylaxis fall into four groups.

Essential

Perhaps the most obvious example is malaria. Areas where this disease is endemic or epidemic are well known, so that people entering such areas would be

Table 8.1 Names, chief indications and dosage schedules for some recently introduced antimicrobial compounds.

Group	Name		Main indications	Adult dosage
	Approved	Proprietary		
Antibacterial agents				
β-Lactams				
(i) penicillins	flucloxacillin	Floxapen	staphylococcal infections	250 mg 6-hourly, oral or i.m.
	amoxycillin	Amoxil	infections of respiratory or lower urinary tract; otitis media	250 mg 8-hourly, oral
	talampicillin	Talpen	infections of respiratory or lower urinary tract; otitis media	250 mg 8-hourly, oral
	carfecillin	Uticillin	certain lower urinary tract infections	500 mg or 1 g, 8-hourly, oral
(ii) cephalosporins	cephalexin	Ceporex Keflex	infections of respiratory or urinary tract	250 mg or 500 mg 6-hourly, oral
	cephradine	Velosef Eskacef	infections of respiratory or urinary tract	250 mg or 500 mg 6-hourly, oral; 500 mg 6-hourly, i.m. or i.v.
	cephazolin	Kefzol	infections of respiratory or urinary tract	500 mg or 1 g 6-hourly, i.m.
Tetracyclines	doxycycline	Vibramycin	respiratory tract infections; non-specific urethritis	200 mg stat 100 mg 24-hourly, oral
	minocycline	Minocin	respiratory tract infections; non-specific urethritis; also infections with anaerobes	200 mg stat 100 mg 12-hourly, oral
Aminocyclitols	spectinomycin	Trobicin	gonorrhoea	♂ 2 g i.m. ♀ 4 g i.m.

Aminoglycosides	tobramycin	Nebcin	serious infections	1–2 mg/kg 8-hourly, i.m. or i.v. Adjust according to blood levels
	amikacin	Amikin	serious infections, especially if gentamicin resistance common	
Ansa compounds	rifampicin	Rifadin Rimactane	tuberculosis	600 mg in single dose daily. Use in combination with another anti-tuberculosis drug
Celesticetins	clindamycin	Dalacin C	infections with staphylococci or anaerobes	150–450 mg, 6-hourly, oral; 600–1200 mg daily, i.m. or i.v.
Antifolate compounds	co-trimoxazole	Septrin Bactrim	infections of urinary or respiratory tracts	trimethoprim 160 mg + sulphamethoxazole 800 mg 12-hourly, oral. Same dosage i.v.
Quinolones	oxolinic acid	Prodoxol	urinary tract infections	750 mg 12-hourly, oral
Nitroimidazoles	metronidazole	Flagyl	anaerobic infections	400 mg 8-hourly, oral
Antifungal agents Chlorimidazoles	clotrimazole	Canesten	infections of skin or nails	1 per cent cream and solution topically
	miconazole	Daktarin	infections of skin or nails	2 per cent cream and powder topically
Fluoropyrimidines	flucytosine	Alcobon	systemic infections with *Candida* spp., *Cryptococcus neoformans*, funguria	500 mg 6-hourly, oral

foolish not to take an agent such as pyrimethamine. *Plasmodium falciparum* strains may show drug resistance, and this must be taken into account when choosing the prophylactic agent.

Another example already referred to is that of giving penicillin before tooth extraction in patients suffering from rheumatic heart disease. In fact it has recently been pointed out that there is no published evidence that the risk of bacterial endocarditis is reduced by such measures. However, ethical reasons would preclude a trial to quantitate the extent of any reduction, and failure to give prophylaxis might result in accusation of professional negligence if bacterial endocarditis occurred.

Prophylactic chemotherapy before the insertion of hip prostheses and mid-thigh amputation (especially where the blood supply may be precarious, as in diabetes) is mandatory. The danger of gas gangrene occurring after such operations is well known, since, being near the rectum, these areas of skin are frequently colonised by *Clostridium welchii* (part of the normal bowel flora). Thus, the administration of penicillin for five days (to which *Cl. welchii* is highly sensitive), starting immediately before the operation, together with precleansing of the skin with an iodophore, is the correct practice. Since resistance of *Cl. welchii* to penicillin is unknown only hypersensitivity to penicillin would necessitate the choice of an alternative antibiotic.

Other conditions where prophylactic chemotherapy is essential include patients who have suffered from rheumatic fever, those *directly exposed* to patients with meningococcal meningitis, and cystic fibrosis of the lung.

When considering the scheme of prophylaxis the reader should consult detailed recommendations set out in the section on further reading.

Useful

This includes certain conditions where lack of controlled trials leaves some doubt about the actual value of this prophylaxis. The complexity of cardiac surgery has encouraged many surgeons to give a combination of ampicillin and cloxacillin (Ampiclox) during the operation. However, this does not seem a rational choice, since *Staphylococcus albus* may often be the infecting organism, and it is often resistant to both ampicillin and cloxacillin.

In recurrent urinary infection it is apparent that there is a group of patients who, if properly selected, benefit from long-term chemotherapy. This applies particularly to women of child-bearing age and men who have chronic infection of the prostatic bed following prostatectomy.

CSF rhinorrhoea is a condition which is generally treated by chemoprophylaxis. Benzylpenicillin or ampicillin is used since both are effective against streptococci, pneumococci, and those anaerobes which colonise areas above the diaphragm.

Strangely, there appears to be no controlled study regarding the prophylaxis of gonorrhoea. The usual procedure is to give an appropriate antibiotic to a patient who has been at risk. In doing this the danger of masking syphilis without eradicating it must be borne in mind. Another indication which has been discussed repeatedly as a useful indication for prophylaxis is premature rupture of the membranes. In appropriate circumstances the administration of an antibiotic which crosses the membranes must be considered. This is yet another example of the importance of understanding the pharmacokinetics of the chosen antibiotic.

Two further examples are the use of isoniazid alone in tuberculosis prophylaxis, and the use of metronidazole to prevent infections caused by anaerobes after gynaecological procedures or appendicectomy.

Doubtful

It has been claimed that a multiple drug regime is valuable following the aggressive chemotherapy of malignancies (and especially leukaemia). Unfortunately such studies are uncontrolled and therefore particularly difficult to assess.

Another doubtful indication is the preoperative antibiotic 'preparation' of the bowel before surgery. However, it is extremely doubtful whether complete sterilisation of the large bowel is possible, and we are unaware of any published data where proper cultural conditions have shown bowel sterilisation to have been achieved.

In general surgical practice it is very doubtful whether the widespread use of pre- or postoperative antibiotic prophylaxis does anything but harm. Nevertheless, antibiotics are widely used in both circumstances. However, two important exceptions should be noted. One is where perforation of the gastrointestinal tract has occurred, and the other is the use of metronidazole to prevent infections with anaerobic bacteria after pelvic surgery.

In elective surgery, extraordinary claims have been made to justify the value of prophylactic antibiotics. Many of these reports are quite ridiculous since they are not based on randomised clinical trials; in addition, bacteriological studies have often been completely inadequate. An important exception is surgery on the lower limb, which has already been discussed in detail. In general, however, by avoiding prophylactic chemotherapy the patient is less likely to become infected by an antibiotic-resistant organism.

In the compromised patient the administration of antimicrobial agents has been shown clearly to increase the danger of infection by opportunistic organisms.

The problem seems to be that clinicians must be persuaded that anticipation and rapid diagnosis of infection will yield better results than the understandable albeit useless endeavour to prevent infection by the use of antibiotics. Furthermore, the use of multiple antimicrobial agents in chemotherapy is likely to result in infection due to highly resistant microbes.

Useless

Bowel sterilisation. Ammonia produced in the gut and then absorbed is believed to be important in causing hepatic coma.

A variety of drugs has been given in order to prevent ammonia production, but unfortunately this has sometimes caused serious toxicity. For example, when neomycin was given orally in doses of 4 to 8 g daily, absorption occurred to a sufficient extent to cause deafness. Also, with regard to 'sterilisation' of the bowel with neomycin, it should be borne in mind that the MIC of *B. fragilis* (which is present in large numbers in the bowel) is of the order of 5000 µg/ml.

With the appreciation of this problem there has been a tendency to revert to the use of tetracycline, although its value has declined because of the observed decrease in the sensitivity of bowel organisms. It is also well known that if tetracycline reaches a sufficient concentration, it is itself hepatotoxic, and under *no circumstances* should it be given by the intravenous route. Survey of the literature shows that from both the metabolic and microbiological point of view it is difficult to justify prophylactic chemotherapy for gut sterilisation.

Respiratory infections. A number of controlled studies have cast serious doubt on the once widespread practice of giving continuous prophylaxis in chronic bronchitis. In those at risk it is probably better to give the patient a supply of tetracycline with instructions to take the drug if he develops a coryza — especially if there are signs of it 'going to the chest'. He should also report to his doctor as soon as possible if this occurs.

There is a tendency to give prophylactic antibiotics to unconscious patients in order to prevent respiratory infections. This practice is bad. Not only is the incidence of infections unchanged, but when infection does occur it is due to resistant bacteria.

CONTROL OF SPECIFIC ORGANISMS

Staphylococcal Infections

Although strains of *Staphylococcus aureus* are now less frequent causes of epidemics of infection, the clinical importance of this organism remains undisputed. It is still a common cause of postoperative wound sepsis (especially in 'clean' surgery), osteomyelitis, and skin infections and abscesses. It is now rarely seen in renal and urinary tract infections, although it may complicate prostatectomy, and is also relatively infrequent as a cause of deep-seated abscesses. A large range of antibiotics is available for the treatment of staphylococcal infections. In general in both hospital and domiciliary practice, most strains are resistant to penicillin, but sensitivity to the newer penicillinase-resistant compounds such as cloxacillin, flucloxacillin and methicillin is universal, except, as mentioned previously, in a few confirmed geographical areas. The reason for these isolated pockets of resistant organisms is unknown, but is unrelated to antibiotic-destroying enzymes such as the β-lactamases. Prevention of staphylococcal infections in hospitals is dependent on the evaluation of nasal and skin carriage in the patient, and possibly in the hospital staff. There is considerable divergence of opinion about the relative importance of these two sources of infection. It is probably true to day that, except in special units where staff with nasal carriage of staphylococci should be excluded, it is impossible to prevent the carrier state in the hospital staff, and preventative measures should only be taken where it can be shown that an increase in the number of carriers has occurred. In screening carriers for staphylococci it is usually only necessary to examine swabs from the anterior nares and to exclude staphylococcal lesions. It should also be remembered that staphylococcal carriage may occur in the axilla, groin, or perianal region. Treatment of staphylococcal carrier states is by the local use of antibiotic or antiseptic creams to the anterior nares and other appropriate carrier sites, associated with antiseptic talcum powders to the axillae and perineum. Naseptin (neomycin and chlorhexidine) is most commonly used, and is not associated with development of neomycin sensitivity.

Fusidic acid (Fucidin) ointment is a valuable alternative, although widespread use of this antibiotic is associated with the development of resistant strains, which is an excellent reason for avoiding its use. It should therefore only be employed in domiciliary practice, and even there should normally be reserved for patients who have failed other treatments.

In general practice, familial staphylococcal infection is a problem, and is probably more common than expected by previous reports. It is necessary to examine all members of a household, as asymptomatic carrier states are common. Parenteral antibiotic therapy is not usually necessary, unless the primary infections are severe, or involve the face. Eradication of the carrier state can usually be achieved with nasal antibiotic ointment and antiseptic talcum powders prescribed for 14 days, but a second course of treatment may be necessary in some cases. In cases where the staphylococcal infections are recurrent and local antibiotic therapy does not work, it has been shown that the nasal strain of *Staph. aureus* can be replaced by a known non-pathogenic strain.

Streptococcal Infections

In general, streptococci are now not as great a problem in hospital patients as in the past. However, epidemics of infection due to Lancefield Group A haemolytic streptococci occur in ward situations and certain departments of the hospital. In obstetric and neonatal practice, infections due to Lancefield Group B haemolytic streptococci carry a high morbidity and are an important cause of neonatal meningitis. Cross-infection from mother to infant occurs most frequently through contamination of the infant from the vaginal flora during birth, although it may occur as cross-infection from infant to infant in the nursery. Other superficial infections, for example of the eye, umbilicus, and skin, may occur early in the neonatal period. Postpartum infection of the uterus, vagina or episiotomy wound can occur in the mother, and frequently necessitates antibiotic therapy. In many hospitals preventative measures are taken in mothers to eradicate both Group A and B haemolytic streptococci prior to delivery. At a recent congress the use of povidone iodine (Betadine) was reported to be effective. In nursing staff asymptomatic pharyngeal carriage can be detected by routine screening procedures, and antibiotic treatment can be given. However, it is debatable whether these measures are economically worthwhile or prevent infection.

In general practice Lancefield Group A haemolytic streptococci are responsible for less than 25 per cent of cases of tonsillitis. Antibiotic treatment, usually with penicillin, for 10 days is necessary for eradication. But where the symptoms are mild and the streptococcus is thought to play an opportunistic role, it is doubtful whether any antibiotic therapy is justified. An exception is made in the case of patients who have suffered from rheumatic fever, where a 10-day course of benzylpenicillin is mandatory. Shorter courses of treatment result in a high incidence of relapse of the organism. In patients, especially children, with recurrent episodes of tonsillitis, it is usually worthwhile to examine the other members of the patient's family, as a high incidence, up to 40 per cent, of asymptomatic carriers are found. Treatment of these carriers results in eradication of infection from the family.

In glomerulonephritis of streptococcal aetiology, the usefulness of antibiotic treatment is unresolved. Whilst the antibiotic therapy will eradicate the bacteria, the liberation of excessive quantities of streptococcal antigen may result in more severe renal damage. In any event there is no evidence that penicillin therapy alters the natural history of acute glomerulonephritis.

Strains of Group A haemolytic streptococci are still highly sensitive to penicillin, and no evidence of resistance has ever been substantiated. The incidence of susceptibility of streptococci to tetracycline, however, has considerably diminished, and in most areas of the country less than 50 per cent of strains are sensitive to even the new more active tetracycline derivatives. Other haemolytic streptococci, e.g. Group B, show a wider spectrum of resistance, many strains being less susceptible to benzylpenicillin, although usually sensitive to ampicillin. For patients hypersensitive to penicillins, erythromycin remains the best alternative where oral therapy is possible. Cephalosporins, fusidic acid, or clindamycin can be used systemically, if justified by the clinical conditions, but the now well-established cross-sensitivity of cephalosporins and penicillins makes this alternative method of treatment hazardous.

Anaerobic Infections

Over the last few years a large increase has been reported in the isolation rate of infections due to anaerobic bacteria, particularly non-sporing Gram-negative bacilli such as bacteroides and fusobacteria. Although these organisms were first characterised in the late nineteenth century, many laboratories failed to isolate them, and the recent increase in isolation rate is partly due to greater care taken in the collection and transport of the specimens, and selective laboratory culture. *Bacteroides fragilis* account for a high proportion of the bacterial population of the faeces, and on a theoretical basis alone these organisms should be present in the majority of infections secondary to intestinal diseases, although the picture may be distorted by the relative ease with which this organism can be grown when compared with other anaerobes. Other anaerobic bacteria such as *Bacteroides oralis, B. melaninogenicus* and *Fusobacterium* spp. are commonly found in the mouth and genital tract, and are implicated widely in infections of these regions. In the past, surgical practice has been solely to drain abscesses related to the intestinal tract, without additional antibiotic therapy. However, it has been shown that the rate of complications following intra-abdominal abscesses is high, and this can be considerably modified by the use specific and appropriate antibiotic therapy.

Penicillin is still the drug of choice for anaerobic infections of the mouth, as all the causative bacteria (especially fusobacteria) are susceptible, but in infections arising from the intestinal tract the commonest organism isolated is *B. fragilis*, which is resistant to this antibiotic. Many strains of *B. fragilis* are sensitive to sulphonamides, tetracycline, erythromycin, and chloramphenicol, but over the last few decades there has been a steady increase in resistance. Tetracycline, although still showing a bimodal pattern of sensitivity, is less effective, as over 60 per cent of strains are resistant to easily achievable blood and tissue concentrations. However, newer compounds such as minocycline show more activity, and may be useful in therapy. Erythromycin can be given, although the difficulties associated with its systemic administration limit its usefulness.

The chemotherapeutic substances with the greatest activity against *B. fragilis* are clindamycin and metronidazole. Clindamycin can be given orally and by intramuscular injection, and has been used with considerable success. However there are reports of pseudomembranous enterocolitis following its use, and its administration should be monitored carefully. It is strange that the incidence varies greatly in different centres, and various explanations, such as the triggering action of certain intestinal viruses, have been put forward to explain this anomaly. Gastrointestinal side-effects such as diarrhoea occur, especially in patients receiving clindamycin after intestinal tract surgery. In many cases the diarrhoea resolves whilst the patient is still receiving the antibiotic, and the side-effect *may* be primarily related to the surgery, or other antibiotics, such as ampicillin or amoxycillin, which are frequently given in combination with clindamycin. Metronidazole and many other nitro-compounds have a marked activity against bacteroides, and are consistently bactericidal. Further reports are awaited before a proper evaluation can be made.

MANAGEMENT OF SPECIFIC DISEASES

It clearly is impossible, in an article such as this, even to attempt to cover all aspects of chemotherapy in a systematic manner. Instead, we have chosen to give brief descriptions of some of the particular problems involved in two serious diseases, meningitis and endocarditis. It is hoped that these considerations will serve to emphasise once again the importance of liaison between clinician and microbiologist, as well as the way in which some knowledge of the likely microbial aetiology, the range of activity of antimicrobial agents and their basic pharmacokinetics can lead to logical antibiotic treatment.

Meningitis

As in the case of all microbial diseases, appropriate laboratory investigations should be carried out before starting treatment. If the fluid is turbid and polymorphonuclear leucocytes are seen in a stained smear, a bacterial cause is likely.

However, the presence of an 'aseptic' meningitis where CSF counts are low but contain a significant number of polymorphs may be suggestive of bacterial aetiology, especially if the patient has been given antibiotics or is extremely ill.

Treatment must be started as soon as possible. Even an experienced worker may not always be able to find bacteria in a Gram film. However, when a tentative identification of the pathogen can be made, this will help in the selection of the antibiotic(s). Cultures are made but it is never justified to wait for identification by this means. Clinical examination may be helpful, and in a meningitis patient with a purpuric rash the cause is likely to be the meningococcus (although rarely such a rash may be caused by other organisms).

Chemotherapy of pyogenic meningitis

Where the cause is bacterial but unknown, chloramphenicol should be given. It is prudent to begin treatment with the succinate by the intramuscular or intravenous route. For an adult the initial dose should be 0.5 to 1.0 g, followed by subsequent doses of 0.5 g. After a day ot two when the patient is better a change to the oral route is justified. In all cases the dose is given 6-hourly.

If the diagnosis is known, more specific antimicrobial treatment is indicated.

Meningococcal meningitis. Sulphonamide-resistant strains are known to be widespread in North America and in some areas in Britain 5 to 10 per cent resistance has been reported. Since sulphonamide is still considered the treatment of choice, a good plan is to begin with penicillin and sulphonamide. If the strain is found to be sulphonamide-sensitive the penicillin can be discontinued. Initially the sulphonamide should be given parenterally (sulphadimidine sodium 1.5 g 6-hourly) and when the patient improves sulphadimidine 1.5 g 6-hourly by mouth.

Haemophilus influenza meningitis. This species is second only to meningo-coccus as a cause of bacterial meningitis and is often found in children. Nearly all cases are due to capsular type b. Either ampicillin or chloramphenicol should be given. Much debate has taken place about the relative merits of the two substances. However, with the emergence of ampicillin-resistant strains and the good results found with chloramphenicol the latter is preferred. The dose is the same as for meningococcal meningitis in adults, but for children the parenteral dose is 2.5 mg/kg, followed by the same oral dose when the child is better (*N.B.* Modification of the dose is needed in the neonate or premature infant.)

Pneumococcal meningitis. This form of meningitis is more likely to prove fatal than other common forms of purulent meningitis. It is often associated with poor general health. The possibility of it resulting from middle-ear disease must always be remembered. The treatment is with benzyl penicillin in very large doses. Because of the inflammation of the meninges, which allows free transfer of penicillin into the CSF, intrathecal penicillin is not needed.

Staphylococcal meningitis. Because of the danger of infection by β-lactamase-producing strains, initial treatment should be by cloxacillin 2 g 6-hourly. If the organism is subsequently found to be sensitive to benzylpenicillin, this antibiotic should be substituted.

Other causes. Listeria spp. meningitis should be treated with parenteral ampicillin.

Chloramphenicol remains the drug of choice for meningitis caused by Gram-negative bacilli, but initially some physicians add gentamicin to the treatment regime, because of the associated septicaemia.

Tuberculous meningitis. Because of the insidious onset of this illness the prognosis is dictated by making an early diagnosis.

However effective the treatment, delay in diagnosis is disastrous, since irreversible brain damage will remain.

Treatment should be started with intramuscular streptomycin 1 g daily, together with rifampicin 450 to 600 mg daily and isoniazid 10 mg/kg daily.

There are still protagonists of intrathecal streptomycin, but the unpleasantness of, and the danger of maintaining meningeal irritation by, repeated lumbar punctures, together with the lack of convincing evidence of improved prognosis, argue against this form of treatment.

Infective Endocarditis

It is unfortunate that, despite the development of a greatly expanded number of antimicrobial agents during the last 15 years, the prognosis in bacterial endocarditis is not as satisfactory as might be hoped. At the same time there has been a profound change in the aetiology in recent years which has further complicated the therapeutic approach. There is no condition in which collaboration between the clinician and the microbiologist is so vital. Lack of such collaboration is likely to result in an unhappy outcome.

Acute infective endocarditis

This is often caused by *Staph. aureus* but many other microorganisms can be responsible and produce a similar clinical picture. β-Haemolytic streptococci, *Strept. pneumoniae*, gonococci, brucellae, bacteroides, and candida are but a few examples.

Acute endocarditis usually develops secondarily to infection elsewhere, and detection of this focus is of great importance in planning treatment.

The treatment of acute endocarditis is complicated and the reader is referred to specialised texts for details. Unfortunately antimicrobial therapy in acute endocarditis is substantially less effective than in the subacute forms.

Subacute bacterial endocarditis

This disease is one in which cure depends upon the correct use of bactericidal antibiotics. The difficulty doubtless stems from the protection to bacteria given by growth in the platelet/fibrin vegetation, which cannot be penetrated by phagocytes.

Prosthetic valve endocarditis

Antimicrobial therapy alone rarely succeeds. Infection may be due to a wide range or organisms including *Candida, Staph. epidermidis,* and *Aspergillus.*

Isolation of the infecting organism is, of course, vital in planning treatment. Even where suitable antibiotics are available, the dose needed may prove too toxic to allow proper use.

Often it is impossible to cure the infection with drugs alone. In such cases an attempt is made to contain the infection, the prosthesis and vegetations removed and the prosthesis replaced by a new one. After surgery, intensive chemotherapy is given, on the basis of culture of the vegetations around the prosthesis and the results of blood culture.

Duration of treatment

Until recently treatment has continued for several months, but there are reports of satisfactory results having been obtained with an intensive course lasting only three weeks. This shorter course of therapy is not yet regarded as standard practice. However, this latter period should be regarded as a minimum, and on no account should treatment be stopped when an immediate clinical response is obtained. In some varieties of endocarditis such as those due to *Staph. epidermidis* or *Staph. aureus* experience has shown that treatment should always be continued for two to three months; shorter courses of treatment are very often followed by relapse. Shorter courses of treatment are usually successful with highly sensitive strains of *Strept. viridans*, especially when diagnosis has been made at an early stage.

Because of the lack of natural defences, bacteriostatic antibiotics do not eliminate the infection, so that relapse occurs when treatment is inadequate, or is stopped too soon. Even with bactericidal antibiotics high dosage is needed, and the minimal inhibitory concentration (MIC) of the infecting organisms needs to be taken into account in planning the dose. Another important property of the antimicrobial agent is its ability to diffuse through the platelet/fibrin mass.

The penicillins have been found to be by far the most valuable agents when the infection is due to *Strept. viridans* or *Strept. faecalis*. Ampicillin is preferred by some workers, but the cephalosporins are all inferior to benzylpenicillin, and so must not be used. When penicillins cannot be used because other organisms are present that are not sensitive, or when the patient is allergic to penicillin, the outcome is, in general, less satisfactory. Even when the organism causing the endocarditis is *Strept. viridans*, with an MIC as low as 0.025 µg/ml or less, penicillin must be given in a dose of at least 2 million units (2.2 g daily), at 6-hourly intervals. Most physicians prefer to give benzylpenicillin by intramuscular injection. For *Strept. faecalis*, or less sensitive strains of *Strept. viridans* (MICs of 1–2 µg/ml), doses of 20 to 50 million units (12–30 g) may be needed. It is also wise to delay renal excretion by giving probenecid 0.5 g 6-hourly. It is usually necessary to prescribe an aminoglycoside such as gentamicin in addition to the penicillin, as a total bactericidal effect is then achieved. When strains are more resistant most (but not all) physicians supplement the treatment with 1.0 g streptomycin per day.

If very large doses of penicillin are used, continuous intravenous infusion is needed because the pain caused by intramuscular injection of large amounts of benzylpenicillin is intolerable.

FURTHER READING

PHARMACOKINETICS

Gibaldi, M. & Perrier, D. (1975) *Pharmacokinetics.* New York: Dekker.

Wagner, J. G. (1971) *Biopharmaceutics and Relevant Pharmacokinetics.* Hamilton, Ill.: Drug Intelligence Publications.

DRUG RESISTANCE

Ayliffe, G. A. J. (1972/73) Control of antibiotic resistance in bacteria. *Prevent,* **1,** 43–48.

Lowbury, E. J. L., Ayliffe, G. A. J., Geddes, A. M. & Williams, J. D. (1975) *Control of Hospital Infection.* London: Chapman and Hall.

Microbiology — 1974 (1975) Washington: American Society of Microbiology.

LABORATORY DIAGNOSIS
Emond, R. T. D. (1974) *A Colour Atlas of Infectious Diseases.* London: Wolfe.
Stratford, B. C. (1976). *An Atlas of Medical Microbiology.* Oxford: Blackwell.
Thomas, W. A. R. (ed.) (1971) *Calling the Laboratory.* Edinburgh: Churchill Livingstone.

PROPHYLAXIS
British Medical Journal (1973) Editorial: Prophylactic antibiotics in caesarian section. *British Medical Journal*, 2, 675–677.
Garrod, L. P. (1975) Chemoprophylaxis. *British Medical Journal*, iv, 561–565.
Lancet (1976) Editorial: Prophylactic povidone iodine. *Lancet*, i, 73–74.
Lancet (1976) Editorial: Prophylaxis of bacterial endocarditis. Faith, hope and charitable interpretations. *Lancet*, i, 519–520.

ANTIMICROBIAL AGENTS
Binda, G., Domenichini, E., Gottardi, A., Orlandi, B., Ortelli, E., Pacini, B. & Fowst, C. (1971) Rifampicin. *Arzneimittel-Forschung*, 21, 1907–1977.
Drugs (1975) Focus on amoxycillin. *Drugs*, 9, No. 2.
Garrod, L. P., Lambert, H. P. & O'Grady, F. (ed.) (1973) *Antibiotic and Chemotherapy*, 4th edn. Edinburgh: Churchill Livingstone.
Gentamicin: Review and Commentary on Selected World Literature (1974) New Jersey: Schering Corp.
Goodman, L. S. & Gilman, A. (eds) (1975) *The Pharmacological Basis of Therapeutics*, 5th edn. New York: Macmillan.
Jawetz, E., Melnick, J. L. & Adelberg, E. A. (1974) *Review of Medical Microbiology*, 11th edn. Los Altos, California: Lange.
Journal of Antimicrobial Chemotherapy (1975) Cephalexin and cephaloridine. *Journal of Antimicrobial Chemotherapy*, 1, No. 3. Supplement.
Journal of Infectious Diseases (1973) Cefazolin. *Journal of Infectious Diseases*, 128, October Supplement.
Journal of Infectious Diseases (1973) Trimethoprimsulphamethoxazole. *Journal of Infectious Diseases*, 128, November Supplement.
Opuscula Medica (1974) Doxycycline. *Opuscula Medica*, 33, Supplement.
Postgraduate Medical Journal (1974) Clotrimazole. *Postgraduate Medical Journal*, 50, July Supplement.
Today's Drugs (1970) London: British Medical Association.
Wagman, G. H. & Weinstein, M. J. (1975) Antimicrobial agents. *Annual Reports in Medicinal Chemistry*, 10,109–119.

TREATMENT
Beeson, P. B. & Ridley, M. (ed.) (1963) *Bacterial Endocarditis.* London: Beecham Research Laboratories.
British Journal of Hospital Medicine, 12 (4) (1974), passim.
British Journal of Hospital Medicine, 14 (5) (1975), passim.
British Medical Journal (1976) Leading article: Chemotherapeutic routes in meningitis. *British Medical Journal*, i, 977–978.
Brumfitt, W. & Asscher, A. W. (eds) (1973) *Urinary Tract Infection.* London: Oxford University Press.
Hoeprich, P. D. (ed.) (1972) *Infectious Diseases.* Hagerstown, Md.: Harper & Row.
Journal of Infectious Diseases (1969) Symposium on pyelonephritis. *Journal of Infectious Diseases*, 120 (1), 1–140.
Kass, E. H. (ed.) (1969) *Preventive Approaches to Chronic Diseases.* New York: Milbank Memorial Fund.
Kaye, D. (ed.) (1976) *Infective Endocarditis.* University Park Press.
Kucers, A. & Bennet, N. McK. (1975) *The Use of Antibiotics.* London: Heinemann.
Lancet (1976) Editorial: Diagnosis and prognosis in pyogenic meningitis. *Lancet*, ii, 1277–1278.
May, J. R. (1972) *Chemotherapy of Chronic Bronchitis.* London: English Universities Press.
Stamey, T. A. (1972) *Urinary Infections.* Baltimore: Williams & Wilkins.
Utz, J. P. (1976) Chemotherapy for the systemic mycoses. *British Journal of Hospital Medicine*, 15, 112–121.
Wrong, O. (ed.) (1968) *Fourth Symposium on Advanced Medicine.* London: Pitman.

9
THE TREATMENT OF PHOBIC AND OBSESSIONAL STATES

M. S. Lipsedge

There has been considerable progress in the treatment of phobic and obsessional disorders over the past 15 years. While the most solid advances have been in the refinement of psychological methods (the so-called behaviour therapies or 'behavioural psychotherapies') there have also been promising developments in physical methods of treatment, both pharmacological and surgical. The therapeutic advances have been accompanied by renewed interest in the phenomenology of these conditions (e.g. Rachman, 1973; Walker and Beech, 1969; Reed, 1968).

PHOBIAS

The monograph *Fears and Phobias* by Marks (1969) provides the most comprehensive review of this topic. He defined a phobia as a special form of fear which is out of proportion to the demands of the situation, cannot be explained or reasoned away, is beyond voluntary control, and leads to avoidance of the feared situation. Phobias can be broadly classified into three major groups, specific phobias, agoraphobia, and social phobias. Specific phobics are morbidly afraid of, for example, certain animals such as dogs or spiders, or of a limited number of clearly defined situations or events, such as heights or thunderstorms.

The most common and distressing phobic disorder in psychiatric practice is the agoraphobic syndrome; its prevalence in the general community is estimated at 6.3/1000 (Agras, Silvester and Oliveau, 1969) and it accounts for 50 to 60 per cent of patients with phobias who are referred to hospital psychiatrists. Agoraphobia consists of a cluster of fears starting in adult life which centre around going out alone and entering any place from which escape may be difficult or embarrassing, such as crowded supermarkets or lifts. Both open and enclosed public places are avoided and the patients (usually women) have a wide range of 'situational anxiety' together with much general or 'free-floating' anxiety. Compared with monosymptomatic phobics, agoraphobics tend to be introverted and have high neuroticism scores (Gelder, Marks and Wolff, 1967) and their palmar skin resistance, which is a measure of anxiety (Lader, 1967) shows significantly more spontaneous fluctuations.

In addition to free-floating anxiety, agoraphobia is often accompanied by depression, depersonalisation, and obsessions. Agoraphobia often begins during a panic attack when the patient becomes afraid of returning to the same or similar places for fear of triggering off further panic attacks (Lader and Marks, 1971).

The phobia may become so severe that the patient is permanently house-bound and always insists on being accompanied by at least one member of the family.

It is not known why some patients who have marked free-floating anxiety with frequent panic attacks, do not develop agoraphobia. The suggestion that differences in conditionability could account for this has not been supported by experiments on eye-blink conditioning (Martin, Marks and Gelder, 1969).

There is a third but less clearly defined group of phobics who suffer from social anxieties. They have a morbid fear of confronting strangers or authority figures, or of making a fool of themselves in public by blushing, trembling, or vomiting. Social phobics have psychophysiological characteristics more similar to those of agoraphobics than monosymptomatics but they have not been so intensively studied.

The damaging effect on personal and family life of being house-bound is obvious. The monosymptomatic phobias may appear more trivial but they can cause as much distress as agoraphobia. A patient with an intense fear of feathers may be unable to leave his house because of the possibility of casual contact with them. Social phobias can also lead to isolation and severe impairment of performance at work. Patients may become dependent on alcohol, barbiturates, or benzodiazepine tranquillisers to deal with the panic attacks which arise in certain situations.

Some forms of sexual dysfunction in both men and women have many of the features of a true phobic state (heterophobia) with disproportionate situational anxiety and avoidance and a similar response to one of the newer forms of psychological treatment (Friedman and Lipsedge, 1971).

OBSESSIONAL NEUROSIS

The symptoms of obsessional neurosis can be divided into ruminations and rituals. Obsessional ruminations include distressing ideas, obscene or blasphemous associations, morbid impulses, and an urge to count or recite repeatedly. Black (1974) quotes Schneider's definition of obsessions as 'contents of consciousness which when they occur, are accompanied by the experience of subjective compulsion and which cannot be got rid of, though on quiet reflection they are recognised as senseless'. Obsessional rituals include hand-washing, checking, and hoarding. The rituals may be triggered off by the ruminations or may occur in response to physical contact with an object that is perceived as dangerous. There is no constant relationship between ruminations and rituals and they can occur independently.

Obsessional neurosis is relatively uncommon. Kringlen (1965) found an incidence of 2.5 per cent in a psychiatric in-patient population. The prognosis is poor: he found that of a total of 82 patients, only 21 were either asymptomatic or improved after 13 to 20 years.

Obsessional symptoms may appear for the first time during the course of a depressive illness (Lewis, 1934). Of 346 cases of depressive psychosis without premorbid obsessions, 25 per cent were found to exhibit obsessions throughout the duration of the depressive episode (Gittleson, 1966). When the obsessions are symptoms of an affective disorder the obsessional illness tends to run a cyclical course. Obsessional symptoms have also been observed after encephalitis lethargica.

An important, and often difficult, differential diagnosis is between obsessional neurosis and schizophrenia. Lewis (1966) has pointed out that the only difference between obsessions and many schizophrenic phenomena towards which the patient retains insight and which he regards as alien, is that the obsessional recognises that the compulsion comes from within his own mind whereas the schizophrenic feels that the compulsion is imposed from without. The development of schizophrenia in obsessional patients is a relatively rare occurrence. Only 3 of a series of 91 obsessional neurotics followed up for between 13 and 20 years developed schizophrenia. (Kringlen, 1965).

The Measurement of Phobic and Obsessional Symptoms

The accurate assessment of response to the treatment of the neuroses requires valid and reliable methods for measuring the severity of symptoms. Satisfactory self-rating and observer-rating scales using visual analogues have been used in a number of trials of systematic desensitisation (Gelder and Marks, 1966) and flooding (Watson et al, 1971). Rachman, Hodgson and Marks (1971) have devised a number of simple behavioural tests to establish the parameters of approach to a feared ('contaminated') object or situation. They have measured the distance the patient maintains from a contaminant and the time taken to approach it. Mechanical devices may also be used. In one study (Lipsedge, 1974) the subjects operated a hand-held compressed air apparatus which controlled the approach of feared objects, thus allowing accurate measurement of avoidance behaviour. Marks (1975) warns that avoidance tests in the experimental situation may be a poor guide to the patient's performance outside hospital. Chronically disabled patients may be persuaded to enter their phobic situation or to desist from rituals during a brief test but this behaviour may not persist outside the clinic. Of 12 severely compulsive patients who failed a behavioural test before treatment, all passed the test after two hours of exposure though improvement on other scales was highly variable (Lipsedge, 1974).

Gillan and Rachman (1974) attributed the failure of their avoidance tests to provide consistent data to their inability to devise a way of enforcing uniformity on the variations in fear encountered in 32 phobic patients.

The measurement of obsessional symptoms presents a number of problems. The wide range of symptoms makes comprehensive questionnaires unwieldy. Flexible individual measures tend to be unreliable for comparisons of individual patients and of group studies. In one study on obsessional ruminations (Stern, Lipsedge and Marks, 1973) it proved difficult to persuade the patients to complete self-rating scales. Prolonged rumination occurred before completing each rating. Often excessive vaccillation was followed by no rating. When completed, ratings were often destroyed for fear of an error. Certain ratings were deemed impossible by some patients but not by others and so flexibility had to be adopted; even then not all patients could complete some measures.

The Leyton Obsessional Inventory (Cooper, 1970) has been used in clinical trials of clomipramine (Rack, 1973; Rigby, Clarren and Kelly, 1973) and in

202 RECENT ADVANCES IN MEDICINE

studies of flooding in obsessionals. The inventory subjectively assesses both obsessional symptoms and traits by means of a card-sorting procedure. Feelings of resistance and the degree of interference produced by symptoms in day-to-day tasks are also quantified. The Leyton Obsessional Inventory correlated poorly with behavioural tests in the study of flooding in obsessionals by Rachman, Marks and Hodgson (1973), partly because it was originally devised to separate house-proud housewives from normal housewives and obsessional neurotics in a study of family relationships. There are no questions to cover the more bizarre symptoms found in obsessional neurosis and the scores are affected by depression and by cultural factors (for example Irishwomen tend to have higher scores than Englishwomen (Kelleher, 1972)).

Philpott (1975) recommends the use of standard measures of depression and anxiety in addition to assessments of obsessional symptoms. He points out that a simple rank correlation of obsessional and depressive change scores could help to identify the therapeutic effect of physical treatments such as the tricyclic antidepressants and psychosurgery. Social deficits due to obsessional illness, including impairment of work and leisure and the effect on sexual and marital relations and financial functioning, also require standardised assessment.

A new battery of rating scales for obsessional symptoms using the visual analogue technique has been described recently (Philpott, 1975). These scales could be used to monitor changes in symptomatology in individuals or in groups of patients and permit comparisons between trials of treatment. They consist of a clinician's scale and a self-rating scale which are both designed to assess the degree of discomfort and the amount of time spent each day on rituals and ruminations. Two of the patient's most prominent and disturbing rituals or ruminations are selected for measurement, such as washing rituals after use of the lavatory or checking trousers. Instructions to the clinician are appended to these scales to assist in eliciting information in a standardised way. The measures are flexible and have the advantage that they can be modified according to the phenomenology of each patient. An interview check-list provides a method of assessing and recording impairment of daily activity by rituals or ruminations. It consists of a comprehensive list of 64 everyday activities that may trigger off obsessional symptoms (such as using sharp instruments, touching glass, or going to the lavatory). Each item is scored on a four-point scale which acts as a crude measure of the amount of time taken up by each activity. The degree to which the patient avoids certain tasks because of obsessional fears is also assessed and provision is also made for recording whether the activity is carried out in a bizarre fashion.

THE TREATMENT OF PHOBIAS

Systematic desensitisation

Systematic desensitisation is the most common form of behaviour therapy used in treating phobic disorders. In one hospital group (St Francis and Lady Chichester Hospitals, Haywards Heath) systematic desensitisation constituted 80 per cent of all the behaviour modification techniques (Mottahedin and Mayo, 1974); operant conditioning and aversion therapy accounted for only 4 per cent and 2 per cent respectively. Systematic desensitisation was introduced by Wolpe (1958) and the standard procedure comprises the construction of a graded list of situations or objects that provoke anxiety in the patient (this list is referred to as a 'hierarchy'), teaching a technique to induce muscular relaxation (Jacobson, 1938; Schultz and Luth, 1959), and the presentation of frightening scenes in a graded fashion which gradually ascend the scale from the least to the most distressing. The patient signals the slightest degree of tension, discomfort or anxiety at which point he is instructed to relax and returns to an item lower in the hierarchy.

Most studies of the effectiveness of systematic desensitisation have been on American psychology students who volunteer for laboratory experiments on the reduction of specific fears (Rachman, 1971). The relevance of the data derived from analogue research to the management of clinical anxiety has been seriously questioned by Cooper, Furst and Bridger (1969), who have found desensitisation to be less effective with patients than with volunteers. They cite an experiment in which the control group of 'snake phobics' who had been instructed to pretend to be cured were actually able to hold a snake without receiving any treatment. Olley and McAllister (1974) have compared a group of volunteer subjects who had specific phobias with a normal control group and a group of phobic patients. The results indicated significant differences between the volunteers and the patients although they shared a common disabling symptom. The patients were distinguished by their high level of neuroticism, anxiety and general psychiatric symptomatology.

Two large but uncontrolled trials of systematic desensitisation in phobic patients have shown remarkably favourable results. Wolpe (1961) found a response rate of 90 per cent in 39 patients with 'phobias and allied neurotic habits' whom he had treated himself. Response to a median number of 10 treatment sessions was rated on a four-point scale covering symptoms, productivity, interpersonal relations, sexual adjustment, and vulnerability to stress. A study of 20 of these patients after an interval of six months to four years from the end of treatment showed no relapse or emergence of new symptoms ('symptom substitution'). Lazarus (1963) reported significant improvement in 78 per cent of 408 patients treated mainly by systematic desensitisation. In a smaller group of 126 more severely handicapped patients, excluding those with monosymptomatic phobias, 62 per cent were rated as markedly improved or recovered after an average of 14 sessions. Patients with generalised anxiety and panic attacks responded less well to treatment.

In a somewhat more rigorous study Hain, Butcher, and Stevenson (1966) treated 27 patients suffering with anxiety and phobic symptoms. In addition to assessment by the therapist the patients were rated by an independent assessor. Seventy-eight per cent showed an improvement in phobic symptoms after a mean of 19 sessions. A study of 14 patients after an average of one year showed that of those who had improved during treatment, 20 per cent had continued to improve and 47 per cent had maintained their initial improvement.

Meyer and Chesser (1970) have pointed out defects in the methodology of clinical research in behaviour therapy which has failed to include adequate controls. Sampling biases are common, assessment of improvement is often made only by the therapist who conducted treatment, and the reliability of ratings is frequently not reported. Patients who have not completed a certain number of sessions may be excluded from the results and when several therapeutic methods have been used together there may be insufficient control to assess the effect of a particular technique. Inadequate follow-up studies with infrequent assessment of progress have given misleading results because of the fluctuating nature of many neuroses.

Among the most rigorous studies of systematic desensitisation have been the series of controlled prospective trials carried out at the Maudsley Hospital. In their first study, Gelder and Marks (1966) allocated 20 matched in-patients with severe agoraphobia randomly to either systematic desensitisation and graded retraining or brief psychotherapy. Each treatment session lasted 45 minutes and was given three times a week. Of 10 patients in both groups seven had improved after about 20 weeks, but by the time of follow-up at one year both groups had relapsed. Gelder, Marks and Wolff (1967) then compared desensitisation plus graded retraining with individual psychotherapy and with group psychotherapy in three matched groups of patients. Each group of patients comprised between 10 and 16 phobic outpatients who were all assessed before, during, and immediately after treatment, and at follow-up, by both the therapist and an independent assessor. Response to treatment was measured by rating scales covering phobic symptoms, work performance and enjoyment of leisure. Desensitisation was administered one hour weekly for an average of nine months whilst individual psychotherapy was given for one hour weekly for a year; group psychotherapy was continued for 18 months and consisted of weekly sessions lasting $1\frac{1}{2}$ hours. Desensitisation produced a much more rapid reduction in symptoms than psychotherapy. A significant improvement in the behaviour therapy group was found at six months but at 18 months the difference was no longer statistically significant.

Lader, Gelder and Marks (1967) found that those patients who benefited most from desensitisation tended to have low levels of arousal as shown by relatively rapid habituation of the galvanic skin responses, few spontaneous fluctuations in palmar skin conductants, and little 'free-floating' anxiety. Patients with specific phobias (those who responded best to desensitisation) had relatively low levels of arousal or physiological correlates of anxiety. In a cross-over study (1968) Gelder and Marks went on to desensitise seven of the patients who had failed to respond to group psychotherapy. They responded much more rapidly than patients who had not had previous psychotherapy and had a three-fold improvement after four months of behaviour therapy compared with their progress in the previous two years.

Failure to respond to desensitisation correlated with the presence of agoraphobic symptoms and other neurotic features especially generalised anxiety, obsessions, depression and hypochondriasis and poor interpersonal relationships. Although the results with systematic desensitisation in specific phobics have been very satisfactory the prospects of recovery for patients with severe agoraphobia and marked anxiety remained relatively poor. However the recent development of flooding (which is discussed in the next section) has improved the outlook for this severely handicapped group of patients.

Flooding

Interest in the therapeutic potential of flooding or throwing the phobic patient 'in at the deep end' was stimulated by the convergence of clinical research and the work of animal psychologists. Stampfl and Levis (1967) introduced 'implosive therapy' in which the patient was required to imagine intensely distressing scenes based on psychodynamic exploration of his symptoms. The repeated evocation of these scenes led to a reduction in phobic behaviour. The laboratory analogue to this work is seen in the research of Baum (1969, 1970). He induced fears in small animals by the application of classical conditioning techniques and then reversed the 'phobic' behaviour by exposing the animals to intense fear-evoking stimuli and preventing their escape ('response prevention').

Subsequent research with patients has shown that the evocation of psychodynamic cues is a superfluous element in flooding (Marks, Boulougouris and Marset, 1971), which has evolved into a procedure whose essential ingredient consists of exposure of the patient for long periods to those objects or situations which evoke the most intense fear. Current research is attempting to identify the conditions most likely to produce lasting reduction in phobic behaviour. Marks (1974) has listed the experimental variables which need to be tested to develop an effective and economical flooding technique. Flooding may be given:

1. in fantasy or in practice;
2. individually or to groups;
3. at varying speeds;
4. with anxiety heightened or lessened;
5. with frightening cues which are relevant or irrelevant;
6. with differing durations of sessions and of intersession intervals;
7. by tape-recorder or by a therapist.

Some of these variables have already been systematically examined. For example although the deliberate evocation of anxiety was thought to be an essential ingredient of the original implosion treatment, several studies have shown that anxiety during flooding does not facilitate improvement (Marks et al, 1971; Mathews et al, 1974; Watson and Marks, 1971) and the use of sedatives has been shown to enhance the procedure (Gaind, Watson and Marks, 1970; Marks et al 1972; McCormick, 1973). Longer flooding sessions appear more potent than shorter ones but the optimum duration is not known. Stern and Marks (1974) gave agoraphobic out-patients four sessions of long or short flooding in fantasy and in practice. Fantasy sessions were given by tape-recorder and produced minimal arousal with little improvement. Two hours of flooding in practice reduced phobias significantly more than did four half-hour periods of the same procedure in one afternoon. Prolonged group exposure has been shown to be effective in agoraphobics, especially when group cohesion is deliberately fostered (Hand, Lamontagne and Marks, 1974). Patients need to be well motivated and to know what is required of them before undertaking what may be a rather unpleasant form of treatment otherwise they may terminate treatment prematurely. A quarter of a series of 125 obsessive-compulsives who were offered a form of flooding refused behaviour therapy (Marks, Hodgson and Rachman,

1975). Although sessions of imagined confrontation with frightening scenes are less effective than exposure in practice (Stern and Marks, 1973; Watson et al, 1971), patients may find this more acceptable, at least as a preliminary procedure.

Comparison of flooding and systematic desensitisations in 16 patients with severe chronic agoraphobia showed flooding to be significantly superior (Marks et al, 1971) but another study in 36 phobic patients failed to show significant differences between these two procedures although both were more effective than control treatment (Mathews et al, 1974). In the first study (Marks et al, 1971) flooding was more effective in severe generalised phobias but systematic desensitisation produced the greatest change in specific phobias. This is consistent with the observation that systematic desensitisation works well with monosymptomatic phobias and is less effective where there is a high degree of free-floating anxiety (Lang and Lazovic, 1963; Lazarus, 1963; Gelder et al, 1967).

Marks (1973) has developed a unifying theory to account for the effectiveness of the contrasting procedures of flooding and desensitisation. A mechanism of action shared by both methods is exposure of the frightened subject to a phobic situation until he acclimatises or 'adapts' (adaptation is a term used in the literature of learning theory to designate the process of getting rid of undesirable responses to a stimulus by repeated presentations of that stimulus). Systematic desensitisation involves a gradual approach to the phobic situation during the 'counteracting' response of relaxation, while flooding involves a rapid approach. The treatment known as modelling also contains the element of exposure. For example Bandura, Blanchard and Ritter (1968) first required a snake phobic subject to observe a model approaching a snake and then instructed him to carry out the same task. Marks suggests (1975) that exposure variants can be ordered along a continuum of approach to distressing situations. At the flooding end of the spectrum the confrontation is sudden, prolonged and distressing. In systematic desensitisation the exposure to the phobic situation is slow, graded and brief; minimum tension is experienced while a contrasting experience (relaxation) is induced.

THE TREATMENT OF OBSESSIONAL RITUALS

In 1966 Meyer developed a new approach to the psychological treatment of obsessional rituals. The method was partly based on the patients' own accounts of their reasons for carrying out compulsive acts. Many obsessionals report that the execution of rituals reduces the immediate feelings of anxiety evoked by distressing ideas or by contact with potential danger (gas taps, locks, electric switches, etc.). There is, however, a significant minority in whom the ritual actually increases the patient's anxiety (Walker and Beech, 1969). In addition, a proportion of patients say that they feel compelled to carry out their rituals in order to avert eventual disaster to themselves or their families. Meyer (1966) predicted that if the obsessional could be persuaded or forced to remain in feared situations and prevented from carrying out the compulsive acts, he may discover that the anticipated disastrous consequences of failing for example to wash or check repeatedly would not actually occur. The patient's expectations of the calamitous effects of not performing his rituals would be altered and his ritualistic behaviour would cease. He applied this 'modification of expectations' or 'reality testing' approach to two patients with long-standing handwashing rituals, one of whom had failed to benefit from systematic desensitisation. The patients were continuously supervised by nursing staff and were encouraged to handle 'contaminating' objects while excessive washing was prevented. In both patients there was a reduction of ritual behaviour, and this improvement was maintained at follow-up after more than one year (Meyer, 1966).

The same worker subsequently published a detailed account of the treatment of a 25-year-old man with an 11-year history of compulsive handwashing (Meyer and Levy, 1970). This patient was placed under continuous supervision for nine days. The taps in his room were turned off and only appropriate routine washing was permitted. During a brief daily visit the therapist persuaded the patient to handle contaminated objects which usually evoked marked anxiety and the urge to carry out washing rituals. These objects included letters and clothing belonging to the patient's brother, whose presence triggered off handwashing rituals. Whenever the patient reported anxiety or an urge to wash he was diverted with persuasion, encouragement, and recreational activities. This treatment led to total abolition of the compulsive washing which had not recurred 18 months later.

Meyer, Levy and Schnurrer (1974) have subsequently reported on the outcome of a similar method in 15 obsessional patients who had a mean duration of symptoms of $15\frac{1}{2}$ years. The authors have used the term 'apotrepic therapy' (derived from a Greek neologism meaning to turn away, deter or dissuade) to describe the technique, which involved continuous supervision by nurses who were instructed to prevent patients carrying out rituals by distracting them with other activities. As soon as total elimination of rituals under supervision had been achieved, the patients were confronted with situations which had previously provoked rituals and were required to handle feared objects. The patients were still prevented from carrying out the rituals and although the nurses' supervision was gradually withdrawn it was resumed if the patient relapsed. Rituals were assessed on a visual analogue scale (Aitken, 1969) and at the end of treatment two-thirds of the subjects were either free of symptoms or had had a reduction in ritual score of at least 75 per cent. Reassessment at an interval ranging from six months to six years after the end of treatment showed that six patients had maintained their post-treatment level of improvement while two others showed further reduction in rituals without additional treatment. Although there was no control group and the ratings were crude and open to bias, the results in this particular group of severe obsessionals were very encouraging.

Another group of workers have reported a series of partially controlled studies of the effect of modelling and exposure in 20 in-patients with chronic obsessional neurosis (Marks et al, 1975). The patients were given a mean of 15 treatment sessions over a period of three weeks. In both exposure (flooding) and modelling sessions they were encouraged to enter situations which caused distress and which provoked avoidance and compulsive rituals. At the end of each 40–60 minute session the patients were encouraged to refrain from carrying out compulsive acts for increasing periods of time. The authors call this 'self-imposed response prevention' since virtually no supervision was provided between sessions. In flooding sessions the therapist limited his activity to acting in a reassuring manner, while in modelling sessions he encouraged the patient to imitate his own confident handling of the provoking objects.

Subjective reports, independent assessments, and behavioural-avoidance tests showed that both flooding and modelling procedures were significantly superior to a control treatment consisting of relaxation training. While the addition of modelling to flooding did not significantly enhance the results for the group as a whole, it did appear to help some of the patients (Marks et al, 1975). Two years later 14 patients were found to have maintained a significant reduction in their obsessions.

Both the modelling and flooding procedures described in this series of studies share two major therapeutic features with the apotrepic technique, namely confrontation of the patient with situations which evoke anxiety and curtailment of rituals. While the superiority of both modelling and flooding over the control procedure has been well demonstrated, it was not possible to distinguish the separate contributions of exposure and the prevention of rituals.

Boulougouris and Bassiakos (1973) have also reported a marked reduction in longstanding obsessional symptoms following treatment which they call 'prolonged flooding'. The three patients in their study remained well during the nine months follow-up period. The patients were exposed in the presence of the therapist to situations which triggered off discomfort and were not allowed to perform their rituals after touching 'contaminating' objects. They were also flooded 'in fantasy' with images of contaminating objects. The mean total treatment time was 22 hours. There was no base-line period of observation since the first rating was made immediately before beginning the first treatment, and the authors made no attempt to assess the separate effects of guided contamination and ritual curtailment (response prevention).

Mills, Barlow and Baugh (1971) have tried to compare the therapeutic contribution of forced exposure to feared objects, without ritual prevention, with the effect of exposure combined with interruption of rituals. An ingenious technical innovation was the use of an objective measure of the ritual behaviour of the two subjects. Whenever the patient approached the washbasin a cumulative recorder was automatically activated, indicating the frequency and duration of handwashing. In neither case was there a decline in handwashing during exposure alone, but a significant and lasting reduction in compulsive behaviour occurred after the introduction of ritual prevention into the treatment procedure. In a further study (Mills et al, 1973) the same group compared the effects of giving verbal instructions with exposure and with ritual-prevention in a series of five patients with compulsive handwashing or checking rituals. Since exposure to contaminated objects without prevention of rituals produced either no change or even caused an increase in the frequency of washing or checking, they deduced that the curtailment of rituals following exposure was a necessary condition for the eventual elimination of rituals. The opposite conclusion was reached in a small pilot study on short-term effects in obsessional handwashers (Lipsedge, 1974). Patients were allowed to wash for as long as they wanted but were continually re-contaminated throughout the washing procedure. These patients showed the same degree of improvement over one week as did other patients who were contaminated but not allowed to wash.

The role of response prevention during the exposure treatment of obsessionals remains uncertain (Marks et al, 1975). Meyer et al (1974) consider that the critical therapeutic ingredient in the apotropic method may be the supervised prevention of rituals. In contrast to their view that it does not matter how the patient is exposed to the disturbing situation so long as he is actively prevented from carrying out his rituals, Marks et al (1975) suggest that the contribution of response prevention is that it simply serves to prolong the period of exposure to the feeling of contamination or a sense of danger. This issue is of practical importance because of the considerable amount of specialised nursing time required for a programme of continuous individual supervision. A recent case report (Meyer, Robertson and Tatlow, 1975) on the successful domiciliary treatment with minimal supervision of a patient with severe obsessional neurosis gives some support to the belief that intimate contact with contaminants is more important than supervised prevention of inter-session compulsive behaviour.

Primary Obsessional Slowness

Rachman (1974) has described a rare subgroup of obsessionals in whom pathological slowness in the performance of daily tasks is not secondary to checking rituals. Encouraging results were obtained with a combination of prompting, 'shaping' and 'pacing' in 10 such patients. After providing the necessary instructions and modelling the therapist prompted more reasonable and quicker behaviour while the patient was carrying out his task e.g. shaving, washing, dressing. Shaping is a term used to describe the use of graduated tasks whose completion is systematically rewarded. Shaping instructions were used to encourage improvements and discourage errors or persisting slowness. External pacing was provided by the therapist simultaneously performing the same tasks. Once some progress had been achieved the patient was shown how to monitor his own performance.

OBSESSIONAL RUMINATIONS

Recurrent morbid ruminations have been even more resistant to psychological methods of treatment than obsessional rituals, partly because of their inaccessibility to observation and direct manipulation and partly because of incomplete understanding of the phenomenology and psychopathology (Rachman, 1971). Some behaviour therapists have found systematic desensitisation to be effective (Bevan, 1960) but the majority have reported poor results with this technique. For example, Furst and Cooper (1970) failed to extinguish the anxiety aroused by imaginary stimuli in two patients treated with systematic desensitisation. Other behavioural methods recently used to treat ruminations include thought-stopping (Wolpe and Lazarus, 1966; Yamagami, 1971), paradoxical intention (Frankl, 1960), and flooding (Hackman and McLean, 1975). The thought-stopping technique requires the patient to think his obsessive thought deliberately (for example that his child has cancer or that he will commit a dreadful sin).

The therapist then makes a sudden loud ('aversive') noise and shouts 'stop'. This appears to interrupt the induced rumination and the patient is then taught to shout 'stop' each time he deliberately produces his own distressing thoughts. After some practice he whispers 'stop' and eventually uses a subvocal command. Several sessions of rehearsing this procedure have led to marked diminution in the frequency of distressing intrusive ideas (Stern, 1970; Yamagami, 1971).

In a controlled trial of thought-stopping (Stern, Lipsedge and Marks, 1973) four patients improved as much by learning to induce neutral thoughts deliberately as by stopping obsessional thoughts. This suggests that thought-stopping does not work by the specific extinction of the obsessional ideas but operates by providing training in self-regulation (Kanfer and Seindner, 1973) and the acquisition of a problem-solving 'set' which the patient learns to employ in controlling his own troublesome thoughts. The obsessional neurotic's fear of loss of control decreases when he recognises that he is capable of bringing his intrusive thoughts under control (Solyom et al, 1972). This interpretation of thought-stopping as a form of training in self-regulation is supported by the promising results of paradoxical intention (Frankel, 1970) in the treatment of obsessional neurosis (Solyom et al, 1972). Ten subjects were told to dwell deliberately on their intrusive thoughts, to exaggerate the fearful or loathsome ideas, and to endeavour to convince themselves of their validity. After six weekly sessions there had been marked diminution of unwanted thoughts in half the subjects.

Thought-stopping has not yet been systematically compared with imaginary flooding with obsessional themes but a recent study by Hackman and McLean (1975) showed it to be almost as effective as flooding in practice in patients with a mixture of rituals and ruminations. They omitted the relaxation training which is an apparently redundant preliminary procedure in the thought-stopping technique originally described by Wolpe and Lazarus in 1966. Elements common to both thought-stopping and exposure include confrontation with distressing situations or experiences and indoctrination in the belief that surrender to fears reinforces them, while actively confronting fearful stimuli leads to weakening of symptoms (Hackman and McLean, 1975). This emphasis on direct confrontation with distressing situations and ideas contrasts with the approach in systematic desensitisation where the patient is advised to wait until the anxiety is extinguished before attempting to face the situation in real life.

PSYCHOTROPIC DRUGS

Iminodibenzyl drugs

In 1968 it was reported that the tricyclic antidepressant clomipramine (chlorinated imipramine), may be effective in the treatment of obsessional states even when the obsessional symptoms are not secondary to a depressive illness (Van Renynghe de Voxvrie, 1968).

Three years later Lopez-Ibor (1971) described 29 chronic obsessional patients whose symptoms responded to an average of 20 daily intravenous infusions of 300 mg of clomipramine. Since then a number of workers have reported favourably on the use of this drug in the treatment of both obsessional states and phobias (Capstick, 1973; Rack, 1973; Waxman, 1975).

One large series (Marshall and Micev, 1975), included 118 patients with obsessional disorders and phobic anxiety states, who were treated with clomipramine administered as a slow intravenous infusion in daily doses of 300–375 mg for about 15 days (Marshall and Micev, 1973). Eighteen of the patients required more than one course of treatment. The mean improvement, on a four-point scale of disability, was over 70 per cent at the end of the follow-up period which ranged from six months to three years.

Although interpretation of the results of both this study and the clinical trials by Capstick (1973) and Rack (1973), must take into account possible observer bias, the absence of a control group and the placebo effect of hospitalisation for a complicated therapeutic procedure, these pilot investigations have shown the need for adequately controlled trials of clomipramine. A more rigorous assessment of the drug has been carried out by Rigby, Clarren and Kelly (1973), who made psychophysiological measurements before treatment, during a saline infusion, and during an infusion of clomipramine. Two of their 13 patients had obsessional neurosis, and two had social phobias, while the remainder were suffering from anxiety or depression. Although there was some improvement on a global clinical scale, the only statistically significant changes in psychometric scores three months after an average of 16 intravenous infusions of about 280 mg of clomipramine were in the Taylor Manifest Anxiety Scale, and in the 'obsessional trait' score of the Leyton Obsessional Inventory (Cooper, 1970). These disappointing results may have been due, at least in part, to the inclusion of the scores of one atypical patient who had many psychopathic features.

The intravenous administration of clomipramine can cause serious adverse effects. Major epileptic convulsions occurred in four out of a series of 50 patients who had this treatment, and a further two subjects showed minor or psychomotor epileptic phenomena (Dickson, 1973). Haemoglobinuria was noted in 14 of another series of 60 cases, and was attributed to transient haemolytic episodes during the infusions (Rack and Rigby, 1973). Severe hypotensive reactions can occur (Symes, 1973) and Capstick (1973) has recommended the concurrent use of dihydro-ergotamine tartrate. Hypertensive episodes have been reported by Rigby et al (1973), who also found that venous thrombosis occurred after one-third of the infusions. In some of the patients in this series most of the superficial veins of both arms had thrombosed by the end of treatment, despite the use of 21 gauge square scalp vein needles and isotonic saline instead of the more usual 5 per cent dextrose (Rigby et al, 1973).

The potentially hazardous procedure of clomipramine infusion has not yet been subjected to adequately controlled comparison with infusions of either a relatively inert substance or with another of the iminodibenzyl group of drugs. Conclusive comparisons of intravenous and oral clomipramine remain to be published, and although there is ample evidence of the effectiveness of clomipramine as an antidepressant (Syment, 1967; Arfwidsson, 1972), the superiority of this drug over the other tricyclic amines in the treatment of obsessions and phobias has not yet been demonstrated. Freed, Kerr and Roth (1972) carried out an uncontrolled retrospective study of the effect of high doses of imipramine, amitriptyline, desipramine, or dothiepin in 16 obsessional patients with a mean duration of severe refractory illness of 8.6 years. (Eleven patients received 200–300 mg of one of these antidepressants daily without experiencing adverse effects.) A postal follow-up after a minimum of four years of 14 patients who had continued to take a high dose indicated that 12 regarded themselves as significantly improved.

In two double-blind controlled studies Klein found that imipramine reduced agoraphobic panic more than a placebo (Klein, 1964), while a group of school phobics treated with the same drug returned to school more readily than those in a placebo treated group (Gittelmen, Klein and Klein, 1971).

Monoamine oxidase inhibitors

The monoamine oxidase inhibitor (MAOI) group of drugs were recommended for the treatment of anxiety states by Sargant and Dally in 1962, and since then there have been further favourable reports (King, 1962; Sargant and Slater, 1962; Dally, 1967). The current status of the MAOIs has been comprehensively reviewed by Tyrer (Tyrer, 1973; Tyrer, 1976). In a large-scale study of 264 patients, Kelly et al (1970) claimed a highly significant improvement in phobic ratings after one month's treatment, but this trial was criticised (Mawson, 1970) for its lack of a control group and the absence of blind ratings. Since then Tyrer, Candy and Kelly (1973), have carried out a rigorous prospective double-blind controlled trial of phenelzine in a dose of 45 mg daily in 32 patients with social anxiety or agoraphobia. At eight weeks the patients on phenelzine showed significant improvement in comparison to a placebo treated group; the degree of improvement in phobias was similar to that obtained by Gelder, Marks and Wolff (1967), with systematic desensitisation in fantasy. However, when Tyrer and Steinberg (1975) followed up this group of patients, they found that at one year there was no significant difference in phobic ratings between the original phenelzine and placebo patients. Both groups had received further pharmacotherapy or behaviour therapy during the follow-up period. The original placebo subjects were not given MAOI, but they did receive more additional treatment. Although the introduction of this extra therapy introduced a bias against phenelzine, the authors conclude that phenelzine has only the same degree of effectiveness in phobic states as other symptomatic treatments.

There have been few attempts to compare the value of drug treatment and behaviour therapy in phobic states. In a comparison of phenelzine and systematic desensitisation, Solyom et al (1973) found MAOI and behaviour therapy to be equally effective in phobic anxiety. Iproniazid has been compared with systematic desensitisation in 60 severely handicapped agoraphobics (Lipsedge et al, 1973). One-third of the patients had previously failed to respond to less toxic but less potent MAOIs. The effect of iproniazid combined with a programme of graded exposure was greater than that of placebo with the same retraining schedule, and was not enhanced by the addition of systematic desensitisation. Both these studies of MAOIs as well as those of Kelly et al (1970) and Sargant and Slater (1972) report a high relapse rate following drug withdrawal. Tyrer and Steinberg (1975) have made similar observations and conclude that MAOIs effect symptom 'supression', but do not 'cure'. This tendency to relapse on discontinuation of MAOIs may be prevented by more vigorous exposure in practice (Marks, 1974).

THE COMBINATION OF DRUG AND BEHAVIOUR THERAPY

Drugs have been used to facilitate those techniques which involve direct or imagined exposure of phobic individuals to the feared object or situation. These include the barbiturates (methohexitone, thiopentone), propanidid, diazepam, and the beta-adrenergic blocking agents. The safer non-barbiturate sedatives administered orally are generally to be preferred. The routine use of the intravenous route can only be justified where there is no oral equivalent of the anxiolytic drugs or where great flexibility of administration is essential. A drug dissociation effect does not seem to occur and behaviour changes acquired under the influence of a drug appear to carry over into the non-drugged state (Brady, 1968; Liberman and Davis, 1974).

Davison and Valins (1969) asserted that changes in behaviour which the patient thinks he has brought about entirely by his own effort will be more enduring than improvement he attributes to external agents such as drugs. This prediction was not borne out in a careful experiment by Johnson and Gath (1973) who found that the degree of recovery in agoraphobia in response to a combination of behaviour therapy and sedative drug was not reduced if the patient attributed his improvement to the medication rather than to the treatment by exposure.

Drug-assisted systematic desensitisation

Satisfactory results with the ultra-short acting barbiturate methohexitone in subanaesthetic doses are reported by Friedman (1966), Mawson (1970), and Lipsedge et al (1973). Methohexitone has been used to induce profound relaxation during the presentation of a graded series of phobic images. It has the advantage of reducing the amount of time required for treatment (Friedman and Silverstone, 1968). The mean number of weekly 15 minute treatment sessions was only 12 in a series of 124 cases (Friedman and Lipsedge, 1971) compared with a mean of 20 sessions of one hour required to achieve improvement with desensitisation employing progressive muscular relaxation (Marks, 1969). In a controlled cross-over trial Mawson (1970) found that methohexitone-assisted desensitisation was over 50 per cent more effective than progressive muscular relaxation in reducing phobic symptoms.

In a controlled prospective study of severe agoraphobia Lipsedge et al (1973) found that methohexitone-assisted desensitisation was more effective than desensitisation with standard muscular relaxation. There was, however, no saline placebo group.

Yorkston, Sergeant and Rachman (1968) encountered certain complications with methohexitone injections in severely agoraphobic patients; these included muscle twitching, memory impairment, marked sleepiness, and barbiturate dependence. These adverse effects however may have been due to the use of relatively large amounts of methohexitone in intravenous infusions over a period of one hour in doses of up to 400 mg daily for five days. In the technique reviewed by Friedman and Lipsedge (1971) only approximately 35 mg of methohexitone was administered during each weekly session and the complications described by Yorkston et al (1968) were not encountered.

Since the safety of methohexitone for out-patient procedures has been questioned (Leading Article, 1969), the non-barbiturate propanidid (Lader and Greenwood, 1974) has been investigated as an alternative relaxing agent. Earlier Silverstone, Salkind and Lipsedge (1970) compared intravenous methohexitone with propanidid and isotonic saline control in the systematic desensitisation of phobic out-patients. While both methohexitone and propanidid procedures reduced phobic symptoms, complete recovery of a fully alert state was significantly more rapid with propanidid. The relatively safe drug diazepam (Stovner and Endresen, 1965) has also been used as a means of inducing relaxation in systematic desensitisation (Pecknold, 1972).

Drug-assisted exposure in practice

Gain, Watson and Marks (1971) used intravenous propanidid to facilitate the confrontation of phobic patients with feared objects. The drug was administered over a period of 30 minutes and the patients were encouraged to remain in close contact with the phobic objects until the drug effect wore off. The total treatment time was about two hours and the degree of improvement was much greater than that observed in comparable groups of patients who received prolonged exposure without drugs. Marks, Viswanathan and Lipsedge (1972) have also demonstrated enhanced extinction of phobias by prolonged exposure during the transitional phase from drug to non-drug state while the anxiolytic effect of oral diazepam was wearing off. McCormick (1973) obtained similar results in a comparable procedure alliteratively labelled Declining Dose Drug Desensitisation.

Beta-adrenergic blocking drugs

Granville-Grossman and Turner (1966) have described the anxiolytic effect of the beta-blocker propranolol. A double-blind comparison of alprenolol and placebo combined with exposure (Ullrich, Grambach and Peikert, 1972) showed that while the alprenalol-exposure combination markedly reduced the auto-nomic effects of anxiety, it failed to diminish the avoidance behaviour. The greater effect of the drug on anxiety rather than avoidance parallels the experience with the combination of behaviour therapy and an MAOI (Lipsedge et al, 1973) and the more recent work with another beta-blocker (tollamolol) by Silverstone and Bernhadt (1970; personal communication) who found that the drug reduced heart rate, but failed to improve approach to a phobic object.

PSYCHOSURGERY

The most severely disabled patients who have failed to respond to other forms of treatment may benefit from selective stereotactic psychosurgery (Knight, 1972; Schurr, 1973). One of the commonest operations has been subcaudate tractotomy (Knight, 1973), in which a lesion is produced beneath the head of the caudate nucleus by the stereotactic insertion of radioactive yttrium seeds. The aim of the procedure is to interrupt the connections from the agranular cortex of the cingulate, posterior orbital and amygdaloid regions (Bridges and Bartlett, 1973). One group of 134 patients who had undergone subcaudate tractotomy was reviewed at an interval of two and a half to four and a half years after operation (Young and Bridges, 1975). The majority of the 18 patients with obsessional neurosis and the seven patients with phobic anxiety had had symptoms for over six years, and in some cases the duration of illness exceeded 16 years. The patients were assessed by a structured interview, and a close relative was similarly interviewed in a standardised way by a social worker. All the phobic patients had either completely recovered or had only mild residual symptoms, which caused little or no interference with daily life, while half of the 18 obsessionals showed considerable improvement in symptoms, in marital adjustment and in work capacity. Epilepsy requiring anticonvulsant medication occurred in 2.2 per cent of the 134 patients. Although the operation had no socially incapacitating effects on personality, the patients' relations reported undesirable changes in behaviour such as extravagance or volubility in 6.7 per cent. Obsessionals who did poorly had developed their original symptoms at an earlier age (mean 22 years), than those who made a good response to tractotomy; the latter group had a mean age of onset of illness of 33 years. A sudden onset of the obsessional disorder was associated with a better result from surgery than was an insidious onset.

Even better results with psychosurgery in severely incapacitating chronic obsessional neurosis have been described in a prospective study by Kelly and Mitchell-Heggs (1973) following limbic leucotomy. This operation usually consisted of the production of three lesions with a cryogenic probe in the lower medial quadrant of the frontal lobe in addition to two pairs of cingulate lesions. The aim of the operation is to interrupt some connections between the frontal cortex and the limbic system, and to make lesions in one of the main limbic circuits in the anterior cingulate gyrus (Kelly, Richardson and Mitchell-Heggs, 1973).

Selection of the most appropriate localisation for the lesions was made more accurate by continuous physiological monitoring during electrical stimulation of the target zones (Kelly, 1972). At a mean of 17 months following surgery there was clinical improvement in 14 of the 16 patients with obsessional neurosis whose average age at the onset of illness was 21 years. Eleven of these patients (69 per cent) were symptom free or much improved. There was also significant reduction in the preoperative psychometric scores of anxiety, obsessions and neuroticism. Postoperative physiological assessment showed reductions in 'basal' and 'stress' heart rates, systolic blood pressure, and forearm blood flow (Kelly, 1966). There was no evidence of emotional blunting, disinhibition, postoperative epilepsy or excessive weight gain, and intelligence (assessed on the Wechsler Adult Intelligence Scale) was not affected.

The rating of 69 per cent of the obsessional patients as symptom-free or much improved at 17 months is a result superior to that obtained with modified prefrontal leucotomy (25 per cent) and rostral leucotomy (50 per cent), while the changes in anxiety and depression psychometric scores were comparable to those produced by the more extensive 'free-hand' types of operation (Kelly, Walter and Sargant, 1966).

Bridges and Bartlett (1973) have commented on the value of postoperative behaviour therapy. Both flooding (Gaind, Watson and Marks, 1971) and response prevention (Levy and Meyer, 1971) are helpful in the alleviation of residual symptoms. Patients with severe phobic anxiety are more likely to respond to behaviour therapy after psychosurgery (Marks, 1969). While Kelly and Mitchell-Heggs (1973) have also found that rehabilitation including behaviour therapy can be helpful after psychosurgery, they question whether such a programme is essential for a favourable outcome in limbic leucotomy since a proportion of their patients improved although they could not take part in a formal rehabilitation scheme.

There have been few attempts to carry out controlled serial retrospective studies on the effect of psychosurgery. Marks, Birley and Gelder (1966) reviewed the outcome of a modified leucotomy aimed at cutting thalamo-frontal fibres which are thought to play a part in maintaining anxiety (Falconer and Schurr, 1959). They compared the case-notes of 22 patients suffering from severe phobias and generalised anxiety with a control group of patients of similar age and sex who were matched for type, duration and severity of symptoms. The mean duration of illness was 16 years. Two independent assessors carried out blind ratings on the progress of the leucotomised patients and the controls at the end of treatment and after five years. The leucotomised patients had fared significantly better than the controls with respect to phobias and general anxiety, while there was a marked improvement in work adjustment. A poorer outcome was associated with an anxious, shy premorbid personality with depression as a major symptom before operation.

A controlled serial enquiry has also been carried out on the effect of bimedial leucotomy in 24 patients with severe obsessional neurosis (Tan, Marks and Marset, 1971). These patients were compared with a matched group over a five year period. The leucotomy patients did considerably better than controls with respect to obsessions, general anxiety and ability to work. The outcome was not affected by any premorbid personality traits and in contrast to the observation in the agoraphobic series (Marks et al, 1966), the final result was actually better in patients who had been clinically depressed before operation.

CHOICE OF TREATMENT IN CLINICAL PRACTICE

The most straightforward clinical problem is the patient with a single phobia. Prolonged exposure or flooding is the most effective treatment but some patients are so terrified of their phobic object or situation that they require a preliminary course of exposure in fantasy or systematic desensitisation before they will tolerate the presence of a small animal or enter a frightening place such as a lift. They may then progress from imaginary contact with their phobic object to looking at pictures of it before actual confrontation and eventual physical contact. Their progress is enhanced if they can observe the therapist handling the feared object in a confident manner (modelling). It may be helpful to give a small dose of diazepam before the first flooding session, preferably as a syrup because of its more rapid absorption. The therapist needs to build a store of commonly feared objects and have access to both toy and real snakes, mice, dogs, etc. (Zoos are usually prepared to supply spiders when they are 'out of season'.) Ancillary aids such as sound effect records of aircraft noise, birds, and thunderstorms are available from EMI. Patients should be given a programme of graded retraining which involves keeping to a time-table of exposure to feared situations. For example in the case of a flying or car phobic, frequent visits to an airport or sitting in a car and even using a flight or automobile simulator would be required. The patients are instructed to keep a daily record of their progress and this acts as an incentive to confront the particular feared situation.

Occasionally patients become attracted to what was formerly a phobic object. For example a young woman who would faint at the sight of blood or a syringe became a student nurse after spending a few sessions in the blood-transfusion laboratory and casualty department of a general hospital.

Agoraphobics seem to respond best to a combination of MAOI (the safest are isocarboxazid and phenelzine) to reduce the free-floating anxiety, and flooding, preceded if necessary by systematic desensitisation or exposure in fantasy. The flooding can be a group activity since patients benefit from the moral support of fellow-sufferers. The families of agoraphobics should be instructed to act as co-therapists and supervise daily outings over a steadily increasing distance from home.

Social phobics with a high level of general anxiety can also benefit from a course of a MAOI combined with systematic desensitisation to images of the situations they fear such as public speaking and meeting strangers. They also do well with a combination of training in assertiveness and role-playing in which social situations are simulated and they are instructed to play the part of a confident person. Tape recordings and videotapes are useful adjuncts since they provide feedback on the patient's social performance.

A high proportion of obsessional neurotics with rituals of checking or handwashing respond to a programme of exposure with or without response prevention. Occasionally very rapid results can be obtained, as in the case of a security guard who was spending eight hours checking light switches; he was able to reduce his checking time to an acceptable 30 minutes after a single evening of supervision. However, several sessions of exposure are generally required and treatment has to be continued in the patient's own home, which is often the focus of ritual activity since it is perceived as the most vulnerable to imaginary contamination or danger.

Obsessional ruminations are still extremely difficult to treat. Tricyclic antidepressants and even ECT may be necessary to deal with any under-lying depression and then thought-stopping or paradoxical intention may be attempted. The newer forms of psychosurgery should be reserved for the most intractable cases of obsessional neurosis of agoraphobia with a high level of free-floating anxiety.

It is important to enlist the aid of members of the family who often collude with agoraphobia or obsessional rituals and allow the life and economy of the family to be manipulated by the patient's symptoms. Often the relatives are reluctant to be firm with such patients or they actually participate in checking, cleaning or hoarding rituals, because they are afraid that refusal to collude will cause the patient to 'go mad'. This does not occur, nor does so-called symptom substitution which was widely anticipated by the critics of behaviour therapy.

Systematic desensitisation and the newer forms of psychological treatment are extremely time consuming. Marks et al (1975) and Stern (1975) have shown that nurses and medical students can achieve results in adult neurotic disorders comparable to those obtained with similar methods by psychologists and psychiatrists.

REFERENCES

Agras, W. S., Sylvester, D. & Oliveau, D. C. (1969) The epidemiology of common fears and phobias. *Comprehensive Psychiatry*, **10**, 151–156.

Aitken, R. C. B. (1969) Measurement of feelings using visual analogue scales. *Proceedings of the Royal Society of Medicine*, **62**, 989–993.

Arfuidsson, L., d'Elias, G., Laurell, B., Ottosson, J. O., Perris, C. & Persson, G. (1972) Comparison of clorimipramine and imipramine in ambulatory treatment of depression. *Acta Psychiatrica et Neurologica Scandinavica*, **48**, 367–371.

Bandura, A., Blanchard, E. B. & Ritter, B. (1969) The relative efficacy of desensitisation and modelling approaches for inducing behavioural, affective and attitudinal changes. *Journal of Personality and Social Psychology*, **13**, 173–199.

Baum, M. (1969) Extinction of an avoidance response following response prevention. *Canadian Journal of Psychology*, **23**, 1–10.

Baum, M. (1970) Extinction of avoidance responding through response prevention (flooding). *Psychological Bulletin*, **74**, 276–284.

Bevan, J. R. (1960) Learning theory applied to the treatment of a patient with obsessional ruminations. In *Behaviour Therapy and the Neuroses*, ed. Eysenck, H. J. Oxford: Pergamon Press.

Black, A. (1974) The natural history of obsessional neurosis. In *Obsessional States*, ed. Beech, H. R. London: Methuen.

Boulougouris, J. C. & Bassiakos, L. (1973) Prolonged flooding in the cases with obsessional compulsive neurosis. *Behaviour Research and Therapy*, **11**, 227-231.

Brady, J. P. (1968) Drugs in Behaviour Therapy. In *Psychopharmacology: A review of Progress, 1957–1967*, ed. Efron, D. H. Public Health Service Publication No. 1836: Washington, D. C.

Bridges, P. K. & Bartlett, J. R. (1973) The work of a psychosurgical unit. *Postgraduate Medical Journal*, **49**, 855–859.

Capstick, N. (1973) The Graylingwell Study. *Journal of International Medical Research*, **1**, 392–398.

Cooper, J. (1970) The Leyton Obsessional Inventory. *Psychological Medicine*, **1**, 48–64.

Cooper, A., Furst, J. B. & Bridger, W. (1966) A brief commentary on the usefulness of studying fears of snakes. *Journal of Abnormal Psychology*, **74**, 413–414.

Dally, P. (1967) *Chemotherapy of Psychiatric Disorders*. London: Logus Press Ltd.

Davison, G. C. & Valines, S. (1969) Maintenance of self-attributed and drug-attributed behaviour change. *Journal of Personality and Social Psychology*, **11**, 25–33.

Dickson, J. (1973) Neurological and EEG Effects of Clomipramine. *Journal of International Medical Research*, **1**, 449–450.

Falconer, M. A. & Schurr, P. H. (1959) Surgical treatment of mental illness. In *Recent Progress in Psychiatry*, ed. Flemminger, A. & Walk, A., pp. 352–367. London: Churchill.

Frankl, V. E. (1960) Paradoxical intention: A logotherapeutic technique. *American Journal of Psychotherapy*, **14**, 520–535.

Frankl, V. (1970) *The Doctor and the Soul*. London: Souvenir Press.

Freed, A., Kerr, T. A. & Martin, R. (1972) The treatment of obsessional neurosis. *British Journal of Psychiatry*, **120**, 590–591.

Friedman, D. E. (1966). A new technique for the systematic desensitisation of phobic patients. *Behaviour Research and Therapy*, **4**, 139–140.

Friedman, D. E. & Lipsedge, M. S. (1971) Treatment of phobic anxiety and psychogenic impotence by systematic desensitisation employing methohexitone-induced relaxation. *British Journal of Psychiatry*, **118**, 87–90.

Friedman, D. E. & Silverstone, J. T. (1967) Treatment of phobic patients by systematic desentisation. *Lancet*, **i**, 470–472.

Furst, J. B. & Cooper, A. (1970) Failure of systematic desensitisation in 2 cases of obsessive-compulsive neurosis marked by fears of insecticide. *Behaviour Research and Therapy*, **8**, 203–206.

Gain, R., Watson, J. P. & Marks, M. (1971) Some approaches to the treatment of phobic disorders. *Proceedings of the Royal Society of Medicine*, **64**, 1118–1120.

Gelder, M. G. & Marks, I. M. (1966) Severe agoraphobia. A controlled prospective trial of behaviour therapy. *British Journal of Psychiatry*, **112**, 309–319.

Gelder, M. G. & Marks, I. M. (1968) Desensitisation and phobias: a crossover study. *British Journal of Psychiatry*, **113**, 53–73.

Gelder, M. G., Marks, I. M. & Wolf, H. H. (1967) Desensitisation and psychotherapy in the treatment of phobic states. A controlled enquiry. *British Journal of Psychiatry*, **113**, 53–73.

Gillan, P. & Rachman, S. (1974) An experimental investigation of behaviour therapy in phobic patients. *British Journal of Psychiatry*, **124**, 392–401.

Gittelman-Klein, R. & Klein, D. F. (1971) Controlled imipramine treatment of school phobia. *Archives of General Psychiatry*, **25**, 204–207.

Gittleson, N. L. (1966) The fate of obsessions in depressive psychosis. *British Journal of Psychiatry*, **112**, 705–708.

Goktepe, E. O., Young, L. & Bridges, P. K. (1975) A further review of the results of stereotactic subcaudate tractotomy. *British Journal of Psychiatry*, **126**, 270–280.

Granville-Grossman, K. L. & Turner, P. (1966) The effect of propranolol on anxiety. *Lancet*, **i**, 788–790.

Greenwood, M. H. & Lader, M. H. (1974) A controlled comparison of the psychotropic effects of propanidid and methohexitone. *Behaviour Research and Therapy*, **12**, 19–27.

Hackman, A. & McLean, C. (1975) A comparison of flooding and thought stopping in the treatment of obsessional neurosis. *Behavioural Research and Therapy*, **17**, 263–269.

Hain, J. D., Butcher, R. H. G. & Stevenson, L. (1966) Systematic desensitisation therapy: an analysis of results in 27 patients. *British Journal of Psychiatry*, **112**, 295–307.

Hand, I., Lamontagne, Y. & Marks, I. M. (1974) Group exposure (flooding) in vivo for agoraphobics. *British Journal of Psychiatry*, **124**, 588–602.

Jacobson, E. (1938) *Progressive Relaxation.* Chicago: University of Chicago Press.

Johnston, D. & Gath, D. (1973) Arousal levels and attribution effects in diazepam-assisted flooding. *British Journal of Psychiatry*, **123**, 463–466.

Kanfer, F. M. & Seidner, M. L. (1973) Self-control; factors enhancing tolerance of noxious stimulation. *Journal of Personality and Social Psychology*, **25**, 381–389.

Kelleher, M. J. (1972) Cross-national (Anglo-Irish) differences in obsessional symptoms and traits of personality. *Psychological Medicine*, **2**, 33–41.

Kelly, D., Richardson, L. & Mitchell-Heggs, N. (1973) Stereotactic limbic leucotomy: Neurophysiological aspects and operative technique. *British Journal of Psychiatry*, **123**, 133–140.

Kelly, D. & Mitchell-Heggs, N. (1973) Stereotactic limbic leucotomy — a follow-up study of 30 patients. *Postgraduate Medical Journal*, **49**, 865–882.

Kelly, D., Guirguis, W., Frommer, E., Mitchell-Heggs, N. & Sargant, W. (1970) Treatment of phobic states with antidepressants. *British Journal of Psychiatry*, **116**, 387–398.

King, A. (1962) Phenelzine treatment of Roth's calamity syndrome. *Medical Journal of Australia*, **1**, 879–883.

Klein, D. F. (1964) Delineation of two drug-responsive anxiety syndromes. *Psychopharmacologia*, **5**, 397–408.

Knight, G. C. (1972) Psychosurgery today; neurosurgical aspects. *Proceedings of the Royal Society of Medicine*, **65**, 1099.

Knight, G. (1973) Further observations from an experience of 660 cases of stereotactic tractotomy. *Postgraduate Medical Journal*, **49**, 845–854.

Kringlen, E. (1965) Obsessional neurotics. A long-term follow-up. *British Journal of Psychiatry*, **111**, 709–722.

Lader, M. H., Gelder, M. G. & Marks, I. M. (1967) Palmar skin-conductance measures as predictors of response to desensitisation. *Journal of Psychosomatic Research*, **11**, 283–290.

Lader, M. & Marks, I. M. (1971) *Clinical Anxiety.* London: Heinemann.

Lang, P. J. & Lazavic, A. D. (1963) The experimental desensitisation of phobia, *Journal of Abnormal and Social Psychology*, **66**, 519–525.

Lazarus, A. (1963) The results of behaviour therapy in 126 cases of severe neurosis. *Behaviour Research and Therapy*, **1**, 66–79.

Leading article (1969) Intermittent intravenous methohexitone. *British Medical Journal*, **ii**, 525–526.

Lewis, A. (1966) Psychological Medicine. In *Price's Textbook of the Practice of Medicine*, ed. Scott, R. B. London: Oxford University Press.

Lewis, A. J. (1934) Melancholia: a clinical survey of depressive states. *Journal of Mental Science*, **80**, 277–378.

Levy, R. & Meyer, V. (1971).Ritual prevention in obsessional patients. *Proceedings of the Royal Society of Medicine*, **64**, 1115–1118.

Liberman, P. & Davis, J. (1974) *Drugs and Behaviour Analysis.* California.

Lipsedge, M. S. (1974) *Therapeutic Approaches to Compulsive Rituals.* Unpublished M.Phil. dissertation, University of London.

Lipsedge, M. S., Hagioff, J., Huggins, J., Napier, P., Pearce, J., Pike, D. J. & Rich, M. (1973) The management of severe agoraphobia; a comparison of iproniazid and systematic desensitisation. *Psychopharmacologia*, **32**, 67–80.

Lopez-Ibor Aline, J. J. (1971) The pharmacological treatment of obsessive neurosis, anorexia nervosa, delusions of reference and Kleine-Levin Syndrome. *Archives of the Faculty of Medicine*, **20** (2), 93–100.

Marks, I. (1969) *Fears and Phobias* (Reprinted 1975). London, Heinemann.

Marks, I. (1974) Problems in exposure (flooding) research. *British Journal of Psychiatry*, **124**, 103–108.

Marks, I. M. (1974) Psycholopharmacology; the combines use of drug and psychological treatments. Paper presented at the meeting of the American Psychopathological Association, Boston.

Marks, I. M. (1975) Behavioural treatments of Phobic and obsessive-compulsive disorders; a critical appraisal. In *Progress in Behavioural Modification*, Vol. 1, eds. Hersen, M., Eister, R. and Miller, P.

Marks, I. M., Birley, J. L. T. & Gelder, M. G. (1966) Modified leucotomy in severe agoraphobia; a controlled serial inquiry. *British Journal of Psychiatry*, **112**, 757–769.

Marks, I. M., Boulougouris, J. & Marset, P. (1971) Flooding versus desensitisation in phobic disorders. *British Journal of Psychiatry*, **119**, 353–375(a).

Marks, I. M., Hallam, R. S., Philpott, R. & Connolly, J. C. (1975). Nurse therapists in behavioural psychotherapy. *British Medical Journal*, iii, 133–148.

Marks, I. M., Hodgson, R. & Rachman, S. (1975) Treatment of chronic obsessive-compulsive neurosis by in vivo exposure. *British Journal of Psychiatry*, **127**, 349–364.

Marks, I. M., Viswanathan, R. & Lipsedge, M. S. (1972) Enhanced extinction of fear by flooding during waning diazepam effect. *British Journal of Psychiatry*, **121**, 493–505.

Martin, I., Marks, I. M. & Gelder, M. G. G. (1969) Conditioned eyelid responses in phobic patients. *Behaviour Research and Therapy*, 7, 115–124.

Mawson, A. B. (1970) Methohexitone-assisted desensitisation in the treatment of phobias. *Lancet*, i, 1084–1086.

Marshall, W. K. & Micev, V. (1975) The role of intravenous clomipramine in the treatment of obsessional and phobic disorders. *Scottish Medical Journal*, **20**, 49–53.

Mathews, A. M., Johnston, D. W., Shaw, P. M. & Gelder, M. G. (1974) Process variables and the prediction of outcome in behaviour therapy. *British Journal of Psychiatry*, **125**, 256–264.

McCormick, W. O. (1973) Declining-dose drug desensitisation for phobias. *Canadian Psychiatric Association Journal*, **18**, 33–40.

Meyer, V. (1966) Modification of expectancies in cases with obsessional rituals. *Behaviour Research and Therapy*, **4**, 273–280.

Meyer, V. & Chesser, E. S. (1970) *Behaviour Therapy in Clinical Psychiatry.* Penguin, England.

Meyer, V. & Levy, R. (1970) Behavioural treatment of a homosexual with compulsive rituals. *British Journal of Medical Psychology*, **43**, 63–68.

Meyer, V., Levy, R. & Schnurer, A. (1974) The behavioural treatment of obsessive-compulsive disorders. In *Obsessional States*, ed. Beech, H. R. London: Methuen.

Meyer, V., Robertson, J. & Tatlow, A. (1975) Home treatment of an obsessive-compulsive disorder by response prevention. *Journal of Behaviour Therapy and Experimental Psychiatry*, **6**, 37–38.

Micev, V. & Marshall, W. K. (1973) Undesired effects in slow intravenous infusion of clomipramine (anafranil). *Journal of International Medical Research*, **1**, 451–455.

Mills, H. L., Barlow, D. H. & Baugh, J. (1971) An experimental analysis of response prevention in the treatment of obsessive-compulsive behaviour. Paper read at the Association for the Advancement of Behaviour Therapy Meeting, Washington, D.C.

Mills, H. L., Agras, W. S., Barlow, D. W. & Mills, J. R. (1973) Compulsive rituals treated by response prevention. *Archives of General Psychiatry*, **28**, 524–529.

Mottahedin, I. & Mayo, P. R. (1974) Behaviour modification in one psychiatric hospital. *British Journal of Psychiatry*, **124**, 615–620.

Olley, M. & McAllister, H. (1974) A comment on treatment analogous for phobic anxiety states. *Psychological Medicine*, **4**, 463–469.

Pecknoid, J. C., Raeburn, J. & Poser, E. G. (1972) Intravenous diazepam for facilitating relaxation for desensitisation. *Journal of Behaviour Therapy and Experimental Psychiatry*, **3**, 39–41.

Philpott, R. (1975) Recent advances in the behavioural measurement of obsessional illness. Difficulties common to these and other measures. *Scottish Medical Journal,* 20 Supp. 1, 35–42.

Rachman, S. (1971) Obsessional ruminations. *Behaviour Research and Therapy,* 9, 229–235.

Rachman, S. (1971) *The Effects of Psychotherapy.* Oxford: Pergamon Press.

Rachman, S. (1973) Some similarities and differences between obsessional ruminations and morbid preoccupations. *Canadian Psychiatric Association Journal,* 18, 71–74.

Rachman, S. (1974) Primary obsessional slowness. *Behaviour Research and Therapy,* 12, 9–18.

Rachman, S., Marks, I. M. & Hodgson, R. (1971) The treatment of obsessive-compulsive neurotics by modelling and flooding in vivo. *Behaviour Research and Therapy,* 11, 463–471.

Rack, P. H. (1973) Clomipramine in the treatment of obsessive states with special reference to the Leyton Obsessional Inventory. *Journal of International Medical Research,* 1, 397–399.

Rack, P. H. & Rigby, B. P. (1973) Haemoglobinuria following intravenous clomipramine infusions. *Journal of International Medical Research,* 1, 477–479.

Reed, G. F. (1968) Some formal qualities of obsessional thinking. *Psychiatric Clinics* 1, 382–392.

Rigby, B., Clarren, S. & Kelly, D. (1973) A psychological and physiological evaluation of the effects of intravenous clomipramine. *Journal of international Medical Research,* 1, 308–316.

Sargant, W. & Dally, P. J. (1962) Treatment of anxiety states by antidepressant drugs. *British Medical Journal,* 1, 6–9.

Sargant, W. & Slater, E. (1972) *An Introduction to Physical Methods of Treatment in Psychiatry.* Edinburgh and London: Churchill Livingstone.

Schultz, J. H. & Luth, W. (1959) *Autogenic Training.* New York, N.Y.: Grune and Stratton.

Schurr, P. H. (1973) Psychosurgery. *British Journal of Hospital Medicine,* 53–60.

Silverstone, J. T. S., Salkind, M. R. & Lipsedge. (1970) Centrally acting drugs in the deconditioning of phobic symptoms. Presented at 7 CNP Congress, Prague.

Solyom, L., Garze-Perez, J., Ledwidge, D. L. & Solyom, C. (1972) Paradoxical intention in the treatment of obsessive thoughts; a pilot study. *Comprehensive Psychiatry,* 13, 291–297.

Solyom, L., Heseltine, G. F. D., McClure, D. J., Solyom, C., Ledwidge, B. & Steinberg, G. (1973) Behaviour therapy versus drug therapy in the treatment of phobic neurosis. *Canadian Psychiatric Association Journal,* 18, 25–32.

Stamfl, T. G. & Lewis, D. J. (1967) The essentials of implosive therapy; a learning theory-based psychodynamic behavioural therapy. *Journal of Abnormal and Social Psychology,* 72, 496–503.

Stern, R. (1970) Treatment of a case of obsessional neurosis using thought-stopping technique. *British Journal of Psychiatry,* 117, 539.

Stern, R. S. (1975) The medical student as behavioural psychotherapist. *British Medical Journal,* 78–81.

Stern, R. S., Lipsedge, M. S. & Marks, I. M. (1973) Thought-stopping of neutral and obsessive thoughts; a controlled trial. *Behaviour Research and Therapy,* 11, 659–662.

Stern, R. S. & Marks, I. M. (1973) Brief and prolonged flooding; a comparison in agoraphobic patients. *Archives of General Psychiatry,* 28, 270–276 (a).

Stovner, J. & Endresen, R. (1965) Diazepam in intravenous anaesthesia. *Lancet,* ii, 1298–1299.

Symes, M. H. (1973) Cardiovascular effects of clomipramine. *Journal of International Medical Research,* 1, 460–463.

Symes, M. H. (1967) Monochlorimipramine: a controlled trial of a new anti-depressant. *British Journal of Psychiatry,* 113, 671.

Tan, E., Marks, I. M. & Marset, P. (1971) Bimedial Leucotomy in obsessive-compulsive neurosis: a controlled serial enquiry. *British Journal of Psychiatry,* 118, 155–164.

Tyrer, P. (1973) Current status of monoamine oxidase inhibitors in psychiatry. *British Journal of Hospital Medicine,* pp. 795–781.

Tyrer, P. (1976) Towards rational therapy with monoamine oxidase inhibitors. *British Journal of Psychiatry,* 128, 354–360.

Tyrer, P., Candy, & Kelly, D. (1973) A study of the clinical effects of phenelzine and placebo in the treatment of phobic anxiety. *Psychopharmacologia (Berlin),* 32, 237–254.

Tyrer, P. & Steinberg, D. (1975) Symptomatic treatment of agoraphobia and social phobias: a follow-up study. *British Journal of Psychiatry,* 127, 163–168.

Ullrich, R., Grambach, G. & Peikert, V. (1972). Three flooding procedures in the treatment of agoraphobics. Paper presented at the *2nd Annual Conference of the European Association of Behaviour Therapy,* Wexford, Eire.

van Renynghe de Voxrie, G. (1968) Anafranil in obsessive neurosis. *Acta Neurologica et Psychiatrica Belgica,* 68, 787–789.

Walker, V. J. & Beech, H. R. (1969) Mood state and the ritualistic behaviour of obsessional patients. *British Journal of Psychiatry,* 115, 1261–1268.

Watson, J. P., Gaind, R. & Marks, I. M. (1971) Prolonged exposure: a rapid treatment for phobias. *British Medical Journal,* **i,** 13–15.

Watson, J. P. & Marks, I. M. (1971) Relevant and irrelevant fear in flooding — a crossover study of phobic patients. *Behaviour Therapy,* **2,** 275–293.

Waxman, D. (1975) An investigation into the use of anafranil in phobic and obsessional disorders. *Scottish Medical Journal,* **20,** 61–66.

Wolpe, J. (1958) *Psychotherapy by Reciprocal Inhibition.* Stanford University Press.

Wolpe, J. (1961) The systematic desensitisation treatment of neurosis. *Journal of Nervous and Mental Disease,* **132,** 189–203.

Wolpe, J. & Lazarus, A. A. (1966) *Behaviour Therapy and Techniques.* Oxford: Pergamon Press.

Yamagami, T. (1971) The treatment of an obsession by thought-stopping. *Journal of Behaviour Therapy and Experimental Psychiatry,* **2,** 233–239.

Yorkston, N., Sergeant, H. & Rachman, S. (1968) Methohexitone relaxation for desensitising agoraphobic patients. *Lancet,* **ii,** 651–653.

Ullrich, R., Crombach, G., & Peiker, V. (1972) Three flooding procedures in the treatment of agoraphobics. Paper to *2nd European Conference on Behaviour Modification,* Wexford, Eire.

10
SURGERY FOR CORONARY
HEART DISEASE

J. Keith Ross

Surgery for coronary heart disease may be considered under four main headings.

1. Surgery for chronic disabling angina, with or without impaired ventricular function.
2. Surgery for threatened, developing or recently established infarction.
3. Surgery for coronary artery disease associated with chronic valvular heart disease.
4. Surgery for the mechanical consequences of infarction, which can be either early or late.

The common denominator in the first three categories is the surgical method for improving the blood supply to the ischaemic myocardium. In the fourth, this is less fundamental but still complementary to the correction of the mechanical defect concerned.

SURGICAL METHOD

The present acceptance that surgery has a place in the management of coronary artery disease dates from 1967, when the technique of introducing a source of arterial blood directly into a partly or totally occluded coronary artery beyond the site of obstruction first came into use (Effler, Favaloro and Groves, 1970). Before this, surgical procedures had been directed towards augmenting or creating a collateral coronary blood supply, the most important of which was the implantation of the internal mammary artery into the ventricular muscle (Vineberg, 1946). This method has been shown to work (Vineberg, 1975) but it lacks the immediacy of a bypass operation and in practice produces rather fickle results (Balcon et al, 1970). Vineberg's observations, both in the long-term survivors and in autopsy specimens, indicate that this is a valid if rather unpredictable way of introducing an arterial blood supply into ischaemic myocardium, and as such it should still be counted among the available surgical procedures.

Other local direct procedures at the site of the coronary artery obstruction have now been largely abandoned, but endarterectomy combined with bypass grafting has been shown to be effective (Yacoub et al, 1975).

The operation most commonly used is the placing of a reversed segment of long saphenous vein by end-to-side anastomosis between the ascending aorta and the coronary artery distal to the block (Favaloro, 1969; Johnson, Flemma and

Lepley, 1970). The internal mammary artery is also used, either mobilised on its pedicle from the inside of the anterior chest wall (Green, 1972) or as a free graft (Cheanvechai et al, 1975). This method has the advantage of an artery-to-artery anastomosis with near uniformity in size between the recipient artery and the graft, both factors probably contributing to the excellent record of late graft patency which is over 90 per cent at two to three years. Studies of graft flows have shown little important difference in the volumes of blood transmitted down vein and internal mammary artery grafts, and serial angiographic studies have shown that the lumen of the internal mammary artery graft can increase in size with the passage of time (Geha et al, 1975). The method does have technical limitations and it is usual for surgeons who advocate its use to employ saphenous vein grafts as well in many instances (Suzuki, Kay and Hardy, 1973; Geha et al, 1975).

Average flow rates in completed vein grafts (at rest) are between 70 and 80 ml per minute with a slightly lower figure (58 ± 7 ml per minute) for internal mammary artery grafts. When three grafts have been inserted, the total graft contribution to coronary blood flow may therefore be in the region of 200 ml per minute.

Investigation and Diagnosis

The decision to advise surgery for coronary artery disease is based on the findings on coronary arteriography (Sones and Shirey, 1962) and on the functional state of the left ventricle. The latter is assessed angiographically (ejection fraction) (Greene et al, 1967; Bristow, Van Zee and Judkins, 1970); by echocardiography (Feigenbaum, 1975), and by conventional haemodynamic measurements (cardiac index, end diastolic left ventricular pressure) made at cardiac catheterisation. It is likely that assay of regional myocardial blood flow by scintigraphy will become an increasingly important method in the future (Ashburn et al, 1971; Weller et al, 1972; Grames et al, 1974). In the classification of data, in selection for surgery, and in the assessment of patients' progress, it may be helpful to adopt an angiographic scoring system (Friesinger, Page and Ross, 1970) to quantify the severity of the disease.

In the course of routine preoperative investigation, it is important to identify known risk factors which include smoking habits, hypertension, diabetes and disorders of lipid metabolism. Serum enzyme estimations are useful to provide a base-line for postoperative levels, and are particularly important in those with progressive angina. An objective measure of the patient's condition may be estimated by an atrial pacing stress test, thus determining the heart-rate at which angina develops (Sowton et al, 1967; Balcon, Maloy and Sowton, 1968).

SURGERY FOR CHRONIC DISABLING ANGINA

The indication for surgery is anginal pain which has proved unresponsive to full medical treatment, and selection is based on the investigations already outlined.

At this point, it is necessary to examine the known prognosis of the disease untreated surgically and to compare this with the risk of the operation itself, and the possible benefit it can bring in the long term. The three factors to be considered here are pain and its relief, ventricular function, and life expectancy, since surgery alone cannot be expected to influence other known risk factors such as hypertension.

The results are now available of a number of studies of patient populations with angiographically documented coronary artery disease followed up for periods of up to 10 years (Bruschke, Proudfit and Sones, 1973; Humphries et al, 1974; Burggraf and Parker, 1975), all of which show that the extent and severity of the coronary artery disease, as demonstrated angiographically, is the key determinant of survival. In Burggraf and Parker's series, the five-year survival rates for single, double and triple vessel disease were 92, 65 and 55 per cent respectively, with an overall five-year survival figure for the whole group of 73 per cent. The same authors emphasise the good prognosis of single vessel disease, particularly if the right coronary artery is the vessel affected. With minor variations, there is remarkably close agreement between the results of similar series reported from widely separated centres. The Cleveland group first drew attention to the high five-year mortality (57 per cent) in patients with disease of the left main coronary artery (Bruschke, Proudfit and Sones, 1973). The data analysis shows the adverse effect of impaired ventricular function on survival, congestive heart failure reducing the five-year survival to 38 per cent, with abnormal haemodynamic findings or left ventricular asynergy reducing the five-year survival figure to around the 60 per cent level. In this context it is interesting that a past history of infarction is not of prognostic significance, neither is the presence or absence of angina, or its severity when present. Hypertension (blood pressure over 150/90 mmHg or 20/12 kPa) also reduces the five-year survival figure to approximately 60 per cent.

Factors influencing selection

The first requisite for advising surgery for intractable angina is the demonstration of a 75 per cent or greater stenosis affecting one or more major vessels. A previous history of infarction is not a contraindication, nor is the presence of other known risk factors which cannot be influenced by surgery.

Impaired ventricular function has emerged as the most important risk factor. Revascularisation procedures in patients who present in congestive failure, with large dilated hearts, and particularly in those who do not have angina, carry a very high operative mortality (Spencer et al, 1971). A recent analysis of fatalities after vein or artery bypass operations at the Cleveland Clinic underlines the high surgical risk that goes with impaired ventricular function (Loop et al, 1975). Although there is real doubt, therefore, about the value of surgery in this category of patients as a whole, the fact that some can benefit exposes the weakness of a policy which automatically rejects such cases (Mitchel et al, 1975). This approach is justified by the up-dated experience of the group who originally identified the problem (Isom et al, 1975) who can now show a significantly improved two-year survival rate (85 per cent) in these severely ill patients.

Disease of the left main coronary artery, as already pointed out, carries a poor prognosis, and is generally accepted as a strong indication for bypass grafting. In spite of a relatively high mortality related both to investigation and surgery in this group, the long-term survival is significantly improved by surgery (Talano et al, 1975).

SINGLE VESSEL DISEASE

The favourable prognosis in single vessel disease treated conservatively (excluding the left main coronary artery) demonstrated by Burggraf and Parker (1975) with five to six year survival figures of 82 and 98 per cent respectively for the left anterior descending (LAD) and right (R) coronary arteries, challenges the justification for surgical intervention. This would be a more compelling argument if it were not for the fact that surgery is first and foremost for the relief of pain and that operation now carries a risk of 2 per cent or less (Hutchinson et al, 1974; Wisoff et al, 1975). This counter-argument is strengthened by the fact that the operative mortality is concentrated among those now identified as carrying a high risk, and by definition these do not include patients with single vessel disease.

Results of Surgery for Angina

The operative mortality has already been referred to and now varies between 1 and 4 per cent. To this has to be added the risk of coronary and left ventricular angiography, which is now less than 1 per cent.

There is an incidence of perioperative infarction of 2 to 15 per cent, the infarct commonly being in the territory of a grafted vessel (Morton et al, 1975), but not all postoperative deaths are associated with infarction, which is frequently non-fatal.

There is also an incidence of postoperative pulmonary embolism (3 to 7 per cent) which has been reduced since the risk of this complication became clear and the need for anticoagulant therapy appreciated.

Complete pain relief is achieved in 70–75 per cent, and pain is moderated in a further 15 per cent (Alderman et al, 1973; Ullyot et al, 1975). The remaining 10–15 per cent includes the hospital mortality and those who gained no benefit from operation. An important prospective randomised study of coronary bypass surgery for stable angina has shown conclusively that after an average follow-up of two years, surgically treated patients show significantly greater subjective and objective improvement than those managed medically (Mathur and Guinn, 1975). There is some evidence that after an initial period of pain relief in the majority (85 per cent), later follow-up may show a return of symptoms in as many as 40 per cent after two to five years (Tecklenberg et al, 1975). The implication is that progression of the underlying atherosclerosis is responsible for the late symptomatic deterioration, and it remains to be seen whether this pattern is repeated in other carefully observed groups of patients as time goes on.

Improvement in ventricular function after bypass surgery can be demonstrated (Rees et al, 1971; Moran et al, 1973; Rutherford et al, 1972) and here there is a correlation with blood flow down the graft, flows of less than 50 ml per minute making little difference to contractile force. The improvement, because of the variables involved, may be inconsistent, but a return towards normal left ventricular function during mild exercise in approximately 70 per cent of patients has been shown.

Fate of the graft

There is a close correlation between graft patency, pain relief, and ventricular performance, and the fate of the graft itself is fundamental to the outcome. The combined experience from many centres shows that the graft patency rate at two years is 80–85 per cent, and that if the graft is patent at two years, it is likely to remain so. Technical improvements and increasing familiarity with the surgical method have resulted in a reduction in the incidence of stenoses at anastomotic sites and also in the incidence of narrowing in the grafts themselves. It has long been appreciated that the flow down the graft is a critical factor in graft patency, and that flows of less than 40 or 50 ml per minute predispose to early graft occlusion. With improved technique, grafts with flows of less than 50 ml per minute have shown improved patency rates at one year (Campeau et al, 1975). In spite of this, the quality of the distal run-off remains an important factor in determining both early and late graft patency, poor run-off being responsible for one-third of late graft failures. In this context it is interesting that endarterectomy combined with vein bypass grafting results in a graft patency rate identical with bypass grafting alone (Groves, Loop and Silver, 1972; Cheanvechai et al, 1975; Yacoub et al, 1975). Fibrous intimal hyperplasia and medial fibrosis which caused widespread anxiety when they were first described, although known to be part of the adaption of a vein to the stress of 'arterialisation' have not, to date, proved a serious problem. It seems likely that the segmental narrowing noted angiographically in earlier series may have been related to the way the graft was handled at operation as this, too, is now less commonly seen. Recently, it has become clear that another important factor in graft patency is the degree of proximal obstruction in the grafted vessel, the less the proximal obstruction, the more likely the graft is to fail (Rees, 1976).

Changes in the grafted coronary arteries

Progression of obstructive proximal lesions in grafted coronary arteries was first described in 1971 (Aldridge and Trimble, 1971) and a more recent report from the same group showed a 40 per cent incidence of progression of disease proximal to the site of graft insertion compared with a 14 per cent incidence of similar change in non-grafted vessels. Of greater significance was the finding of progression of disease distal to the site of graft entry in only 7 per cent of grafted vessels. Progression of the proximal lesions was not found to affect symptomatic improvement (McLaughlin et al, 1975).

Coronary grafting and improved survival

Because coronary bypass graft procedures are palliative, and because their main application is one of pain relief, there has been a natural reluctance to claim that they also prolong life. Evidence is now emerging that this last claim may be justifiable, and is most obvious in the improved survival of the high-risk group who present with cardiac failure (Isom et al, 1975) or when bypass grafting is added to left ventricular aneurysmectomy (Cooperman et al, 1975). Crude survival figures in mixed groups of patients treated surgically show improved survival when compared with the non-surgical groups already described which are used as a data base for the natural history of the disease (Ullyot et al, 1975).

In an analysis of the results of their coronary bypass surgery, the Stanford group are careful to point out the difficulty of comparing one group of patients with another when trying to identify the effect of treatment on longevity. They also stress how little is known about the problem of myocardial infarction in post-bypass patients while recording an incidence of 5 per cent per annum in their own series, with a mortality of 12.5 per cent in those sustaining infarcts. Actuarial analysis of survival in their patients with multivessel disease suggests the operation influences longevity (75 per cent four-year survival, compared with 60 per cent and 35 per cent for two and three vessel disease untreated). Analysis of the figures for survival after surgery for single and multiple vessel disease failed to show any statistically significant differences between the two groups (Tecklenberg et al, 1975).

SURGERY FOR THREATENED, DEVELOPING OR RECENTLY ESTABLISHED INFARCTION

Unstable Angina

Wood (1961) estimated that 10 per cent of all patients with atherosclerotic heart disease present with a preinfarction syndrome. This syndrome has been given many names, including acute coronary insufficiency, impending myocardial infarction, preinfarction angina, crescendo angina and unstable angina. The essential features are those of progressive pain of recent onset, including pain at rest, without evidence of myocardial infarction. Spencer (1972) defines it as a condition intermediate between chronic angina and acute myocardial infarction, and more recently Chahine (1975) has tried to introduce order into the nomenclature and classification of patients who present in this way, preferring the term 'unstable angina'.

DEFINITION

The following criteria should be satisfied before making a diagnosis of unstable angina:

1. Attacks of pain of increasing severity, duration, and/or frequency, either of recent onset or as an exacerbation of a chronic stable anginal state.
2. Prolonged episodes of angina lasting for not less than 15 to 30 minutes.
3. Rest pain.
4. Pain unrelieved by coronary dilator drugs.
5. Recurrent pain despite in-patient bed rest and treatment.
6. ECG changes indicating ischaemia, but limited to ST and T wave changes.
7. Normal serum enzymes — serum aspartate transaminase (AST), serum alanine transaminase (ALT), and creatine kinase (CK) — on serial estimations.

In addition, significant coronary stenosis should be demonstrated angiographically.

Those with overt infarction, bad angina but not fulfilling the above criteria, severe left ventricular failure, and associated left ventricular aneurysm or valve disease, should be excluded from this category.

The natural history of the untreated condition shows a significant incidence of early infarction, 22 per cent within two months (Wood, 1961) and a further 21 per cent within eight months of the onset of symptoms (Gazes et al, 1973). Between 40 and 70 per cent of the infarcts are fatal. In the series reported by Goodin et al (1973) 71 per cent had progressed to infarction (untreated surgically) and 43 per cent were dead within three months of the onset of progressive pain. In another series comparing the results of medical and surgical treatment, and with rigidly applied criteria, no less than 32 of 35 in the medically treated group sustained infarction, and of these 14 (40 per cent) were fatal within one month of hospital admission (Matloff et al, 1975).

INDICATIONS FOR SURGERY

Although the figures for early infarction and its associated mortality vary according to the precise criteria applied by different workers, it is clear that the patient with unstable angina carries a worse prognosis than his counterpart with pain that is not progressive.

The fact that the pain is severe and cannot be properly controlled pharmacologically is a good indication for surgery, and Hammond and Poirier (1975) make the point that the need for narcotics to control the pain may be a more reliable guide than the duration of attacks when considering surgical intervention.

As with stable angina, if surgery can be shown to result in consistent pain relief with statistically less risk to the patient than medical treatment alone, and if the length as well as the quality of life is improved, then the case for bypass grafting on an urgent or emergency basis is a good one. The case for surgery is strengthened further by considering the nature of the underlying pathology. The patients studied by Lawson et al (1975) who had acute pain of recent onset and no previous symptoms, showed a significantly higher incidence of single vessel disease than those in a parallel group with stable angina, and these patients also showed absence of collateral vessels. With increasing numbers of obstructed vessels, the development of collaterals was seen more often, but still not to the same extent as in the stable angina population. These observations suggest that there is an important time factor operating here, and that both the severity of the symptoms and the lack of collaterals are related to the rate of progression of the proximal obstruction in the affected major arteries, especially in the left anterior descending. The absolute (single vessel obstruction) or relative (multiple vessel obstruction) shortage of collaterals in this group exposes them to a greater risk of infarction and sudden death.

There is a well-documented incidence of complications (severe dysrhythmias, cardiac arrest, hypotension) occurring before or during the investigation of patients with unstable angina, and between the time of cardiac catheterisation and subsequent surgery (Matloff et al, 1975). The obviously increased hazard of investigation in this group may be reduced by the use of the intra-aortic balloon pump during this difficult stage, but this is not essential.

RESULTS

The reported operative mortality varies from zero to 3.4 per cent (Matloff et al, 1975), 6.4 per cent (Cheanvechai et al, 1973), and to 8.3 per cent (Goodin et al,

1973), with a perioperative infarction rate of between 5 and 10 per cent. Abolition of angina is achieved in 80–85 per cent of the survivors in the early months after operation with a high rate of return to work in those of appropriate age. Comparable medically treated patients show a higher incidence of angina (Conti et al, 1975) although the late infarction rate was the same in the medical and surgical groups reported by the same authors. Assessment of the true incidence of late myocardial infarction presents the difficulty already seen in surgery for stable angina, aggravated by the lack of angiographic data in medically managed groups used for comparison. Bonchek et al (1974) record a 5 per cent incidence of late infarction with a minimum follow-up of one year. Most reported series show a small but definite incidence of late infarction, and it will be of some interest to see if this differs materially from the infarction rate after surgery for stable angina when the time comes for this comparison to be made.

Survival statistics favour the surgically-treated patient, to the time limits of present experience, in spite of the evident snags in the interpretation of the data. Thus, actuarial analysis of the data of Matloff et al (1975) over three years shows sustained improved survival in the surgically compared with the medically treated group, and with both the 'high risk' and 'low risk' groups of Gazes et al (1973). Similar results are reported by Lawson et al (1975).

The overall evidence suggests that the combined hospital and late mortality in surgery for unstable angina is significantly less than that for medical treatment alone, and that symptomatic relief is also significantly better in those treated by revascularisation. The improved early survival figures in the surgically treated patients implies that the operation has a protective effect and does prevent infarction within the first three months of onset of symptoms. It remains to be determined whether the incidence of late infarction is altered by surgery (itself complicated by infarction, or not) when compared with those who survive an episode of unstable angina on medical treatment alone (with or without infarction).

Surgery in Acute Infarction

The place for surgery in the management of evolving or very recently established myocardial infarction is less well defined than for unstable angina, and whether or not surgery can be considered in the individual case may well depend on uncontrollable factors such as where the patient happens to be at the time, and the availability of a surgical service. For practical purposes genuinely early revascularisation, for example within six hours of the onset of pain (Berg et al, 1975), restricts the offer of surgery to those who either develop infarcts while in hospital or who are admitted very early in their attack. If the patient should be favourably situated, the next question is whether or not he should be submitted to coronary arteriography and left ventricular angiography at this acute stage in his illness. It seems unlikely that investigation in every case will become a universally accepted policy even if this were logistically possible, and that only those with serious complications (dysrhythmias, cardiogenic shock, persistent pain or dependence on a circulatory assistance device) will be selected for urgent or emergency investigation. The risk inherent in such investigations is difficult to assess from the literature, but it is reasonable to assume that it is higher than for stable angina even if angiography is promptly followed by revascularisation. In spite of these considerations the experience of Berg et al (1975) demands attention regardless of their failure to state their policy regarding the primary decision on selection for investigation or the risk that this carried in their hands. Severely impaired left ventricular function, advanced deterioration or a 'stable and uncomplicated' status were considered by them contraindications to surgery, but of those investigated, 60 per cent (a total of 96 patients) were submitted to vein bypass grafting. All had typical pain, Q waves and S–T injury patterns on ECG, elevation of serum aspartate transaminase, and major coronary lesions with abnormal left ventricular wall movement shown angiographically. The hospital mortality in this group was 5.2 per cent, they report one late death in the 91 survivors (a total mortality of 6.3 per cent) and only five have residual angina. These results are compared with a first-year mortality rate of 30 per cent for comparable medically treated patients. Even with all the usual reservations about such comparisons, the efforts of these workers show what can be achieved by revascularisation surgery in the presence of evolving or fresh infarction.

Mundth (1975) stresses the importance of defining the exact stage reached in the infarction process when trying to identify the role that revascularisation has to play. He confirms that surgery early in the evolution of an infarct carries favourable results, but points out that later, with established muscle necrosis, bypass grafting produces immediate oedema and haemorrhage in the infarcted area and in the peri-infarction zone.

In summary, therefore, it appears that the timing of surgery in this situation is critical, that early intervention in ideal circumstances can bring considerable benefit, and that care must be taken to distinguish those with evolving or early infarction (and salvageable muscle) from those with unstable angina on one hand and full-blown established myocardial necrosis on the other.

Surgery in Cardiogenic Shock

Cardiogenic shock following myocardial infarction is associated with:

1. Arterial systolic pressure less than 90 mmHg (12 kPa)
2. Urine output less than 20 ml per hour
3. Signs of poor peripheral perfusion.

When this triad persists in spite of full medical supportive treatment, death is almost certain, and the hazard of definitive investigation is high.

It was in this situation that the initial clinical experience in the use of intra-aortic balloon pump assistance (IABPA) was gained, the major effort being made by the group at the Massachusetts General Hospital in Boston (Mundth et al, 1973).

The intra-aortic balloon pump

The concept of counter-pulsation was first described by Clauss et al (1961) who showed that by withdrawing blood from one femoral artery in systole and re–infusing it into the other during diastole, left ventricular afterload was reduced and thereby peak left ventricular pressure and myocardial oxygen consumption. The raised mean arterial diastolic pressure enhanced coronary blood flow and the perfusion of other vital organs. The same haemodynamic effects were shown to be produced by placing an inflatable balloon in the upper descending thoracic aorta, timed to inflate during diastole (Moulopoulos, Topaz and Kolff, 1962), and with refinements this concept has progressed to widespread clinical use for support of the acutely failing left ventricle (Donnelly, 1975; *British Medical Journal*, 1976). The balloon catheter is introduced by way of the femoral artery, and deflation of the balloon is triggered by the R wave of the electrocardiogram so that it is never inflated during systole. Coronary diastolic blood flow is augmented, and clinical experience shows that this helps to limit the size of an infarct and to relieve pain. The haemodynamic improvement in cardiogenic shock with the use of IABPA was shown by Dunkman et al (1972) to include the following:

1. Cardiac index increased by 44 per cent
2. Mean arterial pressure increased by 10 per cent
3. Pulmonary capillary wedge pressure reduced by 23 per cent.

The use of IABPA alone was shown to reverse cardiogenic shock in 80 per cent of patients, but it soon became clear that this was only a temporary improvement in the majority, relatively few surviving the withdrawal of circulatory support for later elective revascularisation surgery (Mundth et al, 1973).

Perhaps the most important function of IABPA is to make it possible for these very ill patients to be properly investigated so that those who may benefit from bypass grafting may be sensibly selected for emergency surgery, and to provide a margin of safety pre- and post-operatively. Donnelly (1975) makes the point that it is the duration and not the severity of the cardiogenic shock which should be the important factor in deciding which patients should be selected for IABPA, and suggests that a period of shock lasting 12 hours should probably be regarded as the maximum beyond which patients should not be accepted for this method of treatment.

Given the fact that the majority of patients in this category will be shown to be balloon–dependent (mean arterial pressure less than 60 mmHg or 8 kPa; pulmonary capillary wedge pressure greater than 20 mmHg or 2.7 kPa; cardiac index less than 21 per min per m^2; recurrent pain with temporary stopping of IABPA) selection for emergency revascularisation depends on the findings on coronary arteriography and left ventriculography. The Boston experience suggests that approximately 50 per cent are selected for surgery on these grounds and that of these, approximately 50 per cent will survive (Mundth, 1975).

SURGERY FOR CORONARY ARTERY DISEASE ASSOCIATED WITH CHRONIC VALVULAR HEART DISEASE

Evaluation of the usefulness of revascularisation procedures combined with either aortic or mitral valve replacement is difficult because statistics are lacking for patients with known coronary artery disease who have been treated by valve replacement only. Indirect evidence from autopsy material (Coleman and Soloff,

1970) implies an increased risk when valve lesions are treated in the presence of unrecognised or untreated coronary artery disease. The difficulty is increased because of the lack of general agreement on the indications for coronary arteriography before valve replacement. Some believe it should be a routine procedure, particularly in aortic valve disease (Linhart and Wheat, 1967; Oury et al, 1972) while others restrict its application to those with angina (Berndt, Hancock and Harrison, 1973), angina with or without electrocardiographic evidence of previous infarction (Assad-Morell et al, 1975) or on an age basis for those over the age of 35 (Hutchinson et al, 1974).

In a study of patients with severe aortic valve disease, Basta et al (1975) found significant coronary artery disease on angiography in 23.5 per cent of patients presenting with angina and none in those who were pain-free. However, the latter group were not all subjected to angiography. They noted a slight but definite preponderance of coronary artery disease in individuals with aortic stenosis, and Berger, Karp and Kouchoukos (1975) also identify the higher risk in the stenotic as opposed to the regurgitant or mixed lesion groups.

In a similar study, Harris et al (1975) found an overall incidence of significant coronary artery disease in 23.2 per cent of the patients investigated. All had aortic stenosis and of those with angina, 32.5 per cent had important coronary artery obstruction. In the pain-free group the incidence was 10.3 per cent, showing that patients who present with severe aortic stenosis but without angina have a small but definite chance of having significant coronary artery disease.

Aortic Valve Surgery

In aortic valve replacement, the experience of the group at the Mayo Clinic shows an operative mortality of 10 per cent for combined valve replacement and coronary bypass grafting, a figure which is significantly higher than in patients without coronary artery disease. The combined early and late mortality in their series was 27 per cent (Assad-Morell et al, 1975). It is the policy of the same authors to confine preoperative coronary arteriography to those with angina or electrocardiographic evidence of previous myocardial infarction, while recognising that the reported incidence of associated aortic valve and coronary artery disease is between 34 and 62 per cent. They advocate bypass grafting particularly for those with severe angina associated with severe proximal coronary narrowing, including the left main coronary artery, but point out the need for further evaluation of the true incidence of postoperative myocardial infarction and late death due to coronary artery disease.

A key factor in surgery for combined aortic and coronary artery disease is the incidence of infarction during or soon after operation, and Berger et al (1975) not only show that the operative mortality for the combined procedure can be the same as for aortic valve replacement alone, but suggest that protection of the myocardium by bypass grafting can reduce both the early mortality and the incidence of postoperative myocardial injury. It is interesting that their incidence of infarction related to operation (22.5 per cent) was independent of the method used to preserve the myocardium during valve replacement (coronary perfusion or hypothermic arrest), although less efficient methods may be associated with a higher incidence of myocardial injury. It is evident that a significant number of these patients with hypertrophied ventricles suffer intra-operative myocardial injury regardless of the preservation technique that is used, and that the incidence of myocardial damage (63 per cent) following combined valve replacement and bypass grafting is higher than that in patients undergoing either procedure alone (Rossiter et al, 1974).

More time is needed, therefore, to complete evaluation of the effect that bypass grafting has on both the hospital and late mortality in these patients. Symptomatic relief, which is good, cannot be used as an indicator since correction of the valve lesion alone can relieve angina.

Mitral Valve Surgery

In mitral valve replacement for rheumatic mitral valve disease (Assad-Morell et al, 1975) the operative mortality (15 per cent) is lower than for postinfarction mitral regurgitation (33 per cent) but the late mortality is high, and, again, probably related to the combined rheumatic and ischaemic myocardial deficit. Mitral valve replacement for postinfarction mitral regurgitation is discussed in detail separately (see page 239).

SURGERY FOR THE MECHANICAL CONSEQUENCES OF INFARCTION

The value of surgery in the management of postinfarction ventricular aneurysm, ventricular septal defect (VSD) and mitral regurgitation is now beyond dispute.

Accurate diagnosis by coronary and left ventricular angiography allows identification and definitive correction of each of these major mechanical defects, whether they occur singly, or in combination, together with planned revascularisation procedures should these be indicated. In spite of the fact that most follow large infarcts, surgical correction in each instance carries an acceptable risk when compared with the results of conservative management, and the functional improvement following operation is rewarding.

Left Ventricular Aneurysm

INCIDENCE AND NATURAL HISTORY

The incidence of left ventricular aneurysm after myocardial infarction varies between 3 and 30 per cent, depending upon the diagnostic criteria adopted, and although some may pursue a benign course, 60 per cent or more cause ventricular failure (Abrams et al, 1963; Mourdjinis et al, 1968) and this is the common mode of presentation. There is also a significant mortality within the first year after the aneurysm develops, with a three-year mortality of 75 per cent (Schlichter, Hellerstein and Katz, 1954; Nagle and Williams, 1974.) The risk of systemic embolism from clot inside the aneurysm is assessed at between 10 and 50 per cent by various authors, and the presence of the aneurysm may be associated with severe recurrent dysrhythmias. Rupture of well-established ventricular aneurysms is a rare but recognised complication.

VENTRICULAR DYSFUNCTION

In this condition, dysfunction of the left ventricle is directly related to the size of the aneurysm, and becomes critical when the aneurysm occupies 20–25 per cent of the ventricular wall (Klein, Herman and Gorlin, 1967). Ventricular function is impaired both by muscle loss and by the increase in cavity size, which in turn increases wall stress and thereby oxygen consumption by the Laplace relation. Paradoxical systolic expansion of the aneurysm also reduces the stroke volume and ejection fraction, but the expansion is more apparent than real when the aneurysm wall is stiff and fibrotic (Parmely et al, 1973). Under these circumstances, paradox is due to elastic stretch at the borders of the aneurysm, but when the wall contains residual muscle, as it can (Klein, Herman and Gorlin, 1967), true paradox contributes significantly to the reduction in cardiac output. True paradox is also seen in the acutely-developing aneurysm soon after infarction when it is commonly associated with the clinical picture of cardiogenic shock.

DIAGNOSIS

The presence of a left ventricular aneurysm may be suspected on clinical grounds by the detection of systolic expansion over the left ventricle in a patient who remains in refractory congestive failure after infarction. This suspicion may be confirmed both by the characteristic shape of the left heart border on the plain chest radiograph, and by the electrocardiogram. Left ventriculography defines the position and extent of the aneurysm, although mural thrombus may conceal its true dimensions, and selective coronary arteriography identifies the occluded vessel responsible for the infarct as well as the state of the remaining vessels.

MANAGEMENT

The indications for surgery are refractory cardiac failure (acute or chronic), systemic embolism and intractable dysrhythmias, with or without associated angina.

The practical problems of surgery for left ventricular aneurysm have been well described by several authors (Cooley et al, 1964; Kluge et al, 1971; Merin et al, 1973; Sbokos, Monro and Ross, 1976). Although aneurysms can involve the postero-inferior wall of the left ventricle and related ventricular septum, the majority arise from the anterolateral free wall of the ventricle in the territory of the occluded anterior descending branch of the left coronary artery. Because this is so, it is rare for the aneurysm to involve the papillary muscles, but not uncommon for the infarct to have involved the adjacent septum and to have caused an associated ventricular septal defect close to the apex. If mitral regurgitation complicates a ventricular aneurysm, it usually indicates occlusion of either the right or circumflex arteries, although an aneurysm in the 'common' site following left anterior descending occlusion can be associated with anterior papillary muscle rupture or dysfunction. If the mitral regurgitation is severe enough to demand valve replacement, this may be carried out using the ventricular approach provided by resection of the aneurysm: similarly, associated ventricular septal defects are readily closed from the left side after aneurysmec-tomy.

RESULTS

The results of surgery for left ventricular aneurysm show that there is a hospital mortality of 10–20 per cent, and that the commonest cause of late death is further myocardial infarction. Saphenous vein bypass grafting is now combined with aneurysmectomy when the preoperative coronary arteriograms show serious disease in the remaining coronary arteries, and there is already evidence to suggest that aneurysmectomy combined with saphenous vein bypass grafting results in improved long-term survival (Cooperman et al, 1975; Assad-Morell et al, 1975). Relief of congestive cardiac failure is immediate, and provided function in the remaining myocardium is good, the improvement is sustained. The combined hospital and late mortality figures are considerably better than those for the disease untreated (Effler et al, 1971).

Acquired Ventricular Septal Defect (VSD)

INCIDENCE AND NATURAL HISTORY

Rupture of the ventricular septum is found in 1.5 to 2.0 per cent of all deaths following myocardial infarction, and septal rupture occurs, typically, between 4 and 15 days after the development of the infarct. 65 per cent die within two weeks, and 80 per cent within two months (Oldham et al, 1969), only 7 per cent surviving for more than one year (Sanders, Kern and Blount, 1956; Lee, Cardon and Slodki, 1962). Approximately one-quarter of the patients die within 24 hours of the development of the VSD.

FUNCTIONAL DISORDER

This is proportional to the size of the infarct and the resulting defect. When the defect is large, the sudden volume overload on the right ventricle causes it to fail, and this can be followed by the development of severe tricuspid regurgitation which in turn causes serious systemic venous hypertension. This may be sufficient, together with the low cardiac output, to precipitate acute renal and hepatic failure. Pulmonary venous hypertension secondary to left ventricular failure, combined with the increased pulmonary blood flow, leads to rapidly developing, refractory pulmonary oedema.

DIAGNOSIS

The differential diagnosis in the patient who develops a systolic murmur after myocardial infarction is between acquired VSD and mitral regurgitation due to acute papillary muscle rupture or dysfunction. Since both conditions precipitate severe right and left heart failure with appropriate physical and radiological findings, bedside diagnosis is often very difficult. In acquired VSD there tends to be a disproportionately severe and rapid rise in right atrial pressure, a systolic thrill is more frequently present, and the murmur more often pansystolic and louder closer to the sternal edge than in mitral regurgitation. Investigation by left ventriculography and selective coronary angiography is essential, although right heart catheterisation, if necessary at the bedside using a flow-guided catheter, will establish the presence of a left-to-right shunt at ventricular level.

During the preoperative period, including investigation, circulatory support and stabilisation may be provided by intra-aortic balloon pump assistance (IABPA) (Buckley et al, 1973) but this loses its effectiveness after 24 hours and surgery should not be delayed.

MANAGEMENT

Patients with acquired VSD may be classified according to the severity of their associated cardiac failure which in turn is related to the size of the defect. The clinical spectrum varies from small defects in which surgery is not indicated, to larger ones which require closure either after a delay period to allow healing of the margins, or on an urgent or emergency basis (Allen and Woodwark, 1966). Although it may be possible to adopt a waiting policy for the four to six weeks or even longer, needed for fibrous tissue to develop round the margins of a large defect, and so produce optimal conditions for suturing, the mortality figures show that by this time well over 50 per cent are dead. There is therefore much to be said for adopting a more aggressive approach when there is any doubt about the effectiveness of supportive medical therapy. In practice, the patient's deterioration frequently compels surgical intervention sooner rather than later. A more positive attitude has been made possible by the refinement of surgical technique which has taken place since Cooley first closed an acquired VSD (Cooley et al, 1957), and which has been stimulated by the need to apply surgical correction to the worst group of patients in whom death is usual within one or two days if the defect is left open. Exponents of early closure of acquired VSD have all made contributions towards overcoming the problem of suturing in and around doubtfully viable heart muscle (Iben et al, 1969; Gonzalez-Lavin and Zajtchuk, 1971; Shumacker, 1972; Graham et al, 1973). It is often necessary to excise areas of infarcted ventricular wall as part of the operative procedure, and when the infarct responsible for the septal defect involves the apex, amputation of the apex has proved a logical and effective method (Daggett et al, 1970). More recently, the whole subject has been well reviewed and a technique described in which the free wall of the right ventricle is used to reinforce the repair, a method which has proved successful and which represents a significant technical contribution (Hill et al, 1975).

RESULTS

It has been shown that surgical closure can improve the two-month post-septal rupture survival figure from 20 per cent to 60 per cent (Oldham et al, 1969). As surgery for this condition will always include very ill patients, a hospital mortality between 25 and 35 per cent is likely to persist. The risk will remain high for the repair of defects high in the septum where, in addition to the technical difficulties, the infarct which has ruptured may also have involved the conduction mechanism.

Mitral Regurgitation

INCIDENCE AND NATURAL HISTORY

Papillary muscle rupture is considered rare after myocardial infarction, but its true incidence is difficult to define, as many who get this complication never reach hospital. Approximately one-third die almost immediately, there is a 50 per cent mortality within 24 hours, and fewer than 20 per cent survive the second week after the onset of mitral regurgitation.

The interval between infarction and papillary muscle rupture is commonly between 2 and 12 days. It is nearly always the posterior papillary muscle which ruptures following an inferior myocardial infarct, and some degree of necrosis in this muscle has been described in 20 per cent of infarcts on the diaphragmatic surface of the heart (Sanders, Neubuerger and Ravin, 1957). Infarction may also be limited to the papillary muscles themselves (Andersen and Fischer-Hansen, 1973).

CLINICAL PRESENTATION

Appreciation of the whole clinical spectrum of postinfarction mitral regurgitation depends upon an understanding of the anatomy of the papillary muscles and how they may be involved by the infarct (Yacoub, 1975). Each muscle has several 'heads', each of which controls a limited area of cusp tissue belonging to one or both cusps. As each muscle is supplied by at least two main vessels, complete rupture of either is rare, but the posterior muscle has the poorer blood supply and is therefore more often affected.

In practice, three clinicopathological syndromes may be recognised:

1. Acute rupture of the whole or part of one papillary muscle (as described above)
2. Subacute but progressive mitral regurgitation caused by stretching of the papillary muscle(s) in or near the wall of a developing left ventricular aneurysm
3. Chronic mitral regurgitation due to partial rupture or stretching of one or both papillary muscles (papillary muscle dysfunction).

In the first group, commonly presenting within a week or 10 days of infarction, the clinical picture is of cardiogenic shock and pulmonary oedema of sudden onset: untreated, this progresses to death within 24–48 hours. There is an associated early and mid-systolic murmur which fades in late systole due to the rapid equalisation of the left atrial and left ventricular pressures. The fact that the blowing murmur is well heard at the apex may help to distinguish it from the more common parasternal murmur of acquired VSD. Experimental studies have emphasised the importance of the myocardial factor in this syndrome and the part it plays in depressing the response to acute mitral regurgitation, a factor which does not apply in spontaneous chordal rupture or that secondary to infective endocarditis (Omoto, Buckley and Austen, 1972).

The second category includes those whose mitral regurgitation has a more insidious onset but which becomes progressively worse and presents about six weeks after infarction with a steadily enlarging heart and relentless ventricular failure.

Patients in the third category present much later, months or even years after infarction, with classical physical signs of mitral regurgitation, a proportion also having left ventricular aneurysms.

MANAGEMENT AND RESULTS

Those who survive the catastrophe of acute partial or complete papillary muscle rupture to enter hospital select themselves for immediate investigation and emergency mitral valve replacement. This was first successfully achieved in Boston (Austen et al, 1965) and later the same group were able to report five such cases with one hospital death (Austen et al, 1968). The two postoperative deaths reported by Yacoub (1975) illustrate two of the common hazards in this group, which are of infection developing in the oedematous lungs and of renal failure following the preoperative period of cardiogenic shock.

The second group, with progressive mitral regurgitation and progressively severe cardiac failure, has proved to carry a very high operative risk (Glancy et al, 1973) which is an expression of the fact that the mitral regurgitation reflects extensive damage to the left ventricular muscle. Both Yacoub's cases in this category died after operation with a low cardiac output and all five in another series treated postoperatively by intra-aortic balloon pump assistance died after mitral valve replacement (Buckley et al, 1973).

The early results of mitral valve replacement for those in the third group with chronic mitral regurgitation, combined with revascularisation procedures when necessary, are encouraging (Yacoub, 1975). This is the only one of the three categories in which it may be possible to conserve the mitral valve by reconstructing rather than replacing it. It is, however, difficult to compare the results from different centres because authors tend to describe their overall results in postinfarction mitral regurgitation and thus include many of the less favourable cases already described. It is clear that the operative mortality tends to be higher than that for isolated mitral valve replacement for rheumatic disease, and that the protective value of saphenous vein grafting in reducing the incidence of fatal late infarction has yet to be defined (Assad-Morell et al, 1975). It is certain that the quality of long-term survival is directly related, as in surgery for left ventricular aneurysm and acquired VSD, to the degree of left ventricular impairment present preoperatively.

REFERENCES

Abrams, D. L., Edelist, A., Luria, M. H. & Miller, A. J. (1963) Ventricular aneurysm: a reappraisal based on a study of 64 consecutive autopsied cases. *Circulation,* **27,** 164.

Alderman, E. L., Matlof, H. J., Wexler, L., Shumway, N. E. & Harrison, D. C. (1973) Results of direct coronary artery surgery for treatment of angina pectoris. *New England Journal of Medicine,* **288,** 535.

Aldridge, H. E. & Trimble, A. S. (1971) Progression of proximal coronary artery lesions to total occlusion after aortocoronary saphenous vein bypass grafting. *Journal of Thoracic and Cardiovascular Surgery,* **62,** 7.

Allen, P. & Woodwark, G. (1966) Surgical management of postinfarction ventricular septal defects. *Journal of Thoracic and Cardiovascular Surgery,* **51,** 346.

Anderson, J. A. & Fischer-Hansen (1973) Isolated acute myocardial infarction of papillary muscles of the heart: clinicopathological study of nine cases. *British Heart Journal,* **35,** 781.

Ashburn, W. L., Braunwald, E., Simon, A. L., Peterson, K. L. & Gault, J. H. (1971) Myocardial perfusion imaging with radioactive-labeled particles injected directly into the coronary circulation of patients with coronary artery disease. *Circulation,* **44,** 851.

Assad–Morell, J. L., Connolly, D. C., Brandenburg, R. O., Giuliani, E. R., Schattenberg, T. T., Pluth, J. R., Barnhorst, D. A., Wallace, R. B. & Danielson, G. K. (1975) Aorta-coronary artery saphenous vein bypass grafts isolated and combined with other procedures. *Journal of Thoracic and Cardiovascular Surgery*, **69**, 841.

Austen, W. G., Sanders, C. A., Averill, J. H. & Friedlich, A. L. (1965) Ruptured papillary muscle: report of a case with successful mitral valve replacement. *Circulation*, **32**, 597.

Austen, W. G., Sokol, D., De Sanctis, R. W. & Sanders, C. A. (1968) The surgical treatment of papillary muscle rupture complicating myocardial infarction. *New England Journal of Medicine*, **278**, 1137.

Balcon, R., Leaver, D., Ross, D. N. Ross, J. K. & Sowton, E. (1970) Clinical evaluation of internal mammary artery implantation. *Lancet*, **1**, 440.

Balcon, R., Maloy, W. C. & Sowton, E. (1968) Clinical use of atrial pacing test in angina pectoris. *British Medical Journal*, **iii**, 91.

Basta, L. L., Raines, D., Najjar, S. & Kiosches, J. M. (1975) Clinical, haemodynamic and coronary angiographic correlates of angina pectoris in patients with severe aortic valve disease. *British Heart Journal*, **37**, 150.

Berg, R., Kendall, R. W., Duvoisin, G. E., Ganji, J. H., Rudy, L. W. & Everhart, F. J. (1975) Acute myocardial infarction, a surgical emergency. *Journal of Thoracic and Cardiovascular Surgery*, **70**, 432.

Berger, T. J., Karp, R. B. & Kouchoukos, N. T. (1975) Valve replacement and myocardial revascularisation: results of combined operations in 59 patients. *Circulation*, **51, 52**, Suppl. I, 1–126.

Berndt, T., Hancock, E. W. & Harrison, D. C. (1973) Combined aortic valve replacement and coronary artery bypass graft surgery. (abstr.) *Circulation*, **48** (Suppl. IV–74).

Bonchek, L. I., Rahimtoola, S. H., Anderson, R. P., McAnulty, J. A., Rosch, J., Bristow, J. D. & Starr, A. (1974) Late results following emergency saphenous vein bypass grafting for unstable angina. *Circulation*, **50**, 972.

Bristow, J. D., Van Zee, B. E. & Judkins, M. P. (1970) Systolic and diastolic abnormalities of the left ventricle in coronary artery disease: studies in patients with little or no enlargement of ventricular volume. *Circulation*, **42**, 219.

British Medical Journal (1976) Help for the Left Ventricle (editorial). **i**, 3.

Bruschke, V. G., Proudfit, W. L. & Sones, F. M. (1973) Progress study of 590 consecutive non-surgical cases of coronary disease: followed 5–9 years. I. Arteriographic correlations. *Circulation*, **47**, 1147.

Buckley, M. J., Mundth, E. D., Daggett, W. M., Gold, H. K., Leinbach, R. C. & Austen, W. G. (1973) Surgical management of ventricular septal defects and mitral regurgitation complicating acute myocardial infarction. *Annals of Thoracic Surgery*, **16**, 598.

Burggraf, G. W. & Parker, J. O. (1975) Prognosis in coronary artery disease: Angiographic, haemodynamic and clinical factors. *Circulation*, **51**, 146.

Campeau, L., Crochet, D., Lesperance, J., Bourassa, M. G. & Grondin, C. M. (1975) Postoperative changes in aortocoronary saphenous vein grafts revisited. Angiographic studies at two weeks and at one year in two series of consecutive patients. *Circulation*, **52**, 369.

Chahine, R. A. (1975) Unstable angina. The problems of definition. *British Heart Journal*, **37**, 1246.

Cheanvechai, C., Irarrazaval, M. J., Loop, F. D., Effler, D. B., Rincon, G. & Sones, F. M. (1975) Aorto-coronary bypass grafting with the internal mammary artery. *Journal of Thoracic and Cardiovascular Surgery*, **70**, 278.

Cheanvechai, C., Effler, D. B., Loop, F. D., Groves, L. K., Sheldon, W. C., Razavi, M. & Sones, F. M. (1973) Emergency myocardial revascularisation. *American Journal of Cardiology*, **32**, 901.

Cheanvechai, C., Groves, L. K., Reyes, E. A., Shirey, E. K. & Sones, F. M. (1975) Manual coronary endarterectomy: clinical experience in 315 patients. *Journal of Thoracic and Cardiovascular Surgery*, **70**, 524.

Clauss, R. H., Birtwell, W. C., Albertal, G., Lunzer, S., Taylor, W. J., Fosberg, A. M. & Harken, D. E. (1961) Assisted circulation: 1. The arterial counterpulsator. *Journal of Thoracic and Cardiovascular Surgery*, **41**, 447.

Coleman, E. H. & Soloff, L. A. (1970) Incidence of significant coronary artery disease in rheumatic valvular heart disease. *American Journal of Cardiology*, **25**, 401.

Conti, C. R., Gilbert, J. B., Hodges, M., Hutter, A. M., Kaplan, E. M., Newell, J. B., Resnekov, L., Rosati, R. A., Ross, R. S., Russell, R. O., Schroeder, J. S. & Wok, M. (1975) Unstable angina pectoris: randomised study of surgical VS medical therapy. National cooperative unstable angina pectoris study group. *American Journal of Cardiology*, **35**, 129.

Cooley, D. A., Belmonte, B. A., Zeis, L. B. & Schnur, S. (1957) Surgical repair of ruptured intraventricular septum following acute myocardial infarction. *Surgery*, **41**, 930.

Cooley, D. A., Hallman, G. L. & Henly, W. S. (1964) Left ventricular aneurysm due to myocardial infarction. Experience with 37 patients undergoing aneurysmectomy. *Archives of Surgery*, **88**, 114.

Cooperman, M., Stinson, E. B., Griepp, R. B. & Shumway, N. E. (1975) Survival and function after left ventricular aneurysmectomy. *Journal of Thoracic and Cardiovascular Surgery*, **69**, 321.

Daggett, W. M., Burwell, L. R., Lawson, D. W. & Austen, W. G. (1970) Resection of acute left ventricular aneurysm and ruptured interventricular septum after myocardial infarction. *New England Journal of Medicine*, **283**, 1507.

Donelly, R. J. (1975) The intra-aortic balloon pump. *The Current Status of Cardiac Surgery*, ed. D. B. Longmore, p. 406.

Dunkman, W. B., Leinbach, R. C., Buckley, M. J., Mundth, E. D., Kantrowitz, A. R., Austen, W. G. & Sanders, C. A. (1972) Clinical and haemodynamic results of intra-aortic balloon pumping and surgery for cardiogenic shock. *Circulation*, **46**, 465.

Effler, D. B., Groves, L. K., Sones, F. M. & Shirey, E. K. (1964) Endarterectomy in the treatment of coronary artery disease. *Journal of Thoracic and Cardiovascular Surgery*, **47**, 98.

Effler, D. B., Favaloro, R. G. & Groves, L. K. (1970) Coronary artery surgery utilising saphenous vein graft techniques. *Journal of Thoracic and Cardiovascular Surgery*, **59**, 147.

Favaloro, R. G. (1969) Saphenous vein graft in the surgical treatment of coronary artery disease. *Journal of Thoracic and Cardiovascular Surgery*, **58**, 178.

Feigenbaum, H. (1975) Echocardiographic examination of the left ventricle. *Circulation*, **51**, 1 (editorial).

Friesinger, G. C., Page, E. E. & Ross, R. S. (1970) Prognostic significance of coronary arteriography. *Transactions of the Association of American Physicians*, **83**, 78.

Gazes, P. C., Mobley, E. M., Faris, H. M., Duncan, R. C. & Humphries, G. B. (1973) Preinfarctional (unstable) angina — a prospective study — ten-year follow-up. *Circulation*, **48**, 331.

Geha, A. S., Krone, R. J., McCormick, J. R. & Baue, A. E. (1975) Selection of coronary bypass. Anatomic, physiological and angiographic considerations of vein and mammary artery grafts. *Journal of Thoracic and Cardiovascular Surgery*, **70**, 414.

Glancy, D. L., Stinson, E. B., Shepherd, R. L., Itscoitz, S. B., Roberts, W. C., Epstein, S. E. & Morrow, A. G. (1973) Results of valve replacement for severe mitral regurgitation due to papillary muscle rupture or fibrosis. *American Journal of Cardiology*, **32**, 313.

Gonzalez-Lavin, L. & Zajtchuk, R. (1971) Surgical considerations in the treatment of acute acquired ventricular septal defect. *Thorax*, **26**, 610.

Goodin, R. R., Inglesby, T. V., Lansing, A. M. & Wheat, M. W. (1973) Preinfarction angina pectoris: a surgical emergency. *Journal of Thoracic and Cardiovascular Surgery*, **66**, 934.

Graham, A. F., Stinson, E. B., Daily, P. O. & Harrison, D. C. (1973) Ventricular septal defects after myocardial infarction. Early operative treatment. *Journal of the American Medical Association*, **225**, 708.

Grames, G. M., Jansen, C., Gander, M. P., Wieland, B. S. & Judkins, M. P. (1974) Safety of the direct coronary injection of radiolabeled particles. *Journal of Nuclear Medicine*, **15**, 2.

Green, G. E. (1972) Internal mammary artery-to-coronary artery anastomosis: three year experience with 165 patients. *Annals of Thoracic Surgery*, **14**, 260.

Greene, D. G., Carlisle, R., Grant, C. & Bunnell, I. L. (1967) Estimation of left ventricular volume by one-plane cineangiography. *Circulation*, **35**, 61.

Groves, L. K., Loop, F. D. & Silver, G. M. (1972) Endarterectomy as a supplement to coronary artery — saphenous vein bypass surgery. *Journal of Thoracic and Cardiovascular Surgery*, **64**, 514.

Hammond, G. L. & Poirier, R. A. (1975) Surgical management for acute coronary insufficiency with three years follow-up. *Journal of Thoracic and Cardiovascular Surgery*, **69**, 625.

Harris, C. N., Kaplan, M. A., Parker, D. P., Dunne, E. F., Cowell, H. S. & Ellestad, M. H. (1975) Aortic stenosis, angina and coronary artery disease. Interrelations. *British Heart Journal*, **37**, 656.

Hill, J. D., Lary, D., Kerth, W. J. & Gerbode, F. (1975) Acquired ventricular septal defects: evolution of an operation, surgical technique, and results. *Journal of Thoracic and Cardiovascular Surgery*, **70**, 440.

Humphries, J. O., Kuller, L., Ross, R. S., Friesinger, G. C. & Page, E. E. (1974) Natural history of ischaemic heart disease in relation to arteriographic findings: a twelve year study of 224 patients. *Circulation*, **49**, 489.

Hutchinson, J. E., Green, G. E., Mekhjian, H. A. & Kemp, H. G. (1974) Coronary bypass grafting in 376 consecutive patients with three operative deaths. *Journal of Thoracic and Cardiovascular Surgery*, **67**, 7.

Iben, A. B., Pupello, D. F., Stinson, E. B. & Shumway, N. E. (1969) Surgical treatment of postinfarction ventricular septal defects. *Annals of Thoracic Surgery*, **8**, 252.

Isom, O. W., Spencer, F. C., Glassman, E., Dembrow, J. M. & Pasternack, B. S. (1975) Long-term survival following coronary bypass surgery in patients with significant impairment of left ventricular function. *Circulation*, **51–52**, Suppl. 1, 1–141.

Johnson, W. D., Flemma, R. J. & Lepley, D. (1970) Direct coronary surgery utilising multiple-vein bypass grafts. *Annals of Thoracic Surgery*, **9**, 436.

Klein, M. D., Herman, M. V. & Gorlin, R. (1967) A haemodynamic study of left ventricular aneurysm. *Circulation*, **35**, 614.

Kluge, T. H., Ullal, S. R., Hill, J. D., Kerth, W. J. & Gerbode, F. (1971) Dyskinesia and aneurysm of the left ventricle: surgical experience in 36 patients. *Journal of Cardiovascular Surgery*, **12**, 273.

Lawson, R. M., Chapman, R., Wood, J., & Starr, A. (1975) Acute coronary insufficiency: an urgent surgical condition. *British Heart Journal*, **37**, 1053.

Lee, W. Y., Cardon, L. & Slodki, S. J. (1962) Perforation of infarcted interventricular septum. *Archives of Internal Medicine*, **109**, 731.

Linhart, J. W. & Wheat, M. W. (1967) Myocardial dysfunction following aortic valve replacement: the significance of coronary artery disease. *Journal of Thoracic and Cardiovascular Surgery*, **54**, 259.

Loop, F. D., Berrettoni, J. N., Pichard, A., Siegel, W., Razavi, M. & Effler, D. B. (1975) Selection of the candidate for myocardial revascularisation: a profile of high risk based on multivariate analysis. *Journal of Thoracic and Cardiovascular Surgery*, **69**, 40.

Mathur, V. S. & Guinn, G. A. (1975) Prospective randomised study of coronary bypass surgery in stable angina: the first 100 patients. *Circulation*, **51–52**, suppl. 1, 1–133.

McLaughlin, P. R., Berman, N. D., Morton, B. C., McLoughlin, M. J., Aldridge, H. E., Adelman, A. G., Goldman, B. S., Trimble, A. S. & Morch, J. E. (1975) Saphenous vein bypass grafting. Changes in native circulation and collaterals. *Circulation*, **51–52**, suppl. 1, 1–66.

Matloff, J. M., Sustaita, H., Chatterjee, K., Chaux, A., Marcus, H. S. & Swan, H. J. C. (1975) The rationale for surgery in preinfarction angina. *Journal of Thoracic and Cardiovascular Surgery*, **69**, 73.

Merin, G., Schattenberg, T. T., Pluth, J. R., Wallace, R. B. & Danielson, G. K. (1973) Surgery for postinfarction ventricular aneurysm. *Annals of Thoracic Surgery*, **15**, 588.

Mitchel, B. F., Alivizatos, P. A., Adam, M., Geisler, G. F., Thiele, J. P. & Lambert, C. J. (1975) Myocardial revascularisation in patients with poor ventricular function. *Journal of Thoracic and Cardiovascular Surgery*, **69**, 52.

Moran, S. V., Tarazi, R. C., Urzua, J. U., Favaloro, R. G. & Effler, D. B. (1973) Effects of aorto-coronary bypass on myocardial contractility. *Journal of Thoracic and Cardiovascular Surgery*, **65**, 335.

Morton, B. C., McLaughlin, P. R., Trimble, A. S. & Morch, J. E. (1975) Myocardial infarction in coronary artery surgery. *Circulation*, **51–52**, suppl. 1, 1–198.

Moulopoulos, S. D., Topaz, S. & Kolff, W. J. (1962) Diastolic balloon pumping (with carbon dioxide) in the aorta. Mechanical assistance to the failing circulation. *American Heart Journal*, **63**, 669.

Mourdjinis, A., Olsen, E., Raphael, M. J. & Mounsey, J. P. D. (1968) Clinical diagnosis and prognosis of ventricular aneurysm. *British Heart Journal*, **30**, 497.

Mundth, E. D., Buckley, M. J., Leinbach, R. C., Gold, H. K., Daggett, W. M. & Austen, W. G. (1973) Surgical intervention for the complications of acute myocardial infarction. *Annals of Surgery*, **178**, 379.

Mundth, E. D. (1975) Discussion following Berg et al (1975).

Nagle, R. E. & Williams, D. O. (1974) Natural history of ventricular aneurysm without surgical treatment. *British Heart Journal*, **36**, 1037P, 1974.

Oldham, H. N., Scott, S. M., Dart, C. H., Fish, R. G., Claxton, C. P., Dillon, M. L. & Sabiston, D. C. (1969) Surgical correction of ventricular septal defect following acute myocardial infarction. *Annals of Thoracic Surgery*, **7**, 193–201.

Omoto, R., Buckley, M. J. & Austen, W. G. (1972) Haemodynamic response to acute mitral regurgitation in dogs with acute and chronic coronary artery disease. *Journal of Thoracic and Cardiovascular Surgery*, **64**, 254.

Oury, J. H., Quint, R. A., Angell, W. W. & Wuerflein, R. D. (1972) Coronary artery vein bypass grafts in patients requiring valve replacement. *Surgery*, **72**, 1037.

Parmely, W. W., Chuck, L., Kivowitz, C., Matloff, J. M. & Swan, H. J. C. (1973) In vitro length-tension relations of human ventricular aneurysms. Relation of stiffness to mechanical disadvantage. *Americal Journal of Cardiology*, **32**, 889.

Rees, G., Bristow, J. D., Kremkau, E. L., Green, G. S., Herr, R. H., Griswold, H. E. & Starr, A. (1971) Influence of aortocoronary bypass surgery on left ventricular performance. *New England Journal of Medicine*, **284**, 116.

Rees, S. (1976) The Watershed. A factor in coronary vein graft occlusion. *British Heart Journal*, **38**, 197.

Rossiter, S. J., Hultgren, H. N., Kosek, J. C., Wuerflein, R. D. & Angell, W. W. (1974) Ischaemic myocardial injury with aortic valve replacement and coronary bypass. *Archives of Surgery*, **109**, 652.

Rutherford, B. D., Gav, G. T., Danielson, G. K., Pluth, J. R., Davis, G. D., Wallace, R. B. & Frye, R. L. (1972) Left ventricular haemodynamics before and soon after saphenous vein bypass graft operation for angina pectoris. *British Heart Journal*, **34**, 1156.

Sanders, R. J., Kern, W. H. & Blount, S. G. (1956) Perforation of the interventricular septum complicating myocardial infarction: report of eight cases, one with cardiac catheterisation. *American Heart Journal*, **51**, 736, 1956.

Sanders, R. J., Neubuerger, K. T. & Ravin, A. (1957) Rupture of papillary muscles: occurrence of rupture of the posterior muscle in posterior myocardial infarction. *Diseases of the Chest*, **31**, 316.

Sbokos, C., Monro, J. L. & Ross, J. K. (1976) The surgical management of left ventricular aneurysm. *Thorax*, **31**, 55.

Schlichter, J., Hellerstein, H. K. & Katz, L. N. (1954) Aneurysm of the heart: a correlative study of 102 proved cases. *Medicine (Baltimore)*, **33**, 43.

Shumacker, H. B. (1972) Suggestions concerning operative management of postinfarction septal defects. *Journal of Thoracic and Cardiovascular Surgery*, **64**, 452.

Sones, F. M. & Shirey, E. K. (1962) Cine coronary arteriography. *Modern Concepts in Cardiovascular Disease*, **31**, 735.

Sowton, G. E., Balcon, R., Cross, D. & Frick, M. H. (1967) Measurement of the angina threshold using atrial pacing. *Cardiovascular Research*, **1**, 301.

Spencer, F. C., Green, G. E., Tice, D. A., Wallsh, E., Mills, N. L. & Glassman, E. (1971) Coronary artery bypass grafts for congestive heart failure: a report of experiences with 40 patients. *Journal of Thoracic and Cardiovascular Surgery*, **62**, 529.

Spencer, F. C. (1972) Bypass grafting for preinfarction angina. *Circulation*, **45**, 1314.

Suzuki, A., Kay, E. B. & Hardy, J. D. (1973) Direct anastomosis of the bilateral internal mammary artery to the distal coronary artery, without a magnifier, for severe diffuse coronary atherosclerosis. *Circulation*, **48**, Suppl. III-190.

Talano, J. V., Scanlon, P. J., Meadows, W. R., Kahn, M., Pifarre, R. & Gunnar, R. M. (1975) Influence of surgery on survival in 145 patients with left main coronary artery disease. *Circulation*, **51-52**, suppl. 1, 1-105.

Tecklenberg, P. L., Alderman, E. L., Miller, D. C., Shumway, N. E. & Harrison, D. C. (1975) Changes in survival and symptom relief in a longitudinal study of patients after bypass surgery. *Circulation*, **51-52**, Suppl. 1, 1-98.

Ullyot, D. J., Wisneski, J., Sullivan, R. W., Gertz, E. W. & Roe, B. B. (1975) Improved survival after coronary artery surgery in patients with extensive coronary artery disease. *Journal of Thoracic and Cardiovascular Surgery*, **70**, 405.

Vineberg, A. M. (1946) Development of anastomosis between coronary vessels and transplanted internal mammary artery. *Canadian Medical Association Journal*, **55**, 117.

Vineberg, A. (1975) Evidence that revascularisation by ventricular-internal mammary artery implants increases longevity. *Journal of Thoracic and Cardiovascular Surgery*, **70**, 381.

Weller, D. A., Adolph, R. J., Wellman, H. N., Carroll, R. G. & Kim, O. (1972) Myocardial perfusion scintigraphy after intracoronary injection of 99-m Tc labeled human albumin microspheres. *Circulation*, **46**, 963.

Wisoff, B. G., Hartstein, M. L., Aintablian, A. & Hamby, R. I. (1975) Risk of coronary surgery: two hundred consecutive patients with no hospital deaths. *Journal of Thoracic and Cardiovascular Surgery*, **69**, 669.

Wood, P. (1961) Acute and subacute coronary insufficiency. *British Medical Journal*, **1**, 1779.

Yacoub, M. H. (1975) Management of postinfarction mitral regurgitation. In *The Current Status of Cardiac Surgery*, ed. Longmore p. 420. Lancaster, England: Medical and Technical Publishing Co. Ltd.

Yacoub, M. H., Fawzy, E., Anyanwu, H. & Towers, M. (1975) Combined gas endarterectomy and coronary artery bypass graft. *Circulation*, **51-52**, suppl. 1, 1-182.

FURTHER READING

The Current Status of Cardiac Surgery. Longmore (Ed) (1975) Lancaster, England: Medical and Technical Publishing Co. Ltd.

Pluth, J. R. & McGoon, D. C. (1974) Current status of heart valve replacement. *Modern Concepts of Cardiovascular Disease*, **43**, 65.

Rider, A. K., Copeland, J. G., Hunt, S. A., Mason, J., Specter, M. J., Winkle, R. A., Bieber, C. P., Billingham, M. E., Dong, E., Griepp, R. B., Schroeder, J. S., Stinson, E. B., Harrison, D. C. & Shumway, N. E. The Status of Cardiac Transplantation, 1975. *Circulation,* **52**, 531, 1975.
Copeland, J. G., Stinson, E. B., Griepp, R. B. & Shumway, N. E. (1975) Surgical treatment of chronic constrictive pericarditis using cardiopulmonary bypass. *Journal of Thoracic and Cardiovascular Surgery,* **69**, 236. (14 Refs.)

11
HYPERLIPIDAEMIA AND CARDIOVASCULAR DISEASE

Barry Lewis

During the past decade several controlled trials have provided suggestive evidence that reduction of plasma lipid concentrations may decrease the incidence of ischaemic heart disease; and it has become clear from many studies that lipid-lowering diets and drugs can induce regression of experimental atherosclerosis in primates.

Although this evidence is incomplete and not entirely consistent it has stimulated a major research interest in hyperlipidaemia and has encouraged clinicians to identify and treat hyperlipidaemic patients. This review is chiefly concerned with recent advances in our knowledge of the regulation of plasma lipid metabolism and its disorders. Among the highlights of the past few years' research have been an improved understanding of the intravascular metabolism of lipoproteins and of lipoprotein interconversions, of the apolipoproteins and their functional and structural roles in lipoprotein formation and metabolism, of the genetics of the hyperlipidaemias and their clinical classification, and of the pathogenesis of the common primary hyperlipidaemias.

THE PHYSIOLOGICAL BACKGROUND

Definitions of normality

No simple answer is available as to what concentrations of serum lipids justify treatment, i.e. what levels constitute the upper limits of normality. 'Norms' for several apparently healthy populations have been published, based on 10th and 90th percentiles (Lewis et al, 1974a; Fredrickson and Levy, 1972; Goldstein et al, 1973).[1] These define statistical cutoff points for particular populations. However there are wide geographical differences in the distributions of serum lipid levels. Not only are mean cholesterol and triglyceride levels lower in Japan, the Eastern Mediterranean countries and Central Africa than in North America, Northern Europe and Australia, but there is little overlap between the frequency distributions for serum cholesterol levels between, for example, Japan and the United States. There can therefore be no universally-applicable normal ranges (Keys, 1970; Keys and Fidanza, 1960). In most populations the sex difference in cholesterol levels is too small to justify separate normal ranges for men and women, but in London (Lewis et al, 1974a) and Stockholm (Carlson and Ericsson, 1975) quite wide sex differences have been reported in serum

---

[1] The distribution of triglyceride values shows marked positive skewing, and that of cholesterol is also somewhat skewed.

triglyceride concentration. Although serum lipid concentrations are low in cord blood, and in early childhood (Godfrey, Stenhouse, Cullen and Blackman, 1972), levels do not show a consistent trend in adults; in many 'developed' populations values continue to increase until the sixth or seventh decade, then declining, but this is not seen in other communities (Shaper and Jones, 1959; Antonis and Bersohn, 1960). There is no consensus as to whether age-adjusted normal ranges should be employed in adults. The adult ranges employed at St Thomas' Hospital, based on 10th and 90th percentiles of a carefully-screened London population (Lewis et al, 1974a), are shown in Table 11.1 (values are for the fasted state).

Table 11.1   Adult reference values of serum cholesterol and triglycerides

	mmol/l
Serum cholesterol	4.5 –6.5
Serum triglyceride (men)	0.70–2.1
Serum triglyceride (women)	0.60–1.5

Apart from age, sex and geographical differences, serum lipid values show seasonal variation (maxima in the winter) (Carlson and Lindstedt, 1969). They are also affected by stresses, e.g. recent major illness such as myocardial infarction. Energy balance affects serum lipid concentrations; triglyceride and to a lesser extent cholesterol levels show a weak positive correlation with increasing degrees of obesity, and usually decrease during weight reduction. To some extent these relationships may be explained by the greater turnover of plasma free fatty acids in obese subjects and by enhanced cholesterol synthesis in adipose tissue. However energy balance is probably of less significance than the effect of changes in consumption of specific nutrients. The serum cholesterol-elevating effect of dietary saturated fats is well known; and dietary cholesterol also tends to increase serum cholesterol levels though with wide individual variation. Polyunsaturated fats decrease serum levels of cholesterol and triglyceride. Very high intakes of all carbohydrates elevate serum triglyceride concentration; this response is usually evanescent. In susceptible individuals alcohol too has a pronounced effect in elevating triglyceride levels.

In addition there is considerable interlaboratory variation (Whitehead, Browning and Gregory, 1973), particularly when manual methods are employed. Prolonged venous occlusion prior to blood sampling increases cholesterol concentration because of haemoconcentration (Koerselman, Lewis and Pilkington, 1961).

In practice, the decision to prescribe lipid-lowering therapy is not based only on serum lipid levels. Other considerations should be the age of the patient, a family history of early-onset atherosclerotic diseases, and the presence of other risk factors such as hypertension. More generally, it must be taken into account that serum cholesterol and triglyceride concentrations confer a graded risk; threshold levels have not been shown to exist below which ischaemic heart disease risk becomes nil. In this sense it is not meaningful to attempt to define 'normal' and 'high' levels.

Although higher serum cholesterol levels, like higher blood pressure, confer a continuously-rising risk of ischaemic heart disease, the graph relating level to risk status is not a straight line. Risk appears to increase more steeply when serum cholesterol levels are in the region of 6.5 mmol/l or more (Stamler, Berkson and Lindberg, 1972).

Plasma Lipid Metabolism

Lipid transport through plasma depends on the packaging of these water-insoluble molecules with specific apoproteins into lipoproteins, which exist in colloidal solution in plasma. Lipoproteins are also present in intestinal lymph (Ockner, Hughes and Isselbacher, 1969) and the smaller lipoproteins are detectable in peripheral lymph too (Reichl et al, 1973).

Plasma lipoproteins are usually defined by ranges of physical properties: the four major classes are high-density lipoprotein (HDL, α-lipoprotein), low-density lipoprotein (LDL, β-lipoprotein) very-low density lipoprotein (VLDL, pre-β lipoprotein) and chylomicra. Each of these classes is polydisperse, comprising particles with a range of molecular diameters, hydrated densities, lipid and protein compositions. It is useful to distinguish two subclasses of LDL: these are a major component LDL$_2$, and a minor one, intermediate density lipoprotein (IDL or LDL$_1$), which is chemically and metabolically intermediate between VLDL and LDL$_2$.

High density lipoprotein (Scanu, 1969)

This is isolated in the ultracentrifuge in the density range 1.063–1.21 g/ml and is a relatively small particle containing on average 50 per cent lipid (Fig. 11.1). It

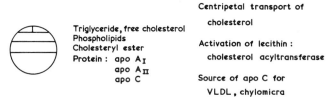

Figure 11.1   High density lipoprotein (α-lipoprotein)

is secreted in nascent form by the liver (Hamilton, 1972) and small intestine and contains free cholesterol and phospholipid, chiefly lecithin, as its major lipid components; nascent HDL is a flattened disc-shaped molecule. HDL proteins include two major components both with C-terminal glutamine, collectively known as apo A; minor components include the group of apoproteins known as apo C, and also apo B, the arginine-rich polypeptide (Alaupovic, 1972; Havel and Kane, 1973) and apo D. The apoproteins serve a partly structural role, and some are of functional importance in activating or inhibiting certain enzymes which play a major role in lipid transport.

The major functions of HDL appear to be a direct role in the centripetal transport of cholesterol from peripheral tissues to the liver (Glomset, 1968), and an indirect role in facilitating triglyceride transport.

Cholesterol is synthesised in most tissues, with the exception of the adult central nervous system. However the major organ for disposal of cholesterol from the body is the liver. Cholesterol which is synthesised in peripheral tissues such as skin, connective tissue and adipose tissue is utilised in formation of cell membranes, and becomes redundant in the course of cell replacement. Plasma HDL readily takes up free cholesterol in vitro (Bondjers and Björkerud, 1974). In HDL, this cholesterol is esterified by the circulating enzyme lecithin : cholesterol acyltransferase (LCAT), by transfer of an unsaturated fatty acid molecule from the 2-position of lecithin (also present in HDL). HDL thus acquires a high proportion of cholesteryl ester. The cholesteryl ester so produced is transported to the liver in HDL, or may be transferred to other lipoproteins in exchange for triglyceride (Gjone and Norum, 1974).

In familial HDL deficiency (Tangier disease), cholesterol accumulates in peripheral tissues, particularly the reticuloendothelial system (Fredrickson, Gotto and Levy, 1972). Familial LCAT deficiency is characterised by virtual absence of cholesteryl esters in plasma; there is often hypercholesterolaemia due to high free cholesterol levels, and hypertriglyceridaemia; and characteristic lesions due to lipid deposition affect particularly the kidney and eye (Gjone and Norum, 1974).

Centrifugal lipid transport
This is mediated by very low density lipoproteins, intermediate density lipoprotein and low density lipoprotein. VLDL, IDL and LDL$_2$ (Figs 11.2, 11.3)

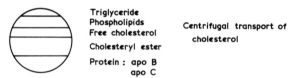

Triglyceride
Phospholipids
Free cholesterol

Cholesteryl ester

Protein : apo B
        apo C

Centrifugal transport of cholesterol

Figure 11.2   Low density lipoprotein (β-lipoprotein, LDL$_2$)

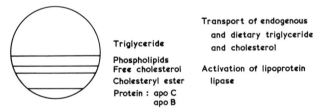

Triglyceride

Phospholipids
Free cholesterol
Cholesteryl ester
Protein : apo C
        apo B

Transport of endogenous and dietary triglyceride and cholesterol

Activation of lipoprotein lipase

Figure 11.3   Very low density lipoprotein (pre-β-lipoprotein)

bear a precursor product relationship, the conversion steps apparently occurring within the plasma compartment. VLDL is a heterogeneous class of large molecules, rich in triglyceride, containing also cholesterol, cholesteryl ester and phospholipid, with about 10 per cent of protein. VLDL is secreted by the liver and to a lesser extent by the small intestinal mucosa, in nascent form (Hamilton, 1972; Bennett et al, 1975). It rapidly converts to its 'mature' form after its secretion, acquiring apolipoprotein C by transfer from HDL; its cholesteryl ester content is probably similarly obtained from HDL (Gjone and Norum, 1974).

VLDL secreted by the liver contains triglyceride of endogenous origin; normally this triglyceride is derived entirely from esterification of free fatty acid (FFA) taken up from plasma by this organ (Havel, 1961; Boberg et al, 1972). Barter, Nestel and Carroll (1972) have shown that, under abnormal circumstances, FFA is partly replaced by other substrates, perhaps including dietary carbohydrate and hepatic triglyceride stores; this occurs in alcoholism, obesity and during the short-term consumption of a very high carbohydrate diet. But normally the hepatic uptake of FFA is the major determinant of endogenous triglyceride secretion, and is principally governed by the plasma FFA concentration, hence by the rate of adipose tissue lipolysis (Carlson, Boberg and Högstedt, 1965).

Most of the uptake of triglyceride from plasma occurs peripherally, particularly in skeletal muscle and adipose tissue. Rössner (1974) has attempted to estimate the proportion of triglyceride taken up by various organs in the fasted state: muscle, adipose tissue, myocardium and splanchnic viscera account for a major proportion of uptake.

Lipoprotein lipase

The enzyme lipoprotein lipase plays a major role in triglyceride uptake, and massive hypertriglyceridaemia develops in subjects in whom it is deficient, a rare genetic disorder (Havel and Gordon, 1960). The enzyme functions at the luminal surface of the capillary endothelium, hydrolysing triglyceride contained in VLDL and chylomicra. The fatty acids so produced largely diffuse into the parenchymal cells (and are oxidised or stored as triglyceride), while the glycerol remains in the plasma. There is evidence that the enzyme is synthesised in the parenchymal cells e.g. adipocytes (at a rate largely independent of functional requirements); and it is transported to its capillary endothelial site of action and simultaneously chemically modified, in response to the nutritional state (Cryer, Davies and Robinson, 1975; Garfinkel and Schotz, 1973). In the fed state, adipose tissue lipoprotein lipase activity increases, diverting circulating triglyceride to this organ for storage; in the fasted state, activity of the enzyme increases in muscle and decreases in adipose tissue.

Dietary fat is incorporated into triglyceride-rich lipoproteins by mucosal cells of the small intestine, and these reach plasma via the thoracic duct. The largest of these particles are chylomicra, defined as having a flotation rate (S_f value) exceeding 400 (Fig. 11.4). A varying proportion of the dietary fat is carried in VLDL of intestinal origin. This closely resembles hepatic VLDL in lipid composition and in content of the various apolipoproteins, but contains somewhat more arginine-rich polypeptide (Dungu, Nicoll and Lewis, in preparation).

Chylomicra are the largest lipoprotein particles, containing chiefly triglyceride and only 1–2 per cent of apoprotein. During the absorption of a large fat load, chylomicra are chiefly responsible for alimentary lipaemia, while the lipaemia following ingestion of 25–50 g fat is due in part to an increase in plasma levels of intestinal VLDL as well as chylomicra.

The metabolism of endogenous and exogenous triglyceride appears to involve a common removal mechanism (Havel, 1965; Brunzell et al, 1973). Whether all circulating triglyceride is initially hydrolysed by lipoprotein lipase is an unresolved and important issue; some recent evidence suggests that this enzyme may not be the obligatory mechanism (Nicoll et al, 1974).

Another lipase of hepatic origin has been described (Krauss, Levy and Fredrickson, 1974); it too can hydrolyse triglyceride present in lipoprotein. Chemically it is identical with extrahepatic lipoprotein lipase apart from its

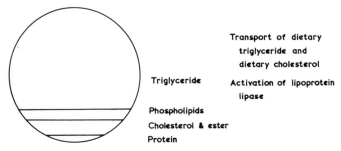

Triglyceride

Phospholipids
Cholesterol & ester
Protein

Transport of dietary
triglyceride and
dietary cholesterol

Activation of lipoprotein
lipase

Figure 11.4   Chylomicrons

carbohydrate moeity (Augustin, Freeze and Brown, 1975). If it has a physio-logical role, this may be the metabolism of the small quantity of triglyceride remaining in chylomicron and VLDL 'remnants' (Redgrave, 1970) after these particles have been exposed to extrahepatic lipoprotein lipase and have lost most of their triglyceride. No state of hepatic lipase deficiency has been described.

Lipoprotein conversion

A current view of the plasma lipoprotein metabolism may now be outlined (Fig. 11.5). VLDL and chylomicra entering plasma rapidly acquire a normal complement of apolipoprotein C by transfer from HDL. One of the C apoproteins, apo C_{II}, is the specific activator of extrahepatic lipoprotein lipase (Havel et al, 1970b; La Rosa et al, 1970) and renders the triglyceride contained in these particles subject to attack by this enzyme. Chylomicra and VLDL are depleted of triglyceride in stepwise fashion (Higgins and Fielding, 1975), partially-delipidated products returning to the circulation before further metabolism occurs. Therefore a series of delipidation products are present in the circulation, progressively decreasing in size and triglyceride content, and relatively enriched in cholesterol. Finally, chylomicron remnants (containing absorbed cholesterol) are produced and are avidly trapped by the liver (Redgrave, 1970). VLDL is converted to IDL, which after further remodelling by unknown mechanisms is converted to LDL_2. This LDL_2 or β-lipoprotein is derived from VLDL, and is not evidently secreted by the liver as such.

Sigurdsson, Nicoll and Lewis (1975) have examined quantitatively this lipoprotein conversion, using labelling of the apoprotein moiety. In normal and hyperlipidaemic subjects, all LDL appears to be derived from VLDL. Normally, at least 90 per cent of VLDL apolipoprotein B reappears in LDL, and this is also true of patients with hyper β-lipoproteinaemia; but in hypertriglyceridaemia, where VLDL production is often increased, about 50 per cent of VLDL is metabolised by a pathway other than conversion to LDL.

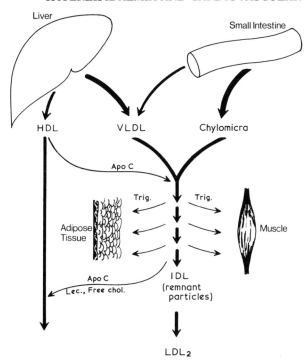

Figure 11.5 Lipoprotein secretion and transformation. Apo C, apolipoprotein C; Free chol, unesterified cholesterol; Lec, lecithin; IDL, intermediate density lipoprotein; Trig, triglyceride

LDL catabolism

The later fate of LDL has long been assumed to involve its uptake and metabolism by the liver. However studies by Sniderman et al (1974) on hepatectomised pigs has yielded the surprising conclusion that much LDL uptake from plasma must be extrahepatic. In 1973 Goldstein and Brown presented the first of a series of papers describing an LDL receptor on the surface of human cultured skin fibroblasts (Brown, Dana and Goldstein, 1973). Binding to this receptor appeared to be responsible for mediating most LDL uptake by this cell line, apart from some non-specific endocytosis. Smooth muscle cells and adipocytes appear to have similar LDL receptors. LDL uptake is followed by lysosomal degradation of apolipoproteins and hydrolysis of cholesteryl esters, and the free cholesterol represses the major rate-limiting enzyme in cholesterol biosynthesis. Thus the LDL receptor regulates LDL catabolism and also cholesterol synthesis in the fibroblast. While this concept is of fundamental importance, current work is suggesting that certain modifications may be necessary. The receptors appear heterogeneous, possibly including several classes with differing binding affinities (Carew, Koschinsky and Steinberg, 1975); and they are less specific than has been supposed, reacting under some circumstances with VLDL, and normal and abnormal HDL (Mahley et al, 1975). It appears that cell surface receptors may play a significant role in regulating LDL degradation and extrahepatic cholesterogenesis.

Hepatic cholesterol synthesis is a major source of this sterol, together with synthesis in the ileum. Absorbed cholesterol (of dietary and endogenous origin) is taken up initially by the liver, in the form of chylomicron remnants. There it exerts feedback regulation of cholesterol synthesis. The liver cholesterol is partly utilised in synthesis of VLDL and HDL; some is excreted as such in bile and a rather smaller proportion (Lewis and Myant, 1967) is converted to bile salts and secreted in the bile. The efficiency of cholesterol homeostasis shows wide species differences, and shows considerable interindividual variation in man (Quintao, Grundy and Ahrens, 1971). The response to high cholesterol intake in man includes repression of cholesterol synthesis and enhanced biliary excretion of cholesterol. Some individuals react to a high cholesterol intake with a negligible rise in plasma cholesterol levels and only modest increase in exchangeable pools of cholesterol, while others show a marked increase in tissue levels and, less often, in plasma cholesterol concentration. Highly efficient regulatory mechanisms have been found in one ethnic group, the Masai, who maintain low plasma lipid levels despite a high milk intake (Ho et al, 1971).

CLASSIFICATION AND DIAGNOSIS OF THE HYPERLIPIDAEMIC STATES

Classifications (Figure 11.6)

Hyperlipidaemia is the common feature of a number of widely disparate genetic and acquired disorders. Their orderly classification presents great difficulty at the present time, for their aetiology and pathogenesis are mostly

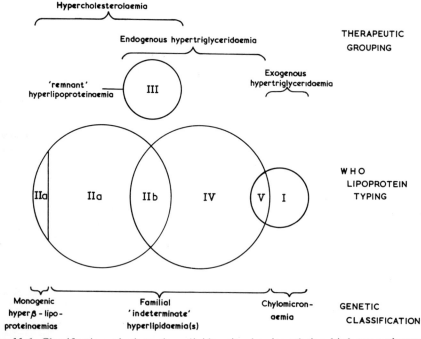

Figure 11.6 Classifications of primary hyperlipidaemias showing relationship between therapeutic groups, WHO lipoprotein types and genetic entities

unknown; only in the rarest disorders have the mechanisms largely been characterised as due to specific enzyme defects, e.g. lipoprotein lipase deficiency. Similarly, genetic classification has been hampered by lack of specific genetic markers.

Fredrickson/WHO classification

The most widely employed classification system for primary hyperlipidaemias is that of Fredrickson, Levy and Lees (1967), which has been slightly extended and modified (Beaumont et al, 1970; Fredrickson and Levy, 1972). This system takes as axiomatic the view that as plasma lipids are transported in complex macromolecules, the lipoproteins, and not in free form, raised lipid levels are the consequence of hyperlipoproteinaemia. Therefore these disorders are best classified (albeit temporarily in the absence of aetiological knowledge) on the basis of the pattern of abnormality of plasma lipoprotein concentrations. Careful analysis of a large series of patients referred for known hyperlipidaemia, and of a number of their affected relatives, suggested the existence of five, and later of six, different 'lipoprotein phenotypes'. In this referral population, the plasma lipoprotein pattern could be classified into six types, I, IIa, IIb, III, IV and V. These corresponded with distinguishable clinical syndromes, and individual-ised dietary and drug treatments have been proposed (Levy, 1972; Strisower, Adamson and Strisower, 1970). Electrophoresis of lipoproteins provides qualitative information on the lipoprotein pattern, and ultracentrifugation with precipitation methods make it possible to quantitate the major lipoprotein classes by measuring their lipid content.

This 6-type classification has not been clearly superseded by a more fundamental system, but it has certain shortcomings (Lewis, 1973; Havel, 1975). Frederickson (1975) has recently questioned the need for electrophoresis of lipoproteins in all cases. Of these shortcomings, the first stems from the fact that it is a classification of serum lipoprotein patterns, rather than of patients (i.e. of genetic defects, metabolic lesions, or clinical syndromes). For example it is clear that a given lipoprotein pattern, e.g. hyper β-lipoproteinaemia, can result from different genetic and metabolic bases (Carter, Slack and Myant, 1971; Goldstein et al, 1973), a primary distinction being into a common 'polygenic' variety and a rarer entity, itself heterogeneous, due to single dominant genes (the monogenic variety). This is probably also true of endogenous hypertriglyceridaemia due to the type IV pattern (Sigurdsson, Nicoll and Lewis, 1976a). On the other hand the hyperlipidaemic members of a particular family, who presumably share the same metabolic lesion, may have different lipoprotein patterns. This is evident from case studies, in which coexistence of type IV and V occur in a given family, or of types III and IV, or of types IIa and IIb, as reviewed by Lewis (1973).

Genetic classification

Further genetic data has come from two large studies of families in which the index patients presented with myocardial infarction (Goldstein et al, 1973; Nikkilä and Aro, 1973). This approach provides a less selected population for study than one obtained by referral of hyperlipidaemic patients to a specialised clinic, and yields five to six times more hyperlipidaemic families than would be expected from an open population survey. Nevertheless some degree of selection still persists. In both Helsinki and Seattle familial aggregation of hyper-lipidaemia proved common in the study population, but it was rare for any one lipoprotein pattern or 'type' to be consistently present in a particular family. The Seattle group has proposed a genetic classification distinguishing five entities on the basis of cholesterol and triglyceride concentrations and the pattern of familial distribution: they describe dominant and polygenic forms of hyper-cholesterolaemia, dominant and sporadic hypertriglyceridaemias, and a common disorder, familial combined hyperlipidaemia (Fig. 11.6). The last named was believed to show dominant inheritance and to manifest variably with elevated levels of cholesterol and triglyceride or of either lipid alone. Slack (1974) has provided reasons for suspecting that the design and execution of this study could have led to bias in favour of overestimating the frequency of dominant inheritance and underestimating polygenic forms of hyperlipidaemia, but this issue has not been resolved.

In Helsinki, Nikkilä and Aro (1973) also found that the commonest form of familial hyperlipidaemia was one in which the lipoprotein pattern was variable ('multiple type hyperlipidaemia'). Elevated levels of cholesterol, triglyceride, or of both lipids were present, the familial distribution being characteristic of polygenic inheritance in this study.

From these studies, and from clinical observation, there is good evidence that a considerable proportion of patients with primary hyperlipidaemia inherit an indeterminate form of lipid abnormality manifesting as an increase of one or other or both lipids. It appears to be of multifactorial aetiology, evidently resulting from multiple genetic determinants interacting with other factors of which diet may well be of major importance. But its genetic basis remains uncertain at present.

In neither of the major genetic studies was the rare disorder of exogenous hypertriglyceridaemia, due to inherited deficiency of lipiprotein lipase, present. Nor have clinical and metabolic studies of these genetically-defined disorders been reported, so that it is not yet possible to describe these entities in full, nor to discuss their therapy.

Therapeutic grouping

A third approach to classification of hyperlipidaemic states has been proposed by Tabaqchali, Chait and Lewis (1974). This is in essence a simplification of the Fredrickson-Levy classification, intended to minimise the number of entities requiring different optimal therapy, and to simplify the laboratory investigation of hyperlipidaemia. A review of the published literature on the management of hyperlipidaemia suggests that there is considerable overlap in the dietary and pharmacological treatments prescribed for types I-V hyperlipoproteinaemias. This implies that for purely therapeutic purposes some rationalisation of existing classifications may be possible. This is supported by the results of a therapeutic trial (Tabaqchali et al, 1974). At least Groups 1 and 2 in this therapeutic classification are clearly heterogeneous, and the approach is clearly a provisional one.

The data base for this classification is as follows:

(a) Clinical examination, with emphasis on the presence and type of xanthomas and on evidence of underlying diseases known to cause hyperlipidaemia.

(b) Two or more cholesterol and triglyceride measurements on serum obtained in the fasted and basal state.

(c) The stored serum test (Havel, 1969). Serum is stored at 4°C for 18 hours, then inspected for lactescence. If present, lactescence may be confined to the upper part of the sample; this indicates the presence of chylomicronaemia, due to exogenous hypertriglyceridaemia. Or opalescence may be diffusely distributed along the tube, an appearance characteristic of endogenous hypertriglyceridaemia. Entirely clear serum may be normal or hypercholesterolaemic, but rarely accompanies substantial hypertriglyceridaemia.

(d) Lipid measurements in accessible first-degree relatives.

(e) Laboratory screening for common causes of secondary hyperlipidaemia, e.g. TSH levels, liver function tests.

As discussed above, electrophoresis of serum lipoproteins is not routinely necessary if the above investigations are performed. It is, however, helpful in distinguishing between hyper β-lipoproteinaemia and hyper α-lipoproteinaemia as causes of mild hypercholesterolaemia, and sometimes in making a presumptive diagnosis of Type III hyperlipoproteinaemia. Nephelometric assessment of triglyceride levels and the use of ultrafiltration to distinguish 'large' and 'medium' sized lipoprotein particles does not add further information to the investigations (a) to (c) above.

Therapeutic Classification

I. Primary

1. Hyper β-lipoproteinaemia. Cholesterol levels are increased, triglyceride levels normal, and serum is clear on inspection (corresponds to type IIa in Fredrickson/Beaumont classification).

2. Endogenous hypertriglyceridaemia, with or without associated hypercholesterolaemia. Stored serum is diffusely lactescent except in the mildest cases (Corresponds to types IIb, III, IV and V).

3. Exogenous hypertriglyceridaemia. There is usually gross hypertriglyceridaemia with relatively slight hypercholesterolaemia. After storage, the turbidity of the serum floats to the upper part of the sample, leaving the subnatant clear or virtually clear. (Corresponds to type I). This type is rare, and most cases present in childhood.

II. Secondary (see p. 264).

PRIMARY HYPERLIPOPROTEINAEMIAS

Primary hyper β-lipoproteinaemia

The prevalence of this disorder depends on the definition chosen. If the upper limit of serum cholesterol concentration is set at 250 mg/100 ml (6.5 mmol/l) then about 10 per cent of men and women living in London are affected (Lewis et al, 1974a). The majority of such patients show relatively weak heritability, the frequency distribution of cholesterol levels in such families being unimodal and shifted to the right; in them polygenic inheritance is postulated, and environmental variables are presumed to interact with these genetic factors. The mechanism or mechanisms of this common form of hyperlipidaemia is unknown.

The gene frequency of the monogenic form of hyper β-lipoproteinaemia has been estimated as 0.2 to 0.5 per cent (Carter et al, 1971; Goldstein et al, 1973). Increased β-lipoprotein levels are present at birth (Kwiterovich, Levy and Fredrickson, 1973), though total serum cholesterol concentration may be normal due to a reciprocal decrease in α-lipoprotein levels.

CLINICAL FEATURES

In this group of disorders, an early onset of ischaemic heart disease and other atherosclerotic disorders is the commonest clinical feature. Among male patients with the monogenic form, overt ischaemic heart disease is present in some 50 per cent by age 50 (Slack, 1969), and a mean life expectation of 21 years has been reported for the rare patients who, most often because of consanguinity are homozygous for the disorder. It is a clinical impression that the vascular risk is not as great in 'polygenic' hyper β-lipoproteinaemia, perhaps because the hypercholesterolaemia is on average less pronounced and because the disorder may not be manifest from birth; the intensity and duration of exposure of the arteries to high β-lipoprotein levels may therefore be less. While the risk to the individual with the polygenic form of hypercholesterolaemia may be less than that due to the monogenic form, the impact of polygenic hypercholesterolaemia on the community is far greater; it is at least 20 times commoner than the monogenic disorder.

Tendon xanthomas are characteristic of hypercholesterolaemia due to a single dominant gene. The homozygous patient and the severely affected heterozygote may develop skin lesions — planar xanthomas on the knees, elbows and buttocks. Corneal arcus and xanthelasmas occurring before age 30 may lead to recognition of either form of hypercholesterolaemia. Aortic or supra-aortic stenosis, and episodes of polyarthritis simulating acute rheumatic fever, occur in homozygotes and also in heterozygotes with cholesterol levels of 12–15 mmol/l.

LABORATORY DIAGNOSIS

This is based on the presence of hypercholesterolaemia with normal triglyceride concentrations. If pronounced, or if accompanied by tendon xanthomas, this is reasonably diagnostic. But occasional patients have mild hypercholesterolaemia due to raised α-lipoprotein levels (Avogaro and Cazzolato, 1975). This is not known to be associated with any untoward consequences and is conceivably protective against ischaemic heart disease (Miller and Miller, 1975). It may be familial. To confirm the presence of hyper β-lipoproteinaemia it is preferable to measure LDL-cholesterol levels quantitatively if methods are available, or to use the qualitative procedure of lipoprotein electrophoresis.

PATHOGENESIS
This has been the elusive goal of active research during the past decade, with many contradictory or negative findings; but kinetic studies using labelled LDL and in vitro studies of lipoprotein and cholesterol metabolism by cultured fibroblasts and other cells have lately shed new light on this disorder. A possible reason for the inconsistencies in published work has been that monogenic hypercholesterolaemia is itself a heterogeneous group of disorders. There is growing support for this possibility.

Cholesterol absorption is normal (Connor and Liu, 1974), and in vivo evidence of overproduction of cholesterol is lacking (Lewis and Myant, 1967; Samuel et al, 1972). Extensive sterol balance studies and measurements of bile acid turnover have been performed to assess the role of impaired catabolism and/or excretion of cholesterol. Subnormal bile acid excretion has been reported (Miettinen and Aro, 1972) and low turnover of cholic acid has been observed. However the sum of the turnovers of the two primary bile acids, cholic acid and chenodeoxycholic acid is only slightly, and not significantly, below normal (Einarsson, Hellström and Kallner, 1974).

The re-injection of autologous LDL after labelling with radioiodine has been employed by Gitlin et al (1958) and more recently by Langer, Strober and Levy (1972) and others in investigating patients with hyper β-lipoproteinaemia. At least 90 per cent of the radiolabelling is on the apolipoprotein B, the major peptide of LDL, which has a half-life of about three days. The disappearance curve can usually be resolved into a fast and a slow exponential, which represent mixing with an extravascular compartment and catabolism, respectively. By use of the Mathews formula, and by calculations of the ratio of urinary to plasma radioactivity, kinetic data have been obtained. Most studies have been of monogenic hyper β-lipoproteinaemia but the genetic basis has not always been clearly defined.

The steady-state synthetic rate of LDL was reported to be normal by Langer, Strober and Levy (1972), while the fractional catabolic rate (FCR) was abnormally slow. The slow FCR could be explained either by a true catabolic defect, or merely because the label was injected into an abnormally-large pool. However reduction of the LDL pool by nicotinic acid, as was studied by Levy and his colleagues (Langer and Levy, 1970) or by plasma exchange (Thompson and Myant, 1975) does not alter the FCR of LDL, suggesting that the FCR of LDL is not dependent upon its pool size. If so, the first explanation is the true one, i.e. that LDL catabolism is impaired in monogenic hyper β-lipoproteinaemia. However, an influence of pool size on FCR cannot fully be excluded until measurements of FCR have been made during acute expansion of the LDL pool; this would determine whether the removal mechanism is saturable when LDL levels are elevated to values pertaining in hyper β-lipoproteinaemia. In the Langer and Levy study, LDL synthetic rates were somewhat higher than in other series. Scott and Hurley (1969) measured LDL turnover and reported increased synthetic rates in a group of hyper β-lipoproteinaemic subjects; these patients were not genetically defined and included some in whom the hypercholesterolaemia was accompanied by hypertriglyceridaemia. Some patients with combined hyperlipidaemia due to raised levels of LDL and VLDL (type IIb) have increased turnover of LDL (Sigurdsson, 1975; Janus et al, 1976). Possibly, therefore, Scott and Hurley's patients were metabolically heterogeneous.

Simons et al (1975) have studied four patients homozygous for familial hyper β-lipoproteinaemia, arguing, as did Lewis and Myant (1967) that such patients should show the metabolic defect in exaggerated form. They reported a pronounced increase in LDL synthetic rate as well as subnormal catabolic rate, suggesting that increased production as well as subnormal removal contributed to the very high LDL concentrations. It is possible, particularly in view of the in vitro data described below, that overproduction of LDL is present in homozygous but not heterozygous patients because of a more complete failure of homeostatic mechanisms in the former.

Perhaps the most remarkable breakthrough in the study of monogenic hyper β-lipoproteinaemia has been the indirect evidence of Goldstein and Brown (1973) suggesting that cultured skin fibroblasts from such patients lack a normal complement of LDL receptors. Their initial finding was that cells from homozygous patients had no receptors, while those from heterozygotes had about one-half the normal number of cell surface receptors. Later (Goldstein et al, 1975) they reported that cells from other homozygotes had grossly subnormal receptor function, perhaps due to low binding affinity of the receptors. These separately-inherited defects were termed receptor-negative and receptor-defective.

Defective or absent receptor function results in impaired uptake ('internalisation') of LDL; Brown and Goldstein have defined two major consequences of this. Firstly LDL degradation by lysosomal enzymes is decreased. Secondly, derepression of cholesterol biosynthesis occurs, i.e. the normal repression, by cholesterol derived from LDL, of the rate-limiting enzyme of cholesterol synthesis (hydroxymethylglutaryl coenzyme A reductase) is lost; synthesis of cholesterol therefore increases.

As a result of impaired LDL catabolism and enhanced cholesterogenesis, LDL levels rise. In heterozygotes, it is conceived that ultimately a steady state is achieved when the concentration of LDL in extracellular fluid has approximately doubled: the high concentration gradient of LDL across the cell membrane compensates for the deficient number or affinity of receptors and leads to normal LDL uptake and degradation and normal cholesterol synthesis. In homozygotes, it may be that a steady state is not fully attained.

It has been questioned whether the fibroblast LDL receptor defect is in itself important in lipoprotein metabolism or whether it is merely an example of defect involving several cell lines. As mentioned above, the existence of receptors has been postulated in other tissues; together with the evidence that LDL catabolism is largely extrahepatic, it seems plausible that LDL catabolism could be accounted for by connective tissue, possibly together with smooth muscle and adipose tissue.

The concepts outlined above are likely to require modification and extension in the light of ongoing research. Studies on leucocytes from heterozygous patients (Fogelman et al, 1975) suggest that in this cell line at least the defect may not be of LDL internalisation but, instead, a failure to retain LDL within the cell; this would account for enhanced cholesterol synthesis, though not necessarily for impaired catabolism of LDL. Recently a family has been described in whom leucocytes had apparently normal receptor function, but the circulating LDL was abnormal in that it was not recognised by the postulated receptors (Higgins, Lecamwasan and Galton, 1975).

The indirect evidence for a defect in cell surface LDL receptors should be interpreted with some caution at the present time. Physiologically, it appears that LDL is not unique in its ability to repress cholesterol synthesis in isolated cells; both VLDL and HDL share this property to some extent, so that the 'receptor' is clearly not entirely specific. Recent studies of fibroblasts from a homozygous patient with familiar hyper β-lipoproteinaemia offer an alternative concept of the underlying defect (Stein et al, 1976). Using methods which permitted separate assessment of cell surface binding and of internalisation of LDL, these investigators concluded that a major defect existed in the process of transferring the lipoprotein from the medium to the cell interior; surface binding was less consistently abnormal.

In general, the concept seems firmly based that a group of dominantly-inherited disorders of LDL uptake by peripheral cells can lead to impaired LDL catabolism and, at least transiently, to increased cholesterol synthesis. However it is not clear how overproduction of cholesterol could lead to increased LDL synthesis without antecedent increase in VLDL production.

The Endogenous Hypertriglyceridaemias and Combined Hyperlipidaemia

Patients falling within this group are clearly heterogeneous, but the great majority appears to be treatable along similar lines. This group appears remarkably common, and overlaps with patients showing the types IIb, III, IV and V hyperlipoproteinaemias as defined by Beaumont et al (1970), and with 'multiple-type hyperlipoproteinaemia' (Nikkilä and Aro, 1973) and with 'familial combined hyperlipidaemia' (Goldstein et al, 1973).

From case-control studies with this group it appears that this is amongst the commonest group of metabolic disorders in patients surviving myocardial infarction. Nevertheless there is considerable controversy, discussed below, concerning the status of hypertriglyceridaemia as a risk factor for ischaemic heart disease.

CLINICAL FEATURES

In this group, obesity is common but by no means invariable. A considerable proportion of patients are glucose-intolerant and hyperinsulinaemic (Reaven et al, 1967; Bierman, 1972). These too are not universal features, and Glueck, Levy and Fredrickson (1969) found glucose intolerance in 52 per cent of patients with endogenous hypertriglyceridaemia due to raised VLDL concentrations (type IV); it was present in 39 per cent of those with the much rarer disorder type III hyperlipoproteinaemia and in 77 per cent of those with the type V pattern. Mild to moderate hyperuricaemia is another frequent association though in many patients the coexistence of hyperuricaemia with endogenous hypertri-glyceridaemia is partly or entirely due to a high alcohol intake.

Endogenous hypertriglyceridaemia was first described in patients in whom dietary carbohydrate appeared to play a role in the pathogenesis (Ahrens et al, 1961). On a low carbohydrate diet made isocaloric by substitution of fat, the hypertriglyceridaemia was much ameliorated though not abolished, and reversion to a higher carbohydrate intake led to a relapse of the hyperlipidaemia. On the other hand few patients show full correction of hypertriglyceridaemia purely in response to carbohydrate restriction (Schonfeld and Kudzma, 1973). Glueck et al (1969) have shown that induction of an abnormal degree of hypertriglyceridaemia in response to a very high carbohydrate diet fed for 10 days, occurs in 50 per cent of patients with elevated VLDL levels. A subgroup of patients with endogenous hypertriglyceridaemia may yet be identified in whom abnormal sensitivity to dietary carbohydrate leads to chronic hypertriglyceridaemia; there is at present no evidence that this is a common entity.

The interface between diabetes mellitus (hypertriglyceridaemia occurs in some 45 per cent of untreated diabetics (Lewis et al, 1972b)) using 90th percentiles for a London population, and primary endogenous hypertriglyceridaemia with glucose intolerance, is unclear. But a recent study by Brunzell et al (1975) has indicated that in patients with familial hypertriglyceridaemia who are also diabetic, the two metabolic disorders are separately inherited.

Other clinical manifestations of the endogenous hypertriglyceridaemia group are confined to patients with pronounced elevation of lipid levels (usually triglyceride concentration exceeds 25 mmol/l). One is the appearance of eruptive xanthomas, sometimes quite acutely, rounded yellow or orange papules often with an erythematous halo. Another is lipaemia retinalis. Perhaps the most frequent, and most significant clinically, are episodes of severe abdominal pain with many local and systemic features suggesting an acute surgical emergency. Laparotomies have inadvertently been performed for such patients, which sometimes reveal no demonstrable lesion. Other patients with severe hypertriglyceridaemia develop abdominal pain which is clearly due to acute pancreatitis. The mechanism of this complication is obscure. Gallstones appear to occur more commonly in patients with endogenous hypertriglyceridaemia (type IV hyperlipoproteinaemia) than in control subjects.

PATHOGENESIS

The mechanism of endogenous hypertriglyceridaemia is still, after some years of research, a matter of controversy. The problem is compounded by the evident heterogeneity of this group of disorders. Unfortunately, methods for investigating the kinetics of endogenous plasma triglyceride are complex, dependent on multiple assumptions, and prone to interpretive difficulties. The first major investigation employed injections of labelled glycerol, which became incorporated into triglyceride. The exponential phase of the decline in triglyceride specific activity was then followed. By this procedure, most patients with endogenous hypertriglyceridaemia show high synthetic rates of VLDL triglyceride, i.e. overproduction appears to be the major mechanism (Olefsky, Reaven and Farquhar, 1974). Similar conclusions have been reached using other methods. The method depends critically on the assumption that input of label into the plasma triglyceride pool is rapid in relation to the rate of clearance of triglyceride from plasma, an assumption which is open to question. The exponential phase of the triglyceride radioactivity curve is followed by a curvilinear phase, and suggests that more than one precursor pool, of differing turnover rates, exists (Grundy et al, 1975). The validity of this procedure is therefore open to question. Other precursor-labelling techniques have suggested that impaired removal of VLDL-triglyceride from plasma is the major mechanism.

Another methodological approach is to catheterise the hepatic vein, and to compare arterial and hepatic-venous triglyceride radioactivity during a constant infusion of labelled fatty acid as precursor (Havel et al, 1970a; Boberg et al, 1972). From the arterio-venous difference and the hepatic blood flow, the splanchnic secretion rate of triglyceride may be calculated; and a variant of the procedure dispenses with radioactivity measurements and their attendant assumptions and is based purely on the arterio-venous concentration difference (Boberg et al, 1972). In essence, these studies have shown a tendency to higher secretion rates in patients with hypertriglyceridaemia but, because of the lack of correlation between serum lipid levels and secretion rates the authors have concluded that differences in input of triglyceride into plasma are unlikely to be the basis of endogenous primary hypertriglyceridaemia. By exclusion, they have attributed this disorder to defective removal of triglyceride from plasma; the mechanism of this removal defect has not been elucidated. In a recent review of the mechanisms of certain disorders of plasma triglyceride metabolism Rössner (1974) has indicated that the experimental error in arterio-venous difference methods is not inconsiderable. The arterio-venous differences measured are remarkably small, and performance of these procedures is a technical tour-de-force of some magnitude.

VLDL TURNOVER

Assessment of VLDL turnover by studying the kinetics of its major apoproteins is substantially more difficult than the measurement of LDL turnover. This is partly because of the multiplicity of apolipoproteins in VLDL, and partly because of diurnal variation in plasma VLDL concentration in normally-fed individuals due to the varying input of intestinal VLDL. After injection of radioiodinated VLDL, therefore, it is necessary to isolate apolipoprotein B from a series of samples of VLDL for specific activity measurement. Apo B is the most appropriate apoprotein because unlike apo C it does not recycle into VLDL; and because the apo B content of a VLDL particle remains constant during its progressive delipidation (Eisenberg et al, 1972), rendering it a suitable marker for metabolism of the molecule as a whole. To maintain constancy of plasma VLDL concentration for the 24 hours of the study, the patient is given a fat free diet, providing about 70 per cent of the normal calorie intake; carbohydrate induction of hypertriglyceridaemia does not occur, at least within the period of observation.

Nicoll, Sigurdsson and Lewis (1975), and Sigurdsson et al (1976a) have developed this procedure for the study of VLDL metabolism in primary and secondary endogenous hypertriglyceridaemic states. The mean synthetic rate of VLDL-apo B is substantially increased in each of these groups compared to normolipidaemic control subjects, and, in the combined material there are positive and highly significant correlations between the synthetic rate and the plasma concentrations of VLDL-apo B and of VLDL-triglyceride. These findings indicate that overproduction of VLDL plays a role in the mechanism of primary endogenous hypertriglyceridaemia, and also in hypertriglyceridaemia due to uncontrolled diabetes and alcoholism. However a minority of patients have VLDL-apo B synthetic rates within the normal range, and in these it is clear that a removal defect without overproduction is the mechanism. An interesting feature of many patients with endogenous hypertriglyceridaemia especially of severe degree, is the low plasma LDL levels. These appear to be due to increased LDL catabolism (Sigurdsson, Nicoll and Lewis 1976b). It therefore appears that patients with primary endogenous hypertriglyceridaemia are metabolically heterogeneous; in some, overproduction of VLDL appears to be responsible alone or together with an accompanying removal defect, while others have hypertriglyceridaemia because of impaired removal. In a disorder so heterogeneous in other respects, this conclusion is not surprising.

Type III hyperlipoproteinaemia

One subgroup of patients, described by Fredrickson et al (1967) as having type III hyperlipoproteinaemia, is almost certainly a discrete entity although recent revisions in its definition have been put forward (see Havel, 1975). These patients commonly have tuberous xanthomas on elbows and knees; and linear xanthomas, seen in the palmar creases, occur most commonly in this form of hyperlipoproteinaemia (though they are not entirely specific). This is endogenous hypertriglyceridaemia and hypercholesterolaemia. Serum is lipaemic. In most patients, lipoprotein electrophoresis reveals a single broad band occupying the β and pre-β region, often with a chylomicron band at the origin. The broad β lipoprotein floats in the VLDL density range; the presence of β-VLDL is most often due to this disorder. A slightly wider definition is based on the abnormal composition of the VLDL density class, in which the cholesterol/triglyceride ratio is elevated. They suggest that the presence of a ratio of VLDL-cholesterol to total serum triglyceride exceeding 0.3 is the preferred criterion for diagnosis; normally it is less than 0.25.

The β-VLDL disorder appears to be dominantly inherited (Morganroth, Levy and Fredrickson, 1975), these recent studies having resolved a previously-controversial issue. Several families have been described in which this disorder, and also endogenous hypertriglyceridaemia due to raised levels of normal VLDL, both occur.

The seemingly-abnormal β-VLDL is likely to be an accumulation of an intermediate lipoprotein class in the conversion of VLDL to LDL, including IDL and the denser end of the VLDL spectrum of molecules. It has a high content of arginine-rich polypeptide, an apoprotein which tends to be associated with cholesteryl esters (Shore, Shore and Hart, 1974; Havel and Kane, 1973). At present there are two views of the mechanism for the accumulation of this intermediate. One based on kinetic studies is that there is marked overproduction of VLDL, leading to saturation of its normal catabolic pathway and to overflow into a secondary delipidation route (Hall et al, 1974). The other suggests that a catabolic defect is responsible; the initial delipidation of VLDL and chylomicra proceeds normally but IDL and chylomicron remnants accumulate in plasma owing to defective hepatic uptake (Gagne, Kushwaha, Albers, Brunzell and Hazzard, 1975).

Occasional patients are seen in whom combined hyperlipidaemia is present, accompanied by tendon xanthomas. There is predominant hypercholesterol-aemia, and on investigating the relatives evidence of dominantly-inherited familial hypercholesterolaemia is obtained (Kwiterovich et al, 1974). Such patients mainly require treatment for the monogenic hypercholesterolaemia. The raised triglyceride levels are often associated with a reversible condition such as obesity, diabetes or alcoholic abuse (Simons et al, 1972).

In patients with very pronounced hypertriglyceridaemia, raised VLDL levels may be accompanied by chylomicronaemia. In such patients it may be presumed that the common mechanism for clearance of triglyceride from plasma is saturated as a result of severe endogenous hypertriglyceridaemia, leading to impairment of chylomicron clearance. This lipoprotein pattern was described by Fredrickson et al (1967) as type V.

Chylomicronaemia, Exogenous Hypertriglyceridaemia

In contrast with groups 1 and 2 this is a rare condition, mostly occurring in infancy or childhood. It presents with acute abdominal pain, or with eruptive xanthomas. The liver and spleen are commonly enlarged. There is gross hypertriglyceridaemia and relatively slight hypercholesterolaemia, due almost entirely to accumulation of chylomicra in plasma. The chylomicronaemia is most easily demonstrated by the stored serum test; the uniquely low density and large diameter of these particles result in their floating towards the meniscus, leaving a clear subnatant.

That the hyperlipidaemia is due to dietary fat-containing particles is demonstrated by providing a low-fat isocaloric diet for five to seven days. With a fat intake of less than 5 g per 24 hours an almost-complete remission occurs within this time. The disorder is due to deficiency or absence of the extrahepatic form of lipoprotein lipase (Krauss et al, 1974). This leads to retention in plasma of chylomicra. It is curious that VLDL levels are normal or at most slightly raised, for VLDL triglyceride too is initially metabolised by lipoprotein lipase. It is possible that normal VLDL concentrations are the result of a very low secretion rate for this lipoprotein class, particularly in children. There is suggestive evidence that the usual age-related rise in serum triglyceride levels is due to changing secretion rate rather than clearance, for the fractional turnover rate of injected triglyceride does not fall significantly during adult life (Lewis et al, 1972a). It is also possible that VLDL, unlike chylomicra, can be metabolised by a lipoprotein lipase-independent pathway (Nicoll, Sigurdsson and Lewis, 1975).

One of the features of patients with lipoprotein lipase deficiency is their low plasma LDL concentrations; total serum cholesterol is usually high in the untreated case, but when chylomicronaemia abates, strikingly low cholesterol levels are often observed.

SECONDARY HYPERLIPIDAEMIAS

Depending upon the pattern of referral, a known underlying cause for hyperlipidaemia may be detected in some 10-20 per cent of patients at a lipid clinic. The most frequent of these are alcoholic abuse, hypothyroidism, diabetes, chronic renal failure, nephrotic syndrome, gout, cholestasis, and exogenous oestrogen administration (e.g. high-oestrogen oral contraceptives). Hyperlipidaemia also occurs in monoclonal and polyclonal hypergammaglobulinaemia, acute porphyria, idiopathic hypercalcaemia, certain forms of glycogen storage disease and in primary carcinoma of the liver. Some of these lead to predominant hypercholesterolaemia and others to predominant hypertriglyceridaemia but in practice the patterns of lipid and lipoprotein abnormality have not been shown to be characteristic of particular secondary hyperlipidaemias except in the instance of obstructive jaundice. Here the elevated levels of free cholesterol and phospholipid are due to the appearance in plasma of an aberrant low-density lipoprotein rich in these lipids, and having apolipoprotein C and albumin as its proteins (Seidel, Alaupovic and Furman, 1969). The molecule is a large, flattened disc, differing from the spherical shape of the normal circulating lipoproteins because it lacks the apolar lipids (cholesteryl esters and triglyceride) which normally constitute the 'core' of the lipoproteins of plasma.

In the great majority of the disorders listed above, secondary hyperlipidaemia is not a consistent feature; some 10–60 per cent of patients with these disorders have elevated lipid levels. It is apparent that hyperlipidaemia occurs as a result of the interaction between the underlying disease on the one hand and other factors which may include nutritional patterns and obesity, additional latent or overt diseases and genetic determinants. For example, it appears that only a minority of alcoholics develop hyperlipidaemia. In those who do, withdrawal of alcohol leads to a characteristically rapid fall in serum triglyceride levels. However lipid levels become entirely normal in only a minority of patients; and often the sometimes-massive lipaemia abates, leaving a persistent mild hypertriglyceridaemia which is regarded as primary (Chait et al, 1972). Most often, therefore, alcohol aggravates a primary abnormality in lipid metabolism. Kudzma and Schonfeld (1971) have recently suggested that this is a rather specific feature of a subgroup of primary endogenous hypertriglyceridaemia. Rather commonly, overt or latent diabetes is also demonstrable in patients with alcoholic lipaemia (Chait et al, 1972).

Abnormal lipoproteins

The composition as well as the concentration of plasma lipoproteins may be altered in secondary hyperlipidaemic states. In hypothyroidism, the commonest patterns are combined hyperlipidaemia and 'pure' hypercholesterolaemia. Rössner (1974) has found that the hypertriglyceridaemia is often due to a high triglyceride content in the LDL density class. The apolipoprotein pattern in hypothyroidism is also of interest in that the concentrations of arginine-rich polypeptide are increased in all lipoprotein classes (Clifford et al, 1975). In pregnancy lipaemia too, there are compositional changes in plasma lipoproteins, with an increase in the triglyceride content of all three density classes (Hillman et al, 1975).

MANAGEMENT OF HYPERLIPIDAEMIAS

The goal in treating hyperlipidaemia is to avert or delay its complications. This is certainly attainable in respect of certain consequences of elevated lipid levels such as acute pancreatitis, and some forms of xanthoma shrink or disappear. The evidence that ischaemic heart disease incidence can be reduced is incomplete but strongly suggestive (Stamler et al, 1972).

The indications for reducing elevated serum lipid concentrations have not been clearly defined. While most would agree that hyperlipidaemia in children and young adults should be corrected, some authorities would not recommend vigorous intervention in the elderly, in whom hyperlipidaemia is less conspicuous as a risk factor. The presence of overt ischaemic heart disease is not a contra-indication; Leren (1966) and others have shown hyperlipidaemia to remain a risk factor for recurrent myocardial infarction, and have reported some reduction in relapse rate when lipid-lowering diets are prescribed.

Where possible, secondary hyperlipidaemia is dealt with by treating the underlying cause. This is entirely effective in some conditions, e.g. hypothyroidism and, most often, in diabetes, but depend on the nature of the primary disorder. The hypertriglyceridaemia of gout does not respond to correction of elevated urate levels by allopurinol or probenecid.

The various categories of primary hyperlipidaemia require different, though overlapping, treatment. Most currently-available therapeutic agents are somewhat non-specific in their effects. As discussed above, three therapeutic groups may be distinguished on present knowledge. There have been few recent advances in this field, and the reader is referred to the symposium edited by Levy (1972) and the monograph by Lewis (1976) for a more detailed account of the subject.

Group 1, hyper β-lipoproteinaemia

In the 'polygenic' or multifactorial form, dietary management is most often effective. Obesity should be corrected as far as possible, and a fat-modified diet is then prescribed. This comprises 35 to 38 per cent fat, in which the ratio of polyunsaturated fatty acids to saturated fatty acids is increased to 1.5–2; cholesterol intake is reduced to less than 300 mg/day. Occasional patients require drug therapy, and clofibrate or small doses of cholestyramine are usually effective.

Patients with monogenic hyper β-lipoproteinaemia are less readily controlled. In addition to a fat modified diet, cholestyramine 16–28 g/day is the drug of choice, and clofibrate 1 g twice daily may be required as additional therapy. Neomycin, D-thyroxine and β-sitosterol have an occasional place in the treatment of this group. An effective but sometimes troublesome combination is cholestyramine with nicotinic acid, the latter in gradually-increasing dosage up to 4–6 g/day. For the rare homozygous patient with extreme hypercholesterolaemia, this drug combination together with diet is often helpful; if this fails, ileal bypass may be effective. The establishment of a portacaval shunt has been dramatically effective, and plasma exchange at intervals of two to three weeks also steeply reduces β-lipoprotein levels; these are best regarded as experimental procedures at present.

Group 2, endogenous hypertriglyceridaemia
   In this heterogeneous group of hypertriglyceridaemias dietary management is emphasised. Most, though by no means all, patients in this category are obese and hyperlipidaemia often shows an indefinite remission or improvement if weight reduction to ideal body weight is attainable. Frequently, long-term treatment by a fat-modified diet produces further reduction in lipid levels. An alternative treatment is by carbohydrate restriction. Medication is best reserved for patients who clearly fail to respons to dietary management. Clofibrate and nicotinic acid are both effective.

Group 3, exogenous hypertriglyceridaemia
   In this rare disorder, impaired clearance of circulating triglyceride is present; on a low fat intake, serum triglyceride levels fall, usually to less than 5 mmol/l but seldom to fully normal levels. However this degree of reduction suffices to cause resolution of xanthomas, and attacks of abdominal pain cease. Initially, fat intake is reduced to 10 per cent of energy intake, and increased to about 15 per cent; in infants and some adults, up to 20 to 25 per cent may be tolerated.

SERUM LIPID ABNORMALITIES AND ATHEROSCLEROSIS

   A wealth of evidence from epidemiology, clinical and experimental studies has established the association between hyperlipidaemia and ischaemic heart disease. In this section I shall discuss the extent to which this body of data indicates a causal role for hyperlipidaemia. There is no doubt that the aetiology of ischaemic heart disease is multifactorial and that hypertension and cigarette smoking play major roles; diabetes also confers vascular risk, partly explained by its association with hypertension and hyperlipidaemia. Obesity has a modest effect in increasing risk, but this appears to be explained entirely on the basis of its strong associations with hypertension, hyperlipidaemia, and diabetes; when these factors, and age and smoking status were taken into account, obesity had no residual risk-factor status in the 7-country study of Keys et al (1972).

Retrospective studies
   The contribution of hyperlipidaemia to the pathogenesis of ischaemic heart disease must be assessed in the knowledge of the many factors which synergistically increase vascular risk. The other general point is that the risk of developing heart disease increases in a graded manner with cholesterol level. There is no 'normal' range or 'upper limit' below which risk disappears. This accounts for the not infrequent finding of apparently normal lipid levels in patients with ischaemic heart disease, particularly in those presenting over the age of 50 to 60 years.
   Many case-control studies have confirmed that mean levels of serum

cholesterol and triglyceride are elevated in ischaemic heart disease; and this is also true of peripheral vascular disease (Greenhalgh et al, 1971). When plasma lipoproteins are quantitatively analysed, levels of VLDL, LDL and less frequently of both lipoproteins may be elevated, and HDL is commonly subnormal (Heinle et al, 1969; Lewis et al, 1974; Carlson and Ericsson, 1975). Combined hyperlipidaemia and hypertriglyceridaemia appear commoner than hypercholesterolaemia (Goldstein et al, 1973; Lewis et al, 1974; Carlson and Ericsson, 1975a and b).

Not only in individuals, but in population groups too a high frequency of ischaemic heart disease is associated with high average levels of cholesterol (Keys, 1970; McGill, 1968) and triglyceride (Bang and Dyerberg, 1972; Lewis, Carlson, Mancini and Micheli, to be published).

Prospective studies

The probability that these associations are causal is increased by the evidence obtained from prospective surveys; in these, one or more characteristics are measured in apparently-healthy individuals, and during a prolonged follow-up period the ability of these characteristics to predict the appearance of ischaemic heart disease is assessed. Hypercholesterolaemia is clearly such a risk factor (Kannell et al, 1971; Carlson and Böttiger, 1972; Wilhelmsen, Wedel and Tibblin, 1972). No single risk factor is predictive of heart disease in an individual, but in a group of individuals the presence of the three major risk factors (hyperlipidaemia, hypertension, and cigarette smoking) has been shown to increase risk some 12-fold compared with a group lacking these characteristics.

There is less unanimity about the risk factor status of hypertriglyceridaemia. The ongoing prospective study in Stockholm indicates that the predictive power of high triglyceride levels is if anything greater that that of cholesterol (Carlson and Böttiger, 1972). A study in Gothenberg initially supported this (Tibblin, 1970) but a recent report suggests that if allowance is made for differences in serum cholesterol level, triglyceride does not show an independent predictive effect (Wilhelmsen, Wedel and Tibblin, 1972).

Risk factors in association

Hypercholesterolaemia is also predictive of further ischaemic events in patients with established heart disease, which has some bearing on the decision to treat elevated cholesterol levels in patients who already have evidence of cardiac ischaemia (Coronary Drug Project Research Group, 1974). In the same study, hypertriglyceridaemia was not similarly predictive. The mathematical tool of multivariate analysis is used in distinguishing whether a risk factor exerts an independent effect or whether its predictive value results from its association with another factor more directly involved in the pathogenesis of atherosclerotic heart disease. Clearly the cholesterol and triglyceride of plasma are metabolically associated in that they are both present in all plasma lipoproteins, and especially in VLDL. To attempt to separate their effects by holding cholesterol levels constant and seeking a predictive power for triglyceride alone might mask the effect of raised VLDL levels. The real problem is whether fasting VLDL and

LDL levels are both independent risk factors, a question which has yet to be addressed because of the formidable volume of laboratory work required. While elevated VLDL levels may result from abnormalities in triglyceride metabolism, there is a real possibility that VLDL may exert an atherogenic effect by virtue of its cholesterol component rather than its quantitatively greater triglyceride moeity. If so this might resolve the apparent discrepancy between the case-control data and certain of the prospective trials.

Further data, also from Carlson's laboratory, has suggested that elevated levels of LDL, VLDL, and especially of both lipoproteins play a role in the pathogenesis of ischaemic heart disease. Carlson, Ekelund and Ericsson (1975) performed lipid studies on a large asymptomatic population and carried out further studies in the top 2 per cent of the frequency distributions. Exercise electrocardiography revealed that ischaemic ST changes were considerably commoner in subjects with several forms of hyperlipoproteinaemia than in subjects with lower lipid levels.

Lipoproteins in the Arterial Intima

The filtration hypothesis of atherogenesis suggests that lipoproteins enter the arterial intima from its luminal surface and that some of the lipid is retained. There is evidence of the presence of LDL (Woolf and Pilkington, 1965) (or of immunologically-similar material) in atheromatous plaques. Two studies have been made of the relation between the amount of lipoprotein present in human arterial intima and that in plasma obtained from the same patients. Smith and Slater (1972) compared LDL levels in autopsy samples of artery with cholesterol concentration in plasma samples obtained at varying times prior to death. They found a close positive correlation. Onitiri et al (1976) assayed apo B and apo C levels (as indices of LDL and VLDL) in intimal samples obtained during cardiovascular surgery, and measured LDL and VLDL levels in simultaneous plasma samples. Arterial LDL levels correlated positively with plasma LDL-cholesterol and with plasma apo B levels, and the arterial apo C concentration showed a similar correlation with plasma VLDL-triglyceride and with plasma apo C levels. It therefore appears that arterial lipoprotein concentrations are determined in part by plasma lipoprotein levels. Arterial apo B levels were markedly elevated in patients with hyper β-lipoproteinaemia and arterial levels of apo C and apo B were increased in those with pre-β-hyperlipoproteinaemia.

These findings concerning VLDL and the arterial wall should be viewed in the light of a recent suggestion by Zilversmit (1973). He has proposed that VLDL is partly delipidated by lipoprotein lipase at the arterial intimal surface. This results in a local high concentration of cholesterol-enriched remnant particles, and it is these rather than the native VLDL which enter the arterial wall.

EXPERIMENTAL EVIDENCE

Induction of atherosclerosis-like lesions has been achieved, in several animal species, since the turn of the century. By feeding high-fat or high-cholesterol diets, marked hyperlipidaemia is induced. These findings support the view that the association of hyperlipidaemia with atnerosclerotic heart disease is causal in nature. A major recent contribution using this experimental model is the demonstration that atherosclerotic lesions, produced by such diets, show marked regression when plasma lipid levels are reduced. The reversibility of vascular lesions has been shown when a plasma lipid-lowering diet is provided, alone (Armstrong and Megan, 1972) or with cholestyramine (Wissler et al, 1975). Even pronounced atherosclerosis shows considerable regression in the primates used.

THERAPEUTIC TRIALS

Comparable evidence concerning human atherosclerotic heart disease has been sought. The design of such trials is a matter of great difficulty. The preferred design would be a controlled trial of the treatment of specific forms of hyperlipidaemia by the optimal therapeutic agents, with due regard to careful randomisation of the participants to a double-blind design. One such trial is in progress; the National Heart and Lung Institute in the USA is investigating the treatment of primary hyper β-lipoproteinaemia. None of the major published trials have selected hyperlipidaemic subjects, nor has the treatment been that of the particular form of hyperlipidaemia. This has necessarily biased against positive results. In most studies the fall in serum lipids has been relatively modest.

The design of most trials so far reported has been to study subjects without regard to their lipid levels. Studies of primary prevention of ischaemic heart disease by a lipid-lowering diet have been reported (e.g. Miettinen et al, 1972); and secondary prevention of relapse in patients with established ischaemic heart disease has been attempted by diet (e.g. Leren, 1966) and by clofibrate, nicotinic acid, oestrogen and D-thyroxine (Coronary Drug Project Research Group, 1975). The primary prevention trials have all shown encouraging reduction in the incidence of new ischaemic events. All these studies have had certain defects in design, differing in each trial; these problems are not such as to have biased towards a positive result. The results of the secondary prevention trials have been less consistent. One of the two dietary trials indicated a reduction in the recurrence rate, and two of the three studies of clofibrate indicated benefit in certain subgroups of patients. In the Drug–Heart study, the trials of D-thyroxine and oestrogen were abandoned because of untoward effects; clofibrate was without benefit, and nicotinic acid in conservative dosage produced some reduction in morbidity from ischaemic heart disease, not attaining statistical significance.

Conclusion

The several lines of evidence summarised in this section, taken together, strongly suggest that hyperlipidaemia is one of the major factors in the pathogenesis of ischaemic heart disease. Certainly this area is under extensive investigation at present. Amongst recent growing points is the suggestion that HDL may be protective against ischaemic heart disease, possibly by facilitating the mobilisation of cholesterol from the arterial wall (Miller and Miller, 1975). The low levels of serum HDL-cholesterol, especially in young patients with ischaemic heart disease (Lewis et al, 1974b) has been referred to. A recent extensive study has confirmed this and has suggested that the HDL concentration in ischaemic heart disease varies independently of the levels of other lipoproteins (Castelli et al, 1975).

REFERENCES

Ahrens, E. H. Jr., Hirsch, J., Oette, K., Farquhar, J. W. & Stein, Y. (1961) Carbohydrate induced and fat induced lipemia. *Transactions of the Association of American Physicians*, **74**, 134–146.

Alaupovic, O. (1972) Conceptual development of classifications of plasma lipoproteins. In *Protides of the Biological Fluids*, vol. 19, pp. 9–19, ed. Peeters, H. Oxford: Pergamon Press.

Antonis, A. & Bersohn, I. (1960) Serum triglyceride levels in South African Europeans and Bantu and in ischaemic heart disease. *Lancet*, **i**, 998–1000.

Armstrong, M. L. & Megan, B. M. (1972) Lipid depletion in atheromatous coronary arteries of rhesus monkeys after regression diets. *Circulation Research*, **30**, 675–680.

Augustin, J., Freeze, H. & Brown, W. V. (1975) Comparison of hepatic triglyceride lipase and lipoprotein lipase from human postheparin plasma. *Circulation*, **51–52**, Suppl. II, 83.

Avogaro, P. & Cazzolato, G. (1975) Familial hyper-HDL-(α)-cholesterolaemia. *Atherosclerosis*, **22**, 63–77.

Bang, H. O. & Dyerberg, J. (1972) Plasma lipids and lipoproteins in Greenlandic west coast Eskimos. *Acta Medica Scandinavica*, **192**, 85–94.

Barter, P. J., Nestel, P. J. & Carroll, K. F. (1972) Precursors of plasma triglyceride fatty acids in humans. *Metabolism*, **21**, 117–124.

Beaumont, J. L., Carlson, L. A., Cooper, G., Fejfar, Z., Fredrickson, D. S. & Strasser, T. (1970) Classification of hyperlipidaemias and hyperlipoproteinaemias. *Bulletin of the World Health Organization*, **43**, 891–915.

Bennett, B., Swift, L., Gray, M. & LeQuire, V. (1975) Intestinal Golgi very low density lipoprotein: a unique lipoprotein subfraction. *Circulation*, **51–52**, Suppl. II, 38.

Bierman, E. L. (1972) Insulin and hypertriglyceridaemia. *Israeli Journal of Medical Sciences*, **8**, 303–307.

Boberg, J., Carlson, L. A., Freyschuss, U., Lassers, B. W. & Wahlquist, M. L. (1972) Splanchnic secretion rates of plasma triglycerides and total and splanchnic turnover of plasma free fatty acids in men with normo- and hypertriglyceridaemia. *European Journal of Clinical Investigation*, **2**, 454–466.

Bondjers, G. & Björkerud, S. (1974) Cholesterol transfer in vitro between the rabbit aorta and serum lipoproteins. In *Atherosclerosis III*, ed. Schettler, G. and Weizel, A., pp. 110–113. Berlin: Springer.

Brown, M. S., Dana, S. E. & Goldstein, J. L. (1973) Regulation of 3-hydroxy-3-methylglutaryl coenzyme A reductase activity in human fibroblasts by lipoproteins. *Proceedings of the National Academy of Sciences, U.S.A.*, **70**, 2162–2166.

Brunzell, J. D., Hazzard, W. R., Motulsky, A. G. & Bierman, E. L. (1975) Evidence for diabetes and genetic forms of hypertriglyceridaemia as independent entities. *Metabolism*, **24**, 1115–1121.

Brunzell, J. D., Hazzard, W. R., Porte, D. & Bierman, E. L. (1973) Evidence for a common, saturable triglyceride removal mechanism for chylomicrons and very low density lipoproteins in man. *Journal of Clinical Investigation*, **52**, 1578–1585.

Carew, T. E., Koschinsky, T. & Steinberg, D. (1975) Binding of low density lipoprotein to pig smooth muscle cells at 0°C. *Circulation*, **51–52**, Suppl. II, 59.

Carlson, L. A., Boberg, J. & Högstedt, B. (1965) Some physiological and clinical implications of lipid mobilisation from adipose tissue. In *Handbook of Physiology*: section 5: Adipose Tissue, chapter 63, pp. 625–644. ed. Cahill, G. F. and Renold, A. E. Washington: American Physiological Society.

Carlson, L. A. & Böttiger, L. E. (1972) Ischaemic heart disease in relation to fasting values of plasma triglyceride and cholesterol. *Lancet*, **i**, 865–868.

Carlson, L. A., Ekelund, L. G. and Olsson, A. G. (1975) Frequency of ischaemic exercise ECG changes in symptom-free men with various forms of primary hyperlipaemia. *Lancet*, **ii**, 1–3.

Carlson, L. A. & Ericsson, M. (1975) Quantitative and qualitative serum lipoprotein analysis, Part 1. *Atherosclerosis*, **21**, 417–433.

Carlson, L. A. & Ericsson, M. (1975) Quantitative and qualitative serum lipoprotein analysis. Part 2. Studies in male survivors of myocardial infarction. *Atherosclerosis*, **21**, 435–450.

Carlson, L. A. & Lindstedt, S. (1969) The Stockholm prospective survey. *Acta Medica Scandinavica,* suppl. 493.

Carter, C. O., Slack, J. & Myant, N. B. (1971) Genetics of hyperlipoproteinaemias. *Lancet,* **1,** 400.

Castelli, W. P., Doyle, J. T., Gordon, T., Haines, C., Hulley, S. B., Kagan, A., McGee, D., Cicic, W. J. & Zukel, W. J. (1975) HDL cholesterol levels in coronary heart disease: a cooperative lipoprotein phenotyping project. *Circulation,* **51-52,** suppl. II, 97.

Chait, A., Mancini, M., February, A. & Lewis, B. (1972) Clinical and metabolic study of alcoholic hyperlipidaemia. *Lancet,* **ii,** 62-64.

Clifford, C., Salel, A. F., Shore, B., Shore, V. & Mason, D. T. (1975) Mechanisms of lipoprotein alterations in patients with idiopathic hypothyroidism. *Circulation,* **51-52,** suppl. II, 18.

Coronary Drug Project Research Group (1974) Factors influencing long-term prognosis after recovery from myocardial infarction — three-year findings of the Coronary Drug Project. *Journal of Chronic Diseases,* **27,** 267-285.

Connor, W. E. & Lin, D. S. (1974) The intestinal absorption of dietary cholesterol by hypercholesterolemic (type II) and normocholesterolemic humans. *Journal of Clinical Investigation,* **53,** 1062-1070.

Coronary Drug Project Research Group (1975) Clofibrate and niacin in coronary heart disease. *Journal of the American Medical Association,* **231,** 360-381.

Cryer, A., Davies, P. & Robinson, D. S. (1975) The control of lipoprotein lipase. In *Blood and Arterial Wall in Atherogenesis and Arterial Thrombosis,* ed. Hautvast, J. G. A. G., Hermus, R. J. J. and van der Haat, F. Leiden: Brill.

Einarsson, K., Hellstrom, K. & Kallner, M. (1974) Bile acid kinetics in relation to serum lipids, body weight and gall bladder disease in patients with various types of hyperlipoproteinaemia. *Journal of Clinical Investigation,* **54,** 1301-1311.

Eisenberg, S., Bilheimer, D., Lindgren, F. & Levy, R. I. (1972). On the apoprotein composition of human plasma very low density lipoprotein subfractions. *Biochimica Biophysica Acta,* **260,** 329-333.

Fogelman, A. M., Edmond, J., Seager, J. & Popjak, G. (1975) Abnormal induction of HMGCoA reductase in leukocytes from subjects with heterozygous familial hypercholesterolemia. *Journal of Biological Chemistry,* **250,** 2045-2055.

Fredrickson, D. S. (1975) It's time to be practical. *Circulation,* **51,** 209-210.

Fredrickson, D. S., Gotto, A. M. & Levy, R. I. (1972) Familial lipoprotein deficiency. In *Metabolic Basis of Inherited Disease,* 3rd edition, Chapter 26. New York: McGraw-Hill.

Fredrickson, D. S. & Levy, R. I. (1972) Familial hyperlipoproteinemia. In *The Metabolic Basis of Inherited Disease,* 3rd edition, ed. Stanbury, J. B., Wyngaarden, J. B. and Fredrickson, D. S. p. 545. New York: McGraw-Hill.

Fredrickson, D. S., Levy, R. I. & Lees, R. S. (1967) Fat transport in lipoproteins — an integrated approach to mechanisms and disorders. *New England Journal of Medicine,* **276,** 32-34, 94-103, 145-156, 215-226, 273-281.

Gagne, C., Kushwaha, R., Albers, J., Brunzell, J. D. & Hazzard, W. R. (1975) Type III hyperlipoproteinemia. *Circulation,* **51-52,** suppl. II. 39.

Garfinkel, A. S. & Schotz, M. C. (1973) Sequential induction of two species of lipoprotein lipase. *Biochimica Biophysica Acta,* **306,** 128-133.

Gitlin, D., Cornwell, D. G., Nakasato, D., Oncley, J. L., Hughes, W. L. & Janeway, C. A. (1958) Studies on the metabolism of the plasma proteins in the nephrotic syndrome. II. The lipoproteins. *Journal of Clinical Investigation,* **37,** 172-184.

Gjone, E. & Norum, K. R. (1974) (Editors) Recent research on lecithin: cholesterol acyl-transferase. *Scandinavian Journal of Clinical Investigation,* **33,** suppl. 137.

Glomset, J. A. (1968) The plasma lecithin: cholesterol acyltransferase reaction. *Journal of Lipid Research,* **9,** 155-167.

Glueck, C. J., Levy, R. I. & Fredrickson, D. S. (1969) Immunoreactive insulin, glucose tolerance and carbohydrate inducibility in types II, III, IV and V hyperlipoproteinemia. *Diabetes,* **18,** 739-747.

Godfrey, R. C., Stenhouse, N. S., Cullen, K. J. & Blackman, V. (1972) Cholesterol and the child. Studies of cholesterol levels of Busselton schoolchildren and their parents. *Australian Paediatric Journal,* **8,** 72-80.

Goldstein, J. L. & Brown, M. S. (1973) Familial hypercholesterolemia: identification of a defect in the regulation of HMG-CoA reductase activity associated with overproduction of cholesterol. *Proceedings of the National Academy of Sciences, U.S.A.,* **70,** 2804-2808.

Goldstein, J. L., Dana, S. E., Brunschede, G. Y. & Brown, M. S. (1975) Genetic heterogeneity in familial hypercholesterolemia. *Proceedings of the National Academy of Sciences, U.S.A.,* **72,** 1092-1096.

Goldstein, J. L., Hazzard, W. R., Schrott, H. G., Bierman, E. L. & Motulsky, A. G. (1973) Hyperlipidemia in coronary heart disease. *Journal of Clinical Investigation*, 52, 1533–1543.

Goldstein, J. L., Schrott, H. G., Hazzard, W. R., Bierman, E. L. & Motulsky, A. G. (1973) Hyperlipidemia in coronary heart disease II. *Journal of Clinical Investigation*, 52, 1544–1568.

Greenhalgh, R. M., Mervart, I., Lewis, B., Calnan, J. S., Rosengarten, D. S. & Martin, P. (1971) Serum lipids and lipoproteins in peripheral vascular disease. *Lancet*, ii, 947–950.

Grundy, S. M., Nestel, P. J., Monell, R., Mok, H., von Bergman, K. & Steinberg, D. (1975) Kinetics of very low density lipoprotein triglycerides following radioglycerol. *Circulation*, 51–52, suppl. II, 39.

Hall, M., III, Bilheimer, D. W., Phair, R. D., Berman, M. & Levy, R. I. (1974) A mathematical model for apoprotein kinetics in normal and hyperlipidemic patients. *Circulation*, 49–50, suppl. II, 114.

Hamilton, R. L. (1972) Synthesis and secretion of plasma lipoproteins. *Advances in Experimental Biology and Medicine*, 26, 7–13.

Havel, R. J. (1961) Conversion of plasma free fatty acids into triglycerides of plasma lipoprotein fractions in man. *Metabolism*, 10, 1031–1034.

Havel, R. J. (1965) Metabolism of lipids in chylomicrons and very-low density lipoproteins. In *Handbook of Physiology*: section 5, chapter 50. Washington: American Physiological Society.

Havel, R. J. (1969) Pathogenesis, differentiation and management of hypertriglyceridemia. *Advances in Internal Medicine*, 15, 117–154.

Havel, R. J. (1975) Hyperlipoproteinemia: problems in diagnosis and challenges posed by the 'type III' disorder. *Annals of Internal Medicine*, 82, 273–274.

Havel, R. J. & Gordon, R. S. (1960) Idiopathic hyperlipemia: metabolic studies in an affected family. *Journal of Clinical Investigation*, 39, 1777–1790.

Havel, R. J. & Kane, J. P. (1973) Primary dysbetalipoproteinemia: predominance of a specific apoprotein species in triglyceride-rich lipoproteins. *Proceedings of the National Academy of Sciences, U.S.A.*, 70, 2015–2019.

Havel, R. J., Kane, J. P., Balasse, E. O., Segel, N. & Basso, L. V. (1970a) Splanchnic metabolism of free fatty acids and production of triglycerides of very low density lipoprotein in normo- and hypertriglyceridemic humans. *Journal of Clinical Investigation*, 49, 2017–2035.

Havel, R. J., Shore, V. G., Shore, B. & Bier, D. M. (1970b) Role of specific glycopeptides of human serum lipoproteins in the activation of lipoprotein lipase. *Circulation Research*, 27, 545–548.

Heinle, R. A., Levy, R. I., Fredrickson, D. S. & Gorlin, R. (1969) Lipid and carbohydrate abnormalities in angiographically-documented coronary artery disease. *American Journal of Cardiology*, 24, 178–186.

Higgins, J. M. & Fielding, C. J. (1975) Lipoprotein lipase: mechanism of formation of triglyceride-rich remnant particles from very-low density lipoproteins and chylomicrons. *Biochemistry*, 14, 2288–2292.

Higgins, M. J. P., Lecamwasan, L. S. & Galton, D. J. (1975) A new type of familial hypercholesterolaemia. *Lancet*, ii, 737–739.

Hillman, L., Schonfeld, G., Miller, J. P. & Wulff, G. (1975) Apolipoproteins in human pregnancy. *Metabolism*, 24, 943–952.

Ho, K. J., Biss, K., Mikkelson, B., Lewis, L. A. & Taylor, C. B. (1971) The Masai of East Africa; some unique biological characteristics. *Archives of Pathology*, 91, 387–410.

Janus, E., Sigurdsson, G., Nicoll, A., Turner, P. & Lewis, B. (1976) The metabolism of very low density lipoprotein (VLDL) and low density lipoprotein (LDL) apolipoprotein B in combined hyperlipidaemia (Type IIb). *Clinical Science and Molecular Medicine*, 51, 8P (abstract).

Kannell, W. B., Castelli, W. P., Gordon, T. & Macnamara, P. M. (1971) Serum cholesterol, lipoproteins and the risk of coronary heart disease. *Annals of Internal Medicine*, 74, 1–12.

Keys, A. (1970) Coronary heart disease in seven countries. *Circulation*, 41, suppl. 1.

Keys, A., Aravanis, C., Blackburn, H., van Buchem, F., Buzina, R., Djordjevic, B. S., Fidanza, F., Karvonen, M. J., Menotti, A., Puddo, V. & Taylor, H. L. (1972) Coronary heart disease: overweight and obesity as risk factors. *Annals of Internal Medicine*, 77, 15–27.

Keys, A. & Fidanza, F. (1960) Serum cholesterol and relative body weight of coronary patients in different populations. *Circulation*, 22, 1091–1102.

Koerselman, H. P., Lewis, B. & Pilkington, T. R. E. (1961) The effect of venous occlusion on the level of plasma cholesterol. *Journal of Atherosclerosis Research*, 1, 85–87.

Krauss, R. M., Levy, R. I. & Fredrickson, D. S. (1974) Selective measurement of two lipase activities in postheparin plasma from normal subjects and patients with hyperlipoproteinemia. *Journal of Clinical Investigation*, 54, 1107–1124.

Kudzma, D. J. & Schonfeld, G. (1971) Alcoholic hyperlipemia: induction by alcohol but not by carbohydrate. *Journal of Laboratory and Clinical Medicine*, 77, 384–395.

Kwiterovich, P. O., Levy, R. I. & Fredrickson, D. S. (1974) Familial hypercholesterolemia (one form of familial type II hyperlipoproteinemia). *Journal of Clinical Investigation*, **53**, 1237–1249.

Kwiterovich, P. O., Levy, R. I. & Fredrickson, D. S. (1973) Neonatal diagnosis of familial type II hyperlipoproteinaemia. *Lancet*, **i**, 118–121.

Langer, T. & Levy, R. I. (1970) Effect of nicotinic acid on beta-lipoprotein metabolism. *Clinical Research*, **18**, 458–464.

Langer, T., Strober, W. & Levy, R. I. (1972) The metabolism of low density lipoprotein in familial type II hyperlipoproteinemia. *Journal of Clinical Investigation*, **51**, 1528–1536.

LaRosa, J. C., Levy, R. I., Herbert, P., Lux, S. E. & Fredrickson, D. S. (1970) A specific apoprotein activator for lipoprotein lipase. *Biochemical and Biophysical Research Communications*, **41**, 57–62.

Leren, P. (1966) The effect of plasma cholesterol lowering diet in male survivors of myocardial infarction: a controlled clinical study. *Acta Medica Scandinavica*, suppl. 466.

Levy, R. I. (1972) (Convenor) Dietary and drug treatment of hyperlipoproteinemia. *Annals of Internal Medicine*, **77**, 267–294.

Lewis, B. (1973) Classification of lipoproteins and lipoprotein disorders. *Journal of Clinical Pathology*, **26**, suppl. 5, 26–31.

Lewis, B. (1976) *The Hyperlipidaemias: Clinical and Laboratory Practice*. Oxford: Blackwell.

Lewis, B., Boberg, J., Mancini, M. & Carlson, L. A. (1972a) Determination of the intravenous fat tolerance test with intralipid by nephelometry. *Atherosclerosis*, **15**, 83–86.

Lewis, B., Chait, A., Wootton, I. D. P., Oakley, C. M., Krikler, D. M., Sigurdsson, G., February, A., Mayrer, B. & Birkhead, J. (1974a) Frequency of risk factors for ischaemic heart disease in a healthy British population. *Lancet*, **i**, 141–146.

Lewis, B., Chait, A., Oakley, C. M., Wootton, I. D. P., Krikler, D. M., Onitiri, A., Sigurdsson, G. & February, A. (1974b). Serum lipoprotein abnormalities in patients with ischaemic heart disease: comparisons with a control population. *British Medical Journal*, **3**, 489–493.

Lewis, B. & Myant, N. B. (1967) Studies in the metabolism of cholesterol in subjects with normal cholesterol levels and in patients with essential hypercholesterolaemia. *Clinical Science*, **32**, 201–213.

Lewis, B., Mancini, M., Mattock, M., Chait, A. & Fraser, T. R. (1972b) Plasma triglyceride and fatty acid metabolism in diabetes mellitus. *European Journal of Clinical Investigation*, **2**, 445–453.

Mahley, R. W., Bersot, T. P., Brown, M. S. & Goldstein, J. L. (1975) Regulation of sterol metabolism in fibroblasts by a swine lipoprotein lacking apo B. *Circulation*, **51–52**, suppl. II, 60.

McGill, H. C., Jr (1968) The geographic pathology of atherosclerosis. *Laboratory Investigation*, **18**, 5–180.

Miettinen, T. A. & Aro, A. (1972) Faecal fat, bile acid excretion and body weight in familial hypercholesterolaemia. *Scandinavian Journal of Clinical and Laboratory Investigation*, **30**, 85–88.

Miettinen, M., Karvonen, M. J., Turpeinen, O., Eluosu, R. & Paavilainen, E. (1972) Effect of cholesterol lowering diet on mortality from coronary heart disease and other causes. *Lancet*, **ii**, 835–838.

Miller, G. J. & Miller, N. E. (1975) Plasma-high-density-lipoprotein concentration and development of ischaemic heart disease. *Lancet*, **i**, 16–19.

Morganroth, J., Levy, R. I. & Fredrickson, D. S. (1975) The biochemical, clinical and genetic features of type III hyperlipoproteinemia. *Annals of Internal Medicine*, **82**, 158–165.

Nicoll, A., Sigurdsson, G. & Lewis, B. (1975) Turnover rate of very low density lipoprotein B peptide in normal subjects and in hyperlipidaemics. *Clinical Science and Molecular Medicine*, **48**, 15P.

Nikkilä, E. A. & Aro, A. (1973) Family study of lipids and lipoproteins in coronary heart disease. *Lancet*, **i**, 954–958.

Ockner, R. K., Hughes, F. B. & Isselbacher, K. J. (1969) Very low density lipoproteins in intestinal lymph. *Journal of Clinical Investigation*, **48**, 2079–2086.

Olefsky, J., Reaven, G. M. & Farquhar, J. W. (1974) Effect of weight reduction on obesity. *Journal of Clinical Investigation*, **53**, 64–76.

Onitiri, A. C., Lewis, B., Bentall, H., Jamieson, C., Wisheart, J. & Faris, I. (1976) Lipoprotein concentrations in serum and in biopsy samples of arterial intima: a quantitative comparison. *Atherosclerosis*, **23**, 513–519.

Quintao, E., Grundy, S. M. & Ahrens, E. H., Jr (1971) Effects of dietary cholesterol on the regulation of total body cholesterol in man. *Journal of Lipid Research*, **12**, 233–247.

Reaven, G. M., Lerner, R. L., Stern, M. P. & Farquhar, J. W. (1967) Role of insulin in endogenous hypertriglyceridemia. *Journal of Clinical Investigation*, **46**, 1756–1767.

Redgrave, T. G. (1970) Formation of cholesteryl ester-rich particulate lipid during metabolism of chylomicrons. *Journal of Clinical Investigation*, **49**, 465–471.

Reichl, D., Simons, L. A., Myant, N. B., Pflug, J. J. & Mills, G. L. (1973) The lipids and lipoproteins of human peripheral lymph with observations on the transport of cholesterol from plasma and tissues into lymph. *Clinical Science and Molecular Medicine*, **45**, 313–329.

Rössner, S. (1974) Studies on an intravenous fat tolerance test. *Acta Medica Scandinavica*, suppl. 564.

Samuel, P., Perl, W., Holtzman, C. M., Rochman, N. D. & Lieberman, S. (1972) Long-term kinetics of serum and xanthoma radioactivity in patients with hypercholesterolemia. *Journal of Clinical Investigation*, **51**, 266–278.

Scanu, A. M. (1969) Serum high density lipoproteins. In *Structural and Functional Aspects of Lipoproteins in Living Systems*, chapter C3, ed. Tria, E. and Scanu, A. M. London: Academic Press.

Schonfeld, G. & Kudzma, D. J. (1973) Type IV hyperlipoproteinemia. A critical reappraisal. *Archives of Internal Medicine*, **132**, 55–62.

Scott, P. J. & Hurley, P. J. (1969) Effect of clofibrate on low-density lipoprotein turnover in essential hypercholesterolaemia. *Journal of Atherosclerosis Research*, **9**, 25–31.

Seidel, D., Alaupovic, P. & Furman, R. H. (1969) A lipoprotein characterizing obstructive jaundice. I and II. *Journal of Clinical Investigation*, **48**, 1211–1223 and **49**, 2396–2407.

Shaper, A. G. & Jones, K. W. (1959) Serum cholesterol, diet and coronary heart disease on Africans and Asians in Uganda. *Lancet*, **ii**, 534–535.

Shore, V. G., Shore, B. & Hart, R. G. (1974) Changes in apolipoproteins and properties of rabbit very low density lipoproteins on induction of cholesteremia. *Biochemistry*, **13**, 1579–1585.

Sigurdsson, G. (1975) Metabolic studies of apolipoprotein B kinetics in human subjects. *Ph.D. thesis*, University of London.

Sigurdsson, G., Nicoll, A. & Lewis, B. (1975) Conversion of very low density lipoprotein to low density lipoprotein: a metabolic study of apolipoprotein B kinetics in human subjects. *Journal of Clinical Investigation*, **56**, 1481–1490.

Sigurdsson, G., Nicoll, A., Reed, P. & Lewis, B. (1975) VLDL metabolism in a patient with primary type I hyperlipoproteinaemia. *Advances in Experimental Medicine and Biology*, **63**, 484.

Sigurdsson, G., Nicoll, A. & Lewis, B. (1976a) Metabolism of VLDL in hyperlipidaemia: measurement of VLDL-apo B kinetics in man. *European Journal of Clinical Investigation*, **6**, 167–177.

Sigurdsson, G., Nicoll, A. & Lewis, B. (1976b) The metabolism of low density lipoprotein in endogenous hypertriglyceridaemia. *European Journal of Clinical Investigation*, **6**, 151–158.

Simons, L., Wahab, S., Chait, A., Kikler, D. M. & Lewis, B. (1972) A study of hyperbeta- and hyperprebeta-lipoproteinaemia. *British Heart Journal*, **34**, 960.

Simons, L. A., Reichl, D., Myant, N. B. & Mancini, M. (1975) The metabolism of the apoprotein of plasma low density lipoproteins in familial hyperbetalipoproteinaemia in the homozygous form. *Atherosclerosis*, **21**, 283–298.

Slack, J. (1969) Risks of ischaemic heart disease in familial hyperlipoproteinaemic states. *Lancet*, **ii**, 1380–1382.

Slack, J. (1974) A comparison of three recent reports on the inheritance of lipid abnormalities in survivors of myocardial infarction. In *Atherosclerosis*, III. pp. 415–418, ed. Schettler, G. and Weizel, A. Berlin: Springer.

Smith, E. B. & Slater, R. S. (1972) Relationship between low density lipoprotein in aortic intima and serum lipid levels. *Lancet*, **i**, 463–469.

Sniderman, A. D., Carew, T. E., Chandler, J. G. & Steinberg, D. (1974) Paradoxical increase in rate of catabolism of low density lipoproteins after hepatectomy. *Science*, **183**, 526–528.

Stamler, J., Berkson, D. M. & Lindberg, H. A. (1972) Risk factors: their role in the etiology and pathogenesis of the atherosclerotic diseases. In *The Pathogenesis of Atherosclerosis*, ed. Wissler, R. W. and Geer, J. C. pp. 41–118. Baltimore: Williams and Wilkins.

Stein, O., Weinstein, D. B., Stein, Y. & Steinberg, D. (1976) Binding, internalization, and degradation of low density lipoprotein by normal human fibroblasts and by fibroblasts from a case of homozygous familial hypercholesterolemia. *Proceedings of National Academy of Science, U.S.A.*, **73**, 14–18.

Strisower, E. H., Adamson, G. & Strisower, B. (1970) Treatment of hyperlipidemic states. *Medical Clinics of North America*, **54**, 1599–1613.

Tabaqchali, S., Chait, A., Harrison, R. & Lewis, B. (1974) Experience with simplified scheme of treatment of hyperlipidaemia. *British Medical Journal*, **i**, 377–380.

Thompson, G. R. & Myant, N. B. (1975) Non-steady state studies of low density lipoprotein turnover. *Circulation*, **51–52**, suppl. II, 39.

Tibblin, G. (1970) Risk factors in coronary heart disease. *Advances in Cardiology*, **4**, 123–133.

Whitehead, T. P., Browning, D. M. & Gregory, A. (1973) A comparative study of the results of analyses of blood serum in clinical chemistry laboratories in the United Kingdom. *Journal of Clinical Pathology*, **26**, 435–440.

Wilhelmsen, L., Wedel, H. & Tibblin, G. (1972) Multivariate analysis of risk factors for coronary heart disease. *Circulation*, **48**, 950–958.

Wissler, R. W., Vesselinovitch, D., Borensztajn, J. & Hughes, R. (1975) Regression of severe atherosclerosis in cholestyramine-treated rhesus monkeys. *Circulation*, **51 and 52**, suppl. II, 16.

Woolf, N. & Pilkington, T. R. E. (1965). The immunohistochemical demonstration of lipoproteins in vessel walls. *Journal of Pathology and Bacteriology*, **90**, 459–463.

Zilversmit, D. B. (1973) A proposal linking atherogenesis to the interaction of endothelial lipoprotein lipase with triglyceride-rich lipoproteins. *Circulation Research*, **33**, 633–638.

12
GLOMERULONEPHRITIS

J. D. Blainey

The widespread use of percutaneous renal biopsy, the development of immunological techniques, and the rapid growth of facilities for treatment of end-stage renal failure have contributed to an explosion of literature on glomerulonephritis in the past 20 years. Before 1955 classification of nephritis was based upon clinical and postmortem observations and resulted in such confusing and meaningless terms as nephritic nephrosis or nephrotic nephritis. The purpose of the present review is to survey some of the numerous histological, immunological, and clinical classifications which have resulted from the application of new diagnostic procedures to large numbers of patients with renal disease, and to attempt an assessment of their relevance to clinical practice.

It is important to emphasise that no classification of glomerulonephritis at the present time is likely to be fully satisfactory, since there is profound ignorance of the causes of the various diseases involved and the evolution of the pathological and immunological changes in the human disorder are still poorly understood. Careful long-term clinical, histological, and immunological studies in well defined groups of patients remain the best method of clarifying the problem since animal models, although helpful to indicate possible mechanisms, are often misleading when applied to man and confusion has arisen from attempts to force clinical data to fit experimental results. It seems probable that further advances will be made in the next decades especially in relating pathological processes to precise forms of individual immunological response and in turn to specific causative factors. Once this step is achieved, treatment will become less haphazard and glomerulonephritis will hopefully cease to be one of the major causes of death and disability in children and young adults.

LABORATORY DIAGNOSIS OF GLOMERULONEPHRITIS

The advance of medical knowledge is firmly based upon improved scientific techniques and in the past 25 years, many valuable diagnostic methods have been developed. A brief review of the merits and limitations in renal disorders is therefore appropriate.

The quantitative measurement of protein in the urine (Bell and Baron, 1968), the estimation of serum proteins, the evaluation of simple renal function tests and the quantitation of urinary cellular deposits remain essential for proper diagnosis and have not changed. Table 12.1 (Hardwicke et al, 1966) shows the basic diagnostic investigations proposed by the Birmingham Renal Group in 1958 which have remained virtually unaltered. Paper test-strip techniques, while valuable for screening purposes, are useless for quantitation and hence for proper diagnosis or evaluation of treatment (Blainey, 1975).

Since the degree of protein loss in the urine is of major diagnostic and functional significance, it is essential that it should be estimated properly and not expressed in some vague system of + units or measured by obsolete methods

Table 12.1   Standard renal function tests

Performed serially
    Total serum protein
    Serum albumin (Specific method)
    Urine protein loss (g/day)   } on 4-hour and
    Creatinine clearance (ml/min)   } 24-hour sample
    Addis count — urinary deposit
    Haematocrit (PCV)
    Serum complement
    Electrophoretic globulin fractions
    Urine fibrin-degradation products (FDP)

Performed once for diagnosis
    Differential protein clearances
        (a) immunochemical
        (b) gel-filtration
    Intravenous pyelogram
    Renal biopsy

such as Esbach's picric acid precipitation. Such grossly inaccurate methods have contributed considerably to the prevailing confusion in classifying glomerulonephritis and should no longer be accepted for publication. The general use of automated techniques for serum protein, albumin and creatinine estimations have removed many of the vagaries of earlier methods with improved standardisation of results between different groups. Immunological methods for the measurement of complement factors (Cameron et al, 1973) and for fibrin degradation products (Merskey, Lalezari and Johnson, 1969) are now well established.

Differential protein clearances

Correlation between the histological changes found on renal biopsy and the relative clearances of six protein molecules of various molecular sizes was first demonstrated by Blainey et al (1960) and Soothill (1962) and has been confirmed by many groups. Although improved immunological methods (Mancini et al, 1965) have made these estimations relatively simple, they are still infrequently performed outside renal centres and are widely misinterpreted. Selective proteinuria, i.e. the loss into the urine of proteins of molecular size closely approximating to the albumin molecule (i.e. transferrin, albumin, α_1-globulin and very small amounts of IgG) is closely related to that type of glomerulo-nephritis in which there is little or no abnormality to be seen in the glomeruli on light microscopy (see below — minimal lesions) and which responds in over 80 per cent of cases (Cameron, Ogg and White, 1973) to steroid therapy. Various methods have been used by different authors to express the results of selectivity measurements, but the ratio

$$\frac{\dfrac{\text{urine IgG concentration (mg/ml)}}{\text{serum IgG concentration (mg/ml)}}}{\dfrac{\text{urine albumin (or transferrin) concentration (mg/ml)}}{\text{serum albumin (or transferrin) concentration (mg/ml)}}}$$

has the advantage of simplicity (Cameron and Blanford, 1966), although the use of only two proteins does introduce errors. By this method it is possible to recognise the patterns of proteinuria (Table 12.2) which correlate broadly with histological changes. Regrettably, the less selective proteinurias show considerable overlap of value for the ratios with histological groups and the method is primarily of value in the diagnosis of the highly selective groups, which predominate in childhood.

Table 12.2 Protein selectivity ratios

	IgG/transferrin	α_2-macroglobulin/ transferrin	Histological changes
Highly selective	<0.15	0	Minimal
Moderately selective	0.15–0.4	0–0.05	Proliferative
Non-selective	>0.4	>0.5	Membranous

Transferrin has often been used as the 'index' protein in preference to albumin because of greater reproducibility of measurement of standards with this protein.

It has been shown that gel-filtration through Sephadex G200 resin separates proteins by their molecular radius and this technique has provided a valuable, if laborious, tool for confirmation of the immunological measurements (Hardwicke, 1965).

Urinary fibrin-fibrinogen degradation products (FDP)

Estimation of FDP in urine has recently been shown to correlate well with the protein selectivity and to provide a simple and useful measurement of selectivity in patients with proteinuria greater than 2 g/l (Ekert et al, 1972; Hall et al, 1975). The fibrin degradation products appear to originate in the serum and to be lost through the damaged glomerular capillary exactly as any other protein of comparable molecular size (Hall et al, 1975). A suggestion that the FDP might reflect the quantity of fibrin deposited on the glomerulus and therefore be an indication of the 'activity' of the disease process in glomerulonephritis has unfortunately not been confirmed; such a measurement would be valuable in the serial assessments of patients on different treatment regimes.

Renal biopsy

Several excellent textbooks have now been published on the appearances of the human kidney in glomerulonephritis and other diseases (Brewer, 1973; Becker, 1968; Heptinstall, 1973) and it is unnecessary to review the many pathological descriptions of light, electron microscopy and fluorescent microscopy in different types of renal disease. As light microscopy still remains the major diagnostic procedure in all but special centres, a brief review of the major histological lesions described with the corresponding changes by more elaborate procedures is shown (Table 12.3). It must be emphasised however that many of these observations are not discrete, unchanging entities but merge into one another in many instances, so that diagnosis and prognosis in the individual patient on purely histological evidence still remains difficult and not always reliable.

THE IMMUNOLOGICAL BASIS OF GLOMERULONEPHRITIS

The experimental studies of Dixon and his colleagues and the widespread use of immunofluorescent examination of renal biopsies have increased our understanding of nephritis. It has been repeatedly shown in animals that two major types of immunological change may be observed in the glomerulus. In the first, which is apparently rare in man, a specific antibody is formed in the host to some fraction of the glomerular basement membrane with the deposition of specific antibasement membrane immunoglobulin in a linear pattern on the basement membrane of the majority of the glomeruli. The further change in glomerular structure which results from this deposition, i.e. cellular proliferation, crescent formation etc. is highly variable even in the same kidney (Wilson and Dixon, 1975) and accounts for some of the confusion in the interpretation of glomerular pathology. In the second type of immunological response in the kidney, antigen–antibody complexes are formed, presumably in the circulation; and because of their size, solubility or other properties, become deposited in the wall of the glomerular capillaries (Germuth and Rodriguez, 1973), where again, they may or may not excite a further secondary cellular reaction or other changes. The characteristic immunopathological change in this type of 'immune-complex' nephritis is the occurrence of deposits of immunoglobulin, with or without complement, fibrin, properdin etc. in various parts of the glomerular membrane (Table 12.3).

In both these major immunological disorders, well studied in the animal model, it is the variability of the secondary response and the absence of information in man on the nature of the antigenic stimulus, that is responsible for much of the confusion. Antiglomerular basement membrane disease is rare in man and occurs most frequently in the usually rapidly progressive renal failure associated with pulmonary haemorrhage, first described by Goodpasture in 1913. Similar linear deposits of immunoglobulin have been observed in systemic lupus erythematosus (Koeffler et al, 1969) and in the perfused donor kidney before renal transplantation. These changes however have not been associated with the presence of either circulating antibodies to glomerular basement membrane, or of antibody which could be eluted from the kidney and are therefore assumed to be non-specific.

Immune Complex Nephritis

A high proportion of renal biopsies examined from human subjects with nephritis shows some kind of granular deposition of IgG, IgM, or IgA (Table

Table 12.3 Histopathology of glomerulonephritis

Definition of lesion (Alternative names)	Light microscopy	Fluorescent microscopy (% positive findings)					Electron microscopy
		IgG	IgA	IgM	C3	Fib	
1. Minimal (lipoid nephrosis)	Normal	0	0	0	0	0	Loss of foot processes of epithelial cells.
2. Membranous (extramembranous) (epimembranous)	Dense spikes (silver-stain) on epithelial aspect GBM beneath foot processes. No cell proliferation.	100	15	15	50	0	As light microscopy. Early dense deposits do not show spike appearances.
3. Diffuse proliferative (acute nephritis) (post-streptococcal nephritis)	Proliferation endothelial and/or epithelial cells (=mesangial cells). Polymorphs. Epithelial cell crescents very occasional or absent.	70	0	0	100	25	Proliferation cells as light microscopy — more suggestive of mesangial proliferation. Electron dense lumps on GBM, swollen split membrane.
4. Diffuse extracapillary g.n. (g.n. with fibrin and crescent formation) (acute rapidly progressive g.n.)	Epithelial cell crescents in over 50% glomeruli. Proliferation of mesangial or epithelial cells. Glomerular necrosis. Fibrin deposits.	50	0	0	20	80	Disruption of capillary walls. Gross glomerular damage.
5. Membrano-proliferative g.n. (mesangiocapillary g.n.) (a) subendothelial deposits (b) dense deposits	(a) Deposits between inner aspect GBM and endothelium. Increased mesangial matrix (lobular pattern). (b) No lesion early cases. Later (especially silver-stain) thick GBM with non-argyrophilic deposits between epithelial and endothelial layers capillary loops. Mesangial and epithelial cells increased. Sometimes epithelial crescents.	70 0	10 10	60 50	100 100	0 10	(a) Mesangial cytoplasm between two layers of modified basement membrane ('tram-tracks'). (b) Amorphous substance in middle layers of basement membrane. Increased mesangial and epithelial cellularity. Epithelial crescents.
6. Focal proliferative g.n. (segmental and focal)	(a) Proliferation endothelial and epithelial cells in portion only of glomerular tuft. Remaining tuft and many other glomeruli normal. Collagen fibrils around proliferation, often adherent to Bowman's capsule. (b) Mesangial cell proliferation.	10	0	10	50	10	As light microscopy, mesangial cell proliferation may predominate.
7. Focal glomerulosclerosis	Local increase mesangial fibrillar material. No cell proliferation. Occluded capillaries and adhesions to Bowman's capsule. Final sclerosis tuft. Tubular atrophy.	15 5	75 5	0 60	50 40	0 5	Fusion of foot processes of epithelial cells. Increase basement membrane like material, extending across capillary lumen with eventual destruction lumen.

12.3) with or without complement deposition. It has perhaps been too readily assumed that because experimental immune complex nephritis (e.g. produced by bovine serum albumin) is associated with antigen–antibody formation and with the deposition of insoluble complexes of immunoglobulin in a granular distribution on the glomerular basement membrane, that all such granular deposits must be associated with immune complex disease. An energetic hunt for possible antigens and the attempted identification of immune complexes has ensued, and while certain types of human nephritis have been conclusively proved to result from this type of reaction, large numbers of patients are seen in whom the sole evidence of immune complex disease rests upon the finding of granular deposits of IgG or other immunoglobulins. This type of confused circular argument does not unfortunately clarify the situation in the individual patient where so often no evidence of any specific antigen–antibody reaction exists.

Post-streptococcal nephritis

Infection with certain types of Group A streptococci, either in the throat or skin, have been known for many years to produce acute glomerulonephritis (Jennings and Earle, 1961). Convincing proof of the antigen–antibody complex reaction was obtained by the finding, early in the acute disease, of streptococcal antigens in the kidney on fluorescent microscopy. It seems likely that these antigens are different from those producing the well-known anti-streptolysin O titre (ASO) (Zabriskie, 1971) and the precise nature of this antigenic material is still in doubt. This difference in the nature of the antigen responsible for the glomerular damage and differences in host antibody responses could well explain the apparent discrepancy between the incidence of glomerulonephritis and ASO titres which has exercised writers for decades. To add to the confusion, evidence has been produced that at least one streptococcal antigen from the inner cell wall shows immunological cross reaction with glomerular basement membrane antigen (Wheeler et al, 1975), an observation which might explain both the localisation of the antigen–antibody complex in the glomerulus and also the occasional occurrence of both granular and linear fluorescence in the same glomerulus. Antibodies to streptococcal membrane antigen have also been observed in the serum of patients with nephritis (Dardenne, Zabriskie and Bach, 1972) quite separately from ASO titres, further confirming the difference in those antigenic reactions. The identification of the immune complex in the serum has been far more difficult, possibly because of early and rapid removal by the kidney and other areas of high reticuloendothelial activity. The mechanism of production of streptococcal nephritis certainly merits renewed investigation because of the relative ease of production of stable streptococcal antigens and because of the well-established human disease.

Systemic lupus erythematosus

The elution of DNA antigens from the granular deposits seen in the mesangial area of the glomerulus in the nephritis associated with systemic lupus, the high titres of circulating anti-DNA antibodies in these patients and the demonstration of DNA antigen in circulating complexes confirms the immune-complex nature of this condition (Germuth and Rodriguez, 1973). The actual lesions of systemic lupus are very variable, ranging from small mesangial deposits of immunoglobulin with slight mesangial cell proliferation only, to significant hypercellularity mainly in the centri-lobular areas. This wide variation in histological appearance may occur between different loops of the capillary in the same glomerulus (i.e. a focal lesion) as well as between different glomeruli, some appearing normal to light microscopy while others show the most severe lesions including necrosis of the loop (Pollak and Pirani, 1974). In the more severe cases of SLE, heavy proteinuria and progressive renal failure may be present and only then are the extensive lesions with 'wire-loop' thickening of the glomeruli observed. In addition to immunoglobulins IgG IgA and IgM, complement fractions and fibrin are also seen in the more severe lesions of the capillary loop, while the earlier lesions are confined to mesangial cells and usually only show IgG deposits. There appears to be little correlation between the levels of circulating DNA antibody and the severity of the lesions in the kidney and it appears that as with other types of immune complex nephritis, factors other than the quantity of antigen or antibody determine the site and severity of the lesions.

Other forms of immune-complex nephritis

Numerous other conditions, with granular deposits in the mesangial areas of the glomerular capillaries or on the glomerular basement membrane, have been described and the relevant antigens isolated (Table 12.4). In few cases have

Table 12.4 Human immune complex glomerulonephritis

Associated pathological condition	Antigen
SLE	DNA, RNA, etc.
Thyroiditis	Thyroglobulin
Colonic carcinoma	Carcino-embryonic antigen
Cryoglobulinaemia	Immunoglobulin
Acute serum sickness	Foreign serum protein, drugs
Poststreptococcal nephritis	Streptococcal antigen
Infected atrio-ventricular shunts	Staphylococcal antigen
Quartian malarial nephrosis	Plasmodium malariae
Subacute bacterial endocarditis	Infecting organism
Hepatitis	Australia antigen
Subacute sclerosing panencephalitis	Measles antigen
Typhoid fever	Salmonella antigen

actual antigen–antibody complexes been identified in the circulation, and the identification of this class of immunological disorder in the kidney depends entirely upon finding antigen or specific antibody or both in the immunoglobulin deposits, or the elution of these from kidney tissue. A careful study of renal clear cell carcinoma by Ozawa et al (1975) has demonstrated both the specificity of the antigen involved and the detailed immunological work needed to establish the relationship between the antigen, the antigen–antibody complex, and the renal lesion. Numerous other renal disorders, associated with such diverse factors as penicillamine, gold, syphilis, schistosomiasis, neoplasms, virus infections, and sarcoidosis have also been assumed to be associated with antigen–antibody complex formation; but as the relevant specific antigens have not been identified, no proof of this type of reaction exists in these patients. There are still unfortunately many patients with granular deposits of immuno-globulin in whom no evidence of any immune-complex formation can be found, possibly because the renal reaction has persisted after the original antigen–antibody reaction has disappeared or as previously suggested, because of the disappearance of the complex into the reticuloendothelial cells.

THE NATURE OF IMMUNE-COMPLEX NEPHRITIS

Much discussion has centred around the apparent frequency of renal involvement in this type of reaction. Antibody production is an almost universal response to an antigenic stimulus and the combination of antigen–antibody may lead to the formation of protein complexes of varying size and solubility. The molecular composition of such complexes therefore depends largely upon the concentration ratio of the two reactants and for any specific immunological system, a certain ratio of antigen to antibody will result in the formation of large, insoluble, highly aggregated immune complexes (optimal proportions precipitation). All other ratios of antigen to antibody will result in smaller soluble complexes or in intermediate partially soluble particles or in mixtures of these three possibilities. The relative amounts of antigen and corresponding antibody in an immune response in a given individual can therefore vary greatly, at different times, i.e. at the beginning or end of a chronic infection and may also vary greatly between different individuals. Germuth and Rodriguez (1973) have shown clearly that the nature of the renal response may vary according to the size and quantity of the immune complexes formed. Thus in experimental bovine serum albumin nephritis small soluble complexes tend to localise within the capillary loops and to give rise to diffuse glomerular changes. Larger, partly soluble complexes localise in the mesangial area and give rise to mesangial cellular proliferation either alone or with local inflammatory changes. The largest insoluble complexes are probably removed by the reticuloendothelial cells and appear unable to produce glomerular localisation. It is thus readily apparent that many conditions in which basic immune processes occur, e.g. bacterial and virus infections, neoplasms, auto-immune disease etc. should in theory be able to produce renal lesions although in practice relatively few conditions have actually been shown to do so.

The formation and deposition of immune complexes, especially IgG or IgM, is accompanied by complement activation, which in turn can result in the liberation of cell or membrane lysins, leucotaxin and other biological factors resulting in inflammatory lesions. The 'classical' cascade of complement activation through at least 11 enzymatic stages is the usual mechanism. It has also been shown however that a second pathway of complement activation involving several other serum proteins including properdin, C3 pro-activator etc. may be activated by immunoglobulin IgA and by certain non-immunological means e.g. bacterial lipopolysaccharides, yeasts, enzymes, etc. (Wilson and Dixon, 1975). Factors present in the serum of patients with low serum complement levels may in themselves activate this alternative pathway and are detected by their ability to activate C3 in normal serum (C3 nephritic factor or

C3NeF). This type of mechanism provides a possible explanation of the progression of renal lesions after the original antigen stimulus has ceased, e.g. following a type 12 streptococcal throat infection when serum complement is low, C3 nephritic factors high (Williams et al, 1972) and when progression of the disease process in the glomeruli continues, with increasing complement and fibrin deposition in the glomeruli. At the same time, however, the original focus of infection has clearly disappeared, other streptococcal antibody titres fall, no streptococcal antigen can be found in the glomeruli but the glomerular damage continues. Further studies of the serum levels of the various complement fractions at different times after the onset of a presumed immune-complex type of nephritis are required to explain this progression of the condition in patients long after the original disorder has disappeared.

Cryoglobulin has also been recognised in the serum in association with various types of nephritis, especially in immune-complex disorders (Adam, Morel-Maroger and Richet, 1973). These cryoprecipitates always contain IgG and are associated with IgM, or less commonly IgA and complement fractions such as C3 or $C1_q$. The presence of these mixed protein aggregates appears to correlate with the activity of the renal disease and they could in themselves act as circulating immune complexes, although without detectable antigen, again providing a possible explanation for the continuation of a disease process over several years when all trace of any antigen has disappeared. Certain types of glomerulonephritis, especially of the membrano-proliferative type (mesangiocapillary) are always associated with low serum complement. Analysis of the serum complement profile and turnover studies suggest that there is evidence of activation of both the classical and alternative pathways of complement breakdown as well as decreased C3 synthesis. Precisely similar abnormalities of complement have been demonstrated in partial lipodystrophy, an inherited abnormality associated with glomerulonephritis. Various other congenital or acquired complement deficiencies have been studied (Peters and Williams, 1975) and are often associated with membrano-proliferative nephritis or systemic disorders resembling SLE. This concept of abnormal complement, or other types of immunological deficiency disorders as a predisposing cause of immune complex disorders has been elaborated by Soothill and Steward (1971), especially in relation to the formation of low avidity antibody in response to virus infections.

CLINICAL, IMMUNOLOGICAL AND PATHOLOGICAL CORRELATIONS

Similar glomerular changes have been delineated in renal biopsies in various centres by the combined efforts of immunologists and histopathologists although variations in terminology for identical lesions still cause confusion (see Table 12.3). Differences in technique of fluorescence microscopy also have led to conflicting reports, especially where reactions are weak or relatively non-specific. Such technical and descriptive problems will be solved eventually by general agreement and standardisation of methods. Correlation of the clinical and biochemical findings in glomerulonephritis is clearly a more difficult problem, since it is unfortunately true that almost every pathological change described in Table 12.3 has now been observed in individual patients with clinical states varying from mild symptomless proteinuria to the nephrotic syndrome and to rapidly progressive renal failure.

Cameron (1975) has emphasised the importance of classifying renal disease at four levels, aetiology and pathogenesis, mediation of injury, morphology, and clinical presentation, and has pointed out the fallacies which have resulted from the confusion of these four different types of observation. Regrettably, information is scanty or non-existent on the aetiology and pathogenesis, or on the mediation of injury in many cases of human nephritis and undisciplined theorising at these levels has caused considerable confusion. Table 12.5 relates the major clinical manifestations of the disease to the most frequently observed morphological changes. This table is incomplete as a clinical guide since it omits the further important factors of biochemical variation e.g. selective or non-selective proteinuria, changes in blood pressure etc., and also omits reference to the clinical course. In a disease process that may continue for 15 years or more (Fig. 12.1) with heavy protein and red cell loss in the urine, but without noticeable deterioration of renal function and with a complete absence of any abnormal physical signs or symptoms, prognosis clearly has to be guarded at the outset. Long-term studies of individual patients with serial clinical and morphological observations have produced reasonable correlations for assessment of the probable outcome of the various forms of treatment proposed in the past 20 years and for ultimate prognosis.

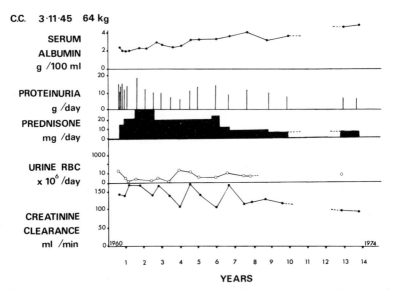

Figure 12.1 Membranoproliferative glomerulonephritis. C. C., male, date of birth 3.11.45. Patient presented with nephrotic syndrome and severe diffuse capillary damage in 1960; 14-year follow-up. Possible initial response to steroids, not maintained. Note continuous heavy proteinuria for 14 years, with high urinary red cell excretion but normal renal function. After first year, symptom free, normotensive and living normal life. Second biopsy in 1967 showed some progression of condition, with glomerular scarring and evidence of activity of condition. Steroid therapy of doubtful value in retrospect

Table 12.5 Clinical manifestations of glomerulonephritis and more commonly related morphological changes on renal biopsy

Syndrome	Clinical features	Variation of syndrome	Usual morphological changes
1. Acute nephritis	Acute onset, Haematuria, Variable proteinuria	Classical acute nephritis, Acute rapidly progressive nephritis, Acute recurrent haematuria, Part of generalised vascular disease	Diffuse proliferative g.n., Diffuse proliferative g.n. with crescents, Focal proliferative g.n., Diffuse proliferative g.n. with crescents
2. Nephrotic	Insidious onset, Oedema, Proteinuria >5.0 g/24h, Serum albumin <20 g/l	No known associated abnormality, Associated with infections, drugs, hypersensitivity, Part of systemic disease (see text for more common associations)	Minimal lesions, Membranous g.n., Membrano-proliferative g.n., Focal glomerulosclerosis, Focal proliferative g.n.
3. Symptomless proteinuria and/or haematuria	Symptomless	No established associated abnormality, Part of systemic disease	No histological abnormality, Focal proliferative g.n., Focal glomerulosclerosis, Membrano-proliferative
4. Chronic renal failure	Symptomless or various features of uraemia	—	Glomerular sclerosis too extensive to establish diagnosis; Diffuse proliferative g.n., Membranous g.n., Membrano-proliferative g.n., Focal glomerulosclerosis, Focal proliferative g.n.

It is clear from Table 12.5 that the clinical classification alone is inadequate for any systematic study of the natural history of glomerulonephritis, since the possible clinical reactions are so limited. Diagnosis, treatment and prognosis therefore must rest upon the morphological changes found on renal biopsy and except in a few clearly defined groups of clinical nephritis, such as the insidious onset of heavy proteinuria in childhood, or those conditions obviously associated with systemic disorders, e.g. systemic lupus erythematosus, a renal biopsy remains the only certain manner of establishing a reasonable diagnosis. The following paragraphs summarise the main findings, response to treatment and prognosis in the different histological groups previously described in Table 12.3.

Minimal change nephrotic syndrome (lipoid nephrosis (Habib and Kleinknecht, 1971; Cameron et al, 1974))

This condition is more common in childhood and is associated with highly selective heavy proteinuria and with a normal appearance of the glomerulus to light microscopy. The loss of foot processes seen on electron microscopy appears to be completely reversible on recovery from the proteinuria. There is no clear evidence of an immunological basis for the condition, although a small minority of cases are associated with sensitivity to specific protein allergies, e.g. pollens, food allergy or drug hypersensitivity. The condition responds rapidly to steroid therapy in over 85 per cent of cases in both children and adults. Other immunosuppressive drugs have been used but have been claimed to produce sterility (Fairly, Barrie and Johnson, 1972). One-third of patients show a remarkable tendency to relapse, often on many occasions but the renal function remains normal and serial renal biopsies show no change (Fig. 12.2).

A small number of both children and adults are refractory to steroid therapy and to immunosuppressive drugs. Difficulty in distinguishing mild focal proliferative lesions (Cameron et al, 1974), or the subsequent development of other lesions e.g. membranous glomerulonephritis or focal glomerulosclerosis, probably explain the majority of such cases, and a second renal biopsy may establish the morphological diagnosis after several months when treatment has apparently failed.

Some patients with this condition, especially those associated with defined allergens, may make a spontaneous recovery without any treatment but clinical trials have shown a significant reduction in the duration of proteinuria and oedema in the majority of patients (Black, Rose and Brewer, 1970). Moderate steroid dosage (e.g. 0.25–0.30 mg prednisone/kg body weight) is unquestionably safer than very high dose regimes but is not always as effective, the diminution of proteinuria and rise of serum albumin taking longer to achieve. The aim of treatment must obviously be to abolish the protein loss, not merely to produce a satisfactory diuresis, since the latter can often be achieved with high protein diets and diuretic alone.

Considerable debate exists as to whether the minimal lesion progresses to other types of morphological glomerular change, such as membranous glomerulonephritis or focal glomerulosclerosis. Certainly occasional patients have been described in whom long-term follow-up studies have apparently shown these progressive changes, but the recognition of the slight early abnormalities of these conditions is extremely difficult, except by electron microscopy, and measurements of protein selectivity are often not performed, or may show anomalies such as in focal glomerulosclerosis (White, Glasgow and Mills, 1973). Several early cases of renal vein thrombosis in the Birmingham series were initially regarded as minimal lesions but after several months developed typical membranous changes. None of these patients however responded to steroid therapy and the protein selectivity changed from selective to non-selective over the first few months of the illness.

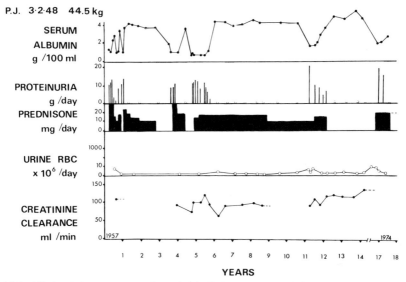

Figure 12.2 Minimal change glomerulonephritis, P. J., male, date of birth 3.2.48. Patient presented in 1957; 17-year follow-up, with six relapses of heavy proteinuria and nephrotic syndrome. Steroid response in all relapses satisfactory. Proteinuria has remained highly selective throughout and repeated biopsy after seven years showed normal glomeruli. Normal renal function and normotensive. No illnesses except during the relapses of proteinuria

Membranous glomerulonephritis (extramembranous or epimembranous nephritis)

The histological changes of this group are now well established on light, fluorescence, and electron microscopy. The very characteristic 'bristles' on silver staining of electron dense material, apparently of the same structure as the membrane itself, appear on the epithelial aspect of the glomerular basement membrane. Granular deposits of IgG are present along the capillary walls in all cases and C3 is present in similar distribution in over 50 per cent. There is never cellular proliferation but the more advanced progressive lesions may show extensive capillary obstruction.

The clinical picture is almost invariably of heavy proteinuria and the nephrotic syndrome. In the 55 cases seen in Birmingham (1958–1970), 50 showed the nephrotic syndrome at some period and a similar incidence is reported by Morel-Maroger and Verroust (1975). The majority of cases do not appear to be associated with any other recognised disorder, but there is a growing list of conditions associated with the same histological and clinical pattern (Rosen,

1971). Table 12.6 lists the present recognised conditions and it seems likely that further study will show more associations. The granular distribution of IgG and the presence of complement strongly suggest an immune-complex disorder, possibly with antigen-antibody complexes of small size that can penetrate the endothelium of the glomerular basement membrane but which get arrested at the epithelial cell surface for unknown reasons.

Although no treatment has been shown to have any effect, considerable argument prevails among nephrologists as to the prognosis of this condition. Row et al (1975) reported a total of 66 patients with complete remission in 25 per cent, persistent proteinuria in 25 per cent, persistent nephrotic syndrome in 25 per cent and death from renal failure in the remaining 25 per cent. Morel-Maroger and Verroust (1975) observed 15 deaths from renal failure out of 47 (32

Table 12.6   Conditions associated with extramembranous nephritis

Renal vein thrombosis	Metals
SLE	Gold
Neoplasia	Mercury
Hodgkin's disease	Drugs
Syphilis	Tridione
Auto-immune thyroiditis	Penicillamine
Sarcoidosis	Australia antigen
Diabetes	Parasitic infestation
Renal tubular antigen	Malaria
	Loiasis

per cent) patients and in the Birmingham series approximately 30 per cent recovered fully, 30 per cent persisted with varying amounts of proteinuria and 30 per cent died from renal failure. Other series have suggested a much higher incidence of progressive renal failure, probably because of different proportions of patients with other associated conditions described above.

The association of membranous nephropathy with renal vein thrombosis has attracted much attention, some writers (Row et al, 1975) regarding the thrombosis as secondary to a pre-existing lesion. That this is not usually the case is shown clearly by patients who were known to have developed heavy proteinuria following trauma, or after extensive deep vein thrombosis (Blainey, Hardwicke and Whitfield, 1954; Rosenman, Pollak and Pirani, 1968) with previously normal renal function. Treatment of the thrombosis with effective anticoagulants, especially the recurrent episodes of thrombosis which occur in the extensive perirenal and periureteric anastomoses, may be life saving.

Diffuse proliferative glomerulonephritis (acute glomerulonephritis)

The main pathological lesion is a diffuse increase in endothelial and mesangial cells, with reduction in the capillary lumen. When very large numbers of polymorphonuclear leucocytes are present in the glomerular tuft, the term 'exudative nephritis' has been used. Eosinophilic humps, electron dense on EM, are seen on the epithelial aspect of the glomerular basement membrane and appear to correspond with the granular deposits of C3 and IgG on immuno-fluorescence.

The majority of patients with proven post-streptococcal glomerulonephritis show this histological pattern (Lewy et al, 1971). Earlier lesions, where biopsies are taken within the first month of the acute illness, usually show more exudative features and are associated with low serum complement levels, frequent presence of cryoglobulins and of C3 splitting activity (C3NeF — see page 292). The reported incidence of streptococcal infections in diffuse proliferative glomerulonephritis varies greatly in different series, presumably because of the difficulty in positive identification of the relevant streptococcal antigen (McCluskey and Baldwin, 1963).

In about 15 per cent this histological lesion is found unrelated to any acute onset or to streptococcal infections (Richet, Chevet and Morel-Maroger, 1973) and associated with symptomless proteinuria or the gradual onset of the nephrotic syndrome.

The prognosis in this condition has generally been regarded as excellent but 15-year follow-up studies by Baldwin (1974) showed that renal failure had developed in 65 per cent of patients, even after a prolonged symptom free interval. This is not the experience in Britain and possibly environmental conditions or the prophylactic use of antibiotics to prevent respiratory re-infections may prevent recurrences of the immune-complex disorder as in rheumatic fever. No adequate study has ever been undertaken on this preventive aspect of acute nephritis, although the greatly diminished incidence of acute nephritis in recent years and the disappearance of so-called 'acute on chronic nephritis' of older textbooks suggest that prompt antibiotic treatment of streptococcal tonsillitis may be important in the prevention of acute glomerulonephritis.

Diffuse proliferative glomerulonephritis with fibrin and crescent formation (diffuse extracapillary glomerulonephritis: acute rapidly progressive nephritis)

This name has been applied to a number of conditions in which numerous epithelial cell crescents (over 50 per cent) are present in Bowman's space. The lesion is thought to arise from proliferation of the cells lining the space and may be so extensive as to obliterate this completely. Glomerular necrosis is often present and proliferation of epithelial, endothelial or mesangial cells may occur in the capillary tufts. Fibrinogen is found in the crescents on immunofluorescence in over 80 per cent of examples, sometimes with IgG and less commonly with C3. On occasions, the immunoglobulin and complement is linear in distribution, indicating an antiglomerular basement membrane disorder.

The clinical pattern is usually one of a rapidly progressive disorder, with a poor prognosis. It often accompanies systemic illness such as subacute bacterial endocarditis, SLE, periarteritis nodosa, severe Henoch–Schönlein purpura or Goodpasture's syndrome but they may be impossible to distinguish from a primary renal disorder. Treatment has usually been unsuccessful, although occasional patients make spontaneous recoveries, and both antilymphocyte antisera (ALG) and plasmapheresis have been used successfully in occasional cases and in those in whom a definite antibody to GBM can be established, either of these methods would appear logical.

Diffuse membrano-proliferative glomerulonephritis (*MPGN*) (mesangiocapillary glomerulonephritis: lobular glomerulonephritis)

Two apparently distinct pathological types have been described (Table 12.3) largely as a result of electron microscopic studies. Electron dense deposits are seen either in the subendothelial layer of the capillary wall or as nodular dense deposits within the middle layers of the glomerular basement membrane itself. Cellular proliferation is variable in both varieties, consisting usually of mesangial and endothelial cells, although epithelial cell crescents in Bowman's space may be present in association with the dense deposit lesions. In both types, immunofluorescent microscopy shows deposits of C3, in the peripheral capillary loops in the subendothelial variety and in the mesangial area in the dense deposit MPGN. Other complement factors $C1_q$ and C4 are found in about 50 per cent of those cases showing subendothelial deposits and IgG IgM or IgA are also frequent. In the dense deposit type, these immunological reactions are consistently absent, suggesting some fundamental differences in the mechanisms in the two groups.

The clinical pattern appears to be similar however, usually with a presentation of symptomless proteinuria, or the nephrotic syndrome. Microscopic haematuria appears constantly at some time, and marked exacerbations of these findings may occur immediately following an acute respiratory infection. The ultimate prognosis appears to be relatively poor, there is no response to steroid therapy, and hypertension often occurs. Those patients who remain normotensive may enjoy remarkably good health for long periods (Fig. 12.1) in spite of proteinuria and haematuria. It has also been observed that the dense deposit MPGN frequently recurs after renal transplantation (Habib et al, 1975).

The abnormalities of complement in this condition are important. The deposits in the glomerular capillaries of C3 and C4 have been described above, and in addition, serum levels of C3 are depressed, while C2, C1 and C4 are normal. A serum factor causing C3 conversion in normal serum, C3NeF and the presence of C3 degradation products are also seen. In dense deposit disease, these changes occur regularly whereas they are much more variable in the course of the disorder associated with subendothelial deposits (Habib et al, 1975). This evidence argues in favour of an immune-complex disease, affecting complement metabolism in several different ways, but there is, at present, little clue as to the nature of the precipitating antigens. Very similar lesions have been observed in association with infected ventriculo-atrial shunts (Moncrieff et al, 1973).

Focal proliferative glomerulonephritis

The essential feature of the various types of focal nephritis is the focal segmental lesion often affecting a few glomeruli only and involving only a part of the glomerular tuft. Electron microscopy usually indicates that the lesions are more extensive than can be seen by light microscopy and the abnormalities are nearly always diffuse on immunofluorescent microscopy.

The glomerular lesions show a combination of epithelial cell proliferation with capsular adhesions or mesangial cell proliferation. Epithelial crescents rarely occur. Electron microscopic evidence suggests that the cellular proliferation is mainly mesangial in origin and not, as originally described, due to endothelial cell proliferation (Churg and Grishman, 1975).

IgA deposits are found in the mesangial area throughout nearly all glomeruli in one group of cases of focal proliferative nephritis, whereas IgG and C3, although present, are less conspicuous. Cl_q and C4 have not been observed in this group. By contrast, other patients appear to have similar focal proliferative lesions, but IgA is not present, and the other immunoglobulins and complement factors have been variously reported (Table 12.3).

The clinical features appear to be the same in the groups with or without IgA deposits and consist of acute episodes of macroscopic haematuria usually occurring within 48 hours of the onset of an acute respiratory infection. Streptococcal infections are not involved and between attacks the urine may be normal. Persistent proteinuria, and more rarely, the nephrotic syndrome may occur. Serum complement factors and IgA levels are normal. The prognosis appears to be good in both adults and children.

Similar focal glomerular changes may be associated with a number of systemic disorders, of which SLE is the most important. IgA is however not usually present, and complement factors C3, C4, Cl_q and properdin are frequently present. The clinical pattern is also usually different but other serological tests for SLE (e.g. anti-DNA antibodies) may be the only method of distinguishing the nature of focal glomerulonephritis if immunofluorescent methods are not available after renal biopsy. Henoch–Schönlein purpura is also associated with focal proliferative lesions especially in adults (Ballard, Eisenger and Gallo, 1970). In children with this disorder diffuse proliferative glomerulonephritis appears to be the commonest lesion in the kidney when deposits of fibrinogen, IgG, IgA, and C3 are widespread.

Focal glomerulosclerosis (focal and segmental hyalinosis)

The typical lesion seen is shrinking or hyalinosis of small portions of the capillary loops with loss of glomerular structure. Electron microscopy reveals an increase of mesangial matrix which obliterates the capillary lumen. There is no cellular proliferation, and the abnormality is difficult to distinguish from the minimal lesions described above, especially in early cases. Further, the abnormality tends to start in the juxta-medullary glomeruli, so that superficial biopsies of outer cortex will not include any obvious lesions.

The condition may be of insidious onset with mild slight symptomless proteinuria, or may present with heavier protein loss and the nephrotic syndrome. In children, steroid resistance in a case of apparent minimal change nephritis often suggests the presence of focal glomerulosclerosis which may be confirmed on repeat biopsy or in the subsequent clinical courses. The proteinuria is generally less selective than in true minimal change lesions and this factor may be crucial in diagnosis (White, Glasgow and Mills, 1973). The course appears to be slowly progressive with the development of chronic renal failure. A recurrence of similar lesions has occurred in patients with this condition after renal transplantation. The difficulty in distinguishing early glomerulosclerosis from minimal change nephritis has naturally led to the speculation that the condition merely represents a progressive variant of that disorder, since little is known of the aetiology of either process. Careful serial studies by White et al (1973) and Habib et al (1973) suggest strongly that the focal sclerosis is a distinct entity, possibly unrelated to any immunological disorder.

The Clinical Significance of Morphological Classifications

The above descriptions and Table 12.4 show clearly the dangers of over-emphasising the detailed pathological findings in different manifestations of glomerulonephritis at the present time. Certain clinical syndromes are now recognised with definite, well defined pathological changes in the glomerulus which have often been followed for sufficiently long periods for a fairly accurate assessment of treatment response and prognosis to be made, although the time scale of improvement or deterioration still remains highly variable and difficult to assess. The correlation of histological changes in the kidney, with electron microscopy and particularly with fluorescent microscopy, has again allowed clearer definition of certain syndromes — e.g. IgA deposits in focal proliferative glomerulonephritis with recurrent haematuria. Further long-term studies are clearly necessary, but the study of 20 908 cases of renal disease at the Hospital Necker (Hamburger, 1975) and the numerous published individual series of patients based upon similar criteria, now present a formidable experience. Glomerulonephritis represents about 12 per cent of all cases of renal disease in Hamburger's experience, although progressive renal failure was due to nephritis in over 50 per cent. The precise frequency of the different types of glomerular lesion varies somewhat in different series and particularly in different parts of the world (Hutt and White, 1975).

Treatment in Glomerulonephritis

Regrettably little progress has been made in the past 25 years in the treatment of glomerulonephritis, although the indications for steroid and other immuno-suppressive therapy have been considerably clarified. General measures, such as the use of diuretics to control oedema and antibiotics to control the ever present dangers of infection in patients with low levels of immunoglobulin and other severe metabolic abnormalities of the nephrotic syndrome, remain as important as ever and must not be neglected in the excitement of attempting to pursue specific remedies. Similarly, the importance of replacing protein losses cannot be overemphasised when it is realised that a patient with the nephrotic syndrome may be losing up to 20 per cent of the total circulating albumin each day. High protein diets remain somewhat unpalatable and unacceptable both to patients and clinicians alike but have a vital place in treatment. The management of hypertension would also appear to be an important factor in the control of the effects of glomerulonephritis, although little real evidence is available that the course of the condition is thereby altered.

The individual disorders in which steroid or other immunosuppressive therapy has been shown to be effective have already been described and are depressingly few in properly controlled trials. The minimal change nephrotic syndrome in children and adults responds satisfactorily and some argument continues as to the relative merits and dangers of steroids or cyclophosphamide. The relapses seem to be better controlled with the latter, especially in children (Barratt et al, 1975), but the possible genetic side-effects are disturbing. Other immunosuppressive drugs have been less effective both in reducing the proteinuria and in affecting the long-term prognosis. Indomethacin has been shown to have a remarkable effect of reducing the proteinuria and urine FDP levels, but the effect is both variable and transitory.

Acute rapidly progressive nephritis has an extremely poor prognosis whether associated with systemic disease such as SLE, polyarteritis, Goodpasture's syndrome or in those patients with no obvious disturbances outside the kidney. Heparin and other anticoagulants have been used in association with steroids and with some success (Brown et al, 1974). In those patients with demonstrable antibasement membrane antibodies in the serum or with linear deposition of fluorescent IgG and complement on the basement membrane, repeated plasmapheresis or the use of specific antilymphocyte globulin has been used successfully to remove the antibody. These conditions are fortunately uncommon and insufficient experience is yet available to evaluate any treatment programme, but if the renal damage is directly mediated by antigen-antibody complexes, or by specific antiglomerular or antitubular antibodies, their removal from the circulation would appear desirable. Unfortunately measurements of serum levels of antibody are difficult and variable and the biopsy immunofluorescent pattern would appear to be the best guide to the choice of anticoagulants and immunosuppression or plasmapheresis.

In spite of treatment however many patients with glomerulonephritis show variable and extremely slow progress to renal failure. The European Dialysis and Transplantation Association reported in 1973 that 56 per cent of the 18 750 patients referred with renal failure were considered to have suffered from glomerulonephritis (Gurland et al, 1973) so even allowing for difficulties in diagnosis in terminal renal failure, this group of conditions remains responsible for considerable morbidity and mortality. For those who progress to renal failure, dialysis treatment presents no special difficulties not seen in any other type of renal failure, and considerable numbers of such patients are currently receiving home or hospital dialysis (Moorhead, 1975).

Renal transplantation was at one time considered to present greater problems in patients with glomerulonephritis because of the potential risk of recurrence of the nephritis in the grafted kidney. Certainly, the more rapidly progressive types of acute nephritis rarely achieve renal transplants, partly because of the high incidence of associated systemic disorders and partly because of the stormy clinical course, often with haemorrhages and severe hypertension so commonly encountered. The incidence of recurrent nephritis after renal transplantation in the more chronic types of glomerulonephritis appears to be surprisingly low, at about 2 per cent of all graft failures (Moorhead, 1975) as compared with 58 per cent failure from rejection. Difficulties in the diagnosis of rejection, both on clinical and renal biopsy evidence as well as the selection factor, may partly invalidate this figure, since a higher incidence of recurrences has been described in rapid progressive nephritis, and in membranoproliferative lesions, especially those associated with electron dense deposits. Hamburger et al (1973) reported recurrence in three patients with focal glomerulosclerosis after transplantation but as the majority of these conditions are very slowly progressive, the fact of occasional recurrence in itself is not a valid reason for refusing a reasonable match renal transplant in the present state of knowledge.

CONCLUSIONS

Considerable progress has been made in the understanding of glomerulo-nephritis since the widespread use of renal biopsy and of specific immunological studies. While the study of long-term clinical patterns will certainly clarify many of the problems of management and diagnosis, many more carefully controlled measurements of immune responses to known antigens, in both the normal population and in those suffering from glomerulonephritis, are required to understand the underlying mechanisms involved. It is already clear that glomerulonephritis occurs as an indirect, almost accidental response to a wide variety of conditions in which the formation of circulating protein complexes of appropriate size is the common factor. Further studies should clearly be devoted to examining the situations which give rise to these complexes and also the means of disposal of these proteins from the circulation by different individuals. This would at present appear to be the most important aspect of the curious and remarkable phenomenon, so typical of glomerulonephritis and other im-munological disorders, of persistence or recurrence of an inflammatory reaction for most of a human life span. Increased knowledge of the mechanism of injury of the glomerulus and the predicted immune response of an individual patient would also be valuable in the selection of suitable treatment, instead of the present rather ineffective and often dangerous use of steroids in the nephrotic syndrome of any cause. This type of information can only be obtained from human studies because of the great species differences in response to antigenic stimuli, and the past 20 years have seen highly encouraging advances in this direction.

REFERENCES

Adam, C., Morel-Maroger, L. & Richet, G. (1973) Cryoglobulins in glomerulonephritis not related to systemic disease. *Kidney International*, 3, 334–341.

Baldwin, D. S. (1974) Natural history of poststreptococcal glomerulonephritis. In *Proceedings of the Vth International Congress Nephrology*. Mexico 1972, pp. 36–60. Basel: Karger.

Ballard, H. S., Eisenger, R. P. & Gallo, G. (1970) Renal manifestations of the Henoch Schönlein syndrome in adults. *American Journal of Medicine*, 49, 328–335.

Barratt, T. M., Berkowsky, A., Osofsky, S. G., Soothill, J. F. & Kay, R. (1975) Cyclophosphamide treatment in steroid sensitive nephrotic syndrome of childhood. *Lancet*, i, 55–58.

Becker, E. L. (1968) *Structural Basis of Renal Disease*. New York: Harper, Row.

Bell, J. L. & Baron, D. N. (1968) Quantitative biuret determination of urine protein. *Proceedings of the Association of Clinical Biochemists*, 5, 63–64.

Black, D. A. K., Rose, G. & Brewer, D. B. (1970) Controlled trial of prednisone in adult patients with the nephrotic syndrome: *British Medical Journal*, 3, 421–426.

Blainey, J. D., Hardwicke, J. & Whitfield, A. G. W. (1954) The nephrotic syndrome associated with thrombosis of the renal veins. *Lancet*, ii, 1208–1211.

Blainey, J. D., Brewer, D. B., Hardwicke, J. & Soothill, J. F. (1960) The nephrotic syndrome, diagnosis by renal biopsy, biochemical and immunological analysis related to steroid therapy. *Quarterly Journal of Medicine*, 29, 235–256.

Blainey, J. D. (1975) Symptomless proteinuria. In *Advanced Medicine Symposium 11*, ed. Lant, A. F. pp. 317–321. London: Pitman.

Brewer, D. B. (1973) *Renal Biopsy*, 2nd edition. London: Arnold.

Brown, C. B., Turner, D., Ogg, C. S., Wilson, D., Cameron, J. S., Chantler, C. & Gill, D. (1974) Combined immunosuppression and anticoagulation in rapidly progressive glomerulonephritis. *Lancet*, ii, 1166–1171.

Cameron, J. S. (1975) A clinician's view of the classification of glomerulonephritis. In *Glomerulonephritis*, ed. Kincaid-Smith, P., Mathew, T. H. and Becker, E. L. pp. 63–79. New York: Wiley.

Cameron, J. S. & Blanford, G. (1966) The simple assessment of selectivity in heavy proteinuria. *Lancet*, ii, 242–247.

Cameron, J. S., Ogg, C. S. & White, R. H. R. (1973) Observations in the minimal change lesions. In *Glomerulonephritis*, ed. Kincaid-Smith, P., Mathew, T. H. and Becker, E. L. pp. 211–216. New York: Wiley.

Cameron, J. S., Vick, R. M., Ogg, C. S., Seymour, W. M., Chantler, C. & Turner, D. R. (1973) Plasma C3 and C4 concentrations in management of glomerulonephritis. *British Medical Journal*, 3, 668–672.

Cameron, J. S., Turner, D. R., Ogg, C. S., Sharpstone, P. & Brown, C. B. (1974) The nephrotic syndrome in adults with minimal change glomerular lesions. *Quarterly Journal of Medicine*, New Series, 43, 461–488.

Churg, J. & Grishman, E. (1975) Ultrastructure of glomerular disease: a review. *Kidney International*, 7, 254–270.

Dardenne, M., Zabriskie, J. & Bach, J. F. (1972) Streptococcal sensitivity in chronic glomerulonephritis. *Lancet*, i, 126–127.

Ekert, H., Barratt, T. M., Chantler, T. & Turner, M. W. (1972) Immunologically reactive equivalents of fibrinogen in sera and urine of children with renal disease. *Archives of Disease in Childhood*, 47, 90–96.

Fairley, K. F., Barrie, J. U. & Johnson, W. (1972) Sterility in testicular atrophy related to cyclophosphamide therapy. *Lancet*, i, 566–570.

Germuth, F. G. & Rodriguez, E. (1973) *Immunopathology of the Renal Glomerulus.* Boston: Little Brown.

Gurland, H. J., Brunner, F. P., Van Dehn, H., Harlen, H., Parsons, F. M. & Schare, K. (1973) Combined report on regular dialysis and transplantation in Europe III. *Proceedings of the European Dialysis and Transplantation Association*, 10, pp. XVII–LVII. London: Pitman Medical.

Habib, R. & Kleinknecht, C. (1971) The primary nephrotic syndrome of childhood. Classification and clinicopathological study of 406 cases. In *Pathology Annual*, ed. Sommers, S. S. pp. 417–474. New York: Appleton Century Crofts.

Habib, R., Kleinknecht, C., Gulder, M. C. & Levy, M. (1973) Idiopathic membranoproliferative glomerulonephritis in children — report of 105 cases. *Clinical Nephrology*, 1, 194–214.

Habib, R., Gubler, M. C., Loirat, C., Maiz, H. B. & Levy, M. (1975) Dense deposit disease: a variant of membranoproliferative glomerulonephritis. *Kidney International*, 7, 204–215.

Hall, C. L., Pejhan, N., Terry, J. M. & Blainey, J. D. (1975) Urinary fibrin-fibrinogen degradation products in nephrotic syndrome. *British Medical Journal*, 1, 419–422.

Hamburger, J., Berger, J., Hinglais, N. & Descamps, B. (1973) New insights into the pathogenesis of glomerulonephritis afforded by a study of renal allografts. *Clinical Nephrology*, 1, 1–7.

Hamburger, J. (1975) Classification of nephropathies with some remarks on the various types of glomerulonephritis, VI International Congress of Nephrology. *Abstracts of Symposia*, pp. 13–14. Florence.

Hardwicke, J. (1965) Estimation of renal permeability to proteins on Sephadex G200. *Clinica Chimica Acta*, 12, 89–96.

Hardwicke, J., Blainey, J. D., Brewer, D. B. & Soothill, J. F. (1966) The nephrotic syndrome. In *Proceedings 3rd International Congress Nephrology*, ed. Washington, Vol. 3, pp. 69–82. Basel: Karger.

Heptinstall, R. H. (1973) *Pathology of the Kidney*, 2nd edition. Boston: Little Brown.

Hutt, M. S. R. & White, R. H. R. (1975) Geographical aspects of glomerulonephritis. In *Recent Advances in Renal Disease*, ed. Jones, N. F. pp. 119–135. Edinburgh: Churchill Livingstone.

Jennings, R. B. & Earle, D. P. (1961) Poststreptococcal glomerulonephritis: histopathologic studies of the acute, subsiding acute and early chronic latent phases. *Journal of Clinical Investigation*, 46, 1525–1557.

Koeffler, D., Agnello, V., Carr, R. T. & Kunkel, H. G. (1969) Variable patterns of immunoglobulin and complement deposition on the kidneys with systemic lupus erythematosus. *American Journal of Pathology*, 56, 305–316.

Lewy, J. E., Salinas-Madrigal, L., Herdson, P. B., Pirani, C. L. & Metcoff, J. (1971) Clinicopathologic correlations in acute poststreptococcal glomerulonephritis. *Medicine*, 50, 453–501.

Mancini, G., Carbonara, A. O. & Heremans, J. F. (1965) Immunochemical quantitations of antigens by single radial immunodiffusion. *Immunochemistry*, 2, 235–254.

McCluskey, R. T. & Baldwin, D. S. (1963) Natural history of acute glomerulonephritis. *American Journal of Medicine*, 35, 213–230.

Merskey, C., Lalezari, P. & Johnson, A. J. (1969) A rapid simple sensitive method for measuring fibrinolytic split products in human serum. *Proceedings of the Society of Experimental Biology and Medicine*, 131, 871–875.

Moncrieff, M. N., Glasgow, E. F., Arthur, L. J. H. & Hargreaves, H. M. (1973) Glomerulonephritis associated with *Staphylococcus albus* in a Spitz-Holter Valve. *Archives of Diseases of Childhood*, 48, 69–72.

Moorhead, J. F. (1975) Chronic renal failure. In *Recent Advances in Renal Disease*, ed. Jones, N. F. pp. 138–151. Edinburgh: Churchill Livingstone.

Morel-Maroger, L. J. & Verroust, P. J. (1975) Clinicopathological correlations in glomerular disease. In *Recent Advances in Renal Disease*, ed. Jones, N. F., pp. 48–85. Edinburgh: Churchill Livingstone.

Ozawa, T., Pluss, R., Lacher, J., Boedecker, E., Guggenheim, W. H. & McIntosh, R. (1975) Endogenous immune complex nephropathy associated with malignancy I. *Quarterly Journal of Medicine*, New Series, 44, 523–541.

Peters, D. K. & Williams, D. G. (1975) Pathogenetic mechanisms of glomerulonephritis. In *Recent Advances in Renal Disease*, ed. Jones, N. F. pp. 90–118. Edinburgh: Churchill Livingstone.

Pollak, V. E. & Pirani, C. L. (1974) Pathology of the kidney in systemic lupus erythematosus, serial biopsy studies and the effect of therapy. In *Lupus Erythematosus*, ed. Dubois, E. L. 2nd edition. University of California Press.

Richet, G., Chevet, D. & Morel-Maroger, L. (1973) Serial biopsies in diffuse proliferative glomerulonephritis in adults. In *Glomerulonephritis*, ed. Kincaid-Smith et al, pp. 363–381. New York: Wiley.

Rosen, S. (1971) Membranous glomerulonephritis: current status. *Human Pathology*, 2, 209–231.

Rosenman, E., Pollak, V. E. & Pirani, C. L. (1968) Renal vein thrombosis: a clinical and pathological study based on renal biopsies. *Medicine*, Baltimore, 47, 269–335.

Row, P. G., Cameron, J. S., Turner, D., Evans, D. J., White, R. H. R., Ogg, C. S., Chantler, C. & Brown, C. B. (1975) Membranous nephropathy. *Quarterly Journal of Medicine*, New Series, 44, 207–239.

Soothill, J. F. (1962) The estimation of eight serum proteins by a gel diffusion precipitin technique. *Journal of Laboratory and Clinical Medicine*, 59, 859–870.

Soothill, J. F. & Steward, M. W. (1971) The immunopathological significance of the hetero-geneity of antibody affinity. *Clinical and Experimental Immunology*, 9, 193–199.

Wheeler, J., Holland, J., Menzies, S. & Blainey, J. D. (1975) Immunological response to glomerular basement membrane and streptococcal antigens in immunised rabbits. *Immunology*, 28, 653–658.

White, R. H. R., Glasgow, E. F. & Mills, R. J. (1973) Focal glomerulosclerosis in childhood. In *Glomerulonephritis*, ed. Kincaid-Smith et al, pp. 231–248. New York: Wiley.

Williams, D. G., Kourilsky, O., Morel-Maroger, L. & Peters, D. K. (1972) C3 breakdown by serum from patients with acute poststreptococcal nephritis, *Lancet*, ii, 260–361.

Wilson, C. B. & Dixon, F. J. (1975) Immunopathological mechanisms of renal disease. *La Ricerca in Clinica laboratorio*, 5, 17–38.

Zabriskie, J. B. (1971) The role of streptococci in human glomerulonephritis. *Journal of Experimental Medicine*, 134, 180_s–192_s.

13
ACCLIMATISATION TO HEAT AND COLD IN MAN

R. Goldsmith

Since the experiments of Blagden (1775), in which subjects were exposed to heat in a brick kiln, studies of man's responses to hot (and cold) climates have continued with enthusiasm, if not with the same degree of imagination and wonderment.

In spite of the colonisation of the tropics by Europeans, ideas about acclimatisation became sunk in a morass of prejudice typified by the flannel binder and cholera belt, worn until very recently by British soldiers (Renbourn, 1957), and the solar topi (Renbourn, 1972) — the status symbol of the tropics. More rigorous studies of acclimatisation of man to extreme environments were spurred on during the 1939–45 war, when men were shipped from equator to Arctic circle and expected to function efficiently on arrival at their new destination. Under these circumstances, the physiological responses and changes brought about by living in extreme climates became of paramount interest. Such studies led to the interesting conclusions that acclimatisation to heat occurred in about 10 days (Macpherson, 1960), and that it was typified by the ability to work in the heat with a lower pulse rate, a lower body temperature and a higher sweat rate — that is, a decreased strain in the face of continuing environmental stress. Arguments persisted as to other effects of acclimatisation, such as changes in blood volume, alterations in peripheral blood flow or endocrine balance (Collins and Weiner, 1968; Rowell, 1974).

Rather less precise evidence was available in man for acclimatisation to cold. Among the factors considered were alterations in heat production, calorie intake, hormone activity, body insulation and vasomotor control, as well as many others (Burton and Edholm, 1955). There was much evidence for acclimatisation to cold in all sorts of animals and there were suggestions that some of these findings could be extrapolated to man. Was not the short tail, found in rats bred in the cold, an example of Bergman's Law? Was not the short squat Eskimo just another example to join the short-tailed rat, ideally suited to the cold, while the elegant long limbs of the Nilhotic people were equivalent to the tails of rats or big ears of pigs bred in hot climates? It is of interest to note that in the book *Man in a Cold Environment* (Burton and Edholm, 1955), of 32 pages devoted to acclimatisation to cold, 15 are about animal experiments!

The last few years have seen a rebirth of interest in various aspects of acclimatisation and some progress in elucidating the nature of changes has been made. The motivations for this renaissance of interest have stemmed largely from military requirements, although growing industrialisation in tropical and polar regions, the settling of desert regions in the Middle East, and the quest for gold in South Africa leading to ever deeper mines have also played their part. The interest sparked off by the International Geophysical Year, and continued since in research in the Antarctic, the development of the Arctic and the adoption by the Human Adaptability Section of the International Biological Program for special study of the circumpolar people have all acted as spurs for the study of acclimatisation to cold (Edholm and Gunderson, 1973).

It is not the purpose of this chapter to review comprehensively all the work that has been published in the last 10–15 years, but rather to present the results from selected studies with a view to suggesting hypotheses to explain observed phenomena. Extensive reviews of various aspects of temperature regulation and acclimatisation may be found in the Annual Review of Physiology (Hammel, 1968; Chafee and Roberts, 1971; Wyndham, 1973) and in more specialised publications (Edholm and Bacharach, 1965; Edholm and Gunderson, 1973; Gunderson, 1974).

DEFINITIONS

What is acclimatisation? How is it related to adaptation, acclimation, or habituation? Hart (1957) defined these in temporal terms; he defined acclimatisation as 'those changes in the responses of an organism produced by continued alterations in the environment', acclimation as 'those changes in a lifetime', and adaptation as 'those occurring during a period of several generations'. The questions that arise from these definitions include: are there, indeed, changes occurring in man over several generations; what environmental factors bring about changes; and do the changes confer an advantage on the organism or may changes that are disadvantageous also be considered under these categories? The imprecision is even more pronounced in defining heat acclimatisation; as a result of work carried out in the United States and elsewhere, acclimatisation to heat was defined as the improved ability to work in the heat (see, for instance, Bass et al, 1955). Thus, the ability to work with minimal strain, i.e. physical fitness, was confused with the ability to control body temperature. For the sake of clarity, it would be logical to adopt a general definition that would be suitable both for cold and hot climates (Eide, 1973).

Extreme climates impose their stresses on man by altering heat balance. The resulting strain is either a gain or loss of body heat, resulting in loss of local or eventually of vital functions and finally endangering survival itself.

Man responds to repeated exposure to a climatic stimulus in a number of ways: most importantly, he does so with his intellect and, as we shall see, this may indeed obviate the need for any other alterations in his responses. These are *behavioural changes* and may be typified by the wearing of specialised clothes or the building of shelter which prevents or minimises exposure to extremes; or the rather less dramatic but often observed reluctance to work in the heat — the lazy native — or the fact that exposure to extreme climates is often related to high energy expenditure (Goldsmith and Hampton, 1967).

Exposure to extreme climates may induce changes in the perception of and responses to sensory stimuli. For instance, the pain of immersing a hand in cold water may disappear if the subject can be persuaded to expose himself to this unpleasant stimulus sufficiently often; the pressor response may also disappear (Eide, 1965). It has frequently been shown that the temperature at which the majority of people are comfortable in a particular situation varies according to the prevailing climate — lower in cold climates and higher in the warm (Adam, 1959; Goldsmith, 1960; Palmai, 1962; Webb, 1964; Lugg, 1965; Nicol, 1974). These findings may be another example of *habituation* — feeling comfortable at skin temperatures previously rated as uncomfortable.

Having discussed behavioural changes and habituation, the remaining physiological changes are ascribed to acclimatisation. Acclimatisation might therefore be defined as the enhanced ability to maintain function in the face of climatic stress (Budd, 1964). The enhancement results from alterations in physiological responses and is often characterised by an improved ability to maintain local or central temperature.

The time courses of the changes may vary so that chronic and acutely acclimatised men may have different responses (Edholm et al, 1964a).

Adaptation is generally reserved either to embrace all changes or to characterise responses that are genetically based. There is as yet very little evidence that there are genetically based physiological responses which endow those who have lived for many generations in extreme climates with a unique survival advantage in the face of climatic stresses. There is little doubt, however, that morphological features have been subject to natural selection, producing people of different build in different climates (Hiernaux, Rudan and Brambati, 1975) which may lead to improved thermoregulation.

ACCLIMATISATION TO HEAT

The Questions

It has been known for a long time that working in the heat results in acclimatisation. During the first exposure to a hot climate, coupled with work, the subject becomes hot and distressed and may, if the exercise is violent enough or the heat stress sufficiently intense, collapse. If exposure is repeated daily, the distress is alleviated and, after a few days, the subject is able to complete a task with relative ease and less discomfort. The physiological findings accompanying these changes in comfort and performance are a reduction in central body temperature and pulse rate and an increase in sweat rate. Other changes, such as a reduction in the sodium and chloride content of sweat (Allan and Wilson, 1971) and changes in plasma volume, have from time to time been noted. The first question that arises is: which are the primary adaptive changes and which merely the sequelae?

As soon as experimenters examined the indigenes of hot countries, the following paradox emerged: people living in hot climates and being natives of those climates generally showed a lack of the classical signs of acclimatisation when they were subjected to tests of working in the heat. This finding has been amply confirmed (Wyndham, Macpherson and Munro, 1964; Wyndham, Metz and Munro, 1964; Wyndham et al, 1964a and b; Fox et al, 1974). How was it then that the work that those natives did in their hot climate did not lead to acclimatisation?

In the early 1960s, when the British Army was withdrawing from its tropical stations, the question arose as to whether it was possible to prepare troops for service in hot countries by artificially acclimatising them at home (Edholm et al, 1962 and 1963). The same sort of question had already been asked by the South African Chamber of Mines about their migrant workers in gold mines. The high incidence of heat illnesses among workers who worked for only six months in the mines before returning to their homes was alarming and expensive (Wyndham, 1965 and 1966). Could artificial heat acclimatisation be carried out before sending these men into the mines? Would heat acclimatisation prevent or reduce casualties resulting from heat illnesses? What would be the most effective method for acclimatising such large numbers of men? The establishment of the Human Adaptability (HA) Section of the International Biological Program (Weiner and Lourie, 1969) revived the question of genetic factors in acclimatisation. Are the races who have lived in the tropics for generations able to withstand heat or control body temperature more efficiently than temperate dwellers? These unanswered queries reopened the assault upon the fundamental problems of heat acclimatisation.

Artificial Acclimatisation

The results of an extensive field and laboratory experiment were reported in 1962, in which the performance in the heat of three groups of soldiers was compared; one artificially acclimatised, one naturally acclimatised, and the last unacclimatised (Edholm et al, 1962). The experimenters set out to obtain answers to the following questions: does artificial acclimatisation confer benefits equal to those of natural acclimatisation? Do naturally or artificially acclimatised troops perform better than the unacclimatised in a simulated battle situation in a hot climate? The experiment failed to produce conclusive answers. The results suggested that there were other factors, such as intelligence, morale and leadership, that almost outweighed the physiological advantages attributable to acclimatisation. However, it was clearly demonstrated that artificial acclimatisation, brought about by a series of daily four-hour exposures to working in the heat, conferred a physiological benefit on the subjects greater than that acquired by natural acclimatisation. The natural acclimatisation had been achieved by the men pursuing a pattern of military training for seven weeks in the same hot climate as that in which the field trial was held. Paradoxically, it also demonstrated that the unacclimatised men, who had done their military training in the cool climate of Scotland, had also acquired some degree of heat acclimatisation. The acclimatisation status of the three groups was assessed at the beginning of the experiment, after their acclimatisation period, and at the end of the experiment by measuring their physiological responses over a four-hour exposure in a hot climate (dry bulb temperature 40°C, relative humidity 57 per cent), during which they worked for two hours and rested for two. On the first occasion, the three groups had similar responses, on the second all had improved, i.e. higher sweat rates, lower pulse rates and body temperature; the artificially

acclimatised were significantly more acclimatised than the naturally acclimatised subjects, who in turn showed a greater degree of acclimatisation than the
so-called unacclimatised. At the end of the field trial no differences remained.
However, it was noted that pulse rate changes were not always related to sweat
rates and temperature levels. It was suggested that physical training could be in
part distinguished from heat acclimatisation.

On a practical level, one of the more important conclusions was that the
discomfort of artificial acclimatisation drained the morale both of soldiers and of
experimenters. If artificial acclimatisation was to become a practical proposition
for such groups, then it was wise to look for other methods. In addition, it was
concluded that if heat acclimatisation was to be studied then its effects must be
separated from those of physical training.

Meanwhile, the position was rather different in the gold mines, where artificial
acclimatisation had been practised for some time and where the social climate
and the motivation of the subjects were different. Here, the procedure of
acclimatisation was standardised and performed above ground (Wyndham,
1965), consisting basically of routines of work and rest in a hot humid climate
simulating the real situation. This made it possible to reduce the period of
acclimatisation from 12 to 8 days without reducing efficiency. The net result was
that heat casualties were drastically reduced, to everyone's benefit. The artificial
acclimatisation of over 250 000 men working in the gold mines (Wyndham and
Strydom, 1969) is perhaps the most successful application to date of physiology
applied to an industrial problem and, in the wake of this achievement, much has
been learned about both the practice and theory of acclimatisation.

Controlled hyperthermia

A technique was evolved in which the work which was thought to be producing
cardiovascular and locomotor training effects (Astrand and Rodahl, 1970) was
separated from acclimatisation. The procedure of controlled hyperthermia (Fox
et al, 1963a) was designed to investigate the nature of acclimatisation to heat and,
at the same time, to suggest practical alternative methods for use in artificial
acclimatisation, so decreasing the discomfort of the subjects and easing the
burden of the experimenters.

In this technique, body temperature is artificially elevated and controlled by
changes in evaporative cooling; the duration of the hyperthermia may be
extended as required. The essential difference between this technique and either
the natural situation or that used heretofore in the laboratory is that the stimulus
to acclimatisation, the elevated body temperature, is held constant throughout
each exposure and from exposure to exposure; whereas in other situations the
body temperature rises throughout each exposure and, on average, falls from one
exposure to the next. The technique of controlled hyperthermia obviates the
need for accurate climatic control, thus making the whole process simpler and
cheaper. Acclimatisation can be carried out without the use of an elaborate
climatic chamber and the process studied under almost ideal controlled
conditions.

The technique of controlled hyperthermia has been refined and adapted in a
number of ways (Allan, Crowdy and Haisman, 1965; Crowdy and Haisman,

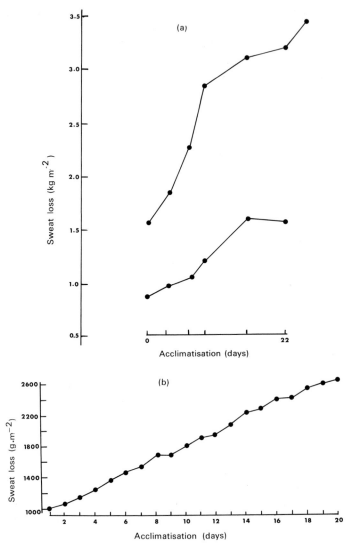

Figure 13.1 (a) The almost exponential change in sweat loss of two subjects tested in six standard four-hour work-in-the-heat tests. The subjects were acclimatised between tests in 16 daily exposures to similar four-hour work-in-the-heat tests. (Reproduced, with permission, from Edholm et al, 1962, *Medical Research Council Report*, **61/827**, 61). (b) The linear change in mean sweat loss of two subjects during 20 daily three-hour controlled hyperthermia sessions — body temperature controlled at 38.5°C. (Reproduced, with permission, from Fox, R. H., 1974, *Heat Loss from Animals and Man*, 286)

1966; Allan and Wilson, 1971; Turk, 1971; Henane and Valatx, 1973; Turk and Worsley, 1974). In the most sophisticated technique, the subject wears an all-enveloping vapour barrier suit and lies on a bed. Body temperature is raised and controlled by covering the subject with an insulating layer and circulating hot air around him at a variable rate and temperature. Control of body temperature is achieved by varying both the volume and temperature of the circulating air, using the convective avenue of heat exchange (Fox et al, 1974). In the original method, body temperature was controlled by evaporative cooling by regulating the supply of dry air to the inside of a vapour barrier suit. Modification

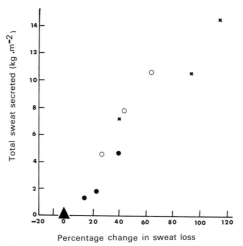

Figure 13.2 The linear ($r = 0.94$) relation between total volume of sweat secreted during acclimatisation by controlled hyperthermia and the percentage increase in sweat loss in standard work-in-the-heat tests. There were nine groups of subjects: the triangular symbol represents the results from untreated controls. Subjects' sweat loss was compared in two-hour work-in-the-heat tests before and after a series of hyperthermia sessions. Between the two tests, the subjects were exposed to 12 consecutive daily hyperthermia sessions of three durations ($\frac{1}{2}$, 1 and 2 hours) and at three levels of controlled body temperature ($\times = 38.5°C$, $\bigcirc = 37.9°C$, $\bullet = 37.3°C$). (Reproduced, with permission, from Fox et al, 1963a, *Journal of Physiology*, **166**, 541)

of the technique has made it possible to measure sweat rate continuously by pumping sweat from the suit, to monitor body temperature at the onset of sweating, and to measure blood flow through the hand or forearm by venous occlusion plethysmography. Most of the variations place the subjects in a hot-wet environment in which hidromeiosis (the reduction in sweating associated with wetting of the skin) is maximised; these methods have been used successfully on both men and women (Fox and Löfsted, 1968; Fox et al, 1969; Bittel and Henane, 1975) and even on rather unsophisticated villagers in New Guinea (Fox et al, 1974).

Sweat capacity
　　The first experiments, using the controlled hyperthermia technique to achieve acclimatisation, showed that the benefits conferred were similar to those using the work-in-the-heat routine (Fox et al, 1963a). If performance was tested by

making men work in the heat before and after a series of exposures, it was found that their abilities to work in the heat had improved, their sweat rates were enhanced and their body temperatures and pulse rates were lower. In all respects, acclimatisation using controlled hyperthermia and work-in-the-heat routines were similar.

When physiological changes during controlled hyperthermia sessions were examined, a rather different picture evolved. Sweat rate rose session by session in an almost linear fashion (Fig. 13.1). Heart rate did not fall and, in those subjects exposed to a high body temperature (37.9°C and 38.5°C), heart rate was higher during the last exposure than it had been in the first. The subjects did not get used to having their body temperatures raised; in fact, the degree of discomfort and irritability seemed to increase rather than decrease. These findings, contrasting with those during repeated work-in-the-heat sessions, may be interpreted as being either primary adaptive or secondary. The primary change is the improved capacity to produce sweat and it was shown to be related to the total amount of sweat secreted. Thus, the concept of sweat gland training evolved (Fig. 13.2).

Further experiments were performed in an attempt to establish the validity of the hypothesis that sweat glands were trained by being made to sweat. It was suggested that if training were a local phenomenon and not due to an increased central drive, inhibiting sweating while raising body temperature should not lead to an increase in the capacity to sweat. On the other hand, stimulating local sweating (without raising central temperature) should lead to enhancement of sweating capacity. (In this context, it is interesting to note that men working on open-hearth furnaces, habitually exposing only one side of their bodies to the intense radiant heat, sometimes complain of excessive sweating of that side of their body.) A number of groups of workers tackled the problem (Fox et al, 1962; Brebner and Kerslake, 1963; Collins, Crockford and Weiner, 1963; Fox et al, 1964); they used different approaches but arrived at the same conclusion. Collins et al (1963) used intradermal injections of mecholyl to 'train' sweat glands and demonstrated that the volume of sweat secreted, resulting from a standard injection, rose following a series of daily injections. Brebner and Kerslake (1963) used presoaking as a method of suppressing sweating and showed that, if subjects were exposed to a series of heat stresses after sweating had been suppressed by presoaking in fresh water, no improvement in sweating capacity occurred. In other words, acclimatisation was prevented by inhibiting the sweating response. Fox and his group (1962) used local heating and cooling of one arm to inhibit or enhance local sweating (Fig. 13.3). They were able to suppress sweating in one arm by cooling it, while the subjects were acclimatised by a series of controlled hyperthermia sessions (Fig. 13.3a). At the conclusion of the acclimatisation period, the sweating capacity of the arms was compared during a further hyperthermia session. The arm that had been cooled had not improved its ability to sweat; on the contrary, when one arm was heated and extra sweating induced, its ability to sweat was enhanced (Fig. 13.3b). Furthermore, it was found possible to improve the sweating capacity of one arm merely by daily immersions in water at 43°C without raising central body temperature at all (Fig. 13.3c). In a further series of experiments, it was shown that, if subjects were pretreated with atropine to inhibit sweating before being subjected to repeated controlled hyperthermia, improvement in the capacity to sweat was also reduced compared with that of untreated controls (Goldsmith, Fox and Hampton, 1967).

The results from one series of experiments (Fox et al, 1967), however, failed to support the hypothesis that improvement in sweating capacity is always related to sweat production. In these experiments, a comparison was made of the acclimatisation effect of controlled hyperthermia in a hot-wet and a hot-dry climate; there were, therefore, hot-dry and hot-wet subjects (Fig. 13.4). The hot-wet situation was the conventional one in which the body temperature was

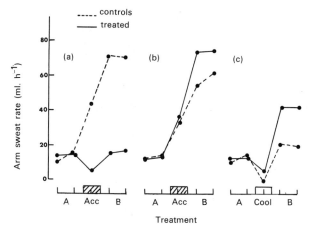

Figure 13.3 Arm sweat rates of three groups of subjects (a), (b) and (c) before (A) and after (B) a period of treatment (Acc. and Cool). The four tests (As and Bs) were identical, consisting of two hours of controlled hyperthermia (body temperature 38.5°C), with the arms enclosed in impervious bags, as they were in all experiments. During period Acc., the subjects were exposed to 15 daily two-hour periods of controlled hyperthermia (37.9°C); the subjects in (c) just sat in a cool room for two hours in the 15 daily sessions (Cool) during these periods. Treated arms were immersed in water — (a) 13°C, (b) and (c) 43°C. Note that in comparing results in (As) and (Bs) in (a), there was no change in the sweat rates of the treated arms, in (c) no change in the controls and all other arms had increased rates. In comparing sweat rates in tests B, in (a) controls had a higher rate and in (b) and (c) rates of treated arms were higher. (Reproduced, with permission, from Fox et al, 1964, *Journal of Physiology*, **171**, 373)

controlled by variable evaporative heat loss. The subjects sat during the acclimatisation period, dressed in all-enveloping vapour barrier suits. The microclimate within the suits was warm and saturated with water vapour and the skin of the subjects wetted throughout each exposure. Body temperature in the hot-dry situation was controlled by variable radiative and convective heat exchange. The hot-dry subjects sat naked in a hot (45–50°C), dry (relative humidity 15–20 per cent) and windy (12 m·s⁻¹) climatic wind-tunnel with their skin remaining totally dry throughout each exposure. An added refinement was that one arm of each hot-dry subject was encased in an impervious bag, so that one area of their body was subjected to a hot-wet climate while the rest was in a hot-dry climate.

As expected, the hot-dry subjects did indeed lose more sweat during the acclimatisation period but, when they were all tested in the conventional hot-wet controlled hyperthermia situation, there was no difference in sweat capacity between the two groups. The authors hypothesised that local training of sweat glands resulted from the metabolic activity of sweat glands, which may be unaffected by the hidromeiosis (Hertig, Riedesel and Belding, 1961; Collins and Weiner, 1962; Brebner and Kerslake, 1964; Brown and Sargent, 1965; Kerslake, 1972; Gonzalez, Pandolf and Gagge, 1974). Hidromeiosis is particularly marked in hot-wet conditions and it has been suggested, although not proven (Dobson, 1962), that it may result from a reabsorption of secreted sweat, causing swelling and blocking of ducts. However, the blocking may not lead to a cessation of the activity of the gland. Fox and his colleagues (1967) demonstrated that

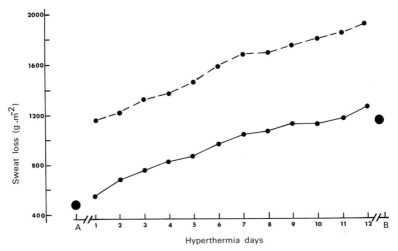

Figure 13.4   Comparison of sweat losses of two groups of subjects acclimatised by being exposed to 12 daily sessions of hyperthermia (body temperature 38.5°C) under hot-wet (solid line) and hot-dry (broken line) conditions. In standard hyperthermia tests in hot-wet conditions (large dots, A and B), sweat loss of the two groups was similar both before and after acclimatisation. (Reproduced, with permission, from Fox et al, 1967, *Journal of Applied Physiology*, **22**, 43)

hidromeiosis also occurred, though less dramatically, in a hot-dry climate and showed that it was reduced by acclimatisation, whether achieved by exposure to hot-wet or hot-dry conditions. Furthermore, they were able to point out an interesting difference between the acclimatisation effects of the two conditions: the hot-wet acclimatised arms showed less hidromeiosis than the hot-dry (Fig. 13.5). How this effect is caused is not clear, although they suggested that maceration of the skin of the hot-wet arms during acclimatisation, leading to partial desquamation, may have played its part. This finding led the authors to suggest that 'this difference between acclimatisation in the two climates could be important in determining subjects' subsequent tolerance to prolonged hot-humid conditions'.

Blood flow

The interpretation of changes in peripheral blood flow resulting from acclimatisation had been rendered difficult by the problem of making measurements against a shifting base line of body temperature. Most measurements had been made in the work-in-the-heat situation in which the body temperature falls from one exposure to the next, while rising within each exposure. Results were conflicting, showing either no change or a decrease due to acclimatisation (see, for instance, Wyndham, 1951; Hellon and Lind, 1955; Whittow, 1961). A comparison of peripheral blood flow before and after acclimatisation using controlled hyperthermia was made, during which blood flows through the hand, forearm, and the skin of the ear and chest were measured (Fox et al, 1963b). The results showed that flow in all these areas was higher after acclimatisation when

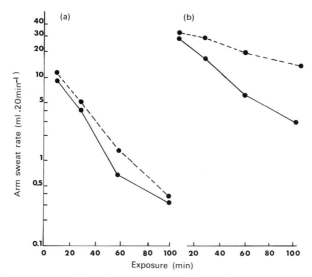

Figure 13.5 Hidromeiosis in differently treated arms of five subjects, showing decline in sweat rate (a) before and (b) after acclimatisation. Sweat rates were measured in standard hot-wet conditions during two hours of controlled hyperthermia (body temperature 38.2°C), before and after acclimatisation. One arm of each subject was acclimatised in hot-wet conditions (broken line), the other in hot-dry (solid line). Note that hidromeiosis declines in both arms as a result of acclimatisation, but more so in the hot-wet acclimatised arms. (Reproduced, with permission, from Fox et al, 1967, *Journal of Applied Physiology*, **22**, 45)

body temperature was elevated. There was some evidence that even at 'normal' temperature forearm blood flow was higher following acclimatisation.

While the increase in blood flow is small (between 10 and 30 per cent) compared with the increase of sweating capacity, it falls into the category of a true acclimatisation phenomenon; it undoubtedly helps to transfer heat from the centre to the periphery, tending to maintain central temperature at a level closer to 'normal' in the face of heat stress.

Central temperature

Many workers have demonstrated that central body temperature measured at rest in a cool climate is lower after heat acclimatisation than before. The mechanisms for the fall are not clear, but it is interesting to speculate whether they may be connected with changes in plasma osmolarity (Senay, 1972; Snellen,

1972; Harrison, 1974; Nielsen, 1974; Harrison, 1975), or with an increase in skin blood flow (Fox et al, 1963). It has been shown (Edholm et al, 1964b; Fox et al, 1966) that the lower temperature is as evident at night with the subject asleep as during the activity of the day, making it unlikely that the lowered body temperature results only from a greater sensitivity of the thermoregulatory mechanisms. Furthermore, the drop in resting body temperature is related to a fall in the body temperature at which sweating is induced, leading to the suggestion that there may be a downward resetting of the set-point temperature (Fox et al, 1963) comparable to the upward resetting during fever. Such a depression of the set-point for temperature elimination would do much to maintain central body temperature at a 'normal' level.

Conclusions

At the beginning of this section, certain questions were posed; the results of the experimental work described suggest some answers.

The changes brought about by acclimatisation may now be classified into primary adaptive and secondary. Among the primary changes are an increased sweating capacity, a higher blood flow through the skin and a fall in resting body temperature. It is suggested that the first may occur as a result of local training of sweat glands, leading to an increased secretion in response to the same central drive, i.e. the same elevation of central temperature. The typical signs and symptoms of acclimatisation, viz. lower heart rate and body temperature and increased comfort, which are so obvious during work, are secondary. Indeed, if body temperature is not allowed to fall then heart rate will be higher and discomfort greater after acclimatisation than before.

Is it possible to acclimatise men artificially in a practical way? The answer undoubtedly is yes. The use of controlled hyperthermia makes the process more acceptable and faster. What is more, if training of the cardiovascular and locomotor system is also desirable, the technique of controlled hyperthermia may be modified so that control of body temperature is achieved by varying the rate of work in a hot climate. This has proved to be a very successful technique for acclimatising large numbers of more or less reluctant troops quickly, efficiently, and with relatively cheap plant. The rather more tedious work-in-the-heat routine takes longer but is, under certain circumstances, very effective, especially as it induces physical conditioning in addition to acclimatisation. In fact, acclimatisation may be achieved by simply taking physical exercise sufficient to cause sweating (Marcus, 1972; Shvartz, Magazanik and Glick, 1974), with the curious consequence that working in the cold may result in heat acclimatisation (Wilkins, 1973).

It is also possible to shed light on the paradox of the unacclimatised native. It seems that the stimulus for acclimatisation is sweating or the activation of sweat glands. If sweating is avoided, then no acclimatisation will ensue. It is at least permissible to speculate that those well adapted to living in hot climates reduce their heat exposure and their energy expenditure to a minimum, resulting in minimal stress and minimal strain. It is only the bustling temperate zone dwellers, who in their native climate must work hard to keep warm, who bring this unwarranted energy to the tropics; they sweat and thus acclimatise. As industrialisation of the developing countries proceeds, replacing self-paced with machine-paced work, the need and the stimulus for heat acclimatisation may well grow.

While studies have shown that there may be differences between chronically and acutely acclimatised individuals, there is little evidence that genetic differences confer any advantage in maintaining body temperature. Chronically acclimatised individuals maintain their body temperature in the face of climatic stress at the same level as the acutely acclimatised, but do so with a smaller sweat loss. The presumptive conclusion is that the distribution of sweating is more even and that less sweat is wasted in dripping. It may be, as has been suggested by Kerslake (1972), that hidromeiosis is an adaptive mechanism, albeit rather inefficient, that prevents the wastage of sweat.

While there seems to be no essential differences between acclimatisation to hot-wet or hot-dry conditions, the minor differences may be ascribed to the consequences of hidromeiosis or to the different stimuli to acclimatisation resulting from exposure to the two conditions. Suppression of sweating, or hidromeiosis, is reduced following acclimatisation, but the reduction is greater in subjects acclimatised in a hot-wet climate. The greater sweat loss in a hot-dry climate (at a fixed central body temperature) does not induce a greater degree of heat acclimatisation but, in a work-in-the-heat routine, the stimulus to acclimatisation (elevation of body temperature) would be relatively less in a hot-dry climate, in which all secreted sweat would be evaporated. On all these counts, therefore, a hot-wet climate would be more efficient for producing acclimatisation to heat.

In summary, some of the difficulties and mysteries of acclimatisation may have become less difficult and less mysterious, and it is possible to build up a detailed descriptive model of acclimatisation to heat, but the essential mechanisms underlying many of the changes still remain obscure.

ACCLIMATISATION TO COLD

Far fewer of the world's population live in cold than in hot regions. Furthermore, the majority of those living in the cold belong to wealthy, technologically highly developed communities, which enables them to modify the cold climate so that they live in a comfortable microclimate. It is, therefore, not surprising that it has been difficult to detect changes of acclimatisation to cold in man similar to those found in animals (Edholm, 1960; Hart, 1960).

Acclimatisation to cold, by definition, is characterised by the enhanced ability to maintain body temperature in the face of cold stress or continued function in spite of loss of body heat. The former may be brought about by better insulation or greater metabolic response; little is known of how it is possible to maintain function at unusually low body temperatures. Whereas in 1960 (Edholm, 1960) it was possible to assert that 'nothing discovered so far would upset the negative hypothesis: that is, that man does not adapt physiologically to cold', in the 1970s this assertion is no longer valid. Budd (1974) states with great conviction that the results from the exploratory work performed in the Australian Antarctic stations 'yielded the important conclusion that man does acclimatise to the cold'. In this section, the aim is to survey some of the evidence that was led to this outspoken conclusion.

Cold exposure

If acclimatisation to cold is to occur, then there must be an exposure to cold. In the heat, the stimulus for acclimatisation is the rise in body temperature; in the cold, it is suggested that it may be cooling of the skin, leading not only to the sensation of cold but to vasomotor responses (Macpherson, 1962). Before seeking the signs of acclimatisation, therefore, one should be sure that the chosen subjects have been exposed to cold. Studies have been carried out to evaluate cold exposure in the natural situation (Milan, 1964; Norman, 1965; Hampton, 1967 and 1969a); they were carried out on men living and working in the Antarctic, which on average is the coldest land on earth. Three separate climates or temperatures were assessed: the first is the met-climate measured by meteorologists in a highly standardised way, as laid down by international agreement. Met-temperature is measured in a Stephenson's screen, shaded and set at a fixed height above the ground; air movement is usually measured atop a 10 m mast. These conditions may be very different from those in which man works and lives. The second is the exposure climate — exposure temperature and air movement are measured at the particular location (indoors or outdoors) of each individual, thus creating an individual climatic profile. The last, and possibly most important, is the subclothing climate measured immediately adjacent to the skin.

The level of the three temperatures for an individual are of course very different, but the daily, weekly, and annual patterns are also at odds. Norman (1961 and 1965) showed that, while monthly averages of met-temperature fell profoundly during the winter, exposure temperatures fell far less and average subclothing temperatures remained steady throughout the year (Fig. 13.6). On average, therefore, man living in a well-heated dwelling adjusts his mode of life and his clothing to maintain a comfortable subclothing temperature. It seems that such people might be less exposed to cold than a poorly-dressed, less well-housed farm worker in England (Goldsmith, 1967). On the other hand, when men do go out of doors then subclothing temperature does fall quite rapidly and, in certain stations, men do spend considerable periods out of doors (Edholm and Lewis, 1964; Budd, 1966).

Certain areas of the body are exposed to cold either because no suitable covering is possible, i.e. face, or because function is impaired by adequate clothing, i.e. hands. There is no evidence that the face acclimatises following cold exposure (Budd, 1974) but there are suggestions that the hands, because of their high exposure, do acclimatise (Goldsmith, 1960; Hellstrøm, 1965).

Another way to assess exposure, or rather the response to it, is to enquire about thermal comfort (Goldsmith, 1960; Palmai, 1962; Budd, 1966; Budd et al, 1969). The results of such studies suggest that thermal discomfort is not at all uncommon in cold climates, in spite of the best clothing. The paradox is that the discomfort is as often occasioned by heat as by cold. In most studies with men outdoors, about one-tenth of the votes cast relate to sensations described as very cold or too cold.

It does seem, therefore, that it is possible to live in the cold and yet not be exposed to it but, if one ventures outdoors, then not only is one likely to feel cold, in spite of the best clothing, but the subclothing temperatures may fall below the values normally associated with comfort.

Metabolic Changes

If man is exposed to cold and responds by changes in metabolism, three possibilities seem to exist: either to raise basal metabolic rate, or to raise or alter the metabolic responses to cold stress.

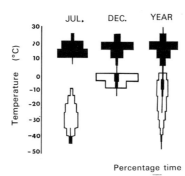

Figure 13.6   Met- and exposure temperatures for one month in summer (December) and one month in winter (July) and a whole year in a station in Antarctica. The solid blocks represent the percentage of time spent at a particular temperature (exposure temperature), the open blocks represent the percentage of time that the met-temperature was at a particular level. Note the concurrence of the two temperatures was only a little greater in December than July. (Reproduced, with permission, from Norman, J. N., 1961, M.D. Thesis)

Early studies (Lewis, Masterton and Rosenbaum, 1961; Wilson, 1965) all seemed to indicate that exposing Caucasians to prolonged living in cold met-climates did not produce any changes in the basal metabolic rate. More recently, however, thanks to careful and persistent work, Japanese workers (Yoshimura et al, 1966; Yoshimura and Yoshimura, 1969; Yurugi, Sasaki and Yoshimura, 1972) have demonstrated a clear seasonal pattern in basal metabolic rate. They have shown that there is a rise of more than 10 per cent between summer and winter, which is uninfluenced by diet and occurs among Japanese living in Japan, in America (Yoshimura and Horvarth, 1967) or in Antarctica (Ohkubo, 1973). It is difficult to reconcile these two sets of findings and it might be suggested that the studies on Caucasians, which were all done on members of polar expeditions, confused the consequences of increasing physical fitness without undue cold exposure. On the other hand, many of the Japanese studies were performed on people living in their 'natural' environments and pursuing their 'normal' work.

It is well established that many mammals respond to cold exposure by altering their metabolic response: shivering is replaced by non-shivering thermogenesis (Carlson and Hsieh, 1970). There now seems to be some evidence that a similar changeover occurs in man. Davis (1961) showed that men, too, altered their metabolic responses following acclimatisation. Acclimatisation was achieved by exposing the men nearly naked for some hours each day in a cold chamber; during the exposures, they remained inactive, experiencing acute discomfort. When tested in a standard cold test after acclimatisation, the men's metabolic rates rose as before but they shivered much less. It was concluded that some 50 per cent of their extra heat production was derived from non-shivering thermogenesis. These men had of course been exposed to the cold in the same way as rats and it is little wonder that such experiments, which require unusual cooperation from subjects, have rarely been repeated. These findings have been confirmed in groups of naturally acclimatised men (Davis and Johnston, 1961; Davis, 1963). demonstrating a seasonal difference in the shivering response of men living in North America.

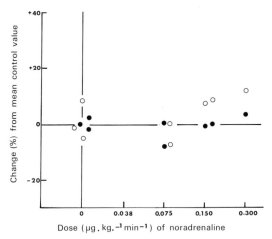

Figure 13.7 The changes in oxygen consumption in response to doses of noradrenaline following acclimatisation to cold in one subject. The solid circles represent the results before acclimatisation and the open circles those after. (Reproduced, with permission, from Budd, G. M. & Warhaft, N., 1966a, *Journal of Physiology*, **186**, 238)

Non-shivering thermogenesis is mediated by the autonomic nervous system; the extra heat is produced by the rapid metabolism of brown fat. It has been shown that the calorigenic effects of infused noradrenaline in man are potentiated by a period of cold exposure (Budd and Warhaft, 1966a; Bodey, 1973), suggesting that man acclimatises in a similar way to other mammals, and that the extra heat production may also result from the breakdown of deposits of brown fat (Fig. 13.7).

The introduction by Scholander et al (1958) of the sleep-in-the-cold test sparked off an extensive investigation of the different ethnic responses to cold. Scholander postulated that sleep was essential for survival and, therefore, that cold adaptation might lead to an improved ability to sleep in the cold. The test consisted of allowing the subject to go to sleep in a cold room (about 3°C) then, after about one hour, removing all but the lightest cover. The unacclimatised response is for the subjects to wake almost at once and then spend the remainder of the night shivering but maintaining central temperature at near normal levels

(Hammel, 1964). In the first experiment, youths were exposed to cold, both during the day and the night in the mountains of Norway, and were compared with unexposed controls. At first, the exposed group slept intermittently because of the discomfort of shivering but, as time passed, they slept and shivered. During the tests, the young men slept in a room at 3°C, using only a light sleeping bag; the exposures during these tests were similar to their nightly exposures in the field. The results showed that the exposed group maintained a higher metabolism and skin temperature than their unexposed controls: this was called metabolic acclimatisation. All the other studies have been performed on so-called primitive men who live in fairly extreme climates, wearing only thin clothing or no clothing at all. The most dramatic differences between their responses and those of urban Caucasians were shown by a group of Australian aborigines, who did not increase their metabolism in spite of falls in peripheral and central temperature. Interpretation of these results is difficult — they could be due to genetic differences or result from extended cold exposures — but the crucial experiments in which there was a comparison of, for instance, urbanised aborigines with their nomadic cousins, have not been done.

Changes in insulation

Response to standard cold stresses in men exposed to polar climates have revealed rather different results. It has been shown repeatedly that after acclimatisation these men maintain central temperature more effectively, without increased rise in metabolic rate. It has been suggested that when man is exposed to the cold he might respond by laying down a thicker layer of insulating subcutaneous fat. Many surveys have shown that body weight and skinfold thickness do rise in the winter in men on polar expeditions (Lewis, Masterton and Rosenbaum, 1960; Wilson, 1960; Easty, 1967; Davies, 1969). The question arises as to whether such changes are a response to the cold or to some other factor (Edholm, 1974). It has been pointed out that, in general, activity is very high during the polar summer and low in winter and it may be that appetite responds only sluggishly to the levels in activity. Nevertheless, the increase in body weight does not occur in all groups, nor does the rise in body weight necessarily relate to a rise in skinfold thickness (Budd, 1974). Furthermore, the rather small changes in skinfold thickness are scarcely enough to have a dramatic effect on insulation.

In a series of experiments (Milan, Elsner and Rodahl, 1961; Budd, 1962 and 1964; Wyndham, Plotkin and Munro, 1964; Budd and Warhaft, 1966b; Wyndham and Loots, 1969), responses to a standard cold stress were examined before and after a long sojourn in a cold climate. The general finding from all these studies indicates that rectal temperatures fall less in the tests after acclimatisation, while oxygen consumption does not rise to higher levels than in the test before acclimatisation (Fig. 13.8). Furthermore, in some tests, an increase in vasoconstrictor tone was shown and Budd (1965) has additionally suggested that there may be an enhancement in counter current heat exchange, also leading to an increased insulation.

In cold climates, hands and faces are exposed to a greater cold stress than the remainder of the body. A number of investigators have examined the response of the hands to cold stress and two opposing views emerge. Men who habitually expose their hands to cold water, like fishermen and fish filleters, show one response, those with less acute local exposure another. The former (Nelms and Soper, 1962; Helmstrøm, 1965) show a less profound vasoconstriction, a more rapid onset and higher level of cold-induced vasodilation when their hands are plunged into ice cold water, compared with unacclimatised controls. These responses would result in better local function of the hand, at the cost of body heat, and occur only as long as central temperature does not fall (Keatinge, 1969). The other group of investigators (Elkington, 1968; Hampton, 1969b) have shown that there is a fall in the 'normal' hand blood flow during acclimatisation.

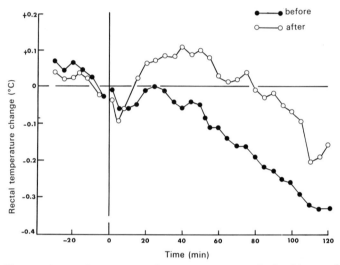

Figure 13.8 Changes in rectal temperature in response to a standard cold stress before (closed circles) and after (open circles) acclimatisation. The results are the means of eight exposures on four subjects. Zero time indicates the commencement of exposure, naked, in a room at 10°C; prior to zero, subjects were in a sleeping bag. (Reproduced, with permission, from Budd, G. M. & Warhaft, N., 1966b, *Journal of Physiology*, **186**, 223)

Furthermore, they have demonstrated that there are alterations in the responses to a cold stress — vasoconstriction becomes more profound while cold-induced vasodilation less prominent. These responses suggest an improvement of insulation which would tend to maintain the level of central body temperature in the face of a local or general threat. The discordant results may be explained by a number of factors. First, there is the question of exposure; the groups that show less profound vasoconstriction are those who habitually expose their hands to cold water or a very cold environment, but the rest of their body may be well protected. Secondly, the studies themselves were rather different: in the former, the responses of the exposed group were compared with unexposed controls and, in the latter, the changing responses of each subject were observed.

Conclusion

Cold acclimatisation does occur in man; it seems to be marked by an increase in basal metabolic rate, an altered metabolic response to cold and improved insulation. There is, however, a group of people — the elderly (Fox et al, 1973) — who may live in a cold climate, with relatively low body temperature; some progress to severe hypothermia occasionally with fatal consequences but the more remarkable finding is that the majority manage tolerably well in spite of their low body temperatures.

It is worth speculating that they may be acclimatising to cold by allowing their body temperatures to fall, with all the metabolic advantages that may accrue from this, without catastrophic loss of function.

Less is known about cold than about heat acclimatisation because it is technically easier to avoid cold exposure; exposure to cold, moreover, elicits greater immediate discomfort, triggering a vigorous intellectual response and, thus, while fuel lasts and cloth is available, the chances of narrowing the gaps in our knowledge are poor. Heat, even in the cold, seems to be the chief climatic stress so that 'man should ever study to keep cool; he makes his inferiors his superiors by heat' — Emerson.

REFERENCES

Adam, J. M. (1959) Subjective sensations and sub-clothing temperatures in Antarctica. *Journal of Physiology*, **145**, 26P.

Allan, J. R. & Wilson, C. G. (1971) Influence of acclimatisation on sweat sodium concentration. *Journal of Applied Physiology*, **30**, 708–712.

Allan, J. R., Crowdy, J. P. & Haisman, M. F. (1965) The use of vapour barrier suit for the practical induction of artificial acclimatisation to heat. I. Winter experiment. *Army Personnel Research Establishment Report*, **4/65**.

Astrand, P. O. & Rodahl, K. (1970) *Textbook of Work Physiology*. New York: McGraw-Hill.

Bass, D. E., Kleeman, C. R., Quinn, H., Henschel, A. & Hegnaver, A. H. (1955) Mechanisms of acclimatisation to heat in man. *Medicine*, **34**, 323–380.

Bittel, J. & Henane, R. (1975) Comparison of thermal exchanges in men and women under neutral and hot conditions. *Journal of Physiology*, **250**, 475–489.

Blagden, C. (1775) Further experiments and observations in an heated room. *Philosophical Transactions of the Royal Society of London*, **65**, Pt. 1, 484–494.

Bodey, A. S. (1973) The role of catecholamines in human acclimatisation to cold: a study of 24 men at Casey, Antarctica. In *Polar Human Biology*, ed. Edholm, O. G. and Gunderson, E. K. E., pp. 141–149. London: Heinemann.

Brebner, D. F. & Kerslake, D. McK. (1963) The effect of soaking the skin in water on the acclimatisation produced by subsequent heat exposure. *Journal of Physiology*. **166**, 13P.

Brebner, D. F. & Kerslake, D.McK. (1964) The true course of the decline in sweating produced by wetting of the skin. *Journal of Physiology*, **175**, 295–302.

Brown, W. S. & Sargent, F. (1965) Hidromeiosis. *Archives of Environmental Health*, **11**, 442–453.

Budd, G. M. (1962) Acclimatisation to cold in Antarctica as shown by rectal temperature response to a standard cold stress. *Nature*, **193**, 886P.

Budd, G. M. (1964) General acclimatisation to cold in men studied before, during and after a year in Antarctica. *Australian National Antarctic Research Expedition Report 70*. Melbourne: Antarctic Division, Department of External Affairs.

Budd, G. M. (1965) Effects of cold exposure and exercise in a wet, cold Antarctic climate. *Journal of Applied Physiology*, **20**, 417-422.

Budd, G. M. (1966) Skin temperature, thermal comfort, sweating, clothing and activity of men sledging in Antarctica. *Journal of Physiology*, **186**, 233–242.

Budd, G. M. (1974) Physiological research at Australian stations in the Antarctic and sub-Antarctic. In *Antarctic Research Series*, ed. Gunderson, E. K. E., Vol. 22, pp. 27–54. Washington DC: American Geophysical Union.

Budd, G. M. & Warhaft, N. (1966a) Cardiovascular and metabolic responses to noradrenaline in man, before and after acclimatisation to cold in Antarctica. *Journal of Physiology*, **186**, 233–242.

Budd, G. M. & Warhaft, N. (1966b) Body temperature, shivering, blood pressure and heart rate during a standard cold stress in Australia and the Antarctica. *Journal of Physiology*, **186**, 216–232.

Budd, G. M., Hicks, K. E., Lugg, D. J., Murray, L. G. & Wigg, D. R. (1969) Thermal discomfort in the Antarctic and sub-Antarctic. *Medical Journal of Australia*, 2, 1285–1288.

Burton, A. C. & Edholm, O. G. (1955) *Man in a Cold Environment*, London: Edward Arnold.

Carlson, L. D. & Hsieh, A. C. L. (1970) *Control of Energy Exchange*. New York: Macmillan.

Chafee, R. R. J. & Roberts, J. C. (1971) Temperature acclimation in birds and mammals. *Annual Reviews of Physiology*, 33, 155–202.

Collins, K. J. & Weiner, J. S. (1962) Observations on arm-bag suppression of sweating and its relationship to thermal sweat gland 'fatigue'. *Journal of Physiology*, 161, 538–556.

Collins, K. J. & Weiner, J. S. (1968) Endocrinological aspects of exposure to high environmental temperatures. *Physiological Reviews*, 48, 785–839.

Collins, K. J., Crockford, G. W. & Weiner, J. S. (1963) The role of glandular activity in the increased sweat response of heat acclimatisation. *Journal of Physiology*, 169, 12P.

Crowdy, J. P. & Haisman, M. F. (1966) The use of a vapour barrier suit for the practical induction of artificial acclimatisation to heat. II. Summer experiment. *Army Personnel Research Establishment Report*. 4/65.

Davies, A. G. (1969) Seasonal changes in body weight and skinfold thickness. *British Antarctic Survey Bulletin*, 19, 75–81.

Davis, T. R. A. (1961) Chamber cold acclimatisation in man. *Journal of Applied Physiology*, 16, 1011–1015.

Davis, T. R. A. (1963) Non-shivering thermogenesis. *Federation Proceedings*, 22, 777–782.

Davis, T. R. A. & Johnston, D. R. (1961) Seasonal acclimatisation to cold in man. *Journal of Applied Physiology*, 16, 231–234.

Dobson, R. L. (1962) The correlation of structure and function in the human eccrine sweat glands. In *Advances in Biology of Skin*, ed. Montague, W., Ellis, R. A. and Silver, A. F., pp. 41–75. Oxford: Pergamon.

Easty, D. (1967) Food intake in Antarctica. *British Journal of Nutrition*, 21, 7–15.

Edholm, O. G. (1960) Polar physiology. *Federation Proceedings*, 19, Suppl. 5, 3–8.

Edholm, O. G. (1974) Physiological research at British Antarctic survey stations. In *Antarctic Research Series*, ed. Gunderson, E. K. E., Vol. 22, pp. 5–26. Washington DC: American Geophysical Union.

Edholm, O. G. & Bacharach, A. L. (1965) *The Physiology of Human Survival*. New York: Academic Press.

Edholm, O. G. & Gunderson, E. K. E. (1973) *Polar Human Biology*. London: William Heinemann.

Edholm, O. G. & Lewis, H. E. (1964) Terrestrial animals in the cold, man in polar regions. In *Handbook of Physiology*, ed. Dill, D. B., Sec. 4, pp. 435–446. Washington DC: American Physiology Society.

Edholm, O. G., Adam, J. M., Cannon, P., Fox, R. H., Goldsmith, R., Shepherd, R. D. & Underwood, C. R. (1962) Study of artificially acclimatised, naturally acclimatised and non-acclimatised troops to exposure to heat. *Medical Research Council Report*, 61, 827P.

Edholm, O. G., Fox, R. H., Adam, J. M. & Goldsmith, R. (1963) Comparison of artificial and natural acclimatisation. *Federation Proceedings*, 22, 709–715.

Edholm, O. G., Fox, R. H., Goldsmith, R., Hampton, I. F. G. & Pillai, K. V. (1964a) A comparison of heat acclimatisation in Indians and Europeans. *Journal of Physiology*, 177, 15–16P.

Edholm, O. G., Fox, R. H., Goldsmith, R., Hampton, I. F. G., Underwood, C. R., Ward, E. J., Wolff, H. S., Adam, J. M. & Allan, J. R. (1964b) The effect of heat on food and water intake on acclimatised and unacclimatised men. *Medical Research Council Report*, 64, 16P.

Eide, R. (1965) The relationship of pain sensation to cold pressor reactions and local cold habituation. *Scandinavian Journal of Clinical Laboratory Investigations*, 17, 584–588.

Eide, R. (1973) The conceptual framework of cold adaptation. In *Polar Human Biology*, ed. Edholm, O. G. & Gunderson, E. K. E., pp. 290–296. London: William Heinemann.

Elkington, E. J. (1968) Finger blood flow in Antarctica. *Journal of Physiology*, 199, 1–10.

Fox, R. H. (1974) *Heat Acclimatisation and the Sweating Response in Heat Loss from Animals and Man*, ed. Monteith, J. L. and Mount, L. E., pp. 277–303. London: Butterworth.

Fox, R. H. & Löfstedt, B. E. (1968) A comparison of thermoregulatory function in men and women. *Journal of Physiology*, 197, 44–45.

Fox, R. H., Goldsmith, R., Hampton, I. F. G. & Lewis, H. E. (1962) The mechanism of the increase in sweating capacity induced by heat acclimatisation. *Journal of Physiology*, 162, 59–60.

Fox, R. H., Goldsmith, R., Kidd, D. J. & Lewis, H. E. (1963a) Acclimatisation to heat in man by controlled elevation of body temperature. *Journal of Physiology*, 166, 530–547.

Fox, R. H., Goldsmith, R., Kidd, D. J. & Lewis, H. E. (1963b) Bloodflow and other thermoregulatory changes with acclimatisation to heat. *Journal of Physiology*, 166, 548–562.

Fox, R. H., Goldsmith, R., Hampton, I. F. G. & Lewis, H. E. (1964) The nature of the increase in sweating capacity produced by heat acclimatisation. *Journal of Physiology,* **171,** 368–376.

Fox, R. H., Goldsmith, R., Hampton, I. F. G. & Hunt, T. J. (1966) The influence of acclimatising man to heat on his temperature regulation at rest in a comfortable environment. *Journal of Physiology,* **183,** 18–19P.

Fox, R. H., Goldsmith, R., Hampton, I. F. G. & Hunt, T. J. (1967) Heat acclimatisation by controlled hyperthermia in hot-dry and hot-wet climates. *Journal of Applied Physiology,* **22,** 39–46.

Fox, R. H., Löfstedt, B. E., Woodward, P. M., Eriksson, E. & Werkstrom, H. (1969) Comparison of thermoregulatory function in men and women. *Journal of Applied Physiology,* **26,** 444–453.

Fox, R. H., Woodward, P. M., Exton-Smith, A. N., Green, M. F., Dennison, D. V. & Wicks, M. H. (1973) Body temperatures in the elderly: A national survey of physiological, social and environmental conditions. *British Medical Journal,* **1,** 200–206.

Fox, R. H., Budd, G. M., Woodward, P. M., Hackett, A. J. & Hendrie, A. L. (1974) A study of temperature regulation in New Guinea people. *Philosophical Transactions of the Royal Society of London,* **268,** 375–391.

Goldsmith, R. (1960) Use of clothing records to demonstrate acclimatisation to cold in man. *Journal of Applied Physiology,* **15,** 776–780.

Goldsmith, R. (1967) Cold exposure of farm and laboratory workers. *Journal of Applied Physiology,* **22,** 47–49.

Goldsmith, R. & Hampton, I. F. G. (1967) Cold exposure in man. In *The Effects of Abnormal Physical Conditions at Work,* ed. Davies, C. N., Davis, P. R. and Tyrer, F. H., pp. 14–24. Edinburgh: E. & S. Livingstone.

Goldsmith, R., Fox, R. H. & Hampton, I. F. G. (1967) Effects of drugs on heat acclimatisation by controlled hyperthermia. *Journal of Applied Physiology,* **22,** 301–304.

Gonzalez, R. R., Pandolf, K. B. & Gagge, A. P. (1974) Heat acclimation and decline in sweating during humidity transients. *Journal of Applied Physiology,* **36,** 419–425.

Gunderson, E. K. E. (1974) *Human Adaptability to Antarctic Conditions.* No. 22. Washington DC: American Geophysical Union.

Hammel, H. T. (1964) Terrestrial animals in the cold: Recent studies of primitive man. In *Handbook of Physiology,* ed. Dill, J. B., Sec. 4, pp. 413–434. Washington DC: American Physiological Society.

Hammel, H. T. (1968) Regulation of internal body temperature. *Annual Review of Physiology,* **30,** 641–710.

Hampton, I. F. G. (1967) Cold exposure during Antarctic journeys with special reference to its effect on the peripheral circulation in man. University of London Ph.D. Thesis.

Hampton, I. F. G. (1969a) Effect of cold exposure in the Antarctic on heat elimination from the hands. *Federation Proceedings,* **28,** 1129–1134.

Hampton, I. F. G. (1969b) Local acclimatisation of the hands to prolonged cold exposure. *British Antarctic Survey Bulletin,* **19,** 9–56.

Harrison, M. H. (1974) Plasma volume change during acute exposure to high environmental temperature. *Journal of Applied Physiology,* **36,** 519–523.

Harrison, M. H. (1975) Plasma volume change during work in a hot environment. *Journal of Physiology,* **245,** 102–103.

Hart, J. S. (1957) Climatic and temperature induced changes in the energetics of homeotherms. *Revue canadienne de biologie,* **16,** 133–174.

Hart, J. S. (1960) Energy metabolism during exposure to cold. *Federation Proceedings,* **19,** Suppl. 5, 15–19.

Hellon, R. F. & Lind, A. R. (1955) Circulation in the hand and forearm with repeated daily exposures to humid heat. *Journal of Physiology,* **128,** 57P.

Hellstrøm, B. (1965) *Local Effects of Acclimatisation to Cold in Man.* Oslo: Universitetsforlaget.

Henane, R. & Valatx, J. L. (1973) Thermoregulatory changes induced during heat acclimatisation by controlled hyperthermia. *Journal of Physiology,* **230,** 255–271.

Hertig, B. A., Riedesel, M. L. & Belding, H. S. (1961) Sweating in hot baths. *Journal of Applied Physiology,* **16,** 647–651.

Hiernaux, J., Rudan, P. & Brambati, A. (1975) Climate and weight/height relationship in sub-Saharan Africa. *Annals of Human Biology,* **2,** 3–12.

Keatinge, W. R. (1969) *Survival in Cold Water.* Oxford: Blackwell.

Kerslake, D. McK. (1972) *The Stress of Hot Environments,* Ch. 7. Cambridge: University Press.

Lewis, H. E., Masterton, J. P. & Rosenbaum, S. (1960) Body weight and skinfold thickness of men on a polar expedition. *Clinical Science,* **19,** 551–561.

Lewis, H. E., Masterton, J. P. & Rosenbaum, S. (1961) Stability of basal metabolic rate on a polar expedition. *Journal of Applied Physiology,* **16,** 397–400.

Lugg, D. J. (1965) Thermal comfort in Antarctica. *Medical Journal of Australia*, 2, 746–750.

Macpherson, R. K. (1960) Physiological responses to hot environments. *Medical Research Council Special Report*, No. 298. London: H.M. Stationery Office.

Macpherson, R. K. (1962) The assessment of the thermal environment. *British Journal of Industrial Medicine*, 19, 151–164.

Marcus, P. (1972) Heat acclimatisation by exercise-induced elevation of body temperature. *Journal of Applied Physiology*, 33, 283–288.

Milan, F. A. (1964) Maintenance of thermal balance in Arctic Eskimos and Antarctic sojourners. In *Antarctic Biology*, ed. Carrick, R., Holdgate, M. and Prepost, J., pp. 529-534. Paris: Hermann.

Milan, F. A., Elsner, R. W. & Rodahl, K. (1961) Thermal and metabolic responses of men in the Antarctic to a standard cold stress. *Journal of Applied Physiology*, 16, 401–404.

Nelms, J. D. & Soper, D. J. G. (1962) Cold vasodilation and cold acclimatisation in the hands of British fish filleters. *Journal of Applied Physiology*, 17, 444–448.

Nicol, J. F. (1974) An analysis of some observations of thermal comfort in Roorkee, India and Bagdad, Iraq. *Annals of Human Biology*, 1, 411–426.

Nielsen, B. (1974) Effects of changes in plasma volume and osmolarity on thermoregulation during exercise. *Acta physiologica scandinavica*, 90, 725–730.

Norman, J. N. (1961) *Man in Antarctica*. Glasgow: M.D. Thesis.

Norman, J. N. (1965) Cold exposure and patterns of activity at a polar station. *British Antarctic Survey Bulletin*, 6, 1–13.

Ohkubo, Y. (1973) Basal metabolism and other physiological changes in the Antarctic. In *Polar Human Biology*, ed. Edholm, O. G. and Gunderson, E. K. E. pp. 161–170. London: Heinemann.

Palmai, G. (1962) Thermal comfort and acclimatisation to cold in a sub-Antarctic environment. *Medical Journal of Australia*, 1, 9–12.

Renbourn, G. T. (1957) The history of the flannel binder and cholera belt. *Medical History*, 1, 211–225.

Renbourn, G. T. (1972) *Materials and Clothing in Health and Disease*. London: H. K. Lewis.

Rowell, L. B. (1974) Human cardiovascular adjustments to exercise and thermal stress. *Physiological Reviews*, 54, 74–159.

Scholander, P. F., Hammel, H. T., Lange Anderson, K. & Løyning, Y. (1958) Metabolic acclimation to cold in man. *Journal of Applied Physiology*, 12, 1–8.

Senay, L. C. (1972) Changes in plasma volume and protein content during exposures of working men to various temperatures before and after acclimatisation to heat separation of the roles of cutaneous and skeletal muscle circulation. *Journal of Physiology*, 224, 61–81.

Shvartz, E., Magazanik, A. & Glick, E. (1974) Thermal responses during training in a temperate climate. *Journal of Applied Physiology*, 36, 572–576.

Snellen, J. W. (1972) Set point in exercise. In *Essays on Temperature Regulation*, ed. Bligh, J. and Moore, R. Amsterdam: North-Holland Publishing.

Turk, J. (1971) Bath and step acclimatisation to heat. 2nd Report. *Army Personnel Research Establishment Report*, 16/71.

Turk, J. & Worsley, D. E. (1974) A technique for rapid acclimatisation to heat for the Army. *Army Personnel Research Establishment Report*, 12/74.

Webb, C. G. (1964) Thermal comfort in a tropical environment. *Nature*, 202, 1193–1194.

Weiner, J. S. & Lourie, J. A. (1969) *Human Biology: A Guide to Field Methods*, IBP Handbook No. 9. Oxford: Blackwell Scientific Publications.

Whittow, G. C. (1961) Flow of blood in the forearm of persons acclimatised to heat. *Nature*, 192, 759–760.

Wilkins, D. C. (1973) Acclimation to heat in the Antarctic. In *Polar Human Biology*, ed. Edholm, O. G. and Gunderson, E. K. E. pp. 171–181. London: Heinemann.

Wilson, O. (1960) Changes in body weight in the Antarctic. *British Journal of Nutrition*, 14, 391–401.

Wilson, O. (1965) Human adaptation to life in Antarctica. In *Biogeography and Ecology in Antarctica*, ed. van Meighem, J., van Oye, P. and Schell, J., Monographs in Biology Vol. 15, pp. 690–752. The Hague: W. Junk.

Wyndham, C. H. (1951) Effect of acclimatisation on circulatory responses to high environmental temperatures. *Journal of Applied Physiology*, 4, 383–395.

Wyndham, C. H. (1965) A survey of the causal factors in heat stroke and their prevention in the gold mining industry. *Journal of the South African Institute of Mining and Metallurgy*, November 125–155.

Wyndham, C. H. (1966) A survey of the research initiated by the Chamber of Mines into clinical aspects of heat stroke. *Proceedings of the Mine Medical Officers Association of South Africa*, 46, 68–80.

Wyndham, C. H. (1973) The physiology of exercise under heat stress. *Annual Review of Physiology*, **35**, 193–220.

Wyndham, C. H. & Loots, H. (1969) Responses to cold during a year in Antarctica. *Journal of Applied Physiology*, **27**, 696–700.

Wyndham, C. H. & Strydom, N. B. (1969) Acclimatising men to heat in a climatic room in mines. *Journal of the South African Institute of Mining and Metallurgy*, **70**, 60–64.

Wyndham, C. H., Macpherson, R. K. & Munro, A. (1964) Reaction to heat of aborigines and Caucasians. *Journal of Applied Physiology*, **19**, 1055–1058.

Wyndham, C. H., Metz, B. & Munro, A. (1964) Reaction to heat of Arabs and Caucasians. *Journal of Applied Physiology*, **19**, 1051–1054.

Wyndham, C. H., Plotkin, R. & Munro, A. (1964) Physiological reactions to cold of men in the Antarctic. *Journal of Applied Physiology*, **19**, 593–597.

Wyndham, C. H., Strydom, N. B., Ward, J. S., Morrison, J. F., Williams, C. G., Bredell, G. A. G., van Rahden, M. J. E., Holdsworth, L. D., van Graan, C. H., Rensburg, A. J. & Munro, A. (1964a) Physiological reactions to heat of bushmen and of unacclimatised and acclimatised Bantu. *Journal of Applied Physiology*, **19**, 885–888.

Wyndham, C. H., Strydom, N. B., Williams, C. G., Morrison, F., Bredel, G. A. G., Peter, J., van Graan, C., Holdsworth, L., van Rensburg, A. & Munro, A. (1964b) Heat reactions of some Bantu tribesmen in southern Africa. *Journal of Applied Physiology*, **19**, 881–884.

Yoshimura, M. & Horvarth, S. M. (1967) Change of basal metabolism in Japanese in the USA. In *Report of the U.S.–Japan Scientific Cooperative Program*, pp. 49–50. Kyoto.

Yoshimura, M. & Yoshimura, H. (1969) Cold tolerance and critical temperature of the Japanese. *International Journal of Biometeorology*, **13**, 163–172.

Yoshimura, M., Yukiyoshi, K., Yoshioka, T. & Takeda, H. (1966) Climatic adaptation of basal metabolism. *Federation Proceedings*, **25**, 1169–1176.

Yurugi, R., Sasaki, T. & Yoshimura, M. (1972) Seasonal variation of basal metabolism in Japanese. In *Advances in Climatic Physiology*, ed. Itoh, S., Ogata, K. and Yoshimura, H., Ch. 24. Tokyo: Igaku Shoin.

14
BILE SALTS AND GALLSTONES

K. W. Heaton

The last ten years have seen astonishing advances in our understanding of bile salts (bile acids) and of their role in health and disease. The interest of clinicians was first aroused when it was discovered that, in ileal disorders and the stagnant loop syndrome, diarrhoea and steatorrhoea are due largely to disturbances of bile salt metabolism. Then followed the realisation that gallstones, the commonest cause of elective abdominal surgery in the West, are a metabolic disease of bile secretion and, soon after, the discovery that some gallstones can be dissolved in situ by feeding a bile acid, chenodeoxycholic acid. Meanwhile, a simple breath test was developed to detect abnormal bile salt metabolism in clinical practice. These advances were made possible by great improvements in analytical techniques, and especially by the use of isotopically labelled bile salts.

The Nature and Formation of Bile

Bile is unique in being both an exocrine secretion and a major excretory pathway. This dual role of bile accounts for its strange composition (Table 14.1).

Table 14.1 Average composition of human hepatic bile (based on data from Burnett, 1965; Thureborn, 1962; Wheeler, 1968)

	Concentration	
	mmol/l	g/l
Organic		
Conjugated bile salts	36	18.0
Phospholipid	9	7.1
Cholesterol	2.5	1.3
Conjugated bile pigment	1.5	0.9
Mucoprotein	trace	0.03–0.30
Inorganic		
Sodium, potassium, chloride	Similar to plasma	
Bicarbonate	27–55	

The main *excretory* substances in bile are the pigments, chiefly bilirubin diglucuronide, and cholesterol. Contrary to popular belief, these are the least abundant of the organic substances in bile, but they are the most blatant troublemakers, being the chief actors in the dramas of jaundice and gallstones. Bile is also an excretory pathway for drugs and hormones. The main *secretory* substances are the conjugated bile salts, and these are by far the most abundant of all the bile solutes. They account not only for the vital detergent properties of bile, in which they are helped by phospholipid, but also for its intensely bitter taste. Bile is of course a watery solution and it is quite dilute, being 95 to 98 per cent water before being concentrated six to ten-fold in the gallbladder. It contains electrolytes in concentrations similar to plasma except that there is about twice as much bicarbonate. The gallbladder mucosa extracts an isotonic solution of sodium chloride and bicarbonate.

The special feature of detergent molecules is their tendency to form clusters in water. Each molecule carries an electrical charge, which is oriented to the surface of the cluster. Such a cluster or micelle is a submicroscopic particle bristling with electrical charges. Hence micelles repel each other and stay in suspension indefinitely, unlike emulsion particles which tend to coalesce. The biliary micelle is negatively charged from the COO⁻ groups at the ends of the bile salt side chains. Its interior contains the bulky steroid moieties of the bile salt molecules. These are hydrophobic or lipid-loving, so that inside the micelle is a micro-droplet of lipid, into which otherwise insoluble lipids can be admitted. In this way, cholesterol, a very insoluble lipid, is held in bile in a stable dispersion. The role of phospholipid (mainly lecithin) is to expand the bile salt micelle and enable it to take up more cholesterol. Thus, the capacity of bile to dissolve cholesterol depends on the concentrations of both bile salts and phospholipids (Carey and Small, 1970).

Bile secretion is the dynamic process whereby this golden micellar solution is transferred across the liver cell membrane into the network of bile canaliculi, and hence into the bile duct system. The motive power for this process comes from the active transport of two solutes, bile salts and sodium, with water following passively. Pressures as high as 20 mmHg (2.7 kPa) can be generated. Many experiments have shown that there is a straight line relationship between bile salt secretion and the volume of bile flow, which shows the importance of bile salts in determining bile flow. However, if the straight line is extrapolated to zero bile salt output, the remaining flow is still substantial. In man, this bile salt-independent fraction probably contributes about 50 per cent of total bile flow (Schersten et al, 1971; Thureborn, 1962). It is mediated by active sodium transport through the action of cyclic AMP and is increased by phenobarbitone therapy (Erlinger and Dhumeaux, 1974).

The rate at which bile salts are secreted by the liver is a measurement of special interest to clinicians since it determines the extent to which newly formed bile is saturated with cholesterol (Redinger and Small, 1972). The physiological reason for this is that, in a given subject, cholesterol is excreted into bile at a virtually constant rate. Therefore, in hepatic bile, the vital ratio bile salt: cholesterol (that is, solubiliser:solute, or detergent:lipid) is governed by the prevailing bile salt secretion rate. A further reason is that as bile salts pass out of the liver cell into the bile canaliculus they tend to take phospholipid with them. Hence the concentration of the co-solubiliser, phospholipid, in hepatic bile is determined by the amount of bile salt being secreted (Fig. 14.1). The clinical implication of all this is that one way to avoid supersaturated bile likely to precipitate cholesterol crystals in one's gallbladder, that is to escape gallstone disease, is to maintain a high bile salt secretion.

The bile duct system is able to modify the composition of bile both by secretion of a bicarbonate-rich fluid and by absorption, but it is uncertain to what extent these processes occur in health.

Functions of Bile Salts in the Intestine

The *raison d'être* of bile salts is to aid the absorption of dietary lipid. When a meal is eaten and the gallbladder contracts, the 2–3 g (4–6 mmol) pool of conjugated bile salt enters the duodenum. Here and in the jejunum, bile salts are present during digestion in a concentration of 5 mmol/l or over, which is well above the critical level necessary for micellar aggregates to form. The chief function of bile salts is to disperse into micellar solution the almost insoluble

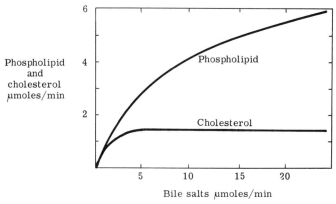

Figure 14.1   Curves showing the relationship between the secretion of bile salts and the output of phospholipid and cholesterol (drawn from the data of Wagner et al, 1973)

products of fat digestion, namely long chain fatty acids and their mono-glycerides, and also other dietary lipids especially the fat-soluble vitamins A, D, E, and K. In the intestine, micelles may be regarded as miniature lipid transporters, ferrying packets of lipid repeatedly to the absorptive membrane of the microvilli. Micellar solubilisation is essential for the absorption of cholesterol and fat-soluble vitamins, but when bile salts are completely absent (as in biliary obstruction or fistula) half the normal dietary load of fat can yet be absorbed. Bile salts also aid fat absorption by helping to emulsify fat before it is split by pancreatic lipase, by activating lipase and lowering its pH optimum, and even by stimulating the formation of chylomicrons in the intestinal mucosa.

Bile salts have antibacterial properties and these may help to explain why bacterial counts in the small intestine are generally below $10^6/l$.

Absorption and Enterohepatic Circulation

Conjugated bile salts have little tendency to diffuse across cell membranes because of their relatively high polarity. Consequently, bile salts remain within the proximal small intestine in relatively high concentration, which allows maximum opportunity for fat absorption. In the terminal ileum the mucosa contains an active transport system which efficiently takes up bile salts and so prevents all but 4 or 5 per cent from entering the bacteria-rich colon. A certain amount of bacterial deconjugation does take place in the terminal ileum, but this is no disadvantage as free (unconjugated) bile acids are quite well absorbed by passive diffusion here and in the proximal colon. Absorbed bile salts are returned to the liver in the portal vein, bound to plasma albumin. The liver extracts bile salts with great avidity, clearing as much as 92 per cent on a single passage. Any deconjugated acids are reconjugated with glycine and taurine in a ratio of about 3 to 1 before being re-secreted into the bile. This completes the enterohepatic circulation.

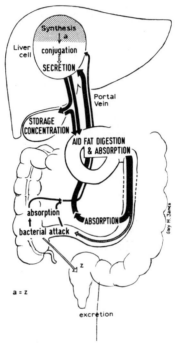

Figure 14.2 The main events in the enterohepatic circulation of bile salts

Because ileal absorption and hepatic clearance are so efficient, the entero-hepatic circulation may be regarded as an almost closed recycling system. It ensures that the concentration of bile salts in peripheral blood is so low that it can only be measured accurately by exquisitely sensitive techniques, such as the recently developed radioimmunoassay (Simmonds et al, 1973). It also ensures that the colon is not exposed to large quantities of bile salts. The purpose of this system is to make maximum use of the small body pool of bile salts. The 2–3 g pool circulates twice or three times during the digestion of a meal, and so six to eight times per day. Therefore each day the small intestine is perfused with about 20 g of detergent to help it to cope with about 100 g of dietary fat. Radioactive studies show that the average bile salt molecule circulates about 20 times before it is lost into the faeces. As a result, only 500 mg of bile salts are lost to the body each day, and have to be replaced by newly synthesised material.

Figure 14.2 shows the main events in the enterohepatic cycle, while Table 14.2 lists the important numbers in bile salt turnover.

Table 14.2   Key numbers in bile salt turnover

Size of circulating pool		4–6 mmol	2–3 g
Number of circulations per day		6–8	
Daily secretion of bile salts		40 mmol/d	20 g/d
Turnover { Excreted in faeces		1 mmol/d	$\frac{1}{2}$ g/d
{ Synthesised by liver			
Fraction of pool turned over per day		0.2	

The Essentials of Bile Salt Metabolism

The two bile salts synthesised by the human liver, cholate and chenodeoxy-cholate, are like nearly all mammalian bile salts in being derivatives of cholanic acid (properly known as 5β-cholanoic acid). They differ only in the fact that cholic acid has a hydroxyl group at the 12 position as well as at the three and seven positions on the steroid ring. In normal European bile, cholate and chenodeoxycholate constitute about 40 per cent and 35 per cent respectively of the bile salts. The other 25 per cent is made up of deoxycholate, with trace amounts of lithocholate. These two bile salts are derived from bacterial action in the colon, and so are called secondary bile salts. In both cases, bacteria have removed, or strictly de-oxygenated, the 7α-hydroxyl group — from cholate to produce deoxycholate, and from chenodeoxycholate to produce lithocholate. The presence of these materials in bile is therefore the end-result of two colonic events, bacterial metabolism and passive absorption of the degradation products. One or both of these events is inhibited by fibre in the diet (Pomare and Heaton, 1973a). The relationships between these four important bile acids are set out in Figure 14.3.

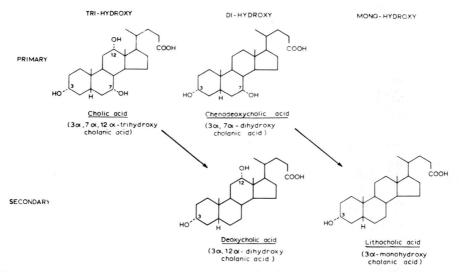

Figure 14.3   The four important primary and secondary bile acids in man, classified by the number of hydroxyl groups on the steroid nucleus

Bile acids are derived from cholesterol; indeed their synthesis is the major pathway of cholesterol catabolism and accounts for about 50 per cent of all cholesterol losses. Synthesis is controlled by a negative feedback system, whereby reabsorbed bile salts reaching the liver inhibit the activity of 7α-hydroxylase, which is the rate-limiting enzyme in the long chain of oxidations and other steps. The final step is conjugation, that is the formation of an amide (peptide) bond between the carboxyl group on the side chain and the amino group of an amino acid, glycine or taurine. Normally, the liver conjugates preferentially with the former, the glycine/taurine conjugation ratio being about 3 to 1.

Methods of Studying Bile Salt Metabolism

Although bile salts are far more important than bile pigments in the mechanisms of the body and its diseases, they are not routinely measured or tested for in clinical practice. This is because assay techniques are time consuming and, until recently, they were non-specific or rather insensitive. The last two deficiencies have now been rectified, but the problem of complexity remains. The main techniques in use now are gas chromatography, enzymic oxidation with measurement of reduced NAD, and radioimmunoassay. The serum bile salt level is a very sensitive indicator of abnormal liver function, especially if a postprandial sample is taken (Kaplowitz, Kok and Javitt, 1973) and, if a simple enough assay technique could be devised, serum bile acids would become a useful supplement to standard liver function tests. A particularly sensitive test could be the intravenous bile acid tolerance test (LaRusso et al, 1975). With the use of radioactively labelled glycocholate or taurocholate (obtainable from the Radiochemical Centre at Amersham) the test would be simple and cost only £5 to £10 a time (LaRusso et al, 1975; Calcraft, LaRusso and Hofmann, 1975).

To obtain detailed information about bile salt metabolism it is usually necessary to analyse bile-rich intestinal contents. Unfortunately this involves intubating the patient followed by extraction and chromatography of the aspirate. This approach has been extremely productive in research on bile salt kinetics and metabolism, usually in combination with the administration of tracer doses of labelled bile salts, but it is too complex for routine clinical use (Hofmann et al, 1970).

Analysis of faecal bile acids is excessively complex if it is done chemically, but is made much simpler by the use of radioactive bile acids. Malabsorption of bile salts is most certainly detected by showing that bile acid radioactivity is excreted more rapidly than normal (Hofmann, 1972). Generally, this involves combustion of a dried aliquot of stool and absorption of the radioactive CO_2 into a counting medium.

An attractively simple technique is to measure the radioactivity in expired air after administration of [^{14}C]glycocholate. This 'breath test' gives information about the rate of deconjugation of bile salts in the intestine, but has certain limitations (see p. 338).

The Toxicity of Bile Salts

If they escape from the confines of the enterohepatic circuit bile salts are toxic to many parts of the body. This is presumably because most organs and tissues are not adapted to the presence of a detergent. The efficiency of the enterohepatic circulation testifies to the importance of keeping bile salts in their place. Disorders which have been blamed on bile salts out of their place include gastric ulcer, oesophagitis, pancreatitis, watery diarrhoea, and pruritus.

Gastric Ulcer and Oesophagitis

A characteristic of gastric ulcer patients is frequent reflux of bile into the stomach. It was suggested by Du Plessis (1965) that bile damaged the gastric mucosa and caused ulceration. However, this theory gained favour only when it was discovered that there is in the gastric mucosa a barrier which normally prevents hydrogen ions from diffusing back into the mucosa, and that bile breaks this barrier (Rhodes, 1972). This theory neatly explains the paradox that, on the one hand hydrochloric acid is essential for ulcers to form ('no acid, no ulcer') and, on the other, that gastric ulcer patients seem to secrete less than the normal amount of acid. It is postulated that, in the presence of bile, much of the acid which is secreted diffuses back into the mucosa, damaging it and causing the gastritis which characteristically surrounds an ulcer. Both bile and acid are necessary. Experimentally, infusing bile into the stomach does not cause gastritis, but infusing bile and acid does so. The components of bile most likely to have this effect are the bile salts. They and other detergents have been shown to be barrier-breakers (Davenport, 1968). In the laboratory, bile salt solutions damage the mucosa, and their effects are proportional both to the bile salt concentration and to the hydrogen ion concentration (Black, Hole and Rhodes, 1971). Similarly, acute gastric erosions could be caused in dogs by inducing local ischaemia, but only if bile salts and hydrochloric acid were present as well (Ritchie, 1975). The ability of aspirin to cause bleeding from the rat gastric mucosa was greatly enhanced by giving conjugated bile acids at the same time (Semple and Russell, 1975). In dogs, stress ulcers can be prevented by administering the bile acid-binding resin cholestyramine (Zike et al, 1973). In view of all this, it is disappointing that, in man, treatment with cholestyramine was found not to aid the healing of gastric ulcers (Black et al, 1971). This may have been because, with intermittent therapy, the resin was present in the stomach for only part of the day.

Besides their direct damaging effect on the mucosa, bile acids in the stomach may be harmful in an indirect way. They have been shown to stimulate the release of gastrin from the gastric antrum and so to increase acid secretion (Bedi et al, 1971).

On the other hand, bile reflux cannot be the whole explanation of gastric ulceration, since not all patients have it and, in those who do, the reflux often persists after the ulcer has healed (Black, Roberts and Rhodes, 1971). Other hypotheses must be considered and Dragstedt's gastric stasis theory has much to commend it (Rhodes, 1972).

More recently, a similar hypothesis has been put forward to explain reflux oesophagitis. Patients with heartburn and hiatus hernia tend to have bile reflux into the stomach (Gillison, Nyhus and Duthie, 1971; Crumplin et al, 1974). In experiments with monkeys, reflux of pure gastric juice into the oesophagus rarely caused damage, whereas when the gastric juice contained bile severe oesophagitis occurred (Gillison et al, 1972). Very recently it has been found that, as with the stomach, the mucosa of the oesophagus possesses a barrier to acid diffusion, and that this is breached by bile salts (Safaie-Shirazi, DenBesten and Zike, 1975). This raises the possibility that acid damages the oesophagus only if bile salts are present to let it into the mucosa. Against the hypothesis, however, is the fact that, in patients complaining of reflux, the regurgitated material is usually quite colourless.

It must be remembered that duodenal juice may contain another detergent besides bile salts, namely lysolecithin. This is produced in the duodenum when the lecithin in bile is partly hydrolysed by the pancreatic enzyme phospholipase A. In experiments, lysolecithin can certainly damage the stomach mucosa (Davenport, 1970). However, even here bile salts could play a role, since they help to activate phospholipase A.

Acute Pancreatitis

Many theories have been advanced for the pathogenesis of acute pancreatitis, and of these the most durable is the reflux of bile into the pancreas. It has recently been strengthened by the remarkable feat of finding gallstones in the stools of 34 out of 36 patients who were recovering from acute pancreatitis (Acosta and Ledesma, 1974). The suggestion here is that, as the stone was passed, there was transient obstruction of the ampulla of Vater, causing bile to reflux into the pancreas. Alternatively, passage of the stone may have damaged the sphincter and made it incompetent. Reflux of duodenal juice could be more damaging than reflux of pure bile, since duodenal juice may contain lysolecithin as well as bile salts (McCutcheon, 1968).

When pure bile salt solutions are injected into the pancreatic ducts of animals, they induce all grades of inflammation and necrosis up to acute haemorrhagic pancreatitis. Dihydroxy bile salts are particularly toxic (Hansson, 1967). A synthetic detergent, lauryl sulphate, produced lesions in the dog pancreas which were morphologically similar to those produced by bile salts, suggesting that the latter act through their detergency (Beck, Sum and Bencosme, 1969). On the other hand, Schmidt and Creutzfeldt (1969) have postulated that bile salts exert their effect by activating phospholipase A, and that it is lysolecithin which actually damages the pancreas.

Some workers doubt that bile reflux is involved in the pathogenesis of acute pancreatitis and stress the possible role of proteases, elastase, and kinins.

The Role of Bile Salts in Cholestasis and Cirrhosis

Cholestasis

This is the ultimate insult to bile salt metabolism. Deprived of all access to the enterohepatic circulation, bile salts are compelled to wander uselessly round the body. Serum bile salt concentrations are raised up to 60 times the normal level (Neale et al, 1971). Probably because of this, bile salt synthesis is markedly depressed. It also tends to be aberrant, for the cholestatic liver may start synthesising exotic bile salts which are normally found only in pigs, toads, or crocodiles! One aberration which has attracted particular attention is the formation by cholestatic infants of an unsaturated, monohydroxy bile salt (Norman and Strandvik, 1973). This is intriguing because in animals cholestasis can be produced by infusing monohydroxy bile salts. Hence, in the clinical situation, it is hard to be sure whether monohydroxy bile salts are the cause or the effect of the cholestasis. In man, the most important monohydroxy bile salt is lithocholate, and a rather elaborate hypothesis was devised by Schaffner and Popper (1969) blaming the tendency of intrahepatic cholestasis to persist upon the synthesis of lithocholate by the obstructed liver. However, supporting evidence has not been forthcoming and high lithocholate levels have not been demonstrated in cholestatic livers. What has been found is quite high levels of the dihydroxy bile salt chenodeoxycholate (Greim et al, 1972). This could be important because, experimentally, dihydroxy bile salts are very toxic to liver microsomes, especially the cytochrome P-450 system, probably through their detergent action. In cholestatic livers there is often some secondary liver cell damage and this tends to be most marked when there are high concentrations of chenodeoxycholate in the liver biopsy.

Urinary bile salts

It has recently been realised that the obstructed liver has an ingenious answer to the problem of getting rid of bile salts from the body. This is to make the bile salt molecule more soluble in water by turning its hydroxyl groups into the much more polar sulphate groups. Sulphated bile salts are cleared into the urine up to 200 times more efficiently than their parent substances (Stiehl, Earnest and Admirand, 1975). This explains the well-known clinical observations that jaundiced urine is frothy and has a lower surface tension so that flowers of sulphur sink in it (Hay's test). Actually, even in complete biliary obstruction the urine contains less than 20 mg (40 μmol) of bile salts in 24 hours (Makino et al. 1975), but in normal urine bile salts are virtually unmeasurable.

Pruritus

This is the most troublesome symptom in cholestasis. It is almost certainly due to retained bile salts deposited in the skin. The correlation between serum bile salt concentration and severity of pruritus is rather poor, but on average serum bile salts are higher in those who itch than those who do not. They are also raised in pregnancy pruritus. The best evidence is that provided by Schoenfield (1969), who reported high concentrations of bile salts on the skin of itching patients and a fall to normal on the day pruritus was relieved. Simply placing a bile salt solution on the skin does not cause pruritus, but it does so rapidly if the solution is placed on an exposed blister base (Kirby, Heaton and Burton, 1974). The most pruritogenic bile salts are the dihydroxy ones.

Malabsorption

The steatorrhoea of cholestasis is due essentially to the absence of bile salt micelles from the intestine. The loss of fat is not of itself very important, but the associated malabsorption of vitamins could well be serious. A prolonged prothrombin time due to vitamin K deficiency is common and, if cholestasis is prolonged, osteomalacia responsive to vitamin D is a well recognised complication. It is customary to blame these disorders on malabsorption due to bile salt deficiency, and there is no doubt that in the absence of bile negligible quantities of fat-soluble vitamins are absorbed (Forsgren, 1969). What is usually overlooked, however, is the fact that there is no known dietary requirement for vitamin K and nutritional deficiency has never been recorded (Davidson and Passmore, 1969), the accepted reason being that naphthoquinones are synthesised by intestinal bacteria and absorbed by the host. Does steatorrhoea prevent this synthesis or absorption? With vitamin D too, there is no established dietary requirement, and the vitamin is synthesised by the skin in adequate amounts when there is normal exposure to daylight. Perhaps in prolonged cholestasis the cause of vitamin D deficiency is not so much malabsorption as the fact that the jaundiced patient is reluctant to go out of his home!

Phenobarbitone in cholestasis

Phenobarbitone, which induces microsomal enzymes, can be of therapeutic value in intrahepatic cholestasis, relieving pruritus and reducing serum bile salts (Stiehl, Thaler and Admirand, 1972). In primary biliary cirrhosis, phenobarbitone could be a useful alternative to cholestyramine, which is not always well tolerated (Earnest, 1972). The action of phenobarbitone is probably due to stimulation of bile flow rather than to a direct effect on bile salts themselves. Experimentally phenobarbitone increases the bile salt-independent fraction of bile flow (Gumucio et al, 1973). Unfortunately, this effect of phenobarbitone cannot be used as a diagnostic test for intrahepatic cholestasis, as it can occur with extrahepatic bile duct obstruction (Metreau et al, 1975). Presumably, the increased bile secretion pressure temporarily overcomes the obstruction.

Disturbances of bile salt metabolism in cirrhosis

In cirrhosis every aspect of bile salt metabolism is disturbed. As one would expect, synthesis is impaired, and consequently the bile salt pool is only half its normal size, with a particular deficiency of cholic acid (Vlahcevic et al, 1972b). Partly because of this, the concentration of bile salts in the small intestine during digestion is low. In fact it is low enough to impair fat absorption, and this probably explains why steatorrhoea is so common in cirrhosis, at least in the non-alcoholic patient (Badley et al, 1970). A contributing factor to the low bile salt concentration is probably the curious tendency of the cirrhotic to secrete copious amounts of excessively dilute bile. It should be added that in alcoholic patients steatorrhoea seems to be related more to chronic pancreatitis and consequent pancreatic exocrine failure than to bile salt deficiency.

The cirrhotic liver has difficulty in clearing bile salts from the blood partly, no doubt, because it is diseased, but also because of portosystemic shunting in patients with portal hypertension. This impaired uptake has been made the basis of two very sensitive liver function tests. One is the two-hour postprandial serum bile salt concentration which, in a series of 26 patients with various liver diseases, was the only test to be abnormal in every case (Kaplowitz et al, 1973). Taking blood postprandially makes the test more sensitive because it ensures that the gallbladder is contracted and so the liver is faced with the job of recycling the whole bile salt pool. The other test is the *intravenous bile acid tolerance* test (Korman et al, 1975). This exploits the fact that, in health, intravenously injected bile salt has a half life in the blood of only two minutes and that, by 12 minutes, the serum concentration has returned to the baseline level. This test has not yet been applied to the routine clinical situation but it meets many of the criteria of an ideal liver function test. It measures directly and specifically the hepatic handling of a physiological substance. Its sensitivity has been proved by the demonstration of a positive result in nine out of 11 patients with biopsy-proven chronic liver disease but normal conventional liver function tests (LaRusso et al, 1975). Its practicality in clinical use will probably rest on the use of radioactively labelled bile salt (Calcraft et al, 1975).

A puzzling and so far unexplained feature of bile salt metabolism in the cirrhotic is a marked reduction in the amount of deoxycholate in bile. It implies that colonic physiology is altered so that either there is less bacterial dehydroxylation of cholate or there is impaired absorption of the deoxycholate formed. In fact there is evidence for both abnormalities (Yoshida et al, 1975), but why the cirrhotic's colon should behave in this way is a mystery.

Bile Salt Diarrhoea (Cholegenic Diarrhoea) and its Causes

It has been known since ancient times that bile had laxative properties. Indeed, Aristotle in the fourth century B.C. regarded bile as 'of no other use than by its acrimony to promote the excretion of the Guts' (Gibson, 1684). For centuries, dried ox bile has been used as a laxative and, even today, it is possible to buy proprietary laxatives containing semi-purified ox bile. The modern concept of a laxative is an agent which inhibits fluid absorption or stimulates fluid secretion by the colon (Binder and Donowitz, 1975), and these properties have been documented more thoroughly with bile salts than with any other laxative. In 1971, Mekhjian, Phillips and Hofmann reported the results of experiments on 20 healthy subjects who had been persuaded to swallow a long tube and retain it until its tip reached the caecum. Test solutions were then perfused into the proximal colon and the effluent was collected by a rectal tube to analyse water and electrolyte changes. When the test solution contained deoxycholate 3 mmol/l or chenodeoxycholate 5 mmol/l, there was not merely inhibition of water absorption but actually net secretion of water, or rather of isotonic sodium chloride. Cholate had no effect even at 10 mmol/l. Normal stool contains deoxycholate in 3–5 mmol/l concentration, but most of it is bound to solid matter. The concentration in stool water is what matters and this is probably much lower in healthy subjects. However, when there is malabsorption of bile salts, the concentration of bile salts in stool water is often over 4 mmol/l, and has been recorded as high as 18 mmol/l (Hofmann and Poley, 1972; Mitchell and

Eastwood, 1972). From this one can predict that malabsorption of bile salts will cause diarrhoea, and this is indeed the case.

Resection or disease of the terminal ileum

This is the model situation for both bile salt malabsorption and cholegenic diarrhoea. There is some dispute as to how much reabsorption remains, some authorities saying virtually none, others claiming that there is significant recirculation of the bile salt which is least polar and so most easily absorbed passively from the jejunum, glycochenodeoxycholate. However, it is generally agreed that faecal bile acid excretion is grossly increased if more than 40 cm ileum is removed, and can be as high as 10 times normal (Hofmann, 1972). Since, in the healthy state, excretion is balanced by new synthesis, this implies that the liver is synthesising far more bile salt than normal. This situation may be seen as the liver attempting to compensate for the loss of the enterohepatic circulation, but it is more accurately described as a disinhibited or de-repressed liver. Loss of bile salt reabsorption means a loss of the negative feedback mechanism controlling bile salt synthesis. The same situation occurs with a biliary fistula, as in continuous T-tube drainage, and when large doses of a bile acid-binding agent such as cholestyramine are fed.

Increased bile salt synthesis has a number of consequences. One is that there is greatly increased catabolism of cholesterol, which is only partly balanced by increased cholesterol synthesis. As a result, the serum cholesterol is low in ileectomy subjects. Indeed the operation of ileal bypass has been used with some success to treat hypercholesterolaemia (Moore, Frantz and Buchwald, 1969; Södal, Gjertsen and Schrump, 1970). Secondly, given time and a functioning gallbladder, the liver can accumulate a reasonable pool of bile salt. In fact, after breakfast the duodenal concentration of bile salts is usually reduced but it is lower still after later meals (van Deest et al, 1968). This largely explains why steatorrhoea is invariable with all but trivial ileal resections, and why it is much worse after ileal than after comparable jejunal resections (Booth, Alldis and Read, 1961). Thirdly, the increased bile salt synthesis has the disadvantage of providing more bile salts to enter and disturb the colon.

The *diarrhoea* of modest ileal resections (up to 100 cm) is characteristically watery and very urgent. It is worse after meals, especially breakfast (when the amount of bile salt available to be malabsorbed is greatest), and it may cause anal soreness. With more extensive resections, the diarrhoea is less watery but there is more steatorrhoea. In these cases, the colonic dysfunction is thought to be due more to unabsorbed fatty acids than to bile acids. The concept of fatty acid diarrhoea rests on two lines of evidence. One is that, with massive ileal resections, diarrhoea is relieved most effectively by prescribing a low fat diet, or a diet in which the normal type of fat (long chain triglycerides) is replaced by medium chain triglycerides (Hofmann and Poley, 1972). The other is that, experimentally long chain fatty acids cause the colonic mucosa to secrete excess fluid; in other words, they are laxatives (Ammon and Phillips, 1973). A famous laxative, castor oil, has as its active ingredient the hydroxylated long chain fatty acid, ricinoleic acid.

The most logical *treatment* of bile acid diarrhoea is to give the bile salt-binding resin, cholestyramine, in a dose of 4 grams (one sachet) with each meal. It acts by reducing the concentration of bile acids in faecal water. Cholestyramine certainly works in most cases but it is not very palatable and it is fortunate that, in practice, many patients do well on codeine phosphate.

To delay the egress of ileal contents is also a function of the ileocaecal valve (better called the ileocaecal sphincter) and if this is resected as part of an ileal resection diarrhoea tends to be much worse. It is particularly bad if the ascending colon is resected as well (Cummings, James and Wiggins, 1973), probably because this is normally the main site of colonic water absorption.

Gallstones are common in patients with resection or extensive disease of the terminal ileum (Heaton and Read, 1969). They probably result from the breakdown in bile salt reabsorption, which reduces the amount of bile salt available to be secreted into bile and so renders the bile supersaturated with cholesterol (Dowling, Bell and White, 1972).

A simplified scheme to explain the main clinical features of bile salt malabsorption is shown in Figure 14.4.

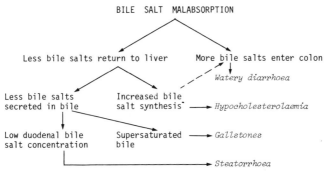

Figure 14.4   A simplified scheme to explain the main clinical features of bile salt malabsorption or interrupted enterohepatic circulation, as seen in patients with resection of the terminal ileum

Postvagotomy diarrhoea

This has long been an enigma, but recent evidence points to bile salt malabsorption as an important cause, at least in the unlucky few who have persistent watery stools after truncal vagotomy and drainage. In seven such patients, the mean faecal bile acid excretion was over three times more than in normal controls (Allan, Gerskowitch and Russell, 1973) and cholestyramine was found to be very effective in controlling the diarrhoea (Allan and Russell, 1975). Why an operation of this sort should cause bile salt malabsorption is quite obscure, but perhaps the most likely explanation is that vagotomy alters the function of the terminal ileum.

Cystic fibrosis

This poses a similar problem. There is now no doubt that children with pancreatic insufficiency secondary to cystic fibrosis have severe bile salt malabsorption (Weber et al, 1973; Weber et al, 1975). Bile acid loss is proportional to faecal fat excretion and improves with pancreatic replacement therapy. This suggests that it is secondary to the malabsorption of fat and nitrogen. The same situation does not occur in coeliac disease, but this may be because in coeliac disease bile salts tend to remain sequestered in a sluggishly contracting gallbladder (Low-Beer et al, 1971).

Two questions of physiology

Can diarrhoea itself cause bile salt malabsorption by rushing bile salt molecules past the active transport sites in the terminal ileum? The answer is probably no. When watery diarrhoea was induced in four volunteers by giving them large volumes of 10 per cent mannitol to drink, there was only a mild decrease in bile salt absorption (Meihoff and Kern, 1968).

Are bile salts physiological laxatives, preventing excessive dehydration of the faeces? Was Aristotle right? The answer is probably yes. When normal subjects are given cholestyramine they do tend to become constipated. In general, too, there is a correlation between the weight of the faeces and their content of bile salts (Woodbury and Kern, 1971). On the other hand, the main natural preventive of constipation, dietary fibre, does not seem to work by increasing faecal bile salts (Findlay et al, 1974).

Tests for cholegenic diarrhoea

How is the clinician to decide whether, in a given patient, diarrhoea is caused by bile salts? The simplest and most direct test, indeed the only conclusive test, is to prescribe cholestyramine 4 g with each meal and see if the diarrhoea is relieved. Ideally, stool weight should be monitored, but usually the clinical response is obvious. The indirect approach is to show that bile salt malabsorption is present. The only practical way to do this is to measure the ^{14}C radioactivity in an aliquot of a 24-hour stool collection after giving an oral dose of [^{14}C]cholic acid. However, this involves homogenising, drying and combusting the stool, trapping the $^{14}CO_2$ and counting in a liquid scintillation spectrometer. A much simpler test is the breath test, but this often gives false negative results (see page 338).

The Stagnant Loop Syndrome

By definition, the stagnant loop or contaminated small bowel syndrome includes any situation where diarrhoea and malabsorption (especially of fat and vitamin B_{12}) are associated with bacterial counts of $10^7/l$ or greater in aspirates from the upper small intestine. The main causes are strictures and blind loops, including diverticulosis of the duodenum and jejunum, and fistulae from the colon to the stomach or small bowel. The bacteria involved are mainly anaerobes such as bacteroides, which are normally present in the colon in counts of 10^{12} to $10^{14}/l$ (Gracey, 1971; Tabaqchali and Booth, 1970). Amongst their many metabolic potentialities, these bacteria are able to deconjugate and dehydroxylate bile salts.

Probably, the most constant feature of the stagnant loop syndrome is the presence of free or unconjugated bile salts within the upper small intestine (Tabaqchali and Booth, 1970; Northfield, Drasar and Wright, 1973). Other tests, including the Schilling test, discriminate poorly between patients with the full syndrome and patients in whom there are raised bacterial counts but no steatorrhoea (Northfield et al, 1973). When antibiotics active against bacteroides are given, such as lincomycin, the free bile acids tend to disappear at the same time as the faecal fat returns to normal. All this suggests that bile salt deconjugation is involved in the pathogenesis of the steatorrhoea.

There are two ways in which bile salt deconjugation could lead to steatorrhoea. Firstly, as proposed by Dawson and Isselbacher in 1960, free bile acids can be toxic to the intestinal mucosa. In the unconjugated state, dihydroxy bile acids in particular have been shown to inhibit every metabolic activity of the mucosa, including one of the steps in fat absorption, namely esterification of free fatty acids (Dietschy, 1967). Some of these effects are artefacts of the laboratory, but recent studies have built up a convincing picture. For example, when three healthy subjects underwent overnight perfusion of the jejunum with a solution containing free deoxycholate in the low concentration of 1 or 2 mmol/l, and then ate a test meal, biopsies of the jejunum showed clear evidence of impaired fat absorption on electron microscopic examination (Shimoda, O'Brien and Saunders, 1974). The changes seen were exactly like those in biopsies from patients with the stagnant loop syndrome. In this syndrome, there is often malabsorption of other nutrients as well as fat, and this may be because enzymes within the mucosal cell and at its microvillous brush border are inhibited by free bile acids. Certainly, adding deoxycholate to the diet produces such enzyme inhibition in rats (Gracey, Houghton and Thomas, 1975).

It was for long thought that the intestinal mucosa is microscopically normal in patients with the stagnant loop syndrome. However, when multiple jejunal biopsies are examined, definite if patchy abnormalities can be seen on light microscopy, while electron microscopy shows that absorptive cells are quite extensively damaged (Ament et al, 1972). Similarly, rats with experimental blind loops have patchy ultrastructural changes in the contaminated small intestine (Gracey, Papadimitriou and Bower, 1974). These changes too could be caused by the toxic action of free bile acids. They have been reproduced in the rat by feeding 25 mg deoxycholate per day for three or four days (Gracey et al, 1973) and by perfusing the small intestine with weak solutions of deoxycholate or chenodeoxycholate (Low-Beer, Schneider and Dobbins, 1970).

While all this evidence supports the role of bile acid toxicity, it is possible that there are other toxic metabolites of anaerobic bacteria as well as free bile acids.

The other way in which bile salt deconjugation could cause steatorrhoea is by leading to detergent deficiency. Free bile acids are of no use in micelle formation because they are precipitated at the relatively acid pH of the upper small intestine. Therefore, when there is extensive deconjugation, the concentration of bile salts in solution could fall to levels at which there are not enough micelles available for fat absorption. Plausible though this theory is, there are patients who have steatorrhoea in the face of plentiful micelles (Ament et al, 1972). A much quoted piece of evidence in favour of detergent deficiency is the fall in faecal fat which occurred when a single patient was fed conjugated bile salts (Tabaqchali, Hatzioannou and Booth, 1967). However, another possible interpretation of this finding is that the extra micelles provided by the fed bile salt dissolved some of the free bile acids. Effectively, this would lower the free bile acid concentration.

A rare but intriguing complication of the stagnant loop syndrome is the formation of *enteroliths* — solid concretions in the lumen of the affected bowel. Typically, these are composed of precipitated free bile acids, especially deoxycholic, with minor amounts of fatty acids (Haslewood, 1967).

The definitive *diagnostic test* is the demonstration that tests of absorption improve after a course of an antibiotic active against anaerobic bacteria. The finding of free bile acids and of high bacterial counts in an aspirate from the small bowel is also direct evidence, but the techniques involved are not generally available. A simple and non-invasive screening test is the glycocholate breath test.

The Radioactive Breath Test

This test, properly known as the [^{14}C] glycocholate or cholylglycine-^{14}C breath test, is the first test involving bile salts to become widely used in clinical practice. It was introduced in 1971 as a means of detecting excessive deconjugation of bile salts (Fromm and Hofmann, 1971). Hence, positive results are obtained in two main circumstances: firstly, when bacteria have access to bile salts more proximally in the gut than normal, which includes bacterial cholangitis as well as stagnant loop syndrome, and secondly, when there is excessive passage of bile salts into the colon, that is with dysfunction of the terminal ileum and consequent malabsorption of bile salts.

The principle of the test is as follows: when glycine-conjugated bile salts, which normally make up about three-quarters of the total in bile, are deconjugated in the intestine, the liberated glycine is either metabolised by bacteria or absorbed and metabolised by the body. In either case, the end products include CO_2, most of which is excreted in the breath. When the glycine is labelled with ^{14}C, radioactive CO_2 is expired at a rate proportional to the rate of bile salt deconjugation. The technique is the same as with other radioactive breath tests. After an overnight fast, the patient is given a liquid test meal to which has been added 5 μCi of cholylglycine-^{14}C (obtainable from the Radiochemical Centre at Amersham). At hourly intervals for four or five hours, the patient blows through dessicating crystals into a molar solution of a CO_2 trapping agent, Hyamine hydroxide. This contains an acid-base indicator which changes colour when 1 ml of Hyamine has taken up 1 mmol of CO_2. The radioactivity in that millimole of CO_2 is measured in a liquid scintillation counter. The result is best expressed as the percentage of the administered dose which is expired per hour, or in the four or five hours of the test. The upper limit of normal is about 1.6 per cent of the dose in 4 hours (Fromm, Thomas and Hofmann, 1973).

Clinically, the main application of this test is in cases of malabsorption where small bowel contamination is suspected. False positive tests, that is abnormal results in malabsorption from other causes, are very uncommon, and only one false negative has been reported in proven stagnant loop syndrome (Parkin et al, 1972). It seems reasonable therefore to use this as a screening test in patients with malabsorption, before deciding whether it is necessary to perform the more invasive and complicated test of small bowel intubation and analysis of the aspirate for free bile acids. The exposure to radiation is negligible.

It is less worthwhile to use the breath test as a screening procedure for ileal dysfunction in cases of diarrhoea without malabsorption. An abnormal test is certainly suspicious since, in one series, positive results were obtained in only 1 out of 18 patients with colitis, and in only 2 out of 30 patients with 'unexplained diarrhoea' (presumably irritable bowel syndrome) (Pedersen, Arnfred and Hess Thaysen, 1973). However, a negative result would have no significance at all, as it is frequently obtained in known ileal disease with documented bile salt malabsorption (Pedersen et al, 1973; Lenz, 1975).

Disappointingly, the breath test is of little value in Crohn's disease. A positive test is hard to interpret because it can mean either ileal dysfunction or bacterial overgrowth due to stricturing and stasis. A negative result is meaningless, at least in unoperated ileal disease since, in a study of 10 such patients, only one was found to have a positive breath test, in spite of the fact that four had active disease and six had documented bile salt malabsorption (Lenz, 1975). This problem can be overcome by combining the breath test with counting of ^{14}C radioactivity in the stool. However, this sacrifices the great advantage of the test, which is its simplicity.

The surprising frequency of negative breath tests in cases of definite bile salt malabsorption is probably explained by rapid transit through the colon, so that bacteria do not have time to detach the labelled glycine or to metabolise it.

Bacterial *cholangitis* is the only other condition in which the breath test is regularly positive (James, Agnew and Bouchier, 1973). Here, deconjugation may be taking place in the biliary tract itself. It is known that obstruction of the common bile duct is commonly accompanied by growth of bacteria in the bile when the cause is gallstones, but rarely so if the cause is a malignant tumour (Scott and Khan, 1967). It would be interesting to know, therefore, if the breath test has any diagnostic value in cases of obstructive jaundice.

An unexpected source of positive breath tests is gynaecological patients who have received pelvic radiotherapy. Of 17 such patients, all but one had an abnormal test (Newman et al, 1973). This was interpreted as evidence of radiation injury to the terminal ileum, and was thought to explain the fact that most of the patients had noticed a permanent change in bowel habit after radiotherapy.

Carcinoma of the Large Intestine

In a comparison of faeces from inhabitants of areas with high and low incidences of colonic cancer, Hill et al (1971) discovered more anaerobic bacteria and more strains able to dehydroxylate cholic acid in samples from high incidence areas (England, Scotland, USA) than from low incidence areas (Uganda, India, rural Japan). Afro-Asian stools contained lower concentrations of bile salts and relatively few highly degraded bile salts. Similarly, in the stools of American vegetarians (who have a reduced incidence of colon cancer) bile acids were present in lower concentration and a less degraded form than in Americans eating an ordinary diet (Reddy and Wynder, 1973). Hill and his colleagues pointed out the structural similarity between bile acids and known carcinogens such as methylcholanthrene, and postulated that colonic cancer is caused by exposure of the mucosa to degraded bile salts. Some at least of the chemical steps necessary to convert bile acids into carcinogens occur when bile acids are incubated with anaerobic bacteria commonly found in the faeces. A key step in this conversion is the desaturation of the steroid ring, that is the introduction of double bonds. Hill et al (1975) found that species of clostridia able to perform this dehydrogenation reaction were present in significantly higher numbers in the faeces of patients with large bowel cancer than in those of patients admitted to hospital with other colonic diseases. The total bile acid concentration was also higher in the faeces of cancer patients. Although these findings seem to support the hypothesis, they could of course be the effect rather than the cause of the disease. The critical evidence would be the finding of these clostridia and of high bile acid concentrations in patients in the precancerous state. Ultimately, this will require massive population surveys, but in the meantime a study was made of a group with an exceptionally high incidence of colon cancer, namely patients with hereditary polyposis coli and, paradoxically, their faeces had a subnormal capacity for degrading steroids (Drasar et al, 1975).

Epidemiological studies suggest a connection between the incidence of colon cancer and the average intake of animal fat and protein (Drasar and Irving, 1973). Some authorities believe that a high fat intake increases bile salt excretion and perhaps also the bacterial degradation of bile acids (Hill, 1974; Wynder and Reddy, 1975). However, the evidence is conflicting for this effect of fat (Ali, Kuksis and Beveridge, 1966) and another crucial factor may well be the stool bulk, which is largely dependent on the intake of distary fibre. In low cancer areas of the world, stool bulk is high (Burkitt, 1971). On a low fibre diet the stools are small and concentrated and any carcinogen within them, bile acid or otherwise, will be present in higher concentration. The slower transit of a small stool may also increase the exposure of the mucosa to carcinogens in the stool (Burkitt, 1971). The effect of fibre on bacterial metabolism in the colon is unknown. Adding bran to the diet reduced the amount of deoxycholate in the bile (Pomare and Heaton, 1973a), but it is not known whether this is due to decreased bacterial formation of deoxycholate or to reduced absorption from the colon.

GALLSTONES

Recent advances have revealed cholelithiasis as a metabolic disease, caused by environmental factors (chiefly diet) and, under favourable circumstances, reversible by medical treatment (Bell, 1974; Swell, Gregory and Vlahcevic, 1974; Bouchier, 1975; Heaton, 1975). Contrary to older beliefs, gallstone formation is not preceded by cholecystitis. In only 2 per cent of cholecystectomies are gallstones absent, and even here they had probably been present previously but were passed in the faeces (Andersson, Bergdahl and Boquist, 1971).

Classification and Composition

The traditional classification into cholesterol, pigment, and mixed stones is based on naked eye appearances, but chemical analysis shows that there is no sharp division but rather a continuous spectrum of stone composition. Since 'mixed' stones usually contain a high proportion of cholesterol, there is a trend to classify simply into cholesterol-rich and pigment.

The term 'pigment stones' is misleading. On chemical analysis they contain only 7 per cent bilirubin, and consist mainly of an amorphous and unidentified residue (Trotman, Ostrow and Soloway, 1974). Most gallstones contain a good deal of calcium salts. On x-ray powder analysis, the average American gallstone is 15 per cent calcium carbonate, whereas English calculi average no less than 30 per cent chalk (Sutor and Wooley, 1971). The significance and origin of this calcium is quite unknown. The same is true of the 'residue' which comprises two-thirds of a pigment stone. The genesis of pigment stones is in fact a complete mystery except in two special circumstances. In haemolytic anaemia, the liver has an excessive load of bilirubin to excrete and biliary levels may exceed the solubility of the pigment. In the Orient, bilirubin-rich stones frequently form in the bile ducts and have been blamed on bacterial infection, often secondary to liver fluke infestation. The mechanism is believed to be deconjugation by *Escherichia coli* glucuronidase and precipitation of the insoluble free bilirubin.

Cholesterol is by far the most important constituent of gallstones in developed countries. It comprises about 60 per cent of the average stone in England, 74 per cent in the USA and 88 per cent in Sweden (Sutor and Wooley, 1971). To a large extent, therefore, the problem of gallstones is the problem of cholesterol precipitation from bile. It is in this area that understanding has advanced recently, and it is with this area that the present review will be mainly concerned.

Epidemiology

Because 70–80 per cent of gallstones are asymptomatic, their exact prevalence can be established only by a cholecystographic survey of the population. This is impracticable, so deductions have to be drawn from autopsy surveys, which are necessarily on a selected sample of the population, and from registers of surgical operations, which are subject to other vagaries besides the incidence of gallstones. In spite of these limitations, it has recently become clear that the old adage describing the typical gallstone sufferer as 'fair, fat, fertile and forty' is largely incorrect.

Race and country

Gallstones are not especially common in fair-skinned races. In the United States, they are as common in Negroes as in Whites (Trotman and Soloway, 1973) and commonest of all in the Indians. In Arizona, no less than 73 per cent of women of the Pima tribe have developed gallstones by the age of 30 (Sampliner et al, 1970). American Indians have been the subject of unusually intense study, and it is not possible to give such precise prevalence figures for any other group. However, it is usually estimated that, at any one time, 10 to 15 per cent of the American population has or has had gallstones. In Europe, cholelithiasis is common in all countries for which statistics are available (Heaton, 1973a). Over the age of 40, stones were present at autopsy in more than half the women in both Malmö and Prague, and in about 30 per cent of the men (Zahor et al, 1974). The equivalent figures for Britain are only slightly lower. The disease has been reported as common in Australia, New Zealand, South Africa, Israel, and Chile (Santiago).

In African Negroes, gallstones are rare except in big cities like Johannesburg. Otherwise the few cases that are seen are pigment stones, probably associated with haemolysis, or are in the most affluent and Westernised members of the population. Similarly, in India gallstones are diagnosed 10 to 20 times more often in social classes I and II than in the lower classes. The same class differences have been noted in Japan (Heaton, 1973a).

Thus, in general, cholelithiasis is a disease of urbanised, economically advanced communities. In developing countries, it is probably becoming commoner. In Tokyo, the overall autopsy incidence rose between 1949 and 1964 from 2.5 per cent to 6.1 per cent (Kameda, 1967). There has been a virtual epidemic of gallstones in Canadian Eskimos who have abandoned their primitive nomadic way of life and adopted Western culture (Schaefer, 1971). In American Negroes, there has been a big change from the early years of this century, when Negroes were widely regarded as immune to gallstones.

Overall, therefore, cholelithiasis is a disease which is acquired with 'civilised' culture, and especially modern affluence, and all races of men are susceptible. Primitive peoples and wild animals do not suffer from it. The only time when a fall in gallstone incidence has been observed was during the Second World War in Europe. Although, of course, accurate statistics are not available, this does suggest that the material standard of living, and especially eating, is a crucial factor.

Age, sex and parity

Cholelithiasis is not, as the adage suggests, especially common in the forties. The prevalence rises steadily with age. However, stones do seem to be asymptomatic more often in the elderly, so that the peak age for gallbladder operations is around 60 years (Holland and Heaton, 1972). The female to male ratio is around two, though it used to be higher. The disease is definitely commoner in women who have been pregnant but, despite the adjective fertile in the adage, it is not at all certain that multiparity increases the risk (Friedman, Kannel and Dawber, 1966).

Cholesterol-rich Gallstones as a Metabolic Disease

The grounds for considering gallstones as a metabolic disease are three-fold — association with other disorders of metabolism, differences in bile composition and in hepatic enzyme activities from control subjects, and reversibility with medical treatment.

Association with other metabolic diseases

Obesity. Gallstone patients are significantly fatter than average, and fat people are excessively prone to cholelithiasis (for references, see Bennion and Grundy, 1975; Zahor et al, 1974).

Diabetes. At autopsy, diabetics have an increased frequency of cholelithiasis, and gallstone patients have twice the expected prevalence of diabetes

(Watkinson, 1967). In life, gallstone patients often have latent diabetes (Braunsteiner et al, 1966). Pima Indians hold the world records for the prevalence of both gallstones and diabetes.

Hypertriglyceridaemia. The fasting plasma triglyceride level is raised in patients with cholelithiasis compared with matched controls (Braunsteiner et al, 1966; Bell et al, 1973). Conversely, patients with type 4 hyperlipidaemia have, by oral cholecystography, a high incidence of gallstones (Einarsson, Hellström and Kallner, 1975). This association may explain the rather weak association between gallstones and coronary heart disease (for references see Heaton, 1973a). Contrary to popular belief, the serum cholesterol level is not raised in gallstone patients.

Obesity, diabetes, and hypertriglyceridaemia are all to a large extent manifestations of overnutrition, and all are most effectively treated by weight reduction. This obviously suggests that gallstones too may be a manifestation of overnutrition.

Ileal dysfunction. The greatly increased frequency of cholelithiasis in patients after ileal resection or with extensive ileal disease is a special case. It is almost certainly the result of interruption of the enterohepatic circulation and consequent deficiency of bile salts (as explained on page 334). Here, clearly, gallstones are a metabolic disease.

Abnormal composition of the bile

In patients with cholesterol-rich gallstones, the gallbladder bile is abnormal in that it is supersaturated with cholesterol in nearly all cases. This is implicit in the long-known fact that crystals of cholesterol can be found in the bile of such patients. Indeed, until quite recently duodenal aspiration and the examination of the aspirate for crystals was used to diagnose gallstones (Hunt, 1956). However, it was 1968 before a method was invented for measuring the saturation of bile with cholesterol. Recognising that this depended on the relative proportions of bile salts, lecithin (phospholipid), and cholesterol, Admirand and Small (1968) made mixtures of these three substances in water in all possible proportions and recorded the presence or absence of crystals or liquid crystals, that is of undissolved material. To display their results they were obliged to use a triangular system of graph-plotting known as triangular co-ordinates. This is illustrated in Figure 14.5, which also shows how the triangle was used to record the physical state of the mixtures. It became clear that cholesterol is safely in solution only if the triple mixture has a composition which places it in the lower left-hand corner of the triangle — the micellar zone. The curved line bounding this zone denotes full saturation with cholesterol. If the composition of a bile sample puts it on this line, that bile has a saturation index (or lithogenic index) of 1.0. If it is in the micellar zone, half-way between the curved line and the base of the triangle, its saturation index is 0.5, whereas if it is an equal distance above the curved line its saturation index as 1.5 (Metzger, Heymsfield and Grundy, 1972). To determine the saturation index of a bile sample it is not, in practice, necessary to plot the results of bile analysis on triangular co-ordinates. An equation is available, into which the molar percentages of cholesterol, lecithin, and bile salt can be entered (Thomas and Hofmann, 1973).

It has been suggested that supersaturated bile should not necessarily be regarded as abnormal, because it is found in a considerable number of normal people, that is subjects with healthy, stone-free gallbladders. It is true that in a Western society, many stone-free people have supersaturated bile — for example 60 per cent of normal Swedes (Nakayama and van der Linden, 1971). However, it is doubtful if the biliary state of such subjects should be regarded as normal, since at least half of them are destined to develop gallstones by the age of 70. In Japan and Africa, where gallstones are uncommon, bile from healthy subjects is very seldom supersaturated. In fact, there is a fairly good correlation between the average saturation of bile and the prevalence of gallstones in a population (Redinger and Small, 1972). As with serum cholesterol concentration, normality

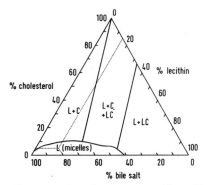

Figure 14.5   Triangular co-ordinates used to plot the composition of bile in terms of its content of cholesterol, lecithin (phospholipid) and bile salts. The point joined by the dotted lines represents a mixture of 5 per cent cholesterol, 15 per cent lecithin and 80 per cent bile salts. A bile sample with this composition lies in the micellar zone and is undersaturated with cholesterol. Bile samples above the curved line are supersaturated and contain crystals or liquid crystals according to the zone they fall into. This diagram is appropriate only for bile samples with a total solute concentration of 5 to 20 per cent. Modified from Admirand and Small (1968). Later studies have indicated that the zone of true cholesterol solubility is somewhat smaller than shown, the area immediately below the curved line being a zone of supersaturation with little tendency to precipitate cholesterol crystals (metastable-labile zone) (Carey and Small, 1973)

should be defined as the level associated with the lowest incidence of the appropriate disease. The Masai of East Africa seem to be totally free of gallstones, and their bile has a saturation index of about 0.5, whereas with European bile the index is usually over 0.8 (Biss et al, 1971). Similarly, bile is very undersaturated in all animal species that have been studied except baboons, and this is the only species which forms gallstones spontaneously and at all commonly.

The fact that supersaturated bile is often present in the absence of gallstones implies that an additional factor must be present in the gallbladder before crystals of cholesterol precipitate out. This factor is probably a nucleating or seeding agent. Its nature is unknown, but likely possibilities are bacteria, desquamated cells, particles of deconjugated bilirubin, and even large glycopro-tein molecules. It must be stressed that none of these will cause cholesterol to crystallise out unless the bile is supersaturated, so the latter must be regarded as the prime cause. When other conditions are right, a crucial factor could be stasis or stratification of bile in the gallbladder (Bouchier, 1975).

The association of gallstones with obesity is explained by the fact that bile saturation is increased in obesity (Bennion and Grundy, 1975). The same is true of ileal resection (Dowling et al, 1972). Bile composition has not been reported in patients with diabetes or hypertriglyceridaemia.

The pathogenesis of supersaturated bile

No credence is given now to the old theory that the gallbladder rendered bile abnormal and so was responsible for gallstone formation. It is possible that, once it is damaged, the gallbladder can absorb bile salts, but in many patients with cholesterol-rich gallstones the gallbladder wall is perfectly normal. It is the liver which is the source of abnormal bile, and the gallbladder should be regarded as the innocent victim of a delinquent liver. Stones form in the gallbladder rather than the bile ducts because only in the gallbladder does bile rest quietly, and time is allowed for crystals to grow and agglomerate.

Theoretically, bile can become supersaturated because there is a deficiency of lecithin. However, there is no evidence that this occurs as a separate event; rather, lecithin secretion into bile is closely dependent upon bile salt secretion. This leaves cholesterol excess and bile salt deficiency as the two possible mechanisms, and in fact both occur.

Cholesterol excess. To measure cholesterol secretion in bile requires a complex technique involving duodenal perfusion and unabsorbable markers, and only two groups of workers have reported their findings in gallstone subjects. In studies of both Indians and Caucasians, Grundy, Metzger and Adler (1972) and Grundy et al (1974) found that gallstone patients secreted nearly twice as much cholesterol per hour as control subjects and concluded that this was a major factor, perhaps the major factor, in the production of supersaturated bile. In these studies, most of the patients were obese and most of the controls were slim. In their investigation of seven Caucasian gallstone patients, Northfield and Hofmann (1975) used controls who were matched for body weight, and they could find no difference in cholesterol secretion between the two groups. This obviously suggests that obesity itself raises cholesterol output into bile. This has now been confirmed by Bennion and Grundy (1975). Moreover, they showed that when a group of very obese men reduced their weight by about 25 per cent their cholesterol secretion fell from 75 to 55 mg/h (0.14–0.18 mmol/h).

This effect of obesity is explained by the fact that in obesity there is a marked increase in the synthesis of cholesterol by the liver. Indeed, the cholesterol production rate is related directly to the weight of body fat (Miettinen, 1971; Nestel, Schreibman and Ahrens, 1973). Liver synthesis of cholesterol is regulated by an enzyme called β-hydroxy-β-methylglutaryl-CoA reductase and, in liver biopsies from gallstone subjects, the activity of this enzyme and the concentration of cholesterol are both greater than in controls (Salen et al, 1975). The activity of this enzyme is reportedly increased by insulin (Nepokroeff et al, 1974) which raises the possibility that the well-known hyperinsulinism of obesity contributes to gallstone formation.

Another factor determining the rate of cholesterol secretion is the amount of chenodeoxycholate (CDC) in the circulating bile salt pool. When this is increased artificially by feeding CDC, there is a fall in cholesterol secretion (Northfield et al, 1975). When it is decreased artificially by feeding deoxycholate, which selectively inhibits CDC synthesis, there is a rise in the saturation index of bile (Pomare and Low-Beer, 1975; Low-Beer and Pomare, 1975). Hence, one determinant of bile cholesterol secretion is the relative amount in bile of a colonic metabolite, deoxycholate.

Bile salt deficiency. The key factor determining the bile salt content of the relaxed gallbladder (in which, presumably, it is easiest for gallstones to form and grow) is the size of the bile salt pool. In patients with presumed cholesterol gallstones, the bile salt pool is only 50 to 60 per cent of its normal size of 2–3 g (4–6 mmol) (Vlahcevic et al, 1970, 1972a; Pomare and Heaton, 1973b). The importance of this is borne out by the fact that the size of the pool correlates very significantly with the saturation index of fasting gallbladder bile (Swell et al, 1974). The cause of the small pool has been much discussed, but it is generally felt that it represents an abnormal suppression of bile salt synthesis. This fits with the fact that the livers of patients with cholelithiasis show decreased activity of the enzyme which controls the rate of bile salt synthesis, 7 α-hydroxylase (Salen et al, 1975).

A key question in gallstone formation, therefore, is why is the synthesis of bile salts suppressed? No generally agreed answer can be given. However, like the other features of this disease, impaired bile salt synthesis can be explained as the result of eating a diet rich in refined, fibre-depleted foods.

A Unifying Dietary Hypothesis for the Aetiology of Cholesterol-rich Gallstones

All the available facts are consistent with the hypothesis that cholesterol-rich gallstones are caused by the consumption of a refined, fibre-depleted diet (Heaton, 1975).

Diet and the epidemiology of gallstones. When modern Western culture is adopted the biggest and most consistent change in eating habits which occurs is the abandonment of staple, starchy carbohydrates such as wheat, rice, maize, potatoes, and cassava, which are eaten with much or all of their fibre intact, and their replacement with refined sugar and highly refined white flour as the main sources of carbohydrate. During the Second World War this trend was temporarily reversed.

Diet and overnutrition. The properties of refined foods are such as to make overnutrition virtually inevitable. Refined foods are designedly more attractive and easier to eat than natural foods. Requiring little or no chewing they are quick to ingest yet do little to distend the stomach and induce satiety (Heaton, 1973b). Hence, refined foods explain the clinical association between gallstones and the diseases of overnutrition — obesity, diabetes, and hypertriglyceridaemia.

Diet and cholesterol excess. Cholesterol excess can be related to refined foods in two ways: through overnutrition and obesity (as already discussed), and through the effect of fibre on the composition of the bile salt pool. When bran was fed to English volunteers, the deoxycholate pool shrank, CDC synthesis increased, and in gallstone patients the saturation index of bile fell (Pomare et al, 1976). The primary effect of bran was presumably to reduce the amount of deoxycholate absorbed from the colon.

Diet and bile salt deficiency.   In laboratory animals, bile salt synthesis is depressed if a semi-synthetic diet is fed. Such a diet invariably contains a great deal of refined carbohydrate (for references, see Heaton, 1972 and 1975).

Diet and experimental gallstones.   Cholesterol-rich gallstones have been induced in at least six mammalian species by feeding abnormal diets. The only factor these diets have in common is a large proportion of refined carbohydrate (Heaton, 1975). In hamsters, such a diet loses its stone-inducing potential if it is supplemented with an artificial bulking agent or if the animal is allowed to eat the straw at the bottom of its cage (Hikasa et al, 1969).

No other coherent theory for the causation of gallstones has been advanced. A deficiency of polyunsaturated fatty acids has been suggested, but this is untenable since feeding these fatty acids seems actually to raise the incidence of gallstones (see below).

Iatrogenic Gallstones

In 1973, Sturdevant, Pearce and Dayton reported that men who, as part of a coronary prevention study, had been persuaded to eat a diet rich in polyunsaturated fatty acids, had an increased frequency of gallstones at autopsy. This was probably because polyunsaturated fatty acids increase the secretion of cholesterol into bile. This indeed is how their hypocholesterolaemic effect is probably achieved (Sodhi et al, 1967).

Similarly, clofibrate increases the flux of cholesterol into bile and doubles the incidence of gallstones (Pertsemlidis, Panveliwalla and Ahrens, 1974; Cooper, Geizerova and Oliver, 1975). Clofibrate may also reduce the size of the bile salt pool. Similar actions have been described with oral contraceptive therapy (Pertsemlidis et al, 1974) and these no doubt explain the two-fold increase in gallstone incidence in women taking the contraceptive pill or taking oestrogens for postmenopausal symptoms (Boston Collaborative Drug Surveillance Program, 1973, 1974).

Medical Therapy of Gallstones

Ever since it was shown that human gallstones dissolve in a dog's gallbladder (Naunyn, 1896) it has been obvious that gallstone formation can be reversed if bile can be rendered unsaturated with cholesterol. This aim is consistently achieved if chenodeoxycholic acid (CDC) is fed in a dose of 15 mg/kg or more daily (Iser et al, 1975). Dissolution of gallstones using CDC therapy was first reported in 1972 by Danzinger and his colleagues at the Mayo Clinic, and in the few years that have passed much has been learnt about the effectiveness, mode of action and safety of this agent. However, its final place in the therapeutic armamentarium is still to be defined.

Obviously, it is only cholesterol-rich stones that are amenable to CDC therapy. In practice, this means selecting radiolucent stones, although even these have a

15 to 20 per cent chance of being pigment stones (Bell et al, 1975; Trotman et al, 1975). The calculi must be in the gallbladder, not the common bile duct, and the gallbladder must opacify normally on oral cholecystography. These conditions are likely to be met in only about 20 per cent of patients awaiting cholecystectomy (Bell, 1974). Since treatment is likely to be prolonged, symptoms must be mild or absent. In most patients, therefore, surgery remains the only appropriate therapy. When surgery is refused or is contraindicated, CDC therapy will sometimes be useful.

Overall, about two-thirds of selected patients can expect dissolution of their stones. Small stones may dissolve within six months whereas large ones can take up to two years. Treatment cost about five pounds sterling per week in 1974. The only common side effect of treatment is diarrhoea, but this is seldom severe at a dose of 1 g daily. Many patients are pleased that their constipation is relieved.

A successfully treated patient is not, unfortunately, a cured patient, since feeding CDC does not remove the underlying metabolic abnormality any more than does vitamin B_{12} therapy in pernicious anaemia. When treatment is stopped, bile becomes supersaturated again and recurrent gallstones have been reported (Mok, Bell and Dowling, 1974; Thistle et al, 1974). Presumably, treatment will have to be lifelong, but there are hopes that intermittent dosage may be possible in prophylaxis.

The rationale for introducing CDC was that expansion of a small bile salt pool should reduce the cholesterol saturation of bile. However, this does not seem to be how CDC works. The bile salt pool is indeed expanded in most cases, but even when it is not altered the bile becomes less saturated (Danzinger et al, 1973). Furthermore, feeding cholic acid expands the bile salt pool but makes no difference to bile saturation (LaRusso et al, 1974). The action of CDC is on the secretion of cholesterol, which is suppressed by CDC but not by cholic acid (Adler et al, 1975; Northfield et al, 1975). The fall in cholesterol secretion probably results from a fall in cholesterol synthesis, and this in turn seems to be due to a specific inhibitory effect of CDC on the rate-limiting enzyme in cholesterol synthesis, HMG-CoA reductase (Pedersen, Arnfred and Hess Thaysen, 1974; Schoenfield, Bonorris and Ganz, 1973). This theory has the virtue of explaining another and unexpected effect of CDC, lowering of the fasting plasma triglyceride level, since the triglyceride level faithfully reflects the rate at which the liver is synthesising cholesterol (Editorial, 1975).

Chenodeoxycholic acid has not been released for general prescription because there have been fears about its possible hepatotoxicity. These arose from the fact that both CDC and its bacterial metabolite lithocholic acid can induce cirrhosis in the rabbit liver. However, there are marked species variations in hepatic sensitivity to CDC. In man, the only evidence of toxicity to date has been transient elevation of serum transaminases in some patients and it has been comforting to learn that liver biopsies show no significant changes, at least when the dose is kept below 1.5 g/day (Bell et al, 1974).

A totally different form of bile salt treatment has been used in patients found to have retained stones in the common bile duct after cholecystectomy. When the T-tube is still in place, this can be used to drip a strong solution of bile salt straight into the common bile duct. Most reported experience has been with

100 mmol/l sodium cholate solution, and this seems to be effective in most cases, usually in 3 to 14 days (Bell, 1974). Severe diarrhoea may be caused, but this can usually be controlled by administration of cholestyramine.

REFERENCES

Acosta, J. M. & Ledesma, C. L. (1974) Gallstone migration as a cause of acute pancreatitis. *New England Journal of Medicine*, **290**, 484-487.

Adler, R. D., Bennion, L. J., Duane, W. C. & Grundy, S. M. (1975) Effects of low dose chenodeoxycholic acid feeding on biliary lipid metabolism. *Gastroenterology*, **68**, 326-334.

Admirand, W. H. & Small, D. M. (1968) The physicochemical basis of cholesterol gallstone formation in man. *Journal of Clinical Investigation*, **47**, 1043-1052.

Ali, S. S., Kuksis, A. & Beveridge, J. M. R. (1966) Excretion of bile acids by three men on corn oil and butter fat diets. *Canadian Journal of Biochemistry and Physiology*, **44**, 1377-1388.

Allan, J. G., Gerskowitch, V. P. & Russell, R. I. (1973) A study of the role of bile acids in the pathogenesis of postvagotomy diarrhoea. *Gut*, **14**, 423-424 (abstract).

Allan, J. G. & Russell, R. I. (1975) Double-blind controlled trial of cholestyramine in the treatment of postvagotomy diarrhoea. *Gut*, **16**, 830 (abstract).

Ament, M. E., Shimoda, S. S., Saunders, D. R. & Rubin, C. E. (1972) Pathogenesis of steatorrhea in three cases of small intestinal stasis syndrome. *Gastroenterology*, **63**, 728-747.

Ammon, H. V. & Phillips, S. F. (1973) Inhibition of colonic water and electrolyte absorption by fatty acids in man. *Gastroenterology*, **65**, 744-749.

Andersson, Å., Bergdahl, L. & Boquist, L. (1971) Acalculous cholecystitis. *American Journal of Surgery*, **122**, 3-7.

Badley, B. W. D., Murphy, G. M., Bouchier, I. A. D. & Sherlock, S. (1970) Diminished micellar phase lipid in patients with chronic non-alcoholic liver disease and steatorrhea. *Gastroenterology*, **58**, 781-789.

Bedi, B. S., Debas, H. T., Gillespie, G. & Gillespie, I. E. (1971) Effect of bile salts on antral gastrin release. *Gastroenterology*, **60**, 256-262.

Beck, I. T., Sum, P. & Bencosme, S. A. (1969) The study of the pathogenesis of bile induced acute pancreatitis in the dog. Experiments with detergent. *Gastroenterology*, **56**, 1247 (abstract).

Bell, G. D. (1974) The present position concerning gallstone dissolution. *Gut*, **15**, 913-929.

Bell, G. D., Dowling, R. H., Whitney, B. & Sutor, D. J. (1975) The value of radiology in predicting gallstone type when selecting patients for medical treatment. *Gut*, **16**, 359-364.

Bell, G. D., Lewis, B., Petrie, A. & Dowling, R. H. (1973) Serum lipids in cholelithiasis: effect of chenodeoxycholic acid therapy. *British Medical Journal*, **iii**, 520-523.

Bell, G. D., Mok, H. Y. I., Thwe, M., Murphy, G. M., Henry, K. & Dowling, R. H. (1974) Liver structure and function in cholelithiasis: effect of chenodeoxycholic acid. *Gut*, **15**, 165-172.

Bennion, L. J. & Grundy, S. M. (1975) Effects of obesity and caloric intake on biliary lipid metabolism in man. *Journal of Clinical Investigation*, **56**, 996-1011.

Binder, H. J. & Donowitz, M. (1975) A new look at laxative action. *Gastroenterology*, **69**, 1001-1005.

Biss, K., Ho, K-J., Mikkelson, B., Lewis, L. & Taylor, C. B. (1971) Some unique biologic characteristics of the Masai of East Africa. *New England Journal of Medicine*, **284**, 694-699.

Black, R. B., Hole, D. & Rhodes, J. (1971) Bile damage to the gastric mucosal barrier: the influence of pH and bile acid concentration. *Gastroenterology*, **61**, 178-184.

Black, R. B., Rhodes, J., Davies, G. T., Gravelle, H. & Sweetnam, P. (1971) A controlled clinical trial of cholestyramine in the treatment of gastric ulcer. *Gastroenterology*, **61**, 821-825.

Black, R. B., Roberts, G. & Rhodes, J. (1971) The effect of healing on bile reflux in gastric ulcer. *Gut*, **12**, 552-558.

Booth, C. C., Alldis, D. & Read, A. E. (1961) Studies on the site of fat absorption. 2. Fat balances after resection of varying amounts of the small intestine in man. *Gut*, **2**, 168-174.

Boston Collaborative Drug Surveillance Programme (1973) Oral contraceptives and venous thromboembolic disease, surgically confirmed gallbladder disease and breast tumours. *Lancet*, **1**, 1399-1403.

Boston Collaborative Drug Surveillance Program (1974) Surgically confirmed gallbladder disease, venous thromboembolism, and breast tumours in relation to postmenopausal estrogen therapy. *New England Journal of Medicine*, **290**, 15-19.

Bouchier, I. A. D. (1975) Gallstones. In *Modern Trends in Gastroenterology-5*, ed. Read, A. E. London: Butterworths.

Braunsteiner, H., Di Pauli, R., Sailer, S. & Sandhofer, F. (1966) Cholelithiasis und latent diabetische Stoffwechsellage. *Schweizerische Medizinische Wochenschrift*, **96**, 44-46.

Burkitt, D. P. (1971) Epidemiology of cancer of the colon and rectum. *Cancer*, **28**, 3–13.

Burnett, W. (1965) The pathogenesis of gallstones. In *The Biliary System*, ed. Taylor, W., pp. 601–618. Oxford: Blackwell.

Calcraft, B., LaRusso, N. F. & Hofmann, A. F. (1975) Development of a simple, safe, bile acid clearance test: the radiocholate clearance test. *Gastroenterology*, **69**, 812 (abstract).

Carey, M. C. & Small, D. M. (1970) The characteristics of mixed micellar solutions with particular reference to bile. *American Journal of Medicine*, **49**, 590–608.

Carey, M. C. & Small, D. M. (1973) Solubility of cholesterol in aqueous bile salt-lecithin solutions. Importance of metastability, lipid concentration and temperature. *Gastroenterology*, **64**, 706 (abstract).

Cooper, J., Geizerova, H. & Oliver, M. F. (1975) Clofibrate and gallstones. *Lancet*, **i**, 1083.

Crumplin, M. K. H., Stol, D. W., Murphy, G. M. & Collis, J. L. (1974) The pattern of bile salt reflux and acid secretion in sliding hiatal hernia. *British Journal of Surgery*, **61**, 611–616.

Cummings, J. H., James, W. P. T. & Wiggins, H. S. (1973) Role of the colon in ileal-resection diarrhoea. *Lancet*, **i**, 344–347.

Danzinger, R. G., Hofmann, A. F., Schoenfield, L. J. & Thistle, J. L. (1972) Dissolution of cholesterol gallstones by chenodeoxycholic acid. *New England Journal of Medicine*, **286**, 1–8.

Danzinger, R. G., Hofmann, A. F., Thistle, J. L. & Schoenfield, L. J. (1973) Effect of oral chenodeoxycholic acid on bile acid kinetics and biliary lipid composition in women with cholelithiasis. *Journal of Clinical Investigation*, **52**, 2809–2821.

Davenport, H. W. (1968) Destruction of the gastric mucosal barrier by detergents and urea. *Gastroenterology*, **54**, 175–181.

Davenport, H. W. (1970) Effect of lysolecithin, digitonin and phospholipase A upon the dog's gastric mucosal barrier. *Gastroenterology*, **59**, 505–509.

Davidson, S. & Passmore, R. (1969) *Human Nutrition and Dietetics*, 4th edition. Edinburgh: Livingstone.

Dawson, A. M. & Isselbacher, K. J. (1960) Studies on lipid metabolism in the small intestine with observations on the role of bile salts. *Journal of Clinical Investigation*, **39**, 730–740.

Dietschy, J. M. (1967) Effects of bile salts on intermediate metabolism of the intestinal mucosa. *Federation Proceedings*, **26**, 1589–1598.

Dowling, R. H., Bell, G. D. & White, J. (1972) Lithogenic bile in patients with ileal dysfunction. *Gut*, **13**, 415–420.

Drasar, B. S., Bone, E. S., Hill, M. J. & Marks, C. G. (1975) Colon cancer and bacterial metabolism in familial polyposis. *Gut*, **16**, 824–825 (abstract).

Drasar, B. S. & Irving, D. (1973) Environmental factors and cancer of the colon and breast. *British Journal of Cancer*, **27**, 167–172.

DuPlessis, D. J. (1965) Pathogenesis of gastric ulceration. *Lancet*, **i**, 974–978.

Earnest, D. L. (1972) The effect of phenobarbital on pruritus and bile salt kinetics in patients with biliary cirrhosis and elevated serum bile salt concentrations. In *Bile Acids in Human Diseases*, ed. Back, P. & Gerok, W. pp. 145–151. Stuttgart: Schattauer.

Editorial (1975) Progress in dissolving gallstones. *British Medical Journal*, **i**, 699–700.

Einarsson, K., Hellström, K. & Kallner, M. (1975) Gallbladder disease in hyperlipoproteinaemia. *Lancet*, **i**, 484–487.

Erlinger, S. & Dhumeaux, D. (1974) Mechanisms and control of secretion of bile water and electrolytes. *Gastroenterology*, **66**, 281–304.

Findlay, J. M., Smith, A. N., Mitchell, W. D., Anderson, A. J. B. & Eastwood, M. A. (1974) Effects of unprocessed bran on colon function in normal subjects and in diverticular disease. *Lancet*, **i**, 146–149.

Forsgren, L. (1969) Studies on the intestinal absorption of labelled fat-soluble vitamins (A, D, E and K) via the thoracic duct lymph in the absence of bile in man. *Acta Chirurgica Scandinavica*, suppl. 399.

Friedman, G. D., Kannel, W. B. & Dawber, T. R. (1966) The epidemiology of gallbladder disease: observations in the Framingham study. *Journal of Chronic Diseases*, **19**, 273–292.

Fromm, H. & Hofmann, A. F. (1971) Breath test for altered bile-acid metabolism. *Lancet*, **ii**, 621–625.

Fromm, H., Thomas, P. J. & Hofmann, A. F. (1973) Sensitivity and specificity in tests of distal ileal function: prospective comparison of bile acid and vitamin B_{12} absorption in ileal resection patients. *Gastroenterology*, **64**, 1077–1090.

Gibson, T. (1684) *The Anatomy of Humane Bodies*, 2nd edition. London: Flesher.

Gillison, E. W., Nyhus, L. M. & Duthie, H. L. (1971) Bile reflux, gastric secretion and heartburn. *British Journal of Surgery*, **58**, 864 (abstract).

Gillison, E. W., de Castro, V. A. M., Nyhus, L. M., Kusakari, K. & Bombeck, C. T. (1972) The significance of bile in reflux osophagitis. *Surgery, Gynecology and Obstetrics*, **134**, 419–424.

Gracey, M. (1971) Intestinal absorption in the 'contaminated small-bowel syndrome'. *Gut,* **12,** 403–410.

Gracey, M., Houghton, M. & Thomas, J. (1975) Deoxycholate depresses small-intestinal enzyme activity. *Gut,* **16,** 53–56.

Gracey, M., Papadimitriou, J. & Bower, G. (1974) Ultrastructural changes in the small intestines of rats with self-filling blind loops. *Gastroenterology,* **67,** 646–651.

Gracey, M., Papadimitriou, J., Burke, V., Thomas, J. & Bower, G. (1973) Effects on small-intestinal function and structure induced by feeding a deconjugated bile salt. *Gut,* **14,** 519–528.

Greim, H., Trülzsch, D., Czygan, P., Rudick, J., Hutterer, F., Schaffner, F. & Popper, H. (1972) Mechanism of cholestasis 6. Bile acids in human livers with or without biliary obstruction. *Gastroenterology,* **63,** 846–850.

Grundy, S. M., Duane, W. C., Adler, R. D., Aron, J. M. & Metzger, A. L. (1974) Biliary lipid outputs in young women with cholesterol gallstones. *Metabolism,* **23,** 67–73.

Grundy, S. M., Metzger, A. L. & Adler, R. D. (1972) Mechanisms of lithogenic bile formation in American Indian women with cholesterol gallstones. *Journal of Clinical Investigation,* **51,** 3026–3043.

Gumucio, J. J., Accatino, L., Macho, A. M. & Contreras, A. (1973) Effect of phenobarbital on the ethynyl estradiol-induced cholestasis in the rat. *Gastroenterology,* **65,** 651–657.

Hansson, K. (1967) Experimental and clinical studies in aetiologic role of bile reflux in acute pancreatitis. *Acta Chirurgica Scandinavica,* suppl. 375.

Haslewood, G. A. D. (1967) *Bile Salts.* London: Methuen.

Heaton, K. W. (1972) *Bile Salts in Health and Disease.* Edinburgh: Churchill Livingstone.

Heaton, K. W. (1973a) The epidemiology of gallstones and suggested aetiology. *Clinics in Gastroenterology,* **2,** 67–83.

Heaton, K. W. (1973b) Food fibre as an obstacle to energy intake. *Lancet,* **ii,** 1418–1421.

Heaton, K. W. (1975) Gallstones and cholecystitis. In *Refined Carbohydrate Foods and Disease. Some Implications of Dietary Fibre,* ed. Burkitt, D. P. and Trowell, H. C. London: Academic Press.

Heaton, K. W. & Read, A. E. (1969) Gallstones in patients with disorders of the terminal ileum and disturbed bile salt metabolism. *British Medical Journal,* **3,** 494–496.

Hikasa, Y., Matsuda, S., Nagase, M., Yoshinaga, M., Tobe, T., Maruyama, I., Shioda, R., Tanimura, H., Muraoka, R., Muroya, H. and Togo, M. (1969) Initiating factors of gallstones, especially cholesterol stones (III) *Archiv Japanische Chirurgie,* **38,** 107–124.

Hill, M. J. (1974) Bacteria and the etiology of colonic cancer. *Cancer,* **34,** 815–818.

Hill, M. J., Crowther, J. S., Drasar, B. S., Hawksworth, G., Aries, V. & Williams, R. E. O. (1971) Bacteria and aetiology of cancer of large bowel. *Lancet,* **i,** 95–100.

Hill, M. J., Drasar, B. S., Williams, R. E. O., Meade, T. W., Cox, A. G., Simpson, J. E. P. & Morson, B. C. (1975) Faecal bile-acids and clostridia in patients with cancer of the large bowel. *Lancet,* **i,** 535–539.

Hofmann, A. F. (1972) Bile acid malabsorption caused by ileal resection. *Archives of Internal Medicine,* **130,** 597–605.

Hofmann, A. F. & Poley, J. R. (1972) Role of bile acid malabsorption in pathogenesis of diarrhoea and steatorrhea in patients with ileal resection. I. Response to cholestyramine or replacement of dietary long chain triglyceride by medium chain triglyceride. *Gastroenterology,* **62,** 918–934.

Hofmann, A. F., Schoenfield, L. J., Kottke, B. A. & Poley, J. R. (1970) Methods for the description of bile acid kinetics in man. In *Methods in Medical Research,* vol. 12, ed. Olson, R. E., pp. 149–180. Chicago: Year Book Medical Publishers.

Holland, C. & Heaton, K. W. (1972) Increasing frequency of gallbladder operations in the Bristol clinical area. *British Medical Journal,* **3,** 672–675.

Hunt, T. (1956) Diseases of the gall-bladder and bile ducts. In *Price's Textbook of the Practice of Medicine,* 9th edition, ed. Hunter, D., pp. 689–700. Oxford: University Press.

Iser, J. H., Dowling, R. H., Mok, H. Y. I. & Bell, G. D. (1975) Chenodeoxycholic acid treatment of gallstones. A follow-up report and analysis of factors influencing response to therapy. *New England Journal of Medicine,* **293,** 378–383.

James, O. F. W., Agnew, J. E. & Bouchier, I. A. D. (1973) Assessment of the ^{14}C-glycocholic acid breath test. *British Medical Journal,* **3,** 191–195.

Kameda, H. (1967) Gallstones, compositions, structural characteristics and geographical distribution. In *Proceedings of 3rd World Congress of Gastroenterology, Tokyo 1966,* vol. 4, pp. 117–124. Basel: Karger.

Kaplowitz, N., Kok, E. & Javitt, N. B. (1973) Postprandial serum bile acid for the detection of hepatobiliary disease. *Journal of the American Medical Association,* **225,** 292–293.

Kirby, J., Heaton, K. W. & Burton, J. L. (1974) Pruritic effect of bile salts. *British Medical Journal,* **4,** 693–695.

Korman, M. G., LaRusso, N. F., Hoffman, N. E. & Hofmann, A. F. (1975) Development of an intravenous bile acid tolerance test. Plasma disappearance of cholyglycine in health. *New England Journal of Medicine*, 292, 1205–1209.

LaRusso, N. F., Hoffman, N. E., Hofmann, A. F. & Korman, M. G. (1975) Validity and sensitivity of an intravenous bile acid tolerance test in patients with liver disease. *New England Journal of Medicine*, 292, 1209–1214.

LaRusso, N. F., Hoffman, N. E., Hofmann, A. F., Northfield, T. C. & Thistle, J. L. (1974) Differing effects of primary bile acid ingestion on biliary lipid secretion in gallstone patients: why chenodeoxycholic acid but not cholic acid dissolves gallstones. *Gastroenterology*, 66, 729 (abstract).

Lenz, K. (1975) An evaluation of the 'breath test' in Crohn's disease. *Scandinavian Journal of Gastroenterology*, 10, 665–671.

Low-Beer, T. S., Heaton, K. W., Heaton, S. T. & Read, A. E. (1971) Gallbladder inertia and sluggish enterohepatic circulation of bile-salts in coeliac disease. *Lancet*, i, 991–994.

Low-Beer, T. S. & Pomare, E. W. (1975) Can colonic bacterial metabolites predispose to cholesterol gallstones? *British Medical Journal*, 1, 438–440.

Low-Beer, T. S., Schneider, R. E. & Dobbins, W. O. (1970) Morphological changes of the small-intestinal mucosa of guinea pig and hamster following incubation in vitro and perfusion in vivo with unconjugated bile salts. *Gut*, 11, 486-492.

Low-Beer, T. S., Wilkins, R. M., Lack, L. & Tyor, M. P. (1974) Effect of one meal on enterohepatic circulation of bile salts. *Gastroenterology*, 67, 490–497.

McCutcheon, A. D. (1968) A fresh approach to the pathogenesis of pancreatitis. *Gut*, 9, 296–310.

Makino, I., Hashimoto, H., Shinozaki, K., Yoshino, K. & Nakayawa, S. (1975) Sulfated and nonsulfated bile acids in urine, serum, and bile of patients with hepatobiliary diseases. *Gastroenterology*, 68, 545–553.

Meihoff, W. E. & Kern, F. (1968) Bile salt malabsorption in regional ileitis, ileal resection and mannitol-induced diarrhea. *Journal of Clinical Investigation*, 47, 261–267.

Mekhjian, H. S., Phillips, S. F. & Hofmann, A. F. (1971) Colonic secretion of water and electrolytes induced by bile acids: persusion studies in man. *Journal of Clinical Investigation*, 50, 1569–1577.

Metreau, J-M., Bismuth, H., Franco, D. & Dhumeaux, D. (1975) Effect of phenobarbital in a case of extrahepatic cholestasis. *Gastroenterology*, 68, 567–571.

Metzger, A. L., Heymsfield, S. & Grundy, S. M. (1972) The lithogenic index — a numerical expression for the relative lithogenicity of bile. *Gastroenterology*, 62, 499–501.

Miettinen, T. A. (1971) Cholesterol production in obesity. *Circulation*, 44, 842–850.

Mitchell, W. D. & Eastwood, M. A. (1972) Faecal bile acids and neutral steroids in patients with ileal dysfunction. *Scandinavian Journal of Gastroenterology*, 7, 29–32.

Mok, H. Y. I., Bell, G. D. & Dowling (1974) Effect of different doses of chenodeoxycholic acid on bile-lipid composition and on frequency of side-effects in patients with gallstones. *Lancet*, ii, 253–257.

Moore, R. B., Frantz, I. D. & Buchwald, H. (1969) Changes in cholesterol pool size, turnover rate and fecal bile acid and sterol excretion after partial ileal bypass in hypercholesteremic patients. *Surgery, St. Louis*, 98–107.

Nakayama, F. & van der Linden, W. (1971) Bile composition: Sweden versus Japan. Its possible significance in the difference in gallstone incidence. *American Journal of Surgery*, 122, 8-12.

Naunyn, B. (1896) *A Treatise on Cholelithiasis*. London: New Sydenham Society.

Neale, G., Lewis, B., Weaver, V. & Panveliwalla, D. (1971) Serum bile acids in liver disease. *Gut*, 12, 145–152.

Neprokoeff, C. M., Lakshmanan, M. R., Ness, G. C., Dugan, R. E. & Porter, J. W. (1974) Regulation of the diurnal rhythm of rat liver β-hydroxy-β-methylglutaryl coenzyme A reductase activity by insulin, glucagon, cyclic AMP, and hydrocortisone. *Archives of Biochemistry and Biophysics*, 160, 387–393.

Nestel, P. J., Schreibman, P. H. & Ahrens, E. H. (1973) Cholesterol metabolism in human obesity. *Journal of Clinical Investigation*, 52, 2389–2397.

Newman, A., Katsaris, J., Blendis, L. M., Charlesworth, M. & Walter, L. H. (1973) Small-intestinal injury in women who have had pelvic radiotherapy. *Lancet*, ii, 1471–1473.

Norman, A. & Strandvik, B. (1973) Excretion of bile acids in extrahepatic biliary atresia and intrahepatic cholestasis of infancy. *Acta Pediatrica Scandinavica*, 62, 253–263.

Northfield, T. C., Drasar, B. S. & Wright, J. T. (1973) Value of small intestinal bile acid analysis in the diagnosis of the stagnant loop syndrome. *Gut*, 14, 341–347.

Northfield, T. C. & Hofmann, A. F. (1975) Biliary lipid output during three meals and an overnight fast. I. Relationship to bile acid pool size and cholesterol saturation of bile in gallstone and control subjects. *Gut*, 16, 1–11.

Northfield, T. C., LaRusso, N. F., Hofmann, A. F. & Thistle, J. L. (1975) Biliary lipid output during three meals and an overnight fast. II. Effect of chenodeoxycholic acid treatment in gallstone subjects. *Gut*, **16**, 12–17.

Parkin, D. M., O'Moore, R. R., Cussons, D. J., Warwick, R. R. G., Rooney, P., Percy-Robb, I. W. & Shearman, D. J. C. (1972) Evaluation of the 'breath test' in the detection of bacterial colonisation of the upper gastrointestinal tract. *Lancet*, **ii**, 777–780.

Pedersen, L., Arnfred, T. & Hess Thaysen, E. (1973) Rapid screening of increased bile acid deconjugation and bile acid malabsorption by means of the glycine-1-(^{14}C) cholylglycine assay. *Scandinavian Journal of Gastroenterology*, **8**, 665–672.

Pedersen, L., Arnfred, T. & Hess Thaysen, E. H. (1974) Cholesterol kinetics in patients with cholesterol gallstones before and during chenodeoxycholic acid treatment. *Scandinavian Journal of Gastroenterology*, **9**, 787–791.

Pertsemlidis, D., Panveliwalla, D. & Ahrens, E. H. (1974) Effects of clofibrate and of an estrogen–progestin combination on fasting biliary lipids and cholic acid kinetics in man. *Gastroenterology*, **66**, 565–573.

Pomare, E. W. & Heaton, K. W. (1973a) Alteration of bile salt metabolism by dietary fibre (bran). *British Medical Journal*, **4**, 262–264.

Pomare, E. W. & Heaton, K. W. (1973b) Bile salt metabolism in patients with gallstones in functioning gallbladders. *Gut*, **14**, 885–890.

Pomare, E. W., Heaton, K. W., Low-Beer, T. S. & Espiner, H. J. (1976) The effect of wheat bran upon bile salt metabolism and upon the lipid composition of bile in gallstone patients. *American Journal of Digestive Diseases*, **21**, 521–526.

Pomare, E. W. & Low-Beer, T. S. (1975) The selective inhibition of chenodeoxycholate synthesis by cholate metabolites in man. *Clinical Science and Molecular Medicine*, **48**, 315–321.

Reddy, B. S. & Wynder, E. L. (1973) Large bowel carcinogenesis: fecal constituents of populations with diverse incidence rates of colon cancer. *Journal of the National Cancer Institute*, **50**, 1437–1442.

Redinger, R. N. & Small, D. M. (1972) Bile composition, bile salt metabolism and gallstones. *Archives of Internal Medicine*, **130**, 618–630.

Rhodes, J. (1972) Etiology of gastric ulcer. *Gastroenterology*, **63**, 171–182.

Ritchie, W. P. (1975) Acute gastric mucosal damage induced by bile salts, acid, and ischemia. *Gastroenterology*, **68**, 699–707.

Safaie-Shirazi, S., DenBesten, L. & Zike, W. L. (1975) Effect of bile salts on the ionic permeability of the esophageal mucosa and their role in the production of esophagitis. *Gastroenterology*, **68**, 728–733.

Salen, G., Nicolau, G., Shefer, S. & Mosbach, E. H. (1975) Hepatic cholesterol metabolism in patients with gallstones. *Gastroenterology*, **69**, 676–684.

Sampliner, R. E., Bennett, P. H., Comess, L. J., Rose, F. A. & Burch, T. A. (1970) Gallbladder disease in Pima Indians. Demonstration of high prevalence and early onset by cholecystography. *New England Journal of Medicine*, **283**, 1358–1364.

Schaefer, O. (1971) When the Eskimo comes to town. *Nutrition Today*, November/December, 8–16.

Schaffner, F. & Popper, H. (1969) Cholestasis is the result of hypoactive hypertrophic smooth endoplasmic reticulum in the hepatocyte. *Lancet*, **ii**, 355–359.

Scherstén, T., Nilsson, S., Cahlin, E., Filipson, M. & Brodin-Persson, G. (1971) Relationship between the biliary excretion of bile acids and the excretion of water, lecithin and cholesterol in man. *European Journal of Clinical Investigation*, **1**, 242–247.

Schmidt, H. Cruetzfeldt, W. (1969) The possible role of phospholipase A in the pathogenesis of acute pancreatitis. *Scandinavian Journal of Gastroenterology*, **4**, 39–48.

Schoenfield, L. J. (1969) The relationship of bile acids to pruritus in hepatobiliary disease. In *Bile Salt Metabolism*, ed. Schiff, L., Carey, J. B. and Dietschy, J. M., pp. 257–265. Springfield: Thomas.

Schoenfield, L. J., Bonorris, G. G. & Ganz, P. (1973) Induced alterations in the rate-limiting enzymes of hepatic cholesterol and bile acid synthesis in the hamster. *Journal of Laboratory and Clinical Medicine*, **82**, 858–868.

Scott, A. J. & Khan, G. A. (1967) The origin of bacteria in bile duct bile. *lancet*, **ii**, 790–792.

Semple, P. F. & Russell, R. I. (1975) Role of bile acids in the pathogenesis of aspirin-induced gastric mucosal hemorrhage in rats. *Gastroenterology*, **68**, 67–70.

Shimoda, S. S., O'Brien, T. K. & Saunders, D. R. (1974) Fat absorption after infusing bile salts into the human small intestine. *Gastroenterology*, **67**, 7–18.

Simmonds, W. J., Korman, M. G., Go, V. L. W. & Hofmann, A. F. (1973) Radioimmunoassay of conjugated cholyl bile acids in serum. *Gastroenterology*, **65**, 705–711.

Södal, G., Gjertsen, K. T. & Schrumpf, A. (1970) Surgical treatment of hypercholesterolemia. *Acta Chirurgica Scandinavica*, **136**, 671–674.

Sodhi, H. S., Wood, P. D. S., Schierf, G. & Kinsell, L. W. (1967) Plasma bile and fecal sterols in relation to diet. *Metabolism*, **16**, 334–344.

Stiehl, A., Earnest, D. L. & Admirand, W. H. (1975) Sulfation and renal excretion of bile salts in patients with cirrhosis of the liver. *Gastroenterology*, **68**, 534–544.

Stiehl, A., Thaler, M. M. & Admirand, W. H. (1972) The effects of phenobarbital on bile salts and bilirubin in patients with intrahepatic and extrahepatic cholestasis. *New England Journal of Medicine*, **286**, 858–861.

Sturdevant, R. A. L., Pearce, M. L. & Dayton, S. (1973) Increased prevalence of cholelithiasis in men ingesting a serum cholesterol lowering diet. *New England Journal of Medicine*, **288**, 24–27.

Sutor, D. J. & Wooley, S. E. (1971) A statistical survey of the composition of gallstones in eight countries. *Gut*, **12**, 55–64.

Swell, L., Cooper Bell, C., Gregory, D. H. & Vlahcevic, Z. R. (1974) The cholesterol saturation index of human bile. *American Journal of Digestive Diseases*, **19**, 261–265.

Swell, L., Gregory, D. H. & Vlahcevic, Z. R. (1974) Current concepts of the pathogenesis of cholesterol gallstones. *Medical Clinics of North America*, **58**, 1449–1471.

Tabaqchali, S. & Booth, C. C. (1970) Bacteria and the small intestine. In *Modern Trends in Gastroenterology* — 4, ed. Card. W. I. and Creamer, B., pp. 143–179. London: Butterworths.

Tabaqchali, S., Hatzioannou, J. & Booth, C. C. (1968) Bile-salt deconjugation and steatorrhoea in patients with the stagnant loop syndrome. *Lancet*, **ii**, 12–16.

Thomas, P. J. & Hofmann, A. F. (1973) A simple calculation of the lithogenic index of bile: expressing biliary lipid composition on rectangular coordinates. *Gastroenterology*, **65**, 698–700.

Thistle, J. L., Yu, P. Y. S., Hofmann, A. F. & Ott, B. J. (1974) Prompt return of bile to supersaturated state followed by gallstone recurrence after discontinuance of chenodeoxycholic acid therapy. *Gastroenterology*, **66**, 789 (abstract).

Thureborn, E. (1962) Human hepatic bile. Composition changes due to altered enterohepatic circulation. *Acta Chirurgica Scandinavica*, suppl. 303.

Trotman, B. W., Ostrow, J. D. & Soloway, R. D. (1974) Pigment versus cholesterol cholelithiasis: comparison of stone and bile composition. *American Journal of Digestive Diseases*, **19**, 585–590.

Trotman, B. W., Petrella, E. J., Soloway, R. D., Sanchez, H. M., Morris, T. A. & Miller, W. T. (1975) Evaluation of radiographic lucency or opaqueness of gallstones as a means of identifying cholesterol or pigment stones. *Gastroenterology*, **68**, 1563–1566.

Trotman, B. W. & Soloway, R. D. (1973) Influence of age, race or sex on pigment and cholesterol gallstone incidence. *Gastroenterology*, **65**, 573 (abstract).

van Deest, B. W., Fordtran, J. S., Morawski, S. G. & Wilson, J. D. (1968) Bile salt and micellar fat concentration in proximal small bowel contents of ileectomy patients. *Journal of Clinical Investigation*, **47**, 1314–1324.

Vlahcevic, Z. R., Bell, C. C., Buhac, I., Farrar, J. T. & Swell, L. (1970) Diminished bile acid pool size in patients with gallstones. *Gastroenterology*, **59**, 165–173.

Vlahcevic, Z. R., Bell, C. C., Gregory, D. H., Buker, G., Juttijudata, P. & Swell, L. (1972a) Relationship of bile acid pool size to the formation of lithogenic bile in female Indians of the Southwest. *Gastroenterology*, **62**, 73–83.

Vlahcevic, Z. R., Juttijudata, P., Bell, C. C. & Swell, L. (1972b) Bile acid metabolism in patients with cirrhosis. II. Cholic and chenodeoxycholic acid metabolism. *Gastroenterology*, **62**, 1174–1181.

Wagner, C. I., Soloway, R. D., Trotman, B. W. & Schoenfield, L. J. (1973) Effects of bile flow and lipid output on composition and cholesterol saturation of bile. *Gastroenterology*, **65**, 575 (abstract).

Watkinson, G. (1967) Relationship between gallstones and other medical diseases. In *Proceedings of 3rd World Congress of Gastroenterology, Tokyo 1966*, vol. 4, pp. 125–130. Basel: Karger.

Weber, A. M., Roy, C. C., Lepage, G., Chartrand, L. & Lasalle, R. (1975) Interruption of the enterohepatic circulation of bile acids in cystic fibrosis. *Gastroenterology*, **68**, 1066 (abstract).

Weber, A. M., Roy, C. C., Morin, C. L. & Lasalle, R. (1973) Malabsorption of bile acids in children with cystic fibrosis. *New England Journal of Medicine*, **289**, 1001–1005.

Wheeler, H. O. (1968) Water and electrolytes in bile. In *Handbook of Physiology*, section 6: Alimentary Canal, vol. V: Bile, digestion, ruminal physiology, pp. 2409–2431, ed. Code, C. F. Washington: American Physiological Society.

Woodbury, J. F. & Kern, F. (1971) Fecal excretion of bile acids: a new technique for studying bile acid kinetics in patients with ileal resection. *Journal of Clinical Investigation*, **50**, 2531–2540.

Wynder, E. L. & Reddy, B. S. (1975) Dietary fat and colon cancer. *Journal of the National Cancer Institute*, **54**, 7–10.

Yoshida, T., McCormick, W. C., Swell, L. & Vlahcevic, Z. R. (1975) Bile acid metabolism in cirrhosis. IV. Characterisation of the abnormality in deoxycholate metabolism. *Gastroenterology*, **68**, 335–341.

Záhoř, Z., Sternby, N. H., Kagan, A., Uemera, K., Vaněček, R. & Vichert, A. M. (1974) Frequency of cholelithiasis in Prague and Malmö. An autopsy study. *Scandinavian Journal of Gastroenterology*, **9**, 3–7.

Zike, W. L., Safaie-Shirazi, S., Paluska, G. & DenBesten, L. (1973) The role of cholestyramine in the prevention of stress ulcers. *Gastroenterology*, **64**, 826 (abstract).

15
HORMONES OF THE GASTROINTESTINAL TRACT

S. R. Bloom

The era of endocrinology began when Bayliss and Starling (1902) at University College Hospital in London were able to show that duodenal acidification caused a flow of pancreatic juice even though all nervous connections were severed. This observation overthrew the Pavlovian theory that the control of digestive function was entirely through nervous reflexes. The word hormone, from a Greek word meaning 'I arouse to activity', was coined specifically to describe the new class of compounds which the responsible substance, termed secretin, was thought to represent. It was proposed that a 'hormone' would be released into the circulation after a physiological stimulus and be carried to act on distant tissues. In spite of this early recognition of the gut hormones, gastrin being discovered by Edkins (1905), it is surprising that they are extremely rarely mentioned in endocrinology textbooks. Indeed so little had been discovered about their physiological role that until recently they often received scanty mention even in physiology reference books.

BACKGROUND

Knowledge of the gut hormones has been increasing very rapidly over the last few years and shows no sign of slowing down. Morphologists have been able to point to a very complex gut endocrine cell system (Solcia et al, 1973). Not only are there a great number of different kinds of endocrine cell but the total mass of endocrine tissue in the gut is considerable. Indeed it has become a recent catch phrase that the gut is the biggest endocrine gland in the body. Matching the progress in morphology, biological chemists have succeeded in isolating not only the classically described gut hormones but also a number of new ones. The era of the physiologist describing normal gut responses and postulating mechanisms to produce them has been overtaken by structural definition of the endocrine cells and chemical isolation of their products. As can be seen in later sections of this review, we now have a number of hormonal peptides coming from defined endocrine cells and circulating in high concentration whose role in physiology is completely unknown. A great effort is now being made by the physiologists to catch up and to lay the foundation for what is to man the most important end product of this research, a better understanding of human pathology.

Methods of study

A lot of knowledge has been obtained in recent years by efficient use of specific antisera to hormones. These can be employed either to measure plasma levels of the hormone by radioimmunoassay or, alternatively, to localise by immuno-cytochemical staining the cells in the mucosa that produce the hormones. Radioimmunoassay for constituents of blood is both inaccurate and imprecise when compared with more classical biochemical assay procedures. It is common knowledge that different laboratories often fail to agree even over such basic facts as the true resting concentration of a hormone, estimates varying by perhaps three or four hundred per cent. There are even arguments as to whether the plasma concentration of a hormone increases or decreases after a given stimulus (Boden, Essa and Owen, 1975). However, no other technique is capable of detecting the extremely low levels at which hormones circulate and it must be accepted that when the methodological problems are overcome, reasonably true answers can be obtained and are capable of accurately predicting physiological events. Three basic problems in radioimmunoassay have been suggested. First there is straightforward laboratory incompetence due to the entry into the field of a number of untrained workers with, for example, the use of unstable standard preparations, samples badly collected with the delicate peptide hormones becoming partially degraded etc. The second source of error, which is fundamental to all antibody-antigen reactions, is the effect of a large number of non-specific influences in plasma on antibody binding. There are many constituents of plasma, that especially when present in high concentration, may cause decreased antibody binding and thus masquerade in a radioimmunoassay as a falsely high hormone level — for example urea or γ-globulins. The third main source of error is the result of a difference between the exact part of the hormone molecule to which the assay antibody binds and thus measures, and the part that is clinically important because it is biologically active. Thus a radioimmunoassay can easily report a high level of a hormone immunologically recognisable, which is in fact biologically inactive, for example prohormone abnormally produced by a tumour or degraded fragments of a hormone in patients with renal failure which are normally removed by the kidney. These three problems in radioimmunoassay are being overcome first by better training, second by better non-specific binding controls, e.g. by use of reference plasma from each individual patient specifically freed from hormone, and third by development of antisera with hormone-binding characteristics very similar to those of the natural cellular binding site which therefore reflect biological potency. Similar problems have arisen with the allied technique of immuno-cytochemistry but as this is a qualitative rather than a quantitative procedure, they have been more readily overcome by use of adequate controls. These include the demonstration of specific quenching of staining only by addition to the slides of a solution of the particular hormone.

Source of hormone

The increasing ease of production of synthetic peptides is now overcoming the enormous problem in supply of gut hormones for use in physiological experimentation and antibody raising. Because the gut endocrine cells are widely scattered, tissue extracts have extremely low concentrations of hormone. This makes purification of significant quantities very difficult. The world production of pure natural cholecystokinin-pancreozymin, for example, is probably less than 1 mg per year and research on it is accordingly very difficult. A large literature has grown up, on the other hand, round gastrin which was the first gut hormone to be made available synthetically (Anderson et al, 1964) and which has been produced in considerable quantities.

Physiology

A vital step in the demonstration that a hormone has a physiological role is to show that infusion of the hormone, giving a level in the circulation similar to that seen after natural stimuli, produces a significant biological response. Much of the early literature has been bedevilled by confusion between effects of a hormone which are likely to occur under physiological conditions and those observed when a very much higher dose is administered. This problem is obviated by measurement of actual plasma levels. The recent use of synthetic hormone fragments, for example with gastrin, gives information on the nature of the hormone receptor interreaction. This is particularly useful when isolated cell or tissue preparations are used. It has been possible to demonstrate that the overlapping action of several gut hormones is not usually due to reaction at the same receptor site, as each hormone can be shown to be independently reacting with its own cellular receptor. The use of isolated cell and tissue techniques to look at the actions of a hormone have, of course, both the advantage of giving a clear understanding of the exact action of the hormone and also very strong disadvantages. Thus, the act of isolating a tissue automatically changes its sensitivity to normal control systems, often by a factor of over a thousand-fold, and this negates any information on the hormone's physiological potency. There is little substitute for whole animal physiology of the classical type in finally deciding what the true effects of a hormone are and whether these are important in overall physiological control.

GASTRIN

Forms and distribution

Although the existence of gastrin had been postulated as early as 1905 (Edkins) it was not finally purified until 1964 (Gregory and Tracy). It was, however, made available synthetically in the same year (Anderson et al, 1964), and this allowed full investigation of its pharmacology. Preparation of synthetic fragments has shown that the full activity of gastrin is exhibited by the last three amino acids (Lin, 1972). The synthetically available pentagastrin (five amino acids, of which four are from gastrin) is widely available for use as a clinical test of gastric acid function. It is perhaps predictable that if only a small part of the molecule is necessary for full biological function, there might be heterogeneity in the rest of the molecule. This is certainly the case with gastrin and Yalow and Berson (1970) showed that the major circulating form of gastrin was not the originally purified material with 17 amino acids but a larger form, big gastrin, subsequently shown to have 34 amino acids (Gregory and Tracy, 1975) (Table 15.1). This big

Table 15.1   Amino acid sequence of porcine CCK-PZ (top two lines) and human big gastrin (bottom two lines)

1	2	3	4	5	6	7	8	9	10	11		12	13	14	15	16
Lys	Ala	Pro	Ser	Gly	Arg	Val	Ser	Met	Ile	Lys		Asn	Leu	Gln	Ser	Leu

17	18	19	20	21	22	23	24	25	26	27		28	29	30	31	32	33
Asp	Pro	Ser	His	Arg	Ile	Ser	Asp	Arg	Asp	Tyr(SO$_3$)	Met	Gly	Trp	Met	Asp	Phe(NH$_2$)	

1	2	3	4	5	6	7	8	9	10	11	12		13	14	15	16	17
Pyro	Leu	Gly	Pro	Gln	Gly	His	Pro	Ser	Leu	Val	Ala		Asp	Pro	Ser	Lys	Lys

18	19	20	21	22	23	24	25	26	27	28	29		30	31	32	33	34
Gln	Gly	Pro	Trp	Leu	Glu	Glu	Glu	Glu	Glu	Ala	Tyr(SO$_3$)	Gly	Trp	Met	Asp	Phe	NH$_2$

gastrin is composed of little gastrin with an additional 17 amino acid N–terminal tail and thus little gastrin can be generated directly from it by splitting with a proteolytic enzyme. More recently still further forms of gastrin have been found in tissue extracts and circulation, including a smaller form, little little gastrin with 14 amino acids, a big big gastrin of comparable size to plasma proteins, and an intermediate big gastrin (Walsh and Grossman, 1975). Although big big gastrin constitutes a significant proportion of the measurable fasting plasma gastrin concentration, it does not change with normal physiological stimuli, for example eating a meal, and has not yet been shown to have any biological activity. Thus only two forms of gastrin are of consequence, firstly the classical gastrin, purified in 1964 (Gregory and Tracy) and now called little gastrin, and secondly big gastrin. In man about two-thirds of the gastrin is found in the antrum of the stomach, while one-third is found in the upper small intestine (Nilsson, Yalow and Berson, 1973). The major form of antral gastrin is little gastrin and the rest is big gastrin. In the upper small intestine the ratios of the two forms are reversed (Berson and Yalow, 1971). Big and little gastrin have an identical spectrum of actions and while little gastrin is slightly more potent, it is also more rapidly cleared from the circulation (Walsh, Debas and Grossman, 1974). Both forms appear to originate from the same cell type, the G cell (McGuigan and Greider, 1971). This cell is easily demonstrated by the technique of indirect immuno-fluorescence using antisera to gastrin and is shown to reside in the middle part of the mucosa.

Physiology

Gastrin is released into the circulation by distension, or addition of peptides and amino acids to the gastric antrum (Blair et al, 1975). In the dog stimulation of the vagal nerve also causes a considerable gastrin rise but in man vagal release is less important (Farooq and Walsh, 1975). The release of gastrin is powerfully inhibited by acid in the stomach (Walsh, Richardson and Fordtran, 1975). This forms a feed-back loop with greater acid production resulting in a smaller gastrin release and thus a reduced stimulus to further acid production, while a low acid output leads to a big release of gastrin. Although the main action of gastrin is to stimulate gastric acid, in high doses it can also stimulate contraction of the gastric musculature and it has been proposed that it might be one of the agents controlling lower oesophageal sphincter pressure (Giles et al, 1969; Castell and Harris, 1970; Grossman, 1974). More recently Johnson and colleagues (1975) in the United States have demonstrated in the rat that atrophy occurs in stomach, pancreas and upper small intestine during intravenous feeding and this can be prevented by simultaneous injections of gastrin in small amounts. It seems possible, therefore, that gastrin is a trophic hormone whose presence is necessary to maintain normal mucosal growth.

Pathology

Plasma gastrin may rise to one hundred times the normal in patients with inadequate gastric acid production, e.g. pernicious anaemia (Ganguli, Cullen and Irvine, 1971). No consequence of this enormously elevated hormone concentration in achlorhydric patients has yet been described. Measurement of the high plasma gastrin (because of the considerably diminished acid output) has been put forward as a possible way of diagnosing carcinoma of the stomach (McGuigan and Trudeau, 1973a), though too many other conditions are associated with hypochlorhydria for this to be very useful. Gastrin measurement is also a simple additional test for pernicious anaemia. A great deal of research has been done on gastrin levels in patients with duodenal ulceration. It is known that these subjects have on average an increased gastric acid output and if the acid is reduced, the duodenal ulcer can be cured. Two possibilities exist, (a) that excessive gastrin release is the cause, and thus drives the stomach to excessive acid production and (b) that another cause exists and that the high gastric acid output would depress the gastrin release, by the feed-back loop mentioned above. The problem seems simple, in the common duodenal ulcer patient gastrin should be either excessively high or, if the second theory is right, below normal. Several groups of workers have unfortunately produced entirely contradictory results (Bloom, 1974a). At the present time the consensus opinion is that the fasting gastrin level may be slightly below normal in duodenal ulcer patients but that postprandially it rises to a higher level (McGuigan and Trudeau, 1973b). It is probably naive to think that duodenal ulcer is caused by a single abnormality and a more likely theory is that it is multifactorial.

Gastrinoma

Although the role of gastrin in common duodenal ulceration is uncertain, in the Zollinger–Ellison (ZE) syndrome the situation is quite clear. Here an endocrine tumour, nearly always pancreatic, produces an excessive quantity of gastrin (Isenberg, Walsh and Grossman, 1973) and thus the clinical syndrome, first described by Zollinger and Ellison (1955), of severe and intractable duodenal ulceration. Detecting this syndrome is important because failure to diagnose it may well prove fatal to the patient. Treatment by conventional ulcer surgery is inevitably followed by a recurrent ulcer and frequently also severe haemorrhage or perforation. The diagnosis is quite simply made by finding a high plasma gastrin level in association with either high gastric acid output or a clinically aggressive duodenal ulcer. Because the measurement of plasma gastrin is easy and the consequences of missing a ZE syndrome considerable, it has now become routine practice in many clinics to measure the plasma gastrin on all patients with aggressive duodenal ulceration. The presence of jejunal ulceration, gastric mucosal hypertrophy or a recurrent ulcer are particular pointers to the presence of the ZE syndrome which also occurs with undue frequency in association with hyperparathyroidism, acromegaly and insulinomas, forming the multiple endocrine adenomatosis syndrome type 1, which is inherited as a dominant characteristic (Levin, 1968).

Plasma gastrin can be measured on a single fasting (as gastrin is normally elevated after a meal) serum or plasma sample and sent to a radioimmunoassay laboratory within 24 hours of collection. In the United Kingdom a Supra-Regional Assay service has been set up to provide facilities for less commonly performed assays. All samples are handled by this service only at the request of the chemical pathologist in each hospital who keeps details of the procedure required, makes the necessary transport arrangements and advises on the indications for the assays. As an alternative to the SAS referral laboratories, several commercial firms sell gastrin assay kits. At the present time, however, these are both expensive and suffer from the fact that considerable expertise is needed to get reliable answers. This is unlikely to occur with occasional one-off samples. A major problem that is now beginning to occur is the reporting of only slightly raised plasma gastrin. The commonest cause for this is that the patient is suffering from mild hypochlorhydria, but cases also occur where the gastric acid output is undoubtedly high. Some of these patients could be suffering from early Zollinger–Ellison syndrome with a relatively small tumour only just beginning to produce systemic effects. To explore this possibility use is made of the intravenous secretin test. One clinical unit per kilogram of pure secretin (Karolinska Institute, Stockholm) is administered intravenously and samples collected basally and at $2\frac{1}{2}$, 5, 10, 15 and 30 minutes. In patients with an early tumour the gastrin level rises, while in those with normal G cells a fall is seen (Schrumpf et al, 1973).

SECRETIN

Chemistry and distribution

Secretin, although discovered in 1902 (Bayliss and Starling) was not finally purified until 1961 (Jorpes and Mutt). Even then the effort was enormous and it took the intestines of some 10 000 pigs to achieve 10 mg of the pure hormone. When its amino acid sequence was worked out it was found to have considerable similarities to that of glucagon and also to two subsequently discovered hormonal peptides, vasoactive intestinal peptide and gastric inhibitory peptide (see below) (Table 15.2) (Bodanszky, Klausner and Said, 1973). These therefore form a hormonal family which may possibly have all evolved from a single precursor hormone. Unlike gastrin there is no smaller part of the amino acid sequence of secretin which is biologically active. This suggests that the tertiary structure of secretin may be important in cellular binding and biological activity. Secretin also differs from gastrin in that there appears to be only a single molecular form (Bryant and Bloom, 1975). The actions of secretin are numerous and shared by the other members of the secretin glucagon family of hormones.

Table 15.2 Amino acid sequence of porcine VIP, secretin, glucagon, and GIP. Boxes show areas of homology

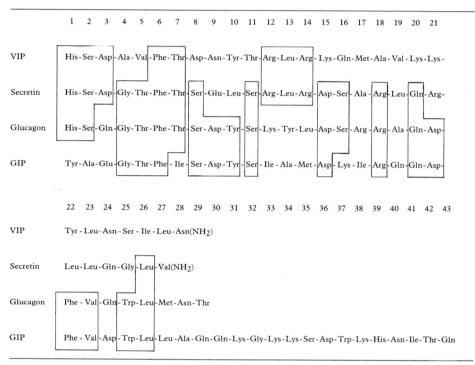

Its most potent effect is stimulating pancreatic bicarbonate juice flow which is physiologically important in neutralising gastric acid in the duodenum. Secretin also directly inhibits gastric acid production, and stimulates insulin release. The secretin-producing cell in the intestinal mucosa has been localised (Polak et al, 1971a) and found to be a cell type previously classified by electron microscopists as the S cell, originally standing for Small granule. Secretin occurs in highest concentration in the duodenal mucosa but significant amounts are found in the jejunum (Bloom, Bryant and Polak, 1975b).

Physiology

The recent development of reliable radioimmunoassays for secretin (Bloom and Ogawa, 1973; Boden et al, 1974; Chey et al, 1975) has at last enabled its physiology to be described convincingly. Only one stimulus releases secretin, that is duodenal or jejunal acidification (Boden et al, 1974; Bloom and Ward, 1974). The pH has to be less than 4.5 for this to happen, which agrees well with previous bioassay data. No release of secretin is seen with protein, fat or carbohydrate in the duodenum (Boden, Essa and Owen, 1975) and, though a recent report claims that secretin is released by alcohol (Straus, Urbach and Yalow, 1975), other laboratories have been unable to confirm this. Buchanan's group in Belfast have shown a considerable rise of secretin during prolonged starvation (Henry, Flanagan and Buchanan, 1975) and suggest it could play a part in metabolic adaptation. This would be an interesting new role for secretin but their finding has also not yet been confirmed by other laboratories. Although the duodenal pH may fall below 4.5 during experimental infusions of hydrochloric acid, it rarely does so under normal circumstances and this may explain why no secretin release has been reported after a normal meal (Bloom, Bryant and Cochrane, 1975a; Chey et al, 1975). The failure of secretin release to be detected in this circumstance had led to the role of secretin as a physiological hormone being challenged. It may be, however, that a very small release of secretin may still be important for stimulation of the pancreatic bicarbonate flow which occurs after a meal, but that this is undetectable with the insensitive assays available at the present time. Half maximal pancreatic bicarbonate output in man is produced by a secretin infusion giving a level of only 22 pmol/l in the plasma (Haecki et al, 1977). It is known that the potency of secretin can be increased four-fold if a significant concentration of cholecystokinin is also present (Petersen and Grossman, 1976). This illustrates the general point that a hormone's potency may be greatly influenced by the circumstances in which this is assessed and it is clear that secretin in the postprandial environment may be very much more potent than when studied in the fasting state. It has now been convincingly shown that the amount of secretin required to produce a physiological inhibition of gastric acid is vastly greater than that ever likely to be released endogenously (Ward and Bloom, 1974). The same is probably also true for the action of secretin in releasing insulin and therefore these two actions of secretin must be considered as pharmacological.

Pathology

As mentioned above, duodenal ulceration is associated with excess acid production and any manoeuvre that reduces acid levels leads to cure of the ulcer. Previously attention has been directed to the rate of gastric acid production but more important is the efficiency of acid neutralisation in the duodenum, where the ulcer is actually found. The most important factor in duodenal acid neutralisation is the pancreatic bicarbonate output, which is controlled by secretin. Thus any failure of secretin release could result in a lower duodenal pH and thus the development of duodenal ulceration. In a series of 23 duodenal ulcer patients studied the secretin release was indeed found to be impaired (Fig. 15.1) (Bloom and Ward, 1975). This appeared to be as great in patients with a short ulcer history as those with a long ulcer history and gave rise to the suggestion that a failure of secretin release could well have been important in the aetiology of the ulcer. Subsequent work, however, has demonstrated that cure of the ulcer by such manoeuvres as vagotomy and pyloroplasty leads to a recovery of secretin release (Ward and Bloom, 1975), making it more likely that the failure in ulcer patients was a secondary phenomenon, perhaps the result of 'duodenitis'. The failure of secretin release is nonetheless of considerable pathophysiological significance as it might well result in a failure of natural healing of a duodenal ulcer by establishing a vicious circle. The more severe the ulcer the less efficient becomes the duodenal neutralisation mechanisms. This is in agreement with the common observation that a remission induced in patients with duodenal ulcer by an intensive period of bed rest and antacids may often last many years.

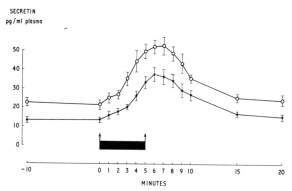

SECRETIN
pg/ml plasma

MINUTES

Figure 15.1   Plasma secretin concentrations in 12 healthy controls (open circles) and 23 patients with duodenal ulcer (solid dots) after intraduodenal infusion of 40 ml of 0.1 M-HCl between 0 and 5 minutes (black bar). Vertical bars indicate the s.e. mean. Taken from Bloom and Ward (1975)

CHOLECYSTOKININ

Chemistry and distribution

Although there was much early work in animals on the easily observed flow of bile, it was not until 1928 that Ivy and Oldberg in the USA postulated the existence of a hormone that caused gallbladder contraction, termed cholecysto-kinin (CCK). On this side of the Atlantic, Harper and Raper (1943) postulated a hormone that stimulated the pancreas to secrete an enzyme-rich juice, and they used the term pancreozymin. When these were both purified they were found to be the same hormone (Jorpes, Mutt and Toczko, 1964). This was found to be 33 amino acids long but it was subsequently shown that the entire biological activity could be seen with the last eight amino acids, and this sequence was in fact more potent than the whole hormone (Debas and Grossman, 1973). CCK thus resembles gastrin in having only a part of its amino acid sequence necessary for full activity (Table 15.1). It was possible to predict from this that multiple forms of CCK would occur, as with gastrin, and in fact a 39 amino acid CCK variant has been found in considerable quantities (Mutt and Jorpes, 1968). The last five amino acids of CCK are identical to the last five amino acids of gastrin suggesting that the two hormones come from a single hormonal family. In agreement with this suggestion high doses of cholecystokinin stimulate gastric acid secretion, and high doses of gastrin stimulate gallbladder contraction and enzyme output from the pancreas. It is of interest that a CCK-like peptide has been found in frog's skin (Dockray and Hopkins, 1975) and has been purified and made available in Italy as a commercial test of pancreatic function. One could imagine that it is present in the frog to cause its predators abdominal pain on ingestion. In man CCK is found in the jejunum and upper ileum (Bloom, 1974b;

Bloom and Bryant, 1973) and has recently been shown to be produced by the previously described I cell (Polak et al, 1975a).

Pharmacology

CCK has been shown to have a wide spectrum of actions, including control of appetite (Gibbs, Falasco and McHugh, 1976), control of pancreatic growth (Johnson, 1976), stimulation of gastrointestinal motor activity, gastric pepsin secretion and brunners gland secretion. It is an extremely potent stimulant of gallbladder contraction and pancreatic enzyme secretion, being equally potent for proteases, lipase, and amylase (Robberecht et al, 1975). It also greatly enhances the action of secretin in stimulating watery bicarbonate juice production (Petersen and Grossman, 1976). Thus secretin and CCK are commonly used in pancreatic function studies and are tending to supersede endogenous stimulation by test meals. A very large literature has developed round the interpretation of pancreatic function tests but while gross degrees of gland dysfunction can easily be detected, pancreatic secretion in the more clinically important early stages of disease shows a considerable overlap with normal. Nevertheless, pancreatic function studies performed using infusions of secretin and CCK are now an established part of the repertoire of most gastrointestinal units, and give important confirmatory evidence of destructive diseases of the pancreas and are a useful way of collecting pancreatic juice for cytology. They are not used more commonly partly because of low diagnostic precision, as mentioned above, partly because they are uncomfortable and expensive in physician time, and partly because the diseases which are thereby detected are frequently not amenable to any treatment. Several endoscopy units are investigating the possibility that direct collection of juice via a pancreatic duct cannula may improve the accuracy of the test but preliminary results are not promising.

Physiology

The physiological role of CCK is difficult to ascertain because no agreement has yet been reached on the hormone's level in the circulation (Thompson et al, 1975; Go and Reilly, 1975). The assay for CCK is fraught with difficulties, not the least being that, as mentioned above, there are probably several forms present in plasma with different biological potencies. Harvey in Bristol has produced some exciting preliminary results demonstrating extremely elevated levels of CCK in patients with pancreatic insufficiency (Harvey et al, 1974). This holds out the possibility that a single fasting blood sample may give more information on the state of pancreatic exocrine function than a morning's examination with a duodenal tube. Unfortunately, CCK seems also to be raised in some other conditions, for example coeliac disease (Low-Beer et al, 1975). To date no other group has been able to confirm these findings (Bloom, 1973).

PANCREATIC POLYPEPTIDE

Chemistry and distribution

In 1968 Kimmel, Pollock and Hazelwood, working on the purification of chicken insulin, noted the presence of a major impurity. This was isolated and found to be a 36 amino acid peptide which was designated avian pancreatic polypeptide (APP). Subsequently Lin and Chance (1972), working in the laboratories of a major USA insulin manufacturer, Eli Lilly, found a similar impurity in bovine pancreatic extracts. A bovine pancreatic polypeptide (BPP) was found and half of the 36 amino acids were identical to APP. Subsequently pancreatic polypeptides were extracted from the pig, sheep and man and were found to differ from BPP in only one or two amino acids (Lin and Chance, 1974). Investigations in the primate have shown that 93 per cent of pancreatic polypeptide (PP) comes from the pancreas with a very small amount being found in the stomach and upper small intestine (Adrian et al, 1976). The PP-producing cells, localised by indirect immunofluorescence, are shown to occur in the pancreas in small clumps lying between the acinar cells, with only a very occasional PP cell being found in the Islets of Langerhans. The PP-producing cell is identical to the previously described D1 cell recognised by electron microscopy listed in the revised Weisbaden classification (Heitz et al, 1976).

Pharmacology and physiology

The pharmacology of PP has been studied using BPP infusions in the dog (Lin and Chance, 1974). The most potent effects were the inhibition of gall bladder and enhancement of choledochal tone, with inhibition of pancreatic enzyme output. These actions being in direct opposition to those of CCK. At slightly higher doses a biphasic action on pancreatic bicarbonate production was seen with an initial stimulation followed by inhibition. A similar effect was noted on gastric secretion where basal secretion could be stimulated but pentagastrin stimulated gastric acid output was inhibited. Still larger doses of BPP caused retching and changes in gastrointestinal tone. Although it was found that chicken APP had a similar aminoacid sequence to that of avian glucagon (Kimmel, Hayden and Pollock, 1975), and caused depletion of hepatic glycogen, this effect was not demonstrable with BPP in the dog, and no change in plasma glucose or insulin was seen. In man a very rapid and large increase in the plasma PP value is observed after eating a meal (Fig. 15.2) (Adrian et al, 1976), the rise being of a similar order of magnitude and speed to that of insulin. Thus the physiology of PP in man could be of considerable interest though to date there have been no reports on the effects of its administration to humans. As the majority of PP is pancreatic in origin and PP levels have been reported to be undetectably low in patients who have undergone total pancreatectomy, the

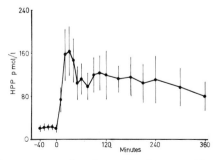

Figure 15.2 Peripheral plasma pancreatic polypeptide after a meal in seven healthy volunteers

postprandial release of PP in man must involve some signal from the gut to the pancreas. This phenomenon is well described for the release of insulin after a meal and the term enteroinsular axis has been coined. One can therefore predict that a similar entero PP axis must exist.

Tumour production

When the assay for human plasma PP levels was first developed an unexpected finding was that PP levels were extremely elevated in patients with endocrine pancreatic tumours (Polak et al, 1976a). Thus patients suffering from insulinomas, gastrinomas, VIPomas (see section on vasoactive intestinal peptide) and glucagonomas were all found to have continuous levels of plasma PP exceeding the peak value obtained in normal subjects after a meal. Histological investigation of the causative pancreatic endocrine tumours demonstrated that they contained large numbers of PP-producing cells and this was equally true of any hepatic metastasis. This then explained the nature of the previously mysterious cells which had been known to occur in these tumours. Extraction of the PP from the tumours demonstrated that it had identical physico-chemical characteristics to normal pancreatic PP and that PP, unlike many other hormones, appeared to exist in only a single molecular form. About one-third of these tumours had few PP cells, low extractable levels and plasma concentrations within the normal range. The clinical picture in these latter patients, however, did not appear to differ from those with high PP levels and thus it is not yet possible to say what the clinical effects, if any, of high PP may be. At the present time the importance of PP production by pancreatic endocrine tumours lies purely in the diagnostic field. As PP circulates in high concentrations and is extremely easy to measure it may be that doubtful or borderline cases of insulinoma or VIPoma, for example, may be more easily diagnosed by measuring their PP production. A routine PP assay used to screen suspected cases should considerably increase the yield of early, and therefore curable, tumours.

PANCREATIC GLUCAGON

In the traditional division of subjects, the acinar tissue of the pancreas is thought of as part of the digestive system, while the Islets of Langerhans are considered under metabolism. Pancreatic glucagon, which is produced by the alpha cells of the islets, is not so neatly pigeon-holed. To begin with it has a very wide spectrum of actions on the gastrointestinal tract and in this respect differs completely from insulin. Secondly, its amino acid sequence places it firmly in the secretin family of gastrointestinal hormones (Table 15.2) and suggests that although it may now have developed a predominantly metabolic role, it probably evolved from a precursor gut hormone. In line with this concept it has recently been shown that in the dog approximately one-third of the pancreatic glucagon is found in the gastric mucosa where alpha cells can be distinctly seen histologically. Thus after pancreatectomy canine plasma pancreatic glucagon levels hardly fall (Sasaki et al, 1975). In the human the situation is different and less than a half per cent of the pancreatic glucagon comes from the mucosa of the gastrointestinal tract. Patients who have undergone a total pancreatectomy have therefore undetectably low pancreatic glucagon concentrations (Barnes and Bloom, 1976). This latter point is of considerable interest to diabetologists as it effectively refutes the theory that diabetes is a bihormonal disease in which glucagon abnormalities are as important as insulin deficiency. Totally pancreatectomised diabetics are without glucagon and have all the normal disease complications.

GI pharmacology

Pancreatic glucagon has a number of extremely powerful actions on the gastrointestinal tract and these have been utilised for diagnostic purposes and also for treatment (Bloom, 1975a). For example glucagon increases coeliac axis blood flow and has been used in angiography. It strikingly dilates the duodenum and has been used for hypertonic duodenography. Glucagon suppresses the output of pancreatic enzymes and juice and has therefore been tried in attacks of acute pancreatitis with initially very promising results, though later surveys are less enthusiastic. Glucagon relaxes the musculature of the small and large bowel and has been used in the treatment of diverticulitis where relief of pain is said to be dramatic. Glucagon also inhibits the production of gastric acid and under some circumstances stimulates small intestinal juice flow.

Glucagonoma

It is not surprising to find that patients suffering from pancreatic endocrine tumours producing glucagon (glucagonomas) (Mallinson et al, 1974) show a number of gastrointestinal manifestations, the most noticeable of which is diarrhoea. A glucagonoma syndrome has now been described consisting of the following seven features: weight loss, anaemia, angular stomatitis, painful glossitis, mild diabetes, a necrolytic migratory erythematous rash, and manifestations of a pancreatic tumour. The description of this syndrome has led to the discovery of several new cases of what was previously thought to be an extremely rare disease. It is clearly important that the disease should not be overlooked, as dramatic recovery of both the diabetes and also a rather unpleasant rash can result.

ENTEROGLUCAGON

History

Enteroglucagon has not yet been purified and because of this its status as a hormone is not secure. It was first discovered in Dallas when Unger et al (1961) found glucagon immuno-reactivity in the intestines as well as the pancreas. They were later able to show that a more specific assay for pancreatic glucagon did not detect this intestinal material which must therefore have had a different amino acid sequence. They also demonstrated that it had a completely different pattern of release into the circulation, stimulants for enteroglucagon inhibiting the release of pancreatic glucagon and vice versa (Unger and Eisentraut, 1967). Attempts to purify enteroglucagon from the intestine showed that it occurred in at least two molecular weight forms, one of molecular weight about 3500 and one rather larger of around 10 000 (Valverde et al, 1968). The failure so far completely to purify the hormone is probably because of its considerable instability. With current techniques it tends to become degraded faster than it can be purified. In the absence of pure hormone, it is not possible to examine the amino acid sequence and say with certainty whether the several peaks of enteroglucagon really form one hormone type. Argument thus occurs as to whether it is reasonable to use the term enteroglucagon at all, implying as it does a single hormone or hormonal family. A scientifically safer, though far more cumbersome, term is 'glucagon-like immunoreactivity of intestinal origin' sometimes shortened to GLI.

Enteroglucagon is found in the human gastrointestinal tract in highest concentrations in the ileum but very significant amounts occur in the colon (Fig. 15.3) (Bloom, Bryant and Polak, 1975b). The enteroglucagon producing cell, or

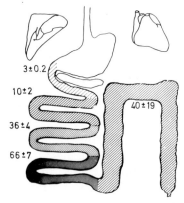

Figure 15.3   Mean concentration of enteroglucagon, in µg per region ± s.e. mean, in four baboon intestines

EG cell, is easily localised and is found in the basal part of the mucosal glands (Polak et al, 1971b). In spite of intensive investigation, only one type of EG cell has been found, which strengthens the concept that enteroglucagon is a single hormone occurring in multiple forms, and is similar in this respect to both gastrin and CCK.

Physiology

Plasma enteroglucagon rises very rapidly after a meal in man (Fig. 15.4) and it has been shown that the two constituents responsible for its release are carbohydrate and long chain tryglycerides (Bottger et al, 1973; Holst, Christiansen and Kuhl, 1976). As it is found relatively low down in the intestine, its release is enhanced by any degree of intestinal hurry and it is very much increased, for example in the dumping syndrome (Fig. 15.5) (Bloom, Royston and Thompson, 1972). Thus one can obtain an extremely good correlation between the speed of gastric emptying and the rise of enteroglucagon (Ralphs et al, 1975). A single case of an enteroglucagon-producing tumour has been reported and the main features of this were increased growth of the mucosa and gross intestinal hypomotility (Gleeson et al, 1971; Bloom, 1972). It is thus possible to speculate that the physiological actions of enteroglucagon may be to act as a long stop.

Unabsorbed food stuffs passing too far down the intestine would stimulate release of an increased amount of enteroglucagon which would lead to a slowing of intestinal transit and an increased growth of the mucosa, enhancing absorption. This hypothesis can only be tested when pure enteroglucagon is available for administration. It was predicted, however, on the basis of this theory that enteroglucagon levels should be elevated after partial gut resection and in the experimental rat this has indeed been found to be the case (Jacobs et al, 1976). Clearly further work is required to see if this also occurs in a number of similar situations in man.

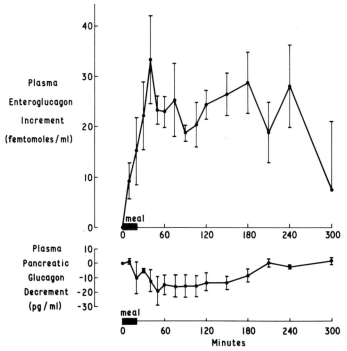

Figure 15.4 The rise of plasma enteroglucagon and fall in pancreatic glucagon after a normal hospital lunch in 10 healthy volunteers. Vertical bars indicate the s.e. mean

GASTRIC INHIBITORY PEPTIDE

Chemistry and distribution

While impure preparations of CCK were found to be powerful inhibitors of gastric acid production, purer preparations of this hormone were less effective. It was therefore postulated that one of the impurities of crude CCK must be a gastric inhibitory peptide (GIP) (Brown, Mutt and Pederson, 1970). GIP was purified by Brown (1971), and it was found capable of inhibiting the effect of histamine, the most powerful known stimulant of gastric acid secretion. Amino acid sequencing showed that it belonged to the glucagon-secretin family of peptides, being the largest member of the group, with 43 amino acids (Table 15.2) (Brown and Dryburgh, 1971). It is found in highest concentrations in the

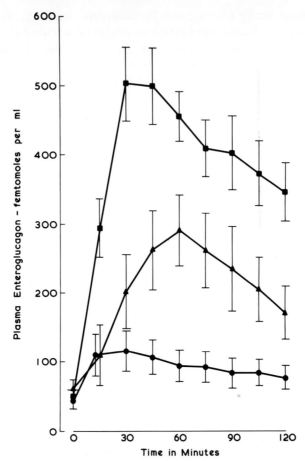

Figure 15.5 Mean rise in plasma enteroglucagon after 100 g oral glucose load in seven preoperative duodenal ulcer patients (solid dots), nine symptom-free patients after vagotomy and pyloroplasty (triangles), and eight patients after vagotomy and pyloroplasty with symptoms of the dumping syndrome (squares). Vertical bars indicate the s.e. mean. Taken from Bloom, Royston and Thompson (1972)

jejenum, though significant amounts are also present in the duodenum and upper ileum (Fig. 15.6) (Bloom et al, 1975b). The GIP-producing cell is most frequently found in the middle zone of the jejunal mucosal glands (Polak et al, 1973).

Physiology

With the development of a plasma radioimmunoassay for GIP, it was soon found to rise very significantly after a meal. The particular constituents which release it most potently are carbohydrate (Fig. 15.7) and fat (Cleator and Gourlay, 1975). As these two substances when placed in the small intestine are known to produce inhibition of gastric acid production, it was early suggested that release of GIP might be the responsible mechanism. Thus GIP was equated with the classically described enterogastrone. By analogy with the other members of the secretin-glucagon family of hormones, it was anticipated that GIP might possibly be an insulin releasing agent. This in fact proved to be the case and GIP caused a profound release of insulin both from isolated Islets of Langerhans and also in vivo (Tze 1975; Turner et al, 1974). Indeed when extracts of whole bowel were chromatographed and each fraction tested for its insulin releasing properties, the fraction with the greatest potency coincided with GIP immunoreactivity. Thus it seemed likely that GIP was the hormone responsible for

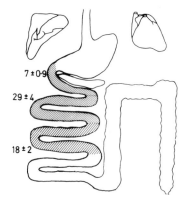

Figure 15.6   Mean concentration of GIP, in μg per region ± s.e. mean, in four baboon intestines

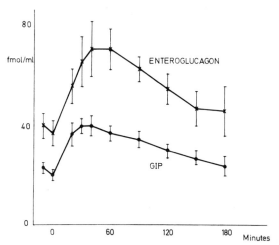

Figure 15.7   Plasma GIP and enteroglucagon concentrations after a 50 g oral glucose load in nine healthy volunteers. Vertical bars indicate s.e. mean

the much greater release of insulin seen when glucose is taken orally than if the same amount of glucose is administered intravenously, the so-called entero-insular axis. Further proof was provided by the demonstration in Montreal by Dupre et al (1973) that an infusion of GIP to man, in a dose giving physiological blood levels, resulted in a dramatic increase in plasma insulin levels.

Pathology

In maturity onset diabetes it is known that the beta cell in the islets contains plenty of insulin but that insulin release is defective. It was clearly possible that this defective release of insulin could be secondary to a failure of GIP release. Surprisingly, however, some studies have shown that GIP release is actually increased in diabetics (Ross et al, 1973) while others have suggested that it is not significantly different from normal (Bloom, 1975b). It has been postulated that GIP release may be increased in states of insulin resistance because of the observation that very high levels occur in extreme obesity (Brown, 1976, personal communication). The role of GIP as an enterogastrone controlling gastric acid output is less well established, little correlation being observed between the release of GIP and inhibition of gastric acid following intraduodenal fat or glucose. It is, nonetheless, one of the factors whose abnormal release could be important in the aetiology of duodenal ulcerations.

MOTILIN

Chemistry and distribution

In 1966 Brown, Johnson and Magee demonstrated that alkalinisation of the duodenum in the dog gave rise to powerful contractions of the isolated canine gastric pouch. They were able to demonstrate that crude duodenal extracts had the same effect, and later a substance was purified from semi-pure secretin preparations and called 'Motilin'. This peptide was shown to have 22 amino acids

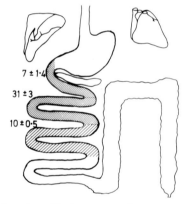

Figure 15.8   Mean concentration of motilin, in μg per region ± s.e. mean, in four baboon intestines

and to differ completely from any known hormone (Brown, Cook and Dryburgh, 1973). Like GIP it is found in highest concentrations in the jejunal mucosa but significant amounts occur in the duodenum and upper ileum (Fig. 15.8) (Bloom et al, 1975b). Its cell of origin has been classified as belonging to the enterochromaffin or EC cell system (Pearse et al, 1974).

Physiology

Motilin has now been synthesised (Wunsch et al, 1973) and the synthetic material, with norleucine substituted for methionine at 13 position to improve stability, has all the actions of the natural material (Strunz et al, 1976). On isolated strips of human stomach and intestine it causes powerful contractions, which are most marked in the antrum and duodenum (Mitznegg et al, 1975).

These effects appear to be direct and do not involve cyclic AMP (Schubert et al, 1975) or the local innervation. Infusion of motilin into human volunteers results in a very significant inhibition of gastric emptying (Ruppin et al, 1975). Further the blood level achieved during such infusions is comparable with the circulating motilin concentration found in normal fasting subjects. It thus seems quite conceivable that motilin is a physiological regulator of the rate of gastric emptying. Recent studies in dogs have shown two other possible effects. Motilin infusions have been found to increase greatly the frequency of the interdigestive myoelectric complex, the so-called housekeeping intermittent waves of contraction that sweep down the gut and are presumed to act to ensure

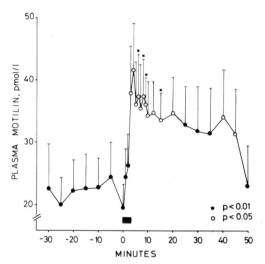

Figure 15.9 Plasma concentration of motilin in six healthy volunteers following intraduodenal instillation of 50 ml of 0.1 M-hydrochloric acid. Vertical lines indicate s.e. mean. Taken from Mitznegg et al (1976)

removal of unwanted secretion and debris (Marik and Code, 1975). Motilin has also been shown to produce phasic pressure changes in the lower oesophageal sphincter at an extremely low and probably physiological dose level (Jennewein et al, 1975). This has given rise to the suggestion that motilin may be a normal regulatory agent for the oesophageal sphincter and studies in man, especially in patients with acid reflux are awaited with interest. It has recently been reported that introduction of acid into the duodenum of volunteers results in a rapid release of motilin (Fig. 15.9) and this would correlate extremely well with the retardation of gastric emptying produced by this stimulus (Mitznegg et al, 1976).

VASOACTIVE INTESTINAL PEPTIDE

History

Professor S. I. Said, a respiratory physiologist, spent a sabbatical year in Stockholm investigating vasodilatory peptides in lung and bowel. He was successful in purifying one of the intestinal peptides, termed vasoactive intestinal peptide or VIP, and was later able to determine its amino acid sequence. It was found to bear a surprising resemblance to that of glucagon and secretin and clearly belonged to the secretin–glucagon family (Table 15.2) (Bodanszky, Klausner and Said, 1973). Subsequent work has shown VIP to be very widely distributed throughout the body occurring in high concentrations not only in the bowel but also in other organs such as the brain (Bryant et al, 1976). Immunofluorescent localisation demonstrates VIP to occur both in discreet endocrine cells in the gastrointestinal mucosa and also in autonomic nerve fibres. The physicochemical characteristics of VIP from the CNS and VIP from the intestine are identical. Thus this hormone appears to straddle the normal division of peripheral hormone and neurotransmitter substance. It adds considerable weight to the theory propounded by Pearse (1969) that endocrine cells have a neuroectodermal origin. Two other hormonal peptides are known to occur both in the CNS and in the gastrointestinal tract, somatostatin and substance P, while a gastrin-like peptide has also been reported in the brain (Vanderhaeghen, Signeau and Gepts, 1975). The old division into control by the nervous system and control by peripheral hormones may be too rigid and indeed the classical definition of a hormone has recently been challenged (Wingate, 1976). It is interesting to speculate that VIP may be illustrating evolution in progress. It is known to possess all the actions of the other members of the secretin–glucagon family and it may thus be the precursor neurotransmitter from which the other hormones have evolved.

Pharmacology and physiology

The pharmacological actions of VIP are very numerous. Like secretin it is a potent stimulator of pancreatic watery bicarbonate juice production and like glucagon it causes hyperglycaemia due to hepatic glycogenolysis (Said and Mutt, 1972). Like GIP it produces a considerable inhibition of gastric acid output (Barbezat and Grossman, 1971) and also stimulates insulin and glucagon release. VIP is an inotropic agent but lowers blood pressure because of its peripheral vasodilatory action. It also greatly stimulated small intestinal juice production and activates mucosal adenylcyclase (Schwartz et al, 1974). Which of these actions, if any, forms the physiological role of VIP is unknown. No significant release of VIP is seen after a meal (Bloom et al, 1975a) neither has any other circumstance been reported when it is released physiologically. It is extremely rapidly cleared from the circulation after injection and it may be that it acts only rarely in its capacity as a circulating hormone. It may, on the other hand, be an important local tissue hormone and thus be a member of the paracrine or local hormone system in addition to its possible role as a neurotransmitter.

VIPomas

One circumstance in which VIP has been found to be extremely raised in the circulation is in the Verner–Morrison syndrome (Fig. 15.10) (Bloom, Polak and Pearse, 1973). This was described in 1958 as a combination of a pancreatic tumour and very severe, indeed lethal watery diarrhoea. It has subsequently been shown that this syndrome can be differentiated from the ZE syndrome where diarrhoea is seen in about a third of the cases, by the finding of extremely low gastric acid output. Removal of the pancreatic tumour produces immediate cure of all symptoms and it was early postulated that the tumour must be producing a hormone (Zollinger, 1975). It was later demonstrated that the tumour contained considerable quantities of VIP and also that the circulating levels of VIP were extremely high (Bloom et al, 1973). No evidence was found of other hormone elevation and in view of the known action of VIP in producing profuse intestinal water secretion, it seemed likely that this hormone was the cause of the syndrome. A recent survey by Verner and Morrison (1974) has shown that approximately half of the pancreatic tumours have metastasised at the time of diagnosis, while in those cases with local tumour a third are so sick at the time of surgery that they die during the postoperative period. Kraft, Thompkins and Zollinger (1970) pointed out that the mean time from onset of symptoms to exploratory laparotomy in the Verner–Morrison syndrome was over three years

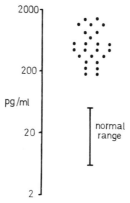

Figure 15.10 Plasma VIP levels in the first received plasma from 24 patients with the Verner–Morrison syndrome

and one may speculate that an earlier diagnosis might well have prevented the development of metastasis in many of these cases. Estimation of a single fasting plasma sample for VIP, available in the United Kingdom through the Supraregional Assay Service, now enables the diagnosis to be made very rapidly. To date, and this is an enviable record that may not be maintained, no diagnostic errors have been made where adequately taken samples for VIP estimation have been available (Bloom and Polak, 1976). For example, cases with diarrhoea due to infection, purgative addiction, ulcerative colitis, Crohn's disease and other less specific diarrhoeas all have very low VIP levels (Fairclough, Bloom and Mitchell, 1976). Thus measurement of plasma VIP is an extremely simple and rapid screening test to pick out this rare but potentially curable cause from other commoner types of diarrhoea. It has recently been noted that although many tumours associated with diarrhoea such as medullary carcinoma of the thyroid and carcinoma of the bronchus are not associated with raised levels of VIP, tumours of the sympathetic chain frequently are. For example ganglioneuro-blastomas which are a common childhood tumour associated with diarrhoea, appear to produce VIP quite frequently (Swift, Bloom and Harris, 1975). VIP measurement is also useful in monitoring treatment and has been used to demonstrate how dramatically successful streptozotocin can be in the chemotherapy of the Verner–Morrison syndrome.

SOMATOSTATIN

History

Somatostatin was first isolated by Guillemin's group at the Salk Institute in California when they were searching for a hormone or factor released by the hypothalamus and controlling pituitary growth hormone (Brazeau and Guillemin, 1974). It is a 14 amino acid polypeptide with a cystine bridge. It has subsequently been prepared synthetically and is now freshly available. After its isolation it was found not only to inhibit the release of growth hormone but also that of TSH (Siler et al, 1974), though no effect whatsoever was seen on the release of LH, FSH or ACTH. More recently it has also been shown to be able to block totally the release of insulin and glucagon produced by any known stimuli (Mortimer et al, 1974; Alberti et al, 1973). As this effect is also seen on isolated islets (Fukimoto, Ensinck and Williams, 1974), it is presumed to be a direct one. The mechanism of action of somatostatin has not yet been elucidated but it apparently acts beyond the cyclic AMP stage and may involve inhibition of hormone release at the cell membrane. Many analogues of somatostatin have been synthesised but so far they all have the same relative potencies for the various target tissues. Somatostatin is very rapidly cleared from the circulation, with a half-life of the order of 1 minute. No analogues have been synthesised which demonstrate any prolongation of action, and to be effective somatostatin must therefore be given by continuous intravenous infusion.

Although somatostatin was originally extracted from the hypothalamus, it has subsequently been found in the rest of the brain and also in considerable concentration in the gastrointestinal tract and pancreas (Arimura et al, 1975). Gel chromatography of pancreatic and brain extracts demonstrate at least two immunoreactive peaks both of which have biological activity. Thus a big somatostatin appears to exist and there is a possibility that a big big somatostatin also occurs (Schally et al, 1975). The somatostatin-producing cell has been localised and found to be identical to the classical D cell known to exist both in the gastrointestinal mucosa and the Islets of Langerhans (Polak et al, 1975b). Somatostatin is also found in nerve cell bodies in the periventricular region of the anterior hypothalamus and more widely in nerve terminals (Hokfelt et al, 1975).

Gastrointestinal pharmacology

In 1974 somatostatin was found to be a potent inhibitor of gastrin release (Fig. 15.11) (Bloom et al, 1974). It was subsequently also found to inhibit gastric acid output (Barros D'Sa, Bloom and Baron, 1975). As this later phenomenon occurred even during pentagastrin infusions, it was concluded that somatostatin must act directly both on the G cell and also independently on the parietal cell. Somatostatin has been found to inhibit pepsin output from the stomach (Gomez-Pan et al, 1975) and it greatly retards gastric emptying (Bloom et al, 1975c). In addition it markedly inhibits the release of motilin, causing a dramatic fall in the resting motilin level (Bloom et al, 1975c). Because of its actions on gastrin release and gastrin target tissues the effect of somatostatin on CCK was investigated. It was found to be a potent inhibitor of gallbladder contraction and also pancreatic enzyme juice production (Creutzfeldt, Lankisch and Folsch, 1975). The effect of somatostatin on secretin-stimulated bicarbonate output is more controversial, however, with some groups showing a very significant reduction (Boden et al, 1975b) and others showing no effect (Bloom, Joffe and Polak, 1975). Somatostatin has also been reported to reduce the output of VIP from VIPomas with a reduction in small intestinal juice production (Lenon et al, 1975).

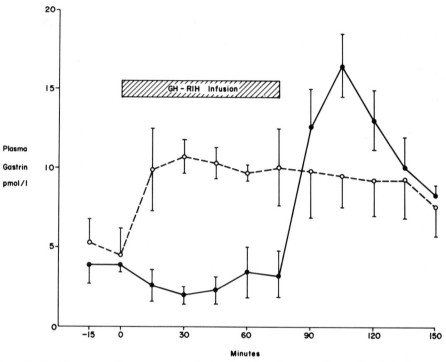

Figure 15.11 Plasma gastrin concentration in four healthy volunteers who ate a breakfast between 0 and 15 minutes. The solid line shows the mean values on a day when a 75 minute 1 mg somatostatin (GH-RIH) infusion was given and dotted lines show a control saline infusion day. Vertical lines indicate s.e. mean. Taken from Bloom et al (1974)

Physiological role

The widespread actions of somatostatin, whose very name implies stopping the whole body, makes it unlikely to be a circulating hormone. In addition relatively high blood levels are required to see its inhibitory effects and it is very rapidly cleared from the circulation. In view of its location both in nerve fibres in the brain and in endocrine cells, a more likely role in the periphery is as a local hormone, a member of the paracrine system. Thus in peripheral tissues this would place it in the same grouping as nerve growth factor, prostaglandins, histamine and epidermal growth factor. If a local hormone action is accepted as likely then one can predict considerable difficulties in working out its physiological role. There are no good techniques presently available for assessing the degree of local release of local hormones and their resulting effects.

The subject is important, however, as excessive somatostatin in the pancreas might give rise to diabetes and deficient somatostatin in the stomach might give rise to hyperacidity and duodenal ulcer formation.

OTHER POSSIBLE HORMONES

A number of other possible hormones have been proposed. Anderson in Sweden was working on a possible factor released from the bulb of the duodenum which inhibits gastric acid, termed bulbogastrone (Anderson, Nilson and Uvnas, 1967). Adelson and Rothman (1975) in California have extracted a substance from the upper small intestine which stimulates pancreatic enzyme production selectively. The substance, termed chymodenin, increases the output of chymotrypsinogen particularly. It has been known for a long time that the enzyme content of pancreatic juice is adjusted according to the nature of the ingested meal and chymodenin may form one of the mechanisms. Harper and colleagues (1974) have proposed that a 'pancreatone' exists in the colonic mucosa which inhibits the output of pancreatic juice. For some years Gregory in ICI has been working to isolate a gastric inhibitory substance from the urine, urogastrone. When he succeeded a year ago, the amino acid sequence turned out to be nearly identical to the epidermal growth factor originally isolated from mouse salivary gland (Gregory, 1975). This substance which is widely distributed throughout the body is a potent inhibitor of gastric acid and may have interesting possibilities both in physiology and therapeutics. If administered to patients with duodenal ulcer, it would inhibit gastric acid and also aid local mucosal healing.

Erspamer's group in Italy has over the years collected a large number of active peptides from amphibian skin. These have been placed into about five groups according to their pharmacological actions. Each group has turned out to have a mammalian counterpart, for example caerulein-like peptides and CCK, physalaemin-like peptides and substance P and the bradykinin-like peptides. One group has not yet had a mammalian counterpart described — the bombesin group of peptides. These peptides, including ranatensin, litorin and alytesin act in the mammal as potent gastrin releasers (Bertaccini et al, 1974) and also cause gallbladder contraction and increased pancreatic enzyme output (Basso et al, 1975). It has been known for some time that substances placed in the intestine can stimulate antral gastrin production and a bombesin-like peptide has been postulated. Recently, using the technique of indirect immunofluorescence, numerous bombesin-producing cells have been seen in the mucosa of the mammalian gastrointestinal tract (Polak et al, 1976b). Knowledge of the exact role of bombesin in human physiology will have to await the development of a plasma radioimmunoassay.

HORMONE INTERREACTION

It is in the nature of the present fragmentary knowledge concerning the gut hormones that they are considered in isolation. Future progress will enable them to be looked at in a more comprehensive manner. It is clear, if one takes as an example gastric acid secretion, that there are a large number of possible controlling influences. There are several stimulants such as gastrin, histamine and acetyl choline and several inhibitors such as somatostatin, secretin, GIP, VIP and urogastrone. The modulating effects of the luminal pH and nutritional content have also to be taken into account. Further there are the powerful effects of the gastric innervation, both sympathetic and parasympathetic, which are subject to unquantifiable psychological influences. In the case of excess gastric acid production, as seen in patients with duodenal ulcer, it is unlikely that a single control system is malfunctioning, the defect is more likely to be a more subtle general imbalance. If a large group of duodenal ulcer patients is investigated one would predict that the mean of all the stimulatory factors would be slightly increased and of all the inhibitory ones slightly reduced. In order to unravel the situation thoroughly it will be necessary to measure and assess each factor individually, an approach somewhat beyond our present technology. The same multi-factorial analysis is likely to be necessary for any other diseases of physiological imbalance, such as spastic colon or functional diarrhoea.

Conclusion

Several new hormones have been recently isolated from the alimentary tract and their cells of origin recognised. Knowledge of their physiology still lags behind, however, and investigation of their pathology has hardly begun. One can predict three areas where in future gut endocrinology will be of importance in human disease. Firstly abnormal production of the gut hormone may cause disease and at present this is only recognised in endocrine tumour situations. Secondly a pre-existing disease may be exacerbated by secondary abnormalities of hormone production, for example it could be that the diarrhoea of ulcerative colitis is the result of a hormone abnormally released by the primary pathology. Thirdly a gut hormone profile, especially following some stimuli such as a standard meal, will be a very useful diagnostic tool for localising in which areas and in what way the gastrointestinal tract is diseased.

REFERENCES

Adelson, J. W. & Rothman, S. S. (1975) Chymodenin, a duodenal peptide: specific stimulation of chymotrypsinogen secretion. *American Journal of Physiology*, **229**, 1680–1686.

Adrian, T. E., Bloom, S. R., Bryant, M. G., Polak, J. M., Heitz, P. & Barnes, A. J. (1976) Distribution and release of human pancreatic polypeptide. *Gut*, **17**, 940–944.

Alberti, K. G. M. M., Christensen, N. J., Christenson, S. E., Hansen, A. A. P., Iversen, J., Lundbaek, K., Seyer-Hansea, K. & Orskov, H. (1973) Inhibition of insulin secretion by somatostatin. *Lancet*, **ii**, 1299–1301.

Anderson, J. D., Barton, M. A., Gregory, R. A., Hardy, P. M., Kenner, G. W., MacLeod, J. K., Preston, J., Sheppard, R. D. & Morley, J. S. (1964) The antral hormone gastrin II. Synthesis of gastrin. *Nature (London)*, **204**, 933–934.

Andersson, S., Nilsson, G. & Uvnas, B. (1967) Effect of acid in proximal and distal duodenal pouches on gastric secretory responses to gastrin and histamine. *Acta physiologica Scandinavica*, **71**, 368–378.

Arimura, A., Sato, H., Dupont, A., Nishi, N. & Schally, A. V. (1975) Somatostatin: abundance of immunoreactive hormone in rat stomach and pancreas. *Science*, **189**, 1007–1009.

Barbezat, G. D. & Grossman, M. I. (1971) Intestinal secretion: stimulation by peptides. *Science*, **174**, 422–423.

Barnes, A. J. & Bloom, S. R. (1976) Pancreatectomised man: a model for diabetes without glucagon. *Lancet*, **i**, 219–222.

Barros D'Sa, A. A. J., Bloom, S. R. & Baron, J. H. (1975) Direct inhibition of gastric acid by growth hormone release inhibiting hormone in dogs. *Lancet*, **i**, 886–887.

Basso, N., Giri, S., Improta, G., Lezoche, E., Melchiorri, P., Percoco, M. & Speranza, V. (1975) External pancreatic secretion after bombesin infusion in man. *Gut*, **16**, 994–998.

Bayliss, W. M. & Starling, E. H. (1902) The mechanism of pancreatic secretion. *Journal of Physiology*, **28**, 325–353.

Berson, S. A. & Yalow, R. S. (1971) Nature of immunoreactive gastrin extracted from tissues of the gastrointestinal tract. *Gastroenterology*, **60**, 215–222.

Bertaccini, G., Erspamer, V., Melchiorri, P. & Sopranzi, N. (1974) Gastrin release by bombesin in the dog. *British Journal of Pharmacology*, **52**, 219–225.

Blair, E. L., Greenwell, J. R., Grund, E. R., Reed, J. D. & Sanders, D. J. (1975) Gastrin response to meals of different composition in normal subjects. *Gut*, **16**, 766–773.

Bloom, S. R. (1972) An enteroglucagon tumour. *Gut*, **13**, 520–523.

Bloom, S. R. (1973) Radioimmunoassay of cholecystokinin-pancreozymin. *Lancet*, **ii**, 1272.

Bloom, S. R. (1974a) Radioimmunoassay of intestinal hormones. *Gut*, **15**, 502–510.

Bloom, S. R. (1974b) Hormones of the gastro-intestinal tract. In *Radioimmunoassay and Saturation Analysis*, ed. Sonksen, P. H., *British Medical Bulletin*, vol. 30, 62–67.

Bloom, S. R. (1975a) Glucagon. *British Journal of Hospital Medicine*, **13**, 150–158.

Bloom, S. R. (1975b) GIP in diabetes. *Diabetologia*, **11**, 334.

Bloom, S. R. & Bryant, M. G. (1973) Distribution of radioimmunoassayable gastrin, secretin, pancreozymin and enteroglucagon in rat, dog and baboon gut. *Journal of Endocrinology*, **59**, XLIV.

Bloom, S. R. & Ogawa, O. (1973) Radioimmunoassay of human peripheral plasma secretin. *Journal of Endocrinology*, **58**, XXIV–XXV.

Bloom, S. R. & Polak, J. M. (1976) VIP measurement in distinguishing Verner-Morrison syndrome and Pseudo Verner-Morrison syndrome. *Clinical Endocrinology*, **5**, 223s–228s.

Bloom, S. R. & Ward, A. S. (1974) Secretin release in man after intraduodenal acid. *Gut*, **15**, 338.

Bloom, S. R. & Ward, A. S. (1975) Failure of secretin release in patients with duodenal ulcer. *British Medical Journal*, **1**, 126–127.

Bloom, S. R., Royston, C. M. S. & Thomson, J. P. S. (1972) Enteroglucagon release in the dumping syndrome. *Lancet*, **ii**, 789–791.

Bloom, S. R., Polak, J. M. & Pearse, A. G. E. (1973) Vasoactive intestinal peptide and water-diarrhoea syndrome. *Lancet*, **ii**, 14–16.

Bloom, S. R., Mortimer, C. H., Thorner, M. O., Besser, G. M., Hall, R., Gomez-Pan, A., Roy, V. M., Russell, R. C. G., Coy, D. H., Kastin, A. J. & Schally, A. V. (1974) Inhibition of gastrin and gastric acid secretion by growth hormone release inhibiting hormone. *Lancet*, **ii**, 1106–1109.

Bloom, S. R., Bryant, M. G. & Cochrane, J. P. S. (1975a) Normal distribution and postprandial release of gut hormones. *Clinical Science and Molecular Medicine*, **49**, 3P.

Bloom, S. R., Bryant, M. G. & Polak, J. M. (1975b) Distribution of gut hormones. *Gut*, **16**, 821.

Bloom, S. R., Ralphs, D. N., Besser, G. M., Hall, R., Coy, D. H., Kastin, A. J. & Schally, A. V. (1975c) Effect of somatostatin on motilin levels and gastric emptying. *Gut*, **16**, 834.

Bloom, S. R., Joffe, S. N. & Polak, J. M. (1975d) Effect of somatostatin on pancreatic and biliary function. *Gut*, **16**, 836–837.

Bodanszky, M., Klausner, Y. S. & Said, S. I. (1973) Biological activities of synthetic peptides corresponding to fragments of and to the entire sequence of the vasoactive intestinal peptide. *Proceedings of the National Academy of Sciences of the USA*, **70**, 382–384.

Boden, G., Essa, N., Owen, O. E. & Reichle, F. A. (1974) Effects of intraduodenal administration of HCl and glucose on circulating immunoreactive secretin and insulin concentrations. *Journal of Clinical Investigation*, **53**, 1185–1193.

Boden, G., Essa, N. & Owen, O. E. (1975a) Effects of intraduodenal amino acids, fatty acids, and sugars on secretin concentrations. *Gastroenterology*, **68**, 722–727.

Boden, G., Sivitz, M. C., Owen, O. E., Essa-Koumar, N. & Landor, J. H. (1975b) Somatostatin suppresses secretin and pancreatic exocrine secretion. *Science*, **190**, 163–165.

Bottger, I., Dobbs, R., Faloona, G. R. & Unger, R. H. (1973) The effects of triglyceride absorption upon glucagon, insulin and gut glucagon-like immunoreactivity. *Journal of Clinical Investigation*, **52**, 2532–2541.

Brazeau, P. & Guillemin, R. (1974) Somatostatin: newcomer from the hypothalamus. *New England Journal of Medicine*, **290**, 963–964.

Brown, J. C. (1971) A gastric inhibitory polypeptide I. The amino acid composition and the tryptic peptides. *Canadian Journal of Biochemistry*, **49**, 255–261.

Brown, J. C. & Dryburgh, J. R. (1971) A gastric inhibitory polypeptide II: the complete amino acid sequence. *Canadian Journal of Biochemistry*, **49**, 867–872.

Brown, J. C., Johnson, L. P. & Magee, D. F. (1966) Effect of duodenal alkalinisation on gastric motility. *Gastroenterology*, **50**, 333–339.

Brown, J. C., Mutt, V. & Pederson, R. A. (1970) A further purification of a polypeptide demonstrating enterogastrone activity. *Journal of Physiology*, **209**, 56–64.

Brown, J. C., Cook, M. A. & Dryburgh, J. R. (1973) Motilin, a gastric motor activity stimulating polypeptide: the complete amino acid sequence. *Canadian Journal of Biochemistry*, **51**, 533–537.

Bryant, M. G. & Bloom, S. R. (1975) Characterisation of the new gastrointestinal hormones. *Gut*, **16**, 840.

Bryant, M. G., Bloom, S. R., Polak, J. M., Albuquerque, R. H., Modlin, I. & Pearse, A. G. E. (1976) Possible dual role for VIP — Gastrointestinal hormone and neurotransmitter substance. *Lancet*, **i**, 991–993.

Castell, D. D. & Harris, L. D. (1970) Hormonal control of gastroesophageal-sphincter strength. *New England Journal of Medicine*, **282**, 886–889.

Chey, W. Y., Rhodes, R. A., Lee, K. Y. & Hendricks, J. (1975) Radioimmunoassay of secretin: further studies. In *Gastrointestinal Hormones*, ed. Thompson, J. C. pp. 269–281.

Cleator, I. G. M. & Gourlay, R. H. (1975) Release of immunoreactive gastric inhibitory polypeptide (IR-GIP) by oral ingestion of food substances. *American Journal of Surgery*, **130**, 128–135.

Creutzfeldt, W., Lankisch, P. G. & Folsch, U. R. (1975) Hemmung der sekretin-und cholezystokinin-pankreozymin-induzierten saft-und enzymsekretion des pankreas und der gallenblasenkontraktion beim menschen durch somatostatin. *Deutsche Medizinische Wochenschrift*, **100**, 1135–1138.

Debas, H. T. & Grossman, M. I. (1973) Pure cholecystokinin: pancreatic protein and bicarbonate response. *Digestion*, **9**, 469–481.

Dockray, G. J. & Hopkins, C. R. (1975) Caerulein secretion by dermal glands in xenopus laevis. *Journal of Cell Biology*, **64**, 724–733.

Dupre, J., Ross, S. A., Watson, D. & Brown, J. C. (1973) Stimulation of insulin secretion by gastric inhibitory peptide in man. *Journal of Clinical Endocrinology and Metabolism*, **37**, 826–828.

Edkins, J. S. (1905) On the chemical mechanisms of gastric secretion. *Proceedings of the Royal Society of London B, Biological Sciences*, **76**, 376.

Fairclough, P. D., Bloom, S. R. & Mitchell, S. J. (1976) Plasma VIP in ulcerative colitis. *Lancet*, **i**, 964.

Farooq, D. & Walsh, J. H. (1975) Atropine enhances serum gastrin response to insulin in man. *Gastroenterology*, **68**, 662–666.

Fujimoto, W. Y., Ensinck, J. W. & Williams, R. H. (1974) Somatostatin inhibits insulin and glucagon release by monolayer cell cultures of rat endocrine pancreas. *Life Sciences*, **15**, 1999–2004.

Ganguli, P. C., Cullen, D. R. & Irvine, W. J. (1971) Radioimmunoassay of plasma-gastrin in pernicious anaemia, achlorhydria without pernicious anaemia, hypochlorhydria and controls. *Lancet*, **i**, 155–158.

Gibbs, J., Falasco, J. D. & McHugh, P. R. (1976) Cholecystokinin-decreased food intake in rhesus monkeys. *American Journal of Physiology*, **230**, 15–18.

Giles, G. R., Mason, M. C., Humphries, C. & Clark, C. G. (1969) Action of gastrin on the lower oesophageal sphincter in man. *Gut*, **10**, 730–734.

Gleeson, M. H., Bloom, S. R., Polak, J. M., HEnry, K. & Dowling, R. M. (1971) An endocrine tumour in kidney affecting small bowel structure motility and absorptive function. *Gut*, **12**, 733–782.

Go, V. L. W. & Reilly, W. M. (1975) Problems encountered in the development of the cholecystokinin assay. *Gastrointestinal Hormones*, pp. 295–299. Austin: University of Texas Press.

Gomez-Pan, A., Reed, J. D., Albinus, M., Shaw, B., Hall, R., Besser, G. M., Coy, D. H., Kastin, A. J. & Schally, A. V. (1975) Direct inhibition of gastric acid and pepsin secretion by growth-hormone release-inhibiting hormone in cats. *Lancet*, **i**, 888–890.

Gregory, H. (1975) The isolation and structure of urogastrone and its relationship to epidermal growth factor. *Nature*, **257**, 325–327.

Gregory, R. A. & Tracy, H. J. (1964) The constitution and properties of two gastrins extracted from hog antral mucosa. *Gut*, **5**, 103–117.

Gregory, R. A. & Tracy, H. J. (1975) The chemistry of the gastrins: some recent advances. In *International Symposium on Gastrointestinal Hormones*, ed. Thompson, J. C. pp. 13–24. Galveston Texas.

Grossman, M. I. (1974) What is physiological? Round 2. *Gastroenterology*, **67**, 766–767.

Haecki, W. H., Belohlavek, D., Bloom, S. R., Demling, L., Domschke, W., Domschke, S., Galariotis, C., Mallinson, C., Mitznegg, P. & Wuensch, E. (1977) Secretin pharmacokinetics and plasma levels for half maximum bicarbonate response in man. *Gut* (in press).

Harper, A. A. & Raper, H. S. (1943) Pancreozymin, a stimulant of the secretion of pancreatic enzymes in extracts of the small intestine. *Journal of Physiology*, **102**, 115–125.

Harper, A. A., Hood, A. J. C., Muskens, J. & Smy, T. R. (1974) Pancreotone: an inhibitor of pancreatic secretion in extracts of ileal and colonic mucosa. *Journal of Physiology*, **253**, 32P.

Harvey, R. F., Dowsett, L., Hartog, M. & Read, A. E. (1974) Radioimmunoassay of cholecystokinin-pancreozymin. *Gut*, **15**, 690–699.

Heitz, P., Polak, J. M., Bloom, S. R. & Pearse, A. G. E. (1976) Identification of the D₁ cell as the source of human pancreatic polypeptide. *Gut*, **17**, 755–758.

Henry, R. W., Flanagan, R. W. J. & Buchanan, K. D. (1975) Secretin: a new role for an old hormone. *Lancet*, ii, 202–203.

Hokfelt, T., Efendic, S., Hellerstrom, C., Johansson, O., Luft, R. & Arimura, A. (1975) Cellular localisation of somatostatin in endocrine-like cells and neurons of the rat with special references to the A₁-cells of the pancreatic islets and to the hypothalamus. *Acta endocrinologica Supplementa*, **80**, 5–41.

Holst, J. J., Christiansen, J. & Kuhl, C. (1976) The enteroglucagon response to intrajejunal infusion of glucose, triglycerides and sodium chloride and its relation to jejunal inhibition of gastric acid secretion in man. *Scandinavian Journal of Gastroenterology*, **11**, 297–304.

Isenberg, J. I., Walsh, J. H. & Grossman, M. I. (1973) Zollinger-Ellison syndrome. *Gastroenterology*, **65**, 140–165.

Ivy, A. C. & Oldberg, E. (1928) A hormone mechanism for gall bladder contraction and evacuation. *American Journal of Physiology*, **86**, 599–610.

Jacobs, L. R., Polak, J. M., Bloom, S. R. & Dowling, R. H. (1976) Does enteroglucagon play a trophic role in intestinal adaptation. *Clinical Science and Molecular Medicine*, **50**, 14–15.

Jennewein, H. M., Hummelt, H., Siewert, R. & Waldeck, F. (1975) The motor-stimulating effect of natural motilin on the lower oesophageal sphincter, fundus, antrum and duodenum in dogs. *Digestion*, **13**, 246–250.

Johnson, L. R. (1976) The trophic action of gastrointestinal hormones. *Gastroenterology*, **70**, 278–288.

Johnson, L. R., Lichtenberger, L. M., Copeland, E. M., Dudrick, S. J. & Castro, G. A. (1975) Action of gastrin on gastrointestinal structure and function. *Gastroenterology*, **68**, 1184–1192.

Jorpes, E. & Mutt, V. (1961) On the biological activity and amino acid composition of secretin. *Acta Chemica Scandinavica*, **15**, 1790–1794.

Jorpes, E., Mutt, V. & Toczko, K. (1964) Further purification of cholecystokinin and pancreozymin. *Acta Chemica Scandinavica*, **18**, 2408–2410.

Kimmel, J. R., Pollock, H. G. & Hazelwood, R. L. (1968) Isolation and characterisation of chicken insulin. *Endocrinology*, **83**, 1323–1330.

Kimmel, J. R., Hayden, L. J. & Pollock, H. G. (1975) Isolation and characterisation of a new pancreatic polypeptide hormone. *Journal of Biological Chemistry*, **250**, 9369–9376.

Kraft, A. R., Thompkins, R. K. & Zollinger, R. M. (1970) Recognition and management of the diarrhoeal syndrome caused by nonbeta islet cell tumours of the pancreas. *American Journal of Surgery*, **119**, 163–170.

Lennon, J. R., Sircus, W., Bloom, S. R., Mitchell, S. J., Polak, J. M., Besser, G. M., Hall, R., Coy, D. H., Kastin, A. J. & Schally, A. V. (1975) Investigation and treatment of a recurrent VIPoma. *Gut*, **16**, 821–822.

Levin, M. E. (1968) Endocrine syndromes associated with pancreatic islet cell tumours. *Medical Clinics of North America*, **52**, 295–345.

Lin, T. M. (1972) Gastrointestinal actions of the C-terminal tripeptide of gastrin. *Gastroenterology*, **63**, 922–923.

Lin, T. M. & Chance, R. E. (1972) Spectrum gastrointestinal actions of a new bovine pancreas polypeptide (BPP). *Gastroenterology*, **62**, 852.

Lin, T. M. & Chance, R. E. (1974) In M. I. Grossman, Candidate hormones of the gut. *Gastroenterology*, **67**, 730–755.

Low-Beer, T. S., Harvey, R. F., Davies, E. R. & Read, A. E. (1975) Abnormalities of serum cholecystokinin and gallbladder emptying in coeliac disease. *New England Journal of Medicine*, **293**, 961–963.

McGuigan, J. E. & Greider, M. H. (1971) Correlative immunochemical and light microscopic studies of the gastrin cell of the antral mucosa. *Gastroenterology*, **60**, 223–236.

McGuigan, J. E. & Trudeau, W. L. (1973a) Serum and tissue gastrin concentrations in patients with carcinoma of the stomach. *Gastroenterology*, **64**, 22–25.

McGuigan, J. E. & Trudeau, W. L. (1973b) Differences in rates of gastrin release in normal persons and patients with duodenal ulcer disease. *New England Journal of Medicine*, **288**, 64–66.

Mallinson, C. N., Bloom, S. R., Warin, A. P., Salmon, P. R. & Cox, B. (1974) A glucagonoma syndrome. *Lancet*, ii, 1–4.

Marik, F. & Code, C. F. (1975) Control of the interdigestive myoelectric activity in dogs by the vagus nerves and pentagastrin. *Gastroenterology*, **69**, 387–395.

Mitznegg, P. Stunz, U., Domschke, W., Wunach, E. & Demling, L. (1975) Analysis of the motor effect of synthetic motilin on animal and human intestinal smooth muscle in vitro. *Archives of Pharmacology Supplement*, **287**, R45.

Mitznegg, P., Bloom, S. R., Domschke, W., Domschke, S., Wunsch, E. & Demling, L. (1976) Release of motilin after duodenal acidification in man. *Lancet*, **i**, 888–889.

Mortimer, C. H., Carr, D., Lind, T., Bloom, S. R., Mallinson, C. N., Schally, A. V., Tunbridge, W. M. G., Yeomans, L., Coy, D. H., Kastin, A. & Besser, G. M. (1974) Growth hormone release inhibiting hormone: effects on circulating glucagon, insulin and growth hormone in normal, diabetic acromegalic and hypopituitary patients. *Lancet*, **i**, 697–701.

Mutt, V. & Jorpes, J. E. (1968) Structure of porcine cholecystokinin-pancreozymin I cleavage with thrombin and with trypsin. *European Journal of Biochemistry*, **6**, 156–159.

Nilsson, G., Yalow, R. S. & Berson, S. A. (1973) *Frontiers in Gastrointestinal Hormone Research*, pp. 95–101. Stockholm: Almquist and Wiksell.

Pearse, A. G. E. (1969) The cytochemistry and ultrastructure of polypeptide hormone-producing cells of the apud series and the embryologic, physiologic and pathologic implications of the concept. *Journal of Histochemistry and Cytochemistry*, **17**, 303–313.

Pearse, A. G. E., Polak, J. M., Bloom, S. R., Adams, C., Dryburgh, J. R. & Brown, J. C. (1974) Enterochromaffin cells of the mammalian small intestine as the source of motilin. *Virchows Archives B Cell Pathology*, **16**, 111–120.

Petersen, H. & Grossman, M. I. (1976) Potentiation between secretin and cholecystokinin (CCK) for pancreatic responses in anesthetised rats. *Gastroenterology*, **70**, 926 (abstract).

Polak, J. M., Bloom, S. R., Coulling, I. & Pearse, A. G. E. (1971a) Immunofluorescent localisation of secretin in the canine duodenum. *Gut*, **12**, 605–610.

Polak, J. M., Bloom, S. R., Coulling, I & Pearse, A. G. E. (1971b) Immunofluorescent localisation of enteroglucagon cells in the gastrointestinal tract of the dog. *Gut*, **12**, 311–318.

Polak, J. M., Bloom, S. R., Kuzio, M., Brown, J. C. & Pearse, A. G. E. (1973) Cellular localisation of gastric inhibitory polypeptide in the duodenum and jejunum. *Gut*, **14**, 284–288.

Polak, J. M., Pearse, A. G. E., Bloom, S. R., Buchan, A. M. J., Rayford, P. L. & Thompson, J. C. (1975a) Identification of cholecystokinin-secreting cells. *Lancet*, **ii**, 1016–1018.

Polak, J. M., Pearse, A. G. E., Grimelius, L., Bloom, S. R. & Arimura, A. (1975b) Growth-hormone release-inhibiting hormone in gastrointestinal and pancreatic D cells. *Lancet*, **i**, 1220–1225.

Polak, J. M., Bloom, S. R., Adruan, T. E., Heights, P., Bryant, M. G. & Pearse, A. G. E. (1976a) Pancreatic polypeptide in insulinomas, gastrinomas, VIPomas and glucagonomas, *Lancet*, **i**, 328–330.

Polak, J. M., Bloom, S. R., Hobbs, S., Solcia, R. & Pearse, A. G. E. (1976b) Distribution of a bombesin-like peptide in the gastrointestinal tract of man. *Lancet*, **i**, 1109–1110.

Ralphs, D. N. L., Bloom, S. R., Lawson-Smith, C. & Thompson, J. P. S. (1975) The relationship between gastric emptying rate and plasma enteroglucagon concentration. *Gut*, **16**, 406.

Robberecht, P., Cremer, M., Vandermeers, A., Vandermeers-Piret, M., Cotton, P., De Neef, P. & Christophe, J. (1975) Pancreatic secretion of total protein and of three hydrolases collected in healthy subjects via duodenoscopic cannulation *Gastroenterology*, **69**, 374–379.

Ross, S. A., Brown, J. C., Dryburgh, J. & Dupre, J. (1973) Hypersecretion of gastric inhibitory polypeptide in diabetes mellitus. *Clinical Research*, **21**, 1029.

Ruppin, H., Domschke, S., Domschke, W., Wunsch, E., Jaeger, E. & Demling, L. (1975) Effects of 13-NLE-motilin in man — inhibition of gastric evacuation and stimulation of pepsin secretion. *Scandinavian Journal of Gastroenterology*, **10**, 199–202.

Said, S. I. & Mutt, V. (1972) Isolation from porcine-intestinal wall of a vasoactive octacosapeptide related to secretin and to glucagon. *European Journal of Biochemistry*, **28**, 199–204.

Sasaki, H., Rubalcava, B., Baetens, D., Blazquez, E., Srikant, C. B., Orci, L. & Unger, R. H. (1975) Identification of glucagon in the gastrointestinal tract. *Journal of Clinical Investigation*, **56**, 135–145.

Schally, A. V., Dupont, A., Arimura, A., Redding, T. W. & Linthicum, G. L. (1975) Isolation of porcine GH-release inhibiting hormone (GH-RIH): The existence of three forms of GH-RIH. *Federation Proceedings*, **34**, 584.

Schrumpf, E., Petersen, H. & Berstad, A. (1973) The effect of secretin on plasma gastrin in the Zollinger-Ellison syndrome. *Scandinavian Journal of Gastroenterology*, **8**, 145–150.

Schubert, E., Mitznegg, P., Strunz, U., Domschke, W., Domschke, S., Wunsch, E., Jaeger, E., Demling, L. & Heim, F. (1975) Influence of the hormone analogue 13-NLE-motilin and of 1-methyl-3-iso-butylxanthine on tone and cyclic 3',5'-AMP content of antral and duodenal muscle in the rabbit. *Life Sciences*, **16**, 263.

Schwartz, C. J., Kimberg, D. V., Sheerin, H. E., Field, M. & Said, S. I. (1974) Vasoactive intestinal peptide stimulation of adenylate cyclase and active electrolyte secretion in intestinal mucosa. *Journal of Clinical Investigation*, **54**, 536–544.

Siler, T. M., Yen, S. S. C., Vale, W. & Guillemin, R. (1974) Inhibition by somatostatin on the release of TSH induced in man by thyrotropin-releasing factor. *Clinical Endocrinology*, **38**, 742–745.

Solcia, E., Pearse, A. G. E., Grube, D., Kobayashi, S., Bussola, G., Cruetzfeldt, W. & Gepts, W. (1973) Revised Wiesbaden classification of gut cells. *Rendic. Gastroenterol.*, **5**, 13–16.

Straus, E., Urbach, H. & Yalow, R. S. (1975) Alcohol-stimulated secretion of immunoreactive secretin. *New England Journal of Medicine*, **293**, 1031–1032.

Strunz, U., Domschke, W., Domschke, S., Mitznegg, P., Wunsch, E., Jaeger, E. & Demling, L. (1976) Gastroduodenal motor response to natural motilin and synthetic position 13 substituted motilin analogues. A comparative in vitro study. *Scandinavian Journal of Gastroenterology*, **11**, 199–204.

Swift, P. G. F., Bloom, S. R. & Harris, F. (1975) Watery diarrhoea and ganglioneuroma with secretion of vasoactive intestinal peptide. *Archives of Disease in Childhood*, **50**, 896–898.

Thompson, J. C., Fender, H. R., Ramus, N. I., Villar, H. V. & Rayford, P. L. (1975) Cholecystokinin metabolism in man and dogs. *Annals of Surgery*, **182**, 496–504.

Turner, D. S., Etheridge, L., Jones, J., Marks, V., Meldrum, B., Bloom, S. R. & Brown, J. C. (1974) The effect of the intestinal polypeptides, IRP and GIP on insulin release and glucose tolerance in the baboon. *Clinical Endocrinology*, **3**, 489–493.

Tze, W. J. (1975) Gastric inhibitory polypeptide (GIP): a potent stimulator of insulin release. *Gastroenterology*, **68**, 621–622.

Unger, R. H., Eisentraut, A., Sims, K., McCall, M. S. & Madison, L. L. (1961) Sites of origin of glucagon in dogs and humans. *Clinical Research*, **9**, 53.

Unger, R. H. & Eisentraut, A. M. (1967) *Hormones in Blood*, 1st edition, ed. Gray, C. H. & Bacharach, A. L. pp. 83–97. New York: Academic Press.

Valverde, I., Rigopoulou, D., Exton, J., Ohneda, A., Eisentraut, A. & Unger, R. H. (1968) Demonstration and characterisation of a second fraction of glucagon-like immunoreactivity in jejunal extracts. *American Journal of Medical Science*, **255**, 415–420.

Vanderhaeghen, J. J., Signeau, J. C. & Geots, W. (1975) A new peptide in the vertebrate central nervous system reacting with antigastrin antibodies. *Nature*, **257**, 604–606.

Verner, J. V. & Morrison, A. B. (1974) Endocrine pancreatic islet disease with diarrhoea. *Archives of Internal Medicine*, **133**, 492–500.

Walsh, J. H. & Grossman, M. I. (1975) Gastrin. *New England Journal of Medicine*, **292**, 1324–1332.

Walsh, J. H., Debas, H. T. & Grossman, M. I. (1974) Pure human big gastrin: immunochemical properties, disappearances half time, and acid stimulating action in dogs. *Journal of Clinical Investigation*, **54**, 477–485.

Walsh, J. H., Richardson, C. T. & Fordtran, J. S. (1975) pH dependence of acid secretion and gastrin release in normal and ulcer subjects. *Journal of Clinical Investigation*, **55**, 462–468.

Ward, A. S. & Bloom, S. R. (1974) The role of secretin in the inhibition of gastric secretion by intraduodenal acid. *Gut*, **15**, 889–897.

Ward, A. S. & Bloom, S. R. (1975) Effect of vagotomy on secretin release in man. *Gut*, **16**, 951–956.

Wingate, D. (1976) The eupeptide system: a general theory of gastrointestinal hormones. *Lancet*, **i**, 529–532.

Wunsch, E., Brown, J. C., Deimer, K. H., Drees, F., Jaeger, E., Musiol, J., Scharf, R., Stocker, H., Thamm, P. & Wendleberger, G. (1973) The total synthesis of norleucine-L3-motilin (preliminary communication). *Zeitschrift für Naturforschung*, **28c**, 235–240.

Yalow, R. S. & Berson, S. A. (1970) Size and charge distinctions between endogenous human plasma gastrin in peripheral blood and heptadecapeptide gastrins. *Gastroenterology*, **58**, 609–615.

Zollinger, R. M. (1975) Diarrhoeogenic tumours of the pancreas. *Australian and New Zealand Journal of Surgery*, **45**, 129–135.

Zollinger, R. M. & Ellison, E. H. (1955) Primary peptic ulceration of the jejunum associated with islet cell tumours of the pancreas. *Annals of Surgery*, **142**, 709–728.

16
THE PROSTAGLANDINS

E. W. Horton

Although work in the prostaglandin field started in the 1930s (see Horton, 1972, for historical background), progress was slow until supplies of pure prostaglandins became available in sufficient quantities for biological investigation. The isolation and chemical characterisation of several prostaglandins in the early 1960s by Bergström et al (1963) was the most significant step. This discovery was coupled with the finding that prostaglandins are distributed widely in animal tissues and not confined, as their name might imply, to tissues of the male reproductive tract.

The discovery of the biosynthetic conversion of arachidonic acid to prostaglandins by sheep seminal vesicle homogenates led to the first large-scale production of prostaglandins for research purposes. This method was gradually superseded by *de novo* chemical synthesis resulting particularly from the brilliant work of E. J. Corey (see Ramwell and Shaw, 1971). Massive quantities of prostaglandins are formed in a marine organism, *Plexaura homomalla*, which, for a while, was harvested for production purposes and used as a valuable alternative to other methods.

The increased availability of prostaglandins enabled biologists throughout the world to investigate their pharmacological properties and possible physiological role. The story is still far from complete and the bewildering diversity of biological actions and interactions has not yet been explained in terms of a single mechanism of action at the cellular level.

Nomenclature

Eight major series of prostaglandins have so far been described (Fig. 16.1). These parent prostaglandins differ in the nature of the substituents on the five-membered ring (except for prostaglandins G and H) and have been designated prostaglandins A to H, inclusive. All are hydroxylated in the 15 position and possess a 13, 14 *trans* double bond. Within each series there are members differing in their degree of unsaturation, possessing either one, two or three double bonds in the side chains. These are indicated by a subscript numeral after the letter (for example, prostaglandins A_1, A_2 and A_3). Those interested in more detailed and precise chemical nomenclature of these compounds should read the excellent article by Nelson (1974).

In this review the abbreviation PG will be used for the word 'prostaglandin' where a specific compound is indicated (e.g. PGE_1, PGE_2, $PGF_{2\alpha}$).

NORMAL BIOCHEMISTRY

Biosynthesis

The enzymatic conversion of arachidonic acid to prostaglandins was demonstrated independently in 1964 by van Dorp (van Dorp et al, 1964) and by Bergström (Bergström, Danielsson and Samuelsson, 1964). The term 'prostaglandin synthetase' has been used to describe the complex of enzymes which catalyzes this conversion. Its occurrence has been demonstrated in most mammalian tissues and also in those of birds, amphibians, fish, and invertebrates (Christ and van Dorp, 1972).

The steps in the biosynthesis are illustrated in Figure 16.2. It seems that substrate for the synthesis is provided by hydrolysis of membrane phospholipids

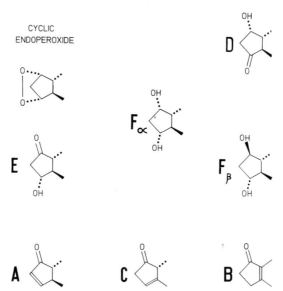

Figure 16.1   Prostaglandin families — differences in the five-membered ring compared. For the full chemical formulae see subsequent figures. Cyclic endoperoxides, PGG$_2$ and PGH$_2$, differ in the 15 position (see Fig. 16.2)

by phospholipase A$_2$, or possibly by the hydrolysis of cholesterol esters which are rich in arachidonic acid, for example in the adrenal glands.

All the major prostaglandins are believed to be formed from arachidonic acid via a highly unstable intermediate, PGG$_2$. Because of its instability, studies on the pharmacology of PGG$_2$ are difficult, but all the evidence suggests that it possesses high biological activity and could itself be concerned in physiological mechanisms before it is converted to the more stable prostaglandins.

PGG$_2$ is important in another respect, it is also an intermediary in the biosynthesis of thromboxane A$_2$ and of prostacyclin. These substances may be thought of as cousins of the prostaglandins. Members of both families originate from common precursor fatty acids but they differ significantly in chemical structure, the prostaglandins having a ring composed of five carbon atoms, whereas the thromboxanes have six atoms in the ring, five carbon and one oxygen (Fig. 16.3). Moreover, thromboxane A₂ has an additional four-membered ring formed by an oxygen bridge. Prostacyclin is also bicyclic, having a furan and a cyclopentane ring. These highly unstable compounds (half-life in aqueous

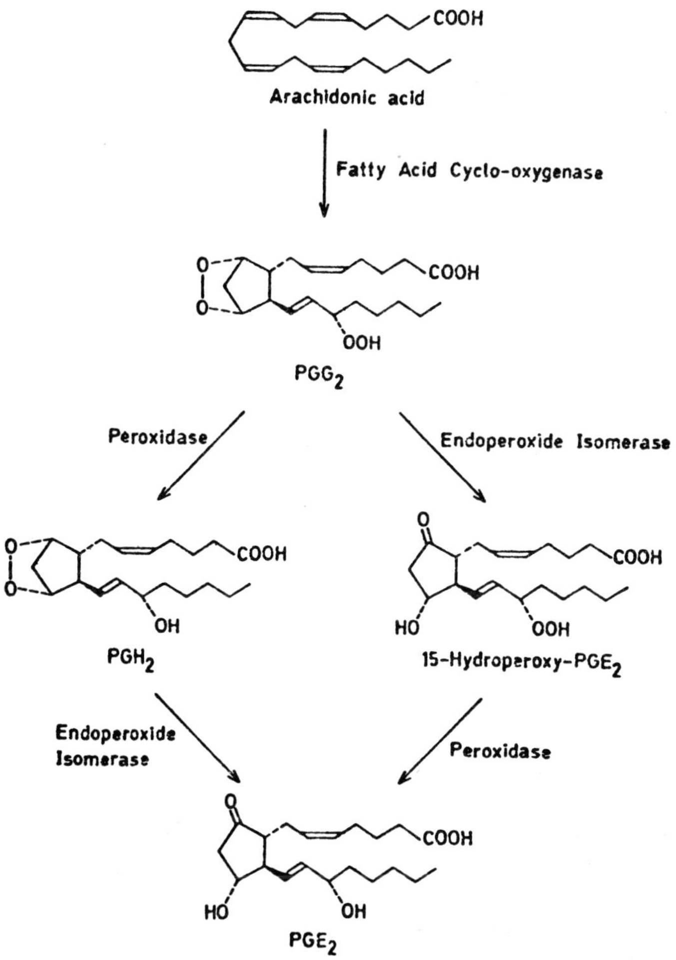

Figure 16.2 Biosynthetic pathway from arachidonic acid to prostaglandin E₂

solution at room temperature around 30 seconds) have great biological potency and almost certainly play a key role in the aggregation of human platelets and in thrombosis.

Many variations on the biosynthetic theme have lately become apparent. Enzymatic interconversion of the major prostaglandins (e.g. PGE₂ to PGF₂α) can occur and many new natural prostaglandins are still being discovered. It is too early to assess the possible biological significance of these observations.

Inhibition of prostaglandin biosynthesis and release

Considerable interest has been aroused by the report of Lewis and Piper (1975) that the anti-inflammatory steroids can inhibit the release of prostaglandins. These workers believe that whereas the non-steroidal anti-inflammatory drugs like aspirin and indomethacin owe their therapeutic effects to the blockade of prostaglandin biosynthesis, the steroids block the release but not the synthesis of prostaglandins. If this mechanism can be confirmed and be shown to be of general application, it may well account for the hitherto puzzling mode of action of the powerful anti-inflammatory glucocorticoids. It is more probable that steroids interfere with release of prostaglandin precursors rather than prostaglandins themselves.

The original discovery by Vane (1971) that aspirin blocks prostaglandin biosynthesis has rapidly led to the further conclusion that this mode of action

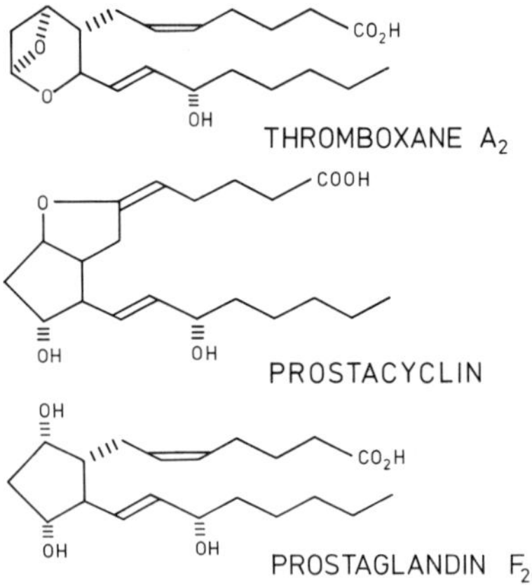

Figure 16.3   The structures of thromboxane A_2, prostacyclin, and prostaglandin $F_{2\alpha}$

accounts for the therapeutic effects of this and related drugs. A symposium was devoted to this important subject in 1973 (Robinson and Vane, 1974) and a voluminous literature has been stimulated by this fundamental discovery. The field was comprehensively reviewed in 1974 (Flower, 1974).

One important concept resulting from this work has been the finding that the prostaglandin synthetase from different sources may have different sensitivities to the actions of various aspirin-like drugs. Thus, paracetamol, which is an antipyretic analgesic with little anti-inflammatory activity has a greater effect on brain synthetase than on the synthetase from spleen. The activity of indomethacin which is both antipyretic and anti-inflammatory is about equally active on enzymes from both sources. This differential sensitivity, which may reflect a distribution of isoenzymes with different pharmacological profiles, has led various groups to consider the possibility of developing drugs with greater selectivity of action. Gryglewski (1974) finds that, in general, potent anti-inflammatory drugs are stronger inhibitors of the bovine seminal vesicular enzyme system than of the rabbit brain enzyme. The possibility that these drugs may have other sites of action should not be forgotten, for example, indomethacin also block prostaglandin metabolism (Bëkhave and Hansin, 1976).

The action of colchicine cannot be accounted for satisfactorily in terms of synthetase inhibition. Indeed, cultured synovial cells *increase* their synthesis of prostaglandins in the presence of colchicine. This effect has now been confirmed in vivo in experiments on the intertarsal joints of the chicken. In spite of the increase in prostaglandin formation, colchicine was found to inhibit the increase in vascular permeability and the migration of leucocytes provoked by injection of urate crystals into the joint (Glatt, Graf and Brune, 1976).

Finally, the possibility that natural fatty acids may act physiologically to inhibit prostaglandin synthetase must be considered. Wolfe and his colleagues reported years ago (see Horton, 1972) that linoleic and linolenic acids had such inhibitory effects. Lands et al (1972) have reported that a 22-carbon unsaturated acid with six double bonds, particularly abundant in brain phospholipids, has potent inhibitory activity, while Hsia et al (1974) have isolated an eicosatetranoic acid from the skin of essential fatty acid deficient rats and shown that it can inhibit prostaglandin synthetase as can linoleic acid, but not palmitic acid.

It is well established that many tumours can synthesise and possibly secrete prostaglandins. A more recent observation of interest is the finding that whereas many tumours can convert linoleic acid to dihomo-γ-linolenic acid and arachidonic acid, themselves the immediate precursors of the prostaglandins, some tumours lack the Δ^6 desaturase enzyme system, thus preventing the conversion of linoleic acid to prostaglandins (Bailey and Dunbar, 1976). Moreover, dietary studies in the cat (Rivers, Sinclair and Crawford, 1975) indicate that this species is unable to desaturate fatty acids, such as linoleic acid, and appears to be dependent upon its dietary intake for a supply of arachidonic acid or other prostaglandin precursors.

Before prostaglandin synthesis can begin, free precursor fatty acids must be made available, possibly from membrane phospholipids. Activation of phospholipase A_2 is, therefore, likely to be the first step in such new synthesis as originally suggested by Kunze and Vogt (1971). Various inhibitors of the phospholipase have now been described, including local anaesthetics such as tetracaine. It can be anticipated that inhibition of this pathway in vivo will throw further light upon the role of prostaglandins and the factors controlling their release. Activation of inactive phospholipase A_2 is likely to be an important mechanism; there is some evidence that the phospholipase A_2 in the thyroid is activated by the thyroid-stimulating hormone, thus promoting the increased synthesis of prostaglandins (Haye, Champion and Jacquemin, 1976).

Metabolism

Isotopic studies have shown that the biological half-life of an injected prostaglandin is very short. For example, a sample of venous blood from a human volunteer collected one minute after the intravenous injection of labelled PGE_2 contained a concentration which indicated that only 4 per cent of the original PGE_2 remained in the circulation. Approximately 40 per cent of the label was present in the form of the principal lung metabolite 13,14-dihydro-15-oxo-PGE_2 (Samuelsson et al, 1971). It is now well established that prostaglandins of the E and F series are very efficiently removed from the circulation on passage through the lungs (Ferreira and Vane, 1967), though others such as prostaglandins of the A series are not taken up in this way (Horton and Jones, 1969).

Autoradiographic studies in mice showed that 15 minutes after the injection of labelled $PGF_{2\alpha}$ or labelled PGE_1 most of the radioactivity was present in the liver, kidney and subcutaneous connective tissue. Prostaglandin metabolites are excreted in the bile and urine; but the biliary metabolites may be reabsorbed from the gut and excreted via the kidney.

The main human urinary metabolite of PGE_2 (Fig. 16.4) is the product of various enzymatic reactions, the most important step being oxidation of the 15 hydroxyl substituent by 15-hydroxy prostaglandin dehydrogenase (PGDH). This enzyme is widely distributed — highest activities being found in lung, spleen and

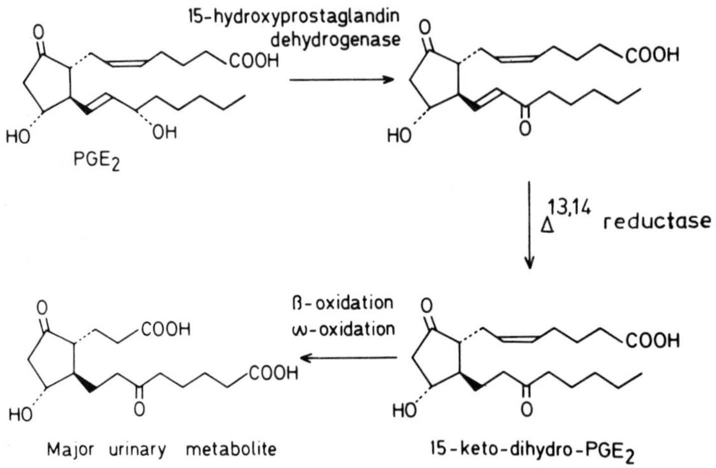

Figure 16.4   Metabolism of prostaglandin E_2 in man

kidney. It is very short-lived, having a half-life of only 45 minutes, and must be replaced by synthesis of new enzyme. The possibility that some diuretics owe their therapeutic efficacy to inhibition of this dehydrogenase, thus slowing down prostaglandin inactivation, has been suggested. Many potent compounds with structures based upon the prostaglandin molecule also inhibit this enzyme. Further therapeutic developments in this area can be anticipated.

METHODS OF DETERMINATION

The advantages and disadvantages of the various ways of measuring prostaglandins have recently been reviewed (Horton, 1976). Basically there are three methods in use, radioimmunoassay, biological assay, and combined gas chromatography-mass spectrometry.

Radioimmunoassay

This method has the immense advantages of high sensitivity, high specificity and the ability to cope with large numbers of samples simultaneously. It has some important limitations. Although antisera with apparently high specificity can be produced, it is never possible to test all substances which could cross-react with the antiserum. Not all prostaglandins and their metabolites are available for such tests; moreover, compounds, as yet unidentified, undoubtedly exist in biological fluids that may cross-react — this possibility should be borne in mind by all users of the technique. A second limitation is the availability of reagents, namely, specific antisera and radioactively-labelled prostaglandin. These are now available for some of the major prostaglandins and their metabolites (for example, the 'lung' metabolite and the main urinary metabolites) but other prostaglandins cannot yet be estimated by this method, for example, PGC, PGD, 19-hydroxy-PGE_2.

An important recent development has been the introduction of a viro-immunoassay for $PGF_{2\alpha}$. The prostaglandin is conjugated chemically to a bacteriophage (T4) which is then added to a colony of *Escherichia coli* in soft agar. The mixture is spread on nutrient agar. The $PGF_{2\alpha}$-modified bacteriophage then infects a bacterium in which it multiplies. Lysis of the bacterial cell after 30 minutes releases hundreds of progeny which re-infect further bacteria. After 12 hours plaques can be seen against a background of dense bacterial growth. If the phage is first incubated with dilute $PGF_{2\alpha}$ antiserum it is neutralised and so cannot form plaques. The assay depends upon preventing this neutralisation with $PGF_{2\alpha}$ itself. A sensitivity of 1 picogram of $PGF_{2\alpha}$ is claimed: moreover the method does not require actively-labelled compounds or a liquid scintillation counter (Andrieu, Mamas and Dray, 1976).

Biological assay

This technique has been used in two ways. The first is used after prior extraction and chromatographic separation of the prostaglandins (Horton and Main, 1967), the second directly measures the prostaglandin content of tissue fluids (blood or saline perfusates) by superfusing a series of tissues in a cascade as developed and exploited so successfully by Vane (1969).

If activity on smooth muscle is detected in a sample of biological fluid, there are very many substances which could be responsible. Most of these substances are either basic or water-soluble, or both. The prostaglandins, as a group, can be separated from them by simple partition of the sample, after mild acidification, with ethyl acetate. Tentative identification of the presence of a prostaglandin is simple. Confirmation, however, requires rigorous chemical analysis.

The cascade technique has the enormous advantage that instant results are obtained and changes in prostaglandin output from an organ can be monitored continuously. On the other hand, it may be impossible to measure absolute levels of prostaglandin concentration and difficulties will arise if more than one prostaglandin is present.

Identification is never conclusive using the cascade technique alone. However, evidence is quickly obtained about the conditions under which the prostaglandin-like substance(s) is released, and the effluent can then be analysed by other techniques giving more definitive answers. The specificity of the method can be enhanced by an appropriate selection of assay tissues and by the use of antagonists to exclude interference from other substances such as adrenaline, 5-hydroxytryptamine, etc.

This method has yielded extremely valuable results. Provided that its limitations are realised, it should continue to find application particularly at the early stages of an investigation.

Combined gas chromatography and mass spectrometry

This is the ultimate tool in the identification of prostaglandins. The technique combines good quantitation with virtually conclusive evidence of identification. A refinement of this technique called multiple ion detection, or tuned ion analysis, makes use of stable isotopes, a deuterated prostaglandin being added to the sample as an internal standard. The mass spectrometer estimates the concentration of the natural prostaglandin in terms of the deuterated form. This method is sensitive and specific. The use of an internal standard introduced early compensates for losses throughout the entire procedure (Samuelsson et al, 1971).

Most workers do not have immediate access to a mass spectrometer. It is, therefore, impractical to suggest the routine use of such methods by everyone. It is, nonetheless, important that those using biological or radioimmune assays should obtain confirmation of identification by submitting some of their samples to rigorous physicochemical analysis.

APPLIED PHYSIOLOGY

Actions of Prostaglandins on the Female Reproductive Tract

ACTIONS ON NON-PREGNANT SMOOTH MUSCLE

One of the earliest indications that the prostaglandins existed came from experiments on the human myometrium. Kurzrok and Lieb (1930) observed that human seminal plasma had profound effects on the contractions of non-pregnant human uterus in vivo. Effects of different prostaglandins on isolated myometrial strips have been observed by many workers, and the great sensitivity of the Fallopian tubes to prostaglandins was reported in a series of investigations by Sandberg (Sandberg, Ingelman-Sundberg and Rydén, 1964).

USE IN PARTURITION

Although prostaglandins of the E series often relax the myometrium in vitro, when given to the pregnant woman these compounds stimulate uterine contractions. This was first discovered by Karim using intravenous infusions of $PGF_{2\alpha}$ in women at term. He suggested that this compound might be useful in initiating parturition. It was soon discovered that PGE_2 is more effective and, in the doses required, lacks some of the adverse effects of $PGF_{2\alpha}$, namely, vomiting and diarrhoea. Since that time there have been numerous clinical investigations throughout the world. The method of administration remained a difficulty until it was shown that PGE_2 is also effective orally. This is now the method of choice in many centres. Extra-amniotic injection of PGE_2 has also been used with success (Calder, Hillier and Embrey, 1976).

USE AS ABORTIFACIENTS

In higher doses, intravenous infusions of prostaglandins can also induce abortion in early or mid-pregnancy. Side-effects are often troublesome, especially with $PGF_{2\alpha}$. Both extra- and intra-amniotic injections have been used successfully to induce abortion and the method of choice appears to be the extra-amniotic injection of PGE_2 during the mid-trimester. In early pregnancy other methods are usually preferred.

Early hopes that the vaginal route of administration might combine simplicity with a minimum of side-effects were not sustained but there has been a recent report that the methyl ester of 15-methyl-$PGF_{2\alpha}$ is well absorbed from the vagina and is a highly effective abortifacient both in first and second trimester pregnancies (Bygdeman et al, 1976).

Csapo (1976) has introduced the technique of Double Prostaglandin Impact, 10 mg $PGF_{2\alpha}$ being injected transcervically, 5 mg at the right and 5 mg at the left side of the extraovular space. In about a third of these patients (100 volunteers) supplementary intravenous infusion was necessary, but the success rate was 99 per cent.

The use of synthetic prostaglandin analogues for the induction of abortion is still at an early stage. It is known, however, that potent compounds such as the 15-methyl analogues which are not metabolised by prostaglandin dehydrogenase can be very effective.

POSSIBLE DEVELOPMENT OF A 'MORNING-AFTER' PILL

The possibility that prostaglandins or their analogues could be used as a post-coital contraceptive ('morning-after Pill') has been discussed for some years. One approach would be to administer the compounds whenever a menstrual period was missed thus inducing menstruation, or, more probably, a very early abortion. The success rate with PGE_2 given by intravenous infusion can be high, but such a method requires hospitalisation and is hardly a practical procedure for widespread use. The intra-uterine route using doses up to 0.5 mg PGE_2 is not universally successful — about 88 per cent success in a series reported by Mackenzie, Hillier and Embrey (1976). Further work with synthetic analogues of prostaglandins may eventually establish a technique which can be used conveniently on a large scale.

ROLE OF PROSTAGLANDINS IN PARTURITION, ABORTION AND DYSMENORRHOEA

The possible involvement of prostaglandins in the physiological events leading up to parturition and in the pathology of abortion has been the subject of much speculation. Certainly the umbilical cord and, to a lesser extent, the amniotic fluid are rich sources of prostaglandins, as shown by Karim (1972). Reports that peripheral venous blood levels of $PGF_{2\alpha}$ are increased immediately before and during uterine contractions of parturition have been the subject of much controversy. If the human lungs can take up and metabolise prostaglandins as effectively as the lungs of some laboratory species, the concentrations reported by Karim must represent an enormous production of $PGF_{2\alpha}$ by the human uterus. There is as yet no agreement about the circulating levels of $PGF_{2\alpha}$

in women at parturition but from experiments in sheep and goats there seems every likelihood that this prostaglandin does have some key function in the processes of childbirth.

This is supported by numerous reports that parturition can be delayed in animals by the administration of drugs such as indomethacin which block the synthesis of the prostaglandins. Moreover, this drug has been used successfully to prevent premature abortion (Wiqvist, Lundström and Gréen, 1976) which evidence together with the known abortifacient properties of the prostaglandins suggest that they may be implicated as causal factors in spontaneous abortion. There is a similar report from this group that dysmenorrhoea is alleviated by indomethacin. In patients with this disorder abnormally high levels of 15-oxo-13,14-dihydro-PGF$_{2\alpha}$ were found and these were reduced by the treatment. Again an involvement of prostaglandins is implied but not yet finally proved.

ACTIONS ON THE CORPUS LUTEUM

The luteolytic effect of PGF$_{2\alpha}$, first reported by Pharriss and Wyngarden (1969) in rats, has been the subject of considerable investigation. In several species, though apparently not in man, there is strong evidence for the existence of a hormone which is released from the uterus towards the end of the oestrous cycle and which, acting locally, causes the corpora lutea in the ovaries to regress. The hormone has been named 'luteolysin'. There is now overwhelming evidence that luteolysin is in fact prostaglandin F$_{2\alpha}$ and the subject has been reviewed recently elsewhere (Horton and Poyser, 1976).

In the veterinary field, practical applications have resulted from the discovery of this luteolytic action. Thus, in horses and cattle which show cyclic behaviour during their breeding season, the life of an established corpus luteum can be terminated by a single injection of PGF$_{2\alpha}$ or of a synthetic analogue. By interrupting the normal cycle in this way, the onset of the next oestrus and ovulation can be timed precisely. The pig is dependent upon functional corpora lutea throughout pregnancy, parturition being preceded by luteal regression. Again an application can be envisaged — the prostaglandin being adminstered to allow farrowing to occur at some predetermined time rather than haphazardly. All these veterinary and agricultural practices are likely to prove labour-saving in a field in which the cost of skilled labour is increasing.

IMPLANTATION AND THE INTRA-UTERINE DEVICE

There is much evidence to support the contention that prostaglandins are also implicated in the processes of ovulation and of implantation. Moreover, the possibility that prostaglandin release may contribute to the mode of action of the intra-uterine device has been proposed — more conclusive evidence is, however, required.

Actions at Adrenergic Nerve Terminals

The variety of different stimuli which can effect prostaglandin release is great. One specific function resulting from such release may be the modulation of transmitter output from adrenergic nerve terminals. Considerable evidence has accumulated in support of such a mechanism. On the other hand, there are discrepancies which may undermine the general acceptance of this hypothesis (see Horton, 1973, 1976 for references).

Early work established that prostaglandin-like substances are released from organs such as adipose tissue and spleen in response to electrical stimulation of their adrenergic nerve supply (Shaw and Ramwell, 1968; Davies, Horton and Withrington, 1968). Moreover, an intra-arterial infusion of adrenaline or noradrenaline causes a similar release (Gilmore, Vane and Wyllie, 1968). The question of the possible biological significance of this prostaglandin release was considered by Davies and Withrington (1968). Clearly a prostaglandin was not the chemical transmitter at adrenergic nerve endings — the evidence for noradrenaline was already overwhelming — moreover, none of this prostaglandins when injected mimicked the effects of adrenergic nerve stimulation. It appeared that prostaglandins E_1 and E_2 had remarkably little pharmacological activity on the dog spleen and failed to modify either the effects of nerve stimulation or the responses to noradrenaline.

Since that time, however, experiments on other organs conducted by Swedish workers, notable amongst whom is Hedqvist, suggest that PGE_2 could have a role at adrenergic terminals since transmitter release in response to nerve stimulation is reduced by PGE_2 infused intra-arterially. Moreover, responses to nerve stimulation are reduced by doses of PGE_2 which do not affect responses of similar magnitude elicited by noradrenaline.

If prostaglandin biosynthesis is blocked using indomethacin or an analogue of arachidonic acid, eicosatetraynoic acid, responses to adrenergic nerve stimulation are enhanced — an observation which is compatible with the view that the inhibitory effect of PGE_2 has been removed. This is further evidence in support of the hypothesis. However, the hypothesis in its present form does not account for the $PGF_{2\alpha}$ which is also released on adrenergic nerve stimulation nor for the negative findings of Davies and Withrington using the dog spleen. One of the weakest links in the story is failure to obtain convincing evidence of the identification of or an accurate estimate of the prostaglandins released from the various organs in which this mechanism is believed to operate.

A drug which would inhibit the release of noradrenaline in response to activation of the sympathetic nervous system could find therapeutic application, for example in the control of hypertension, though it would undoubtedly suffer from the limitations of the conventional adrenergic neurone blocking drugs. It is possible that such a drug could be evolved from the work described above.

Actions on the Central Nervous System

Prostaglandins are widely distributed throughtout the central nervous system. Moreover, prostaglandin-like substances are released from the brain and spinal cord in response to drugs, chemicals or electrical stimulation of neuronal pathways (see Horton, 1969 for references). The variety of effects observed in animals following either intraventricular or systemic administration suggest that prostaglandins act upon many sites within the central nervous system. The important observation that prostaglandins applied micro-iontophoretically can affect the firing of single neurones (Avanzino, Bradley and Wolstencroft, 1966) does not rule out the possibility that some or all the effects observed can be attributed to changes in blood flow to the brain. It is now well documented that some prostaglandins have potent activity on the cerebral vasculature (Yamamoto et al, 1972). Whatever the exact location of the action of prostaglandins, it is clear that their effects differ from one species to another and the differences between different prostaglandins are striking. It is not possible to make any rational generalisation to account for the various actions on the brain, it is possible, however, to catalogue some of the effects which have been observed, namely sedation, stupor, catalepsy and fever (see below) following the injection of PGE_1 or PGE_2 into the lateral ventricle of the brain of the cat. $PGF_{2\alpha}$, in larger doses, by the same route produces none of these effects. Spinal reflexes tend to be potentiated by prostaglandins but inhibition of reflexes is also observed depending upon the species and the type of biological preparation used (see Horton, 1969, for fuller details).

It is well known that the brain is rich in adenylate cyclase. PGE_2 but not $PGF_{2\alpha}$, increases the synthesis of cyclic AMP in slices of rat cortex and potentiates the action of noradrenaline on this system (Berti et al, 1976). Moreover, brain prostaglandin synthetase itself is activated by noradrenaline (and dopamine) in slices of cat cerebral cortex but the increased prostaglandin is mainly $PGF_{2\alpha}$ (Wolfe, Pappius and Marion, 1976). Furthermore, PGE_2 (1 mg/kg) which antagonises leptazol convulsions in mice (Holmes and Horton, 1968a) completely prevents the rise of cerebellar cyclic GMP which occurs in these leptazol-treated animals (Berti et al, 1976). These workers postulate that there may be some relationship between PGE_2 and GABA in controlling cerebellar cyclic GMP levels.

Hoffer, Siggins and Bloom (1969) had previously shown by microiontophoretic studies on single Purkinje cells in the cerebellum that the inhibition of spontaneous firing which can be elicited with noradrenaline is mimicked by cyclic AMP. On the other hand, PGE_2 application restored the firing when given during a noradrenaline administration but failed to antagonise the inhibition produced by cyclic AMP. These workers conclude that the effects of PGE_2 on noradrenaline inhibition could be mediated via the inhibition of adenylate cyclase.

It is quite possible that PGE_2 has different effects on adenylate cyclase in different cells within the brain. It is already known that prostaglandins of the E series can inhibit this enzyme in some tissues (for example, fat) but activate it in others (for example, thyroid).

The role of prostaglandins in the central nervous system and their possible implication in abnormalities of brain function are largely unexplored. There is sufficient evidence to make such an investigation very attractive. By further fundamental studies of this kind it is likely that novel advances in the treatment of mental disease will take place.

FEVER, INFLAMMATION AND PAIN

The discovery by Vane and others (Vane, 1971; Ferreira, Moncada and Vane, 1971; Smith and Willis, 1971) that aspirin and related drugs inhibit the biosynthesis of prostaglandins provides a very plausible explanation for the antipyretic, anti-inflammatory and analgesic effects of this group of drugs (Vane, 1973). It is implicit in such an explanation that prostaglandins have some essential role in the aetiology of fever, inflammation and pain. Much evidence has now accumulated in favour of this hypothesis.

Fever

As first reported by Milton and Wendlandt (1970) PGE_1 and PGE_2 cause a rise in body temperature when injected in submicrogram quantities into the third ventricle of the brain. A PGE-like substance has been identified in cat brain (Horton and Main, 1967) and also in the hypothalamic region of dog brain (Holmes and Horton, 1968b). By measuring the release of prostaglandin from the brain into the ventricular system, it has been established that during fever induced by bacterial pyrogens, levels of a PGE-like substance increase considerably. As the temperature is lowered by one of the antipyretic drugs which also block prostaglandin synthesis, the levels of this PGE also fall (Feldberg, 1975). It has also been suggested that the stupor which may accompany high fever is also attributable to the release of prostaglandins. Whether the cataleptic-like condition which sometimes accompanies such stupor is related to clinical catalepsy is a question needing urgent exploration.

Inflammation

Attempts to find 'the mediator' of inflammation have in the past either been unsuccessful or at most led to equivocal results. It is therefore with caution that one should attempt to attribute to any of the prostaglandins, this complex role. Like so many other naturally-occurring substances, prostaglandins of the E series can mimic the cardinal signs of inflammation by their action on arterioles, capillaries and nerve endings. Moreover, both in experimental inflammation and in a wide variety of clinical conditions which can broadly be classified as inflammatory, the release of prostaglandins or prostaglandin-like material has been demonstrated. These conditions range from eczema and burns to rheumatoid arthritis.

In the laboratory, further evidence for a role of prostaglandins in inflammation has been obtained by immunising animals against PGE or by inhibiting phospholipase A. Both these procedures reduce the inflammatory response to carrageenin (Vane, 1976). It is by no means certain, however, that PGE_2 is the only prostaglandin implicated. The possible involvement of PGE_1, PGD_2, the endoperoxide intermediaries, or even the thromboxanes, cannot at this stage be excluded. There is some evidence that the prostaglandins may originate from leucocytes and that they have a modulator role in the leucocytic lysosome (Weissman, Goldstein and Hoffstein, 1976).

Pain

Prostaglandins are not very effective themselves as pain-producing substances. However, it has now been established that the effects of other pain-producing substances (for example, bradykinin) are greatly enhanced and prolonged by a dose of PGE_2 which itself has no detectable algesic action. It was shown by Lim

(1965) that the analgesic action of aspirin is peripheral, not central. It appears that some kinds of pain are associated with the generation of prostaglandins near to sensory nerve endings. When this formation is reduced by means of a non-narcotic analgesic drug, such as aspirin or paracetamol, the potentiating influence of PGE_2 is removed and the pain is thus alleviated.

Actions on Platelets

Interest in the relationship between prostaglandins and blood platelets was initiated by the observation that PGE_1 (but not PGE_2) is a powerful inhibitor of platelet aggregation. The only other natural prostaglandins to show similar activity are PGD_1 and PGD_2. The mechanism is unknown. A recent finding which may have important therapeutic implications is that prostacyclin formed from PGG_2 by an enzyme in blood vessel endothelium is the most potent inhibitor of aggregation yet discovered.

In contrast, much more is known about the role of other prostaglandins, notably the cyclic endoperoxide intermediates, in the normal process of aggregation which can be induced by thrombin or by ADP. It is well established that aspirin inhibits platelet aggregation and it had been shown that PGE_2 had some activity in potentiating the aggregating actions of ADP. When the cyclic endoperoxides were discovered they were found to be more potent as potentiators of ADP induced aggregation. Moreover, thromboxane A_2, which like the prostaglandins is a product of the cyclic endoperoxides, is an even more potent aggregator (Hamberg, Svensson and Samuelsson, 1974). The formation and release of both endoperoxides and thromboxane A_2 during platelet aggregation has now been demonstrated.

CONCLUDING SUMMARY

Prior to 1960 few biologists and even fewer clinicians were aware of the existence of the prostaglandins. Information then was sparse; now, in contrast, there is an overwhelming literature on the subject, which seems to suggest that prostaglandins are implicated in almost every biological process and that the number of known prostaglandins and their metabolites, already bewilderingly great, is increasing daily. In this final section I shall attempt to highlight those advances which have occurred between 1960 and 1976 which are of special relevance to clinical medicine.

In spite of their name, prostaglandins are not substances peculiar to the male reproductive tract but have been found in almost every kind of tissue in all higher animals so far investigated including man. With a few exceptions, prostaglandins are not stored in cells as such. They are synthesised as they are needed; thus release from an organ can usually be equated with new synthesis. The synthesis of prostaglandins by tissues has at least two important clinical implications. First, the precursors of the prostaglandins are all members of the group of polyunsaturated fatty acids which are essential dietery constituents (although linoleic acid itself is not an immediate precursor of the prostaglandins — it must first be transformed to arachidonic acid). Second, the enzyme which catalyzes the synthesis of prostaglandins is blocked by aspirin and all other non-steroidal anti-inflammatory drugs in common use. This mechanism is believed to account for the mode of action of aspirin in the relief of pain, as an anti-inflammatory drug and as an antipyretic.

Prostaglandins have short biological half-lives — they are rapidly metabolised especially by the lungs. This was an important observation because the lungs are uniquely situated for the removal of drugs from the circulation and because the role of the lungs in metabolising drugs is only now being realised. The final urinary metabolites in man have been identified and these can be measured by radioimmunoassay to determine overall production of prostaglandins by the body. Such estimations do not, of course, give any indication as to where the prostaglandins originated from.

Pharmacological actions of the natural prostaglandins are numerous and new ones continue to be discovered. Some, as in stimulating the pregnant myometrium to contract, have been put to practical clinical application. Others, for example inhibition of gastric secretion, dilatation of the bronchioles, reduction of arterial blood pressure, increase in venous return to the heart, constriction of nasal mucosal vessels, control of the patency of the ductus arteriosus in the new-born, increase in blood flow to vital organs and control of the function of various endocrine glands may have to await the synthesis of unnatural prostaglandins with more selective activity before widespread clinical application will prove feasible. In many instances there is evidence that prostaglandin formation is excessive or unwanted and may contribute to disease processes — fever, pain, inflammation, and cataleptic stupor have been mentioned above. Prostaglandins have also been implicated in platelet aggregation, the spread of bone metastases in breast carcinoma, spontaneous abortion and dysmenorrhoea. In all these instances a selective prostaglandin antagonist would be of great therapeutic interest. At present the best that can be done is to block non-selectively the production of prostaglandins. The price to be paid is simultaneous interference with processes which are beneficial. However, it does seem that in the short term, prostaglandin formation cannot be essential to life since over 95 per cent of the biosynthesis in man can be inhibited without fatality.

Whatever role the prostaglandins, thromboxanes, and prostacyclin may eventually prove to play, it is virtually certain that these natural substances will form the basis for therapeutic advances. The synthesis of prostaglandin-like compounds with more selective activity will provide better drugs (just as the newer corticosteroids have replaced cortisone). The complexities of the field are therefore likely to increase further as such new and exciting drugs become available.

REFERENCES

Andrieu, J. M., Mamas, S. & Dray, F. (1976) Viroimmunoassay of $PGF_{2\alpha}$: a new immunological method of prostaglandin quantitation at the picogram level. In *Recent Advances in Prostaglandin and Thromboxane Research*, vol. 2, p. 863. New York: Raven Press.

Avanzino, G. L., Bradley, P. B. & Wolstencroft, J. H. (1966) Actions of prostaglandins on brain stem neurones. *British Journal of Pharmacology and Chemotherapy*, 27, 157–164.

Bailey, J. M. & Dunbar, L. M. (1976) Synthesis of prostaglandin precursors from labelled essential fatty acids by normal and tumour cells in tissue culture. In *Recent Advances in Prostaglandin and Thromboxane Research*, vol. 2, p. 855. New York: Raven Press.

Bergström, S., Danielsson, H. & Samuelsson, B. (1964) The enzymatic formation of prostaglandin E_2 from arachidonic acid. *Biochimica et biophysica acta*, **90**, 207–210.

Bergström, S., Ryhage, R., Samuelsson, B. & Sjövall, J. (1963) The structure of prostaglandins E_1, $F_{1\alpha}$ and $F_{1\beta}$. *Journal of Biological Chemistry*, **238**, 3555–3564.

Berti, F., Folco, G. C., Fumagalli, R. & Paoletti, R. (1976) Prostaglandins and cyclic nucleotides in the central nervous system. In *Recent Advances in Prostaglandin and Thromboxane Research*, vol. 2, pp. 848–849. New York: Raven Press.

Blackwell, G. J., Flower, R. J., Parsons, M. F. & Vane, J. R. (1975) Factors influencing the turnover of prostaglandin synthetase. *British Journal of Pharmacology*, **53**, 467P.

Bükhave, K. & Hansin, H. S. (1976) The metabolism of ^{3}H-PGE_1 in the pulmonary and peripheral circulation in the rat and the putative inhibition by indomethacin. In *Recent Advances in Prostaglandin and Thromboxane Research*, vol. 2, p. 861. New York: Raven Press.

Bygdeman, M., Borell, U., Leader, A., Lundström, V., Martin, J. N., Eneroth, P. & Gréen, K. (1976) First and second trimester abortion by vaginal administration of 15-(S)-15-methyl $PGF_{2\alpha}$ methyl ester. In *Recent Advances in Prostaglandin and Thromboxane Research*, vol. 2, pp. 693–704. New York: Raven Press.

Calder, A. A., Hillier, K. & Embrey, M. P. (1976) Induction of labour with extra-amniotic PGE_2. In *Recent Advances in Prostaglandin and Thromboxane Research*, vol. 2, p. 994. New York: Raven Press.

Christ, E. J. & Dorp, D. A. van (1972) Comparative aspects of prostaglandin biosynthesis in animal tissues. *Biochimica et biophysica acta*, **270**, 537–545.

Csapo, A. I. (1976) Termination of pregnancy with double prostaglandin impact. In *Recent Advances in Prostaglandin and Thromboxane Research*, vol. 2, pp. 705–718. New York: Raven Press.

Davies, B. N., Horton, E. W. & Withrington, P. G. (1968) The occurrence of prostaglandin E_2 in splenic venous blood of the dog following nerve stimulation. *British Journal of Pharmacology and Chemotherapy*, **32**, 127–135.

Davies, B. N. & Withrington, P. G. (1968) The effects of prostaglandin E_1 and E_2 on the smooth muscle of the dog spleen and on its responses to catecholamines, angiotensin and nerve stimulation. *British Journal of Pharmacology and Chemotherapy*, **32**, 136–144.

Dorp, D. A. van, Beerthius, R. K., Nugteren, D. H. & Vonkeman, H. (1964) The biosynthesis of prostaglandins. *Biochimica et biophysica acta*, **90**, 204–207.

Feldberg, W. S. (1975) Body temperature and fever: changes in our views during the last decade. *Proceedings of the Royal Society, London, B*, **191**, 199–229.

Ferreira, S. H., Moncada, S. & Vane, J. R. (1971) Indomethacin and aspirin abolish prostaglandin release from the spleen. *Nature New Biology*, **231**, 237–239.

Ferreira, S. H. & Vane, J. R. (1967) Prostaglandins: their disappearance from and release into the circulation. *Nature*, **216**, 868–873.

Flower, R. J. (1974) Drugs which inhibit prostaglandin biosynthesis. *Pharmacological Reviews*, **26**, 33–67.

Gilmore, N., Vane, J. R. & Wyllie, J. H. (1968) Prostaglandin released by the spleen. *Nature*, **218**, 1135–1140.

Glatt, M., Graf, P. & Brune, K. (1976) Anti-inflammatory doses of colchicine increase prostaglandin content in inflamed tissue. In *Recent Advances in Prostaglandin and Thromboxane Research*, vol. 2, pp. 111–116. New York: Raven Press.

Gryglewski, R. J. (1974) Structure-activity relationships of some prostaglandin synthetase inhibitors. In *Prostaglandin Synthetase Inhibitors*, ed. Robinson, H. J. and Vane, J. R., pp. 33–52. New York: Raven Press.

Hamberg, M. & Samuelsson, B. (1974) Prostaglandin endoperoxides: novel transformations of arachidonic acid in human platelets. *Proceedings of the National Academy of Sciences of the United States of America*, **71**, 3400–3404.

Hamberg, M., Svensson, J. & Samuelsson, B. (1974) Prostaglandin endoperoxides: a new concept concerning the mode of action and release of prostaglandins. *Proceedings of the National Academy of Sciences of the United States of America*, **71**, 3824–3828.

Haye, B., Champion, S. & Jacquemin, Cl. (1976) Stimulation by TSH of prostaglandin synthesis in pig thyroid slices. In *Recent Advances in Prostaglandin and Thromboxane Research*, vol. 1, pp. 29–34. New York: Raven Press.

Hensby, C. N. (1974) Reduction of prostaglandin E_2 to prostaglandin $F_{2\alpha}$ by an enzyme in sheep blood. *Biochimica et biophysica acta*, **38**, 145–154.

Hoffer, B. J., Siggins, G. R. & Bloom, F. E. (1969) Prostaglandins E_1 and E_2 antagonise norepinephrine effects on cerebellar Purkinje cells: a microelectrophoretic study. *Science, New York*, **166**, 1418–1420.

Holmes, S. & Horton, E. W. (1968a) Prostaglandins and the central nervous system. In *Prostaglandin Symposium of the Worcester Foundation for Experimental Biology*, ed. Ramwell, P. W. and Shaw, J. E., pp. 21–28. New York: Interscience.

Holmes, S. W. & Horton, E. W. (1968b) The identification of four prostaglandins in dog brain and their regional distribution in the central nervous system. *Journal of Physiology, London*, **195**, 731–742.

Horton, E. W. (1969) Hypotheses on physiological roles of prostaglandins. *Physiological Reviews*, **49**, 122–161.

Horton, E. W. (1972) *Prostaglandins: Monographs on Endocrinology*, vol. 7. Heidelberg: Springer-Verlag.

Horton, E. W. (1973) Prostaglandins at adrenergic nerve endings. *British Medical Bulletin*, **29**, 148–151.

Horton, E. W. (1976) The measurement of prostaglandins. In *The Role of Prostaglandins in Inflammation*, ed. Lewis, G. P. Berne: Huber.

Horton, E. W. & Jones, R. L. (1969) Prostaglandins A_1, A_2 and 19-hydroxy A_1; their actions on smooth muscle and their inactivation on passage through the pulmonary and hepatic portal vascular beds. *British Journal of Pharmacology*, **37**, 705–722.

Horton, E. W. & Main, I. H. M. (1967) Identification of prostaglandins in central nervous tissues of the cat and chicken. *British Journal of Pharmacology and Chemotherapy*, **30**, 582–602.

Horton, E. W. & Poyser, N. L. (1976) The uterine luteolytic hormone: a physiological role for prostaglandin $F_{2\alpha}$. *Physiological Reviews*, **56**, 595–652.

Hsia, S. L., Ziboh, V. A. & Synder, D. S. (1974) Naturally-occurring and synthetic inhibitors of prostaglandin synthetase in the skin. In *Prostaglandin Synthetase Inhibitors*, ed. Robinson, H. J. and Vane, J. R., pp. 353–362. New York: Raven Press.

Karim, S. M. M. (1972) Prostaglandins and human reproduction: physiological roles and clinical uses of prostaglandins in relation to human reproduction. In *The Prostaglandins: Progress in Research*, ed. Karim, S.M.M., pp. 71–164. Oxford: MTP.

Kunze, H. & Vogt, W. (1971) Significance of phospholipase A for prostaglandin formation. *Annals of the New York Academy of Science*, **180**, 123–125.

Kurzrok, R. & Lieb, C. (1930) Biochemical studies of human semen. The action of semen on the human uterus. *Proceedings of the Society for Experimental Biology, New York*, **28**, 268–272.

Lands, W. E. M., Le Tellier, P. R., Rome, L. H. & Vanderhoek, J. Y. (1972) Inhibition of prostaglandin biosynthesis. In *Advances in the Biosciences, 9*, ed. Bergström, S. and Bernhard, S., pp. 15–28. Oxford: Pergamon.

Lee, S. C. & Levine, L. (1974) Prostaglandin Metabolism 1: cytoplasmic reduced nicotinamide adenine dinucleotide phosphate dependent and mocrosomal reduced nicotinamide adenide dinucleotide dependent prostaglandin E_1, 9-ketoreductase activities in monkey and pigeon tissues. *Journal of Biological Chemistry*, **249**, 1369–1375.

Lewis, G. P. & Piper, P. J. (1975) Inhibition of release of prostaglandins as an explanation of some of the actions of anti-inflammatory corticosteroids. *Nature*, **254**, 308–311.

Lim, R. K. S. (1965) A revised concept of the mechanism of analgesia and pain. In *Pain: Proceedings of the Henry Ford International Hospital Symposium*, ed. Knighton, R. S. and Dumke, P. R., pp. 117–154. Boston: Little, Brown & Co.

Mackenzie, I. Z., Hillier, K. & Embrey, M. P. (1976) Intra-uterine PGE_2 as an early postconceptional abortifacient. In *Recent Advances in Prostaglandin and Thromboxane Research*, vol. 2, p. 1010. New York: Raven Press.

Milton, A. S. & Wendlandt, S. (1970) A possible role for prostaglandin E_1 as a modulator for temperature regulation in the central nervous system of the cat. *Journal of Physiology, London*, **207**, 76–77P.

Nelson, N. A. (1974) Prostaglandin nomenclature. *Journal of Medicinal Chemistry*, **17**, 911–918.

Pace Asciak, C. R. & Noshat, M. (1976) Mechanism of formation of 6(9)oxy $PGF_{2\alpha}$, deuterium labelled arachidonic acid and endoperoxide studies. In *Recent Advances in Prostaglandin and Thromboxane Research*, vol. 2, pp. 858–859. New York: Raven Press.

Pharriss, B. B. & Wyngarden, C. J. (1969) The effect of $PGF_{2\alpha}$ on the progestogen content of ovaries from pseudopregnant rats. *Proceedings of the Society for Experimental Biology and Medicine*, **130**, 92–94.

Piper, P. J. & Vane, J. R. (1969) Release of additional factors in analphylaxis and its antagonism by anti-inflammatory drugs. *Nature*, **223**, 29–35.

Rivers, J., Sinclair, A. & Crawford, M. A. (1975) Inability of the cat to desaturate essential fatty acids. *Nature*, **258**, 171–173.

Rückrick, M. F., Wendel, A., Schlegel, W., Jackisch, R. & Jung, A. (1976) Molecular and kinetic properties of prostaglandin 15-hydroxy dehydrogenase from human placenta. In *Recent Advances in Prostaglandin and Thromboxane Research*, vol. 1, pp. 153–158. New York: Raven Press.

Samuelsson, B., Granström, E., Gréen, K. & Hamberg, M. (1971) Metabolism of prostaglandins. *Annals of the New York Academy of Science*, **180**, 138–163.

Sandberg, F., Ingelman-Sundberg, A. & Rydén, G. (1964) The effect of prostaglandin E_2 and E_3 on the human uterus and fallopian tubes *in vitro*. *Acta obstetrica gynecologica Scandinavica*, **42**, 269–278.

Schlegel, W. & Greep, R. O. (1976) Kinetic studies on prostaglandin 15-hydroxy dehydrogenase from human placenta. In *Recent Advances in Prostaglandin and Thromboxane Research*, vol. 1, pp. 159–162. New York: Raven Press.

Shaw, J. E. & Ramwell, P. W. (1968) Release of prostaglandin from rat epididymal fat pad on nervous and hormonal stimulation. *Journal of Biological Chemistry*, **243**, 1498–1503.

Smith, J. B. & Willis, A. L. (1971) Aspirin selectively inhibits prostaglandin production in human platelets. *Nature, New Biology*, **231**, 235–237.

Sun, F. F., Armour, S. B. & Bockstanz, V. R. (1976) Studies on the 15-hydroxy prostaglandin dehydrogenase from monkey lung. In *Recent Advances in Prostaglandin and Thromboxane Research*, vol. 1, pp. 163–170. New York: Raven Press.

Tai, H. H. & Hollander, C. S. (1976) Kinetic evidence of a distinct regulatory site on 15-hydroxy prostaglandin dehydrogenase. In *Recent Advances in Prostaglandin and Thromboxane Research*, vol. 1, pp. 171–176. New York: Raven Press.

Thaler-Dao, H., Saintot, M., Baudin, G., Descomps, B. & Crastes de Paulet, A. (1976) The prostaglandin dehydrogenase of human placenta: purification, binding site, regulation. In *Recent Advances in Prostaglandin and Thromboxane Research*, vol. 1, pp. 177–182. New York: Raven Press.

Vane, J. R. (1971) Inhibition of prostaglandin synthesis as a mechanism of action for aspirin-like drugs. *Nature, New Biology*, **231**, 232–235.

Vane, J. R. (1973) Inhibition of prostaglandin biosynthesis as the mechanism of action of aspirin-like drugs. In *Advances in the Biosciences 9*, ed. Bergström, S. and Bernhard, S., pp. 395–411. Oxford: Pergamon.

Vane, J. R. (1969) The release and fate of vasoactive hormones in the circulation. *British Journal of Pharmacology*, **35**, 209–242.

Vane, J. R. (1976) Prostaglandins as mediators of inflammation. In *Recent Advances in Prostaglandin and Thromboxane Research*, vol. 2, pp. 791–802. New York: Raven Press.

Weissman, G., Goldstein, I. & Hoffstein, S. (1976) Prostaglandins and the cyclic nucleotide control of lysosomal enzyme release. In *Recent Advances in Prostaglandin and Thromboxane Research*, vol. 2, pp. 803–814. New York: Raven Press.

Wiqvist, N., Lundström, V. & Gréen, K. (1976) Indomethacin and premature labour. In *Recent Advances in Prostaglandin and Thromboxane Research*, vol. 2, p. 998. New York: Raven Press.

Wolfe, L. S., Pappius, H. M. & Marion, J. (1976) The biosynthesis of prostaglandins by brain. In *Recent Advances in Prostaglandin and Thromboxane Research*, vol. 1, pp. 345–356. New York: Raven Press.

Yamamoto, Y. L., Feindel, L., Wolfe, L. S., Katoh, H. & Hodge, C. P. (1972) Experimental vasoconstriction of cerebral arteries by prostaglandins. *Journal of Neurosurgery*, **37**, 385–397.

FURTHER READING

To attempt to present an exhaustive review of the prostaglandin field, in particular the recent advances in all their many ramifications, is beyond the competence of the present author. I have attempted to highlight a few of the growing points in this exciting field, all too conscious that more has been omitted than included.

The reader is urged to consult the many sources of information now available. The journal *Prostaglandins* includes current scientific articles of interest. A comprehensive bibliography is published at intervals by the Upjohn Company.

A new series published by Raven Press under the general titles *Recent Advances in Prostaglandin and Thromboxane Research* started in 1976 — the first two volumes representing the proceedings of an International Symposium on Prostaglandins held in Florence in 1975.

Proceedings have been published of earlier international symposia held in Vienna (Bergström and Bernhard, 1973), New York (Ramwell and Shaw, 1971), Worcester (Ramwell and Shaw, 1968), Stockholm (Bergström and Samuelsson, 1967) and Bristol (Pickles and Fitzpatrick, 1966). The following monographs provide much useful background information, Euler and Eliasson, 1967; Horton, 1972; Cuthbert, 1972; Karim, 1976; Ramwell, 1974; Robinson and Vane, 1974. A volume of abstracts is published by the Population Information Program.

Finally, some of the intricacies of the interactions and interrelationships between prostaglandins and other natural substances have been the subject of two further conferences. *Prostaglandins, Peptides and Amines* was edited by Mantegazza and Horton (1969) whilst *Prostaglandins and Cyclic AMP* was edited by Kahn and Lands (1973).

Bergström, S. & Bernhard, S. (1973) *Advances in the Biosciences 9.* Braunschweig, W. Germany: Pergamon Press.

Bergström, S. & Samuelsson, B. (1967) *Nobel Symposium 2 Prostaglandins.* Uppsala, Sweden: Almqvist & Wiksell Boktryckeri.

Cuthbert, M. F. (1972) *The Prostaglandins: Pharmacological and Therapeutic Advances.* London: Heinemann.

Euler von, U. S. & Eliasson, R. (1967) *Prostaglandins. Medicinal Chemistry Monographs Vol. 8.* New York–London: Academic Press.

Kahn, R. H. & Lands, W. E. M. (1973) *Prostaglandins and Cyclic AMP Biological Actions and Clinical Applications.* New York: Academic Press, Inc.

Karim, S. M. M. (1976) *The Prostaglandins: Progress in Research.* Oxford: Medical & Technical Pub. Co. Ltd. (Three Volumes).

Mantegazza, P. & Horton, E. W. (1969) *Prostaglandins, Peptides and Amines.* London: Academic Press, Inc.

Pickles, V. R. & Fitzpatrick, R. J. (1966) *Endogenous Substances Affecting the Myometrium.* Memoirs, Society for Endocrinology, vol. 14.

Ramwell, P. W. (1973) *The Prostaglandins, Volume 1.* New York: Plenum Press.

Ramwell, P. W. (1974) *The Prostaglandins, Volume 2.* New York: Plenum Press.

Ramwell, P. W. & Shaw, J. E. (1968) *Prostaglandin Symposium of the Worcester Foundation for Experimental Biology.* New York: John Wiley & Sons Inc.

Ramwell, P. W. & Shaw, J. E. (1971) *Annals of the New York Academy of Sciences: Prostaglandins.* New York: Academy of Sciences.

Robinson, H. J. & Vane, J. R. (1974) *Prostaglandin Synthetase Inhibitors: Their Effects on Physiological Functions and Pathological States.* New York: Raven Press.

17
INFERTILITY

I. D. Cooke   A. K. Thomas

Since 1958 when ovulation was first induced in the human the management of infertility has changed strikingly, so that at present the principal cause of infertility in most clinics is ovulatory failure (Cox, 1975). Although treatment can mostly be offered for anovulation, specific therapy for the male with defective spermatogenesis is rarely available, although the development of sperm banks and donor insemination provide a possible solution. Male-only infertility may account for one-third of all problems (Santomauro, Sciarra and Varma, 1972) but about one-third of couples have defects in both partners. These circumstances require careful evaluation of both partners of an infertile marriage, and with social change in the form of the Abortion Act (1967) subsequently reducing the numbers of babies available for adoption the demand for comprehensive infertility investigation and treatment has increased dramatically. Although components of the investigation and treatment may be organised by the gynaecologist, urologist, or endocrinologist a co-ordinated regime is necessary and is best supervised from a regional infertility clinic. Initial complete investigation of both partners is essential before beginning treatment of either, as multiple factors in either partner or factors in each partner will influence the prognosis. The patients should be aware of this as treatment is often prolonged and requires considerable motivation.

INITIAL INVESTIGATION OF THE COUPLE

Eligibility for investigation

A frequent question posed is when should investigations begin. If no contraception is used 90 per cent of newly married couples will become pregnant within the first eighteen months (Potter and Parker, 1964) so an 18 month waiting period may be used in the young marrieds; however many young couples nowadays are regularly exposed to pregnancy for some time before marriage and this should be taken into account. If a couple, even unmarried, enquires before this time it is worth taking a history and performing routine physical examination (including a pelvic examination of the female) and either reassuring them or directing further investigations to the cause of their underlying anxiety which may be oligomenorrhoea or cryptorchidism. Primary infertility need not be distinguished from secondary infertility, which is infertility following pregnancy even if it ended in abortion, as the cumulative conception rates are no different in each group (Lamb, 1972). The previous pregnancy can guarantee little and in no way influences the routine of investigation. If the wife is over 35 then as long as six months of normal intercourse has occurred, or sooner if the history is suggestive of some abnormality, investigation should be undertaken.

Initial investigation

If a couple presents then the initial investigation of the husband can be restricted to examination of an ejaculated seminal fluid specimen. The wife requires a general physical examination not only to discover any evidence of the disease contributing to the infertility but also to anticipate any problems that may complicate subsequent pregnancy, such as hypertension or valvular heart disease, that could not be adequately investigated by radiological means during a pregnancy. A pelvic examination is important and abnormalities of cervical cytology need to be pursued by a repeat smear, treatment of local inflammatory disease such as trichomonal vaginitis, and punch biopsy of colposcopically defined lesions. An erythrocyte sedimentation rate is helpful as a general screening test, and a mid-stream specimen of urine for asymptomatic bacteriuria is also useful. Basic investigations consist of basal body temperature record for a minimum of two months, and a test of tubal patency. As tubal insufflation has a significant false positive and false negative rate it is preferable to use hysterosalpingography with screening. The timing needs to observe the 10 day rule but an oligomenorrhoeic or amenorrhoeic patient can be advised to abstain from coitus until the examination. The hysterosalpingogram also provides details of the shape of the uterine cavity relevant to histories of abortion. Alternatively if the patient lives at a distance, or historically there is evidence of pelvic inflammatory disease, laparoscopy under general anaesthesia may allow better definition of the tubal disease. However evaluation of the male and of the ovulatory status should be completed before this is done as it is convenient to proceed to definitive surgery of the damaged tubes if appropriate under the same anaesthetic. If the wife presents alone then the husband's seminal fluid analysis should be requested and further investigation of the wife delayed until the result is available. If the husband presents alone and his wife needs to be seen, particularly if he is already known to be oligo- or azoospermic and the question of donor insemination has been raised, documentation of his wife's potential ability to conceive is crucial to a decision to proceed with insemination.

Further investigation and definition of the problem

Two to three months after the first visit the basal temperature record may be reviewed. If the patient has been instructed properly and her technique checked, it should be possible to define obvious anovulation or oligo-ovulation by flat depressed records rather than a regular biphasic pattern. More subtle defects may be inferred when the first part of the record prior to the temperature rise is of less than 10 days' or more than 18 days' duration. A rise of 0.6°C should occur over no more than two days and it should be maintained uniformly elevated for at least 12 days. The pattern may vary from month to month and a definitive diagnosis can only usually be made where clear cut anomalies occur; a diagnosis of other defects needs to be supported by further investigations (see ovarian factors).

The hysterosalpingogram will show any intrauterine pathology such as gross polyps, subendometrial fibroids or synechiae, and congenital abnormalities such as a bicornuate or subseptate uterus. Tubal patency may be noted and the delayed film after 20 minutes should show any local adhesions preventing widespread distribution of the water-soluble contrast and producing loculation. If tubal occlusion is present it may be proximal at the uterine cornua or distal at the fimbrial end of the tubes when degrees of dilatation may be seen in a single or in bilateral hydrosalpinges (see uterine and tubal factors).

If the seminal fluid analysis is abnormal the technique of collecting the whole of the ejaculate should be questioned, particularly if the volume is small. If the motility is low then the time lapse between ejaculation and examination needs to be ascertained, particularly in the winter. If the specimen is of poor quality but has been reliably collected and delivered to the laboratory it should be repeated after 70 days as the sperm generation cycle is 69–72 days. In the interim the husband should be sought for a detailed history and physical examination although the basic history of past and present health, drugs, occupation, and coital activity should be obtainable from the wife (see male factors).

If ovulation appears to be normal then an endometrial biopsy, if timed by the basal temperature record for the second half (luteal or secretory phase) of the cycle, should support this observation, but it is no longer thought to be definitive (see ovarian factors). It may be done by aspiration biopsy in the conscious patient as an out-patient procedure when she attends the clinic rather than by attempting to predict the secretory phase date for it to be done as an in-patient under anaesthesia. Minor anatomical variants such as an acutely anteverted or retroverted uterus, a very small cervix and cervical canal, or even a very anxious patient unable to relax may be better served by examination under anaesthesia where dilatation of the cervix may be initially employed. Endometrial culture to exclude tuberculosis is now usually only done in immigrants, in patients with a history of tuberculosis or ectopic gestation, where the ESR is elevated, or in some parts of the country where a significant incidence of the disease still occurs.

The postcoital test (Sims–Hühner or PCT) is a useful functional assessment of fertility. There seems to be little point in using it as the first investigation as its constituents have not been examined and although a good quality test may be reassuring a poor quality test achieves little and nothing further is gained by repeating it. The PCT examines motility of ejaculated sperm in endocervical mucus. It looks critically at the act of coitus and the interaction of cervical mucus and ejaculated sperm, provided that the ejaculated sperm are known to be of good quality when examined independently, and that ovulation is thought to occur so that the timing can be arranged by the basal temperature record to obtain optimum preovulatory cervical mucus. If the sperm and ovulation are known to be abnormal then the test will be poor and does nothing to help. Absent sperm may uncover a psychosexual problem such as impotence or frigidity or a defect in coital technique. A retroverted uterus results in the cervix being directed upwards and forward away from the posterior forniceal pool of semen. If a postcoital test reveals sperm in the posterior fornix but none in the endocervical canal the retroversion itself may be implicated, but would need to be confirmed by repeating the PCT after the uterus had been anteverted using a Hodge–Smith pessary. Defective follicular maturation and ovulation may be identified by poor quality mucus, or mucus antibodies may rarely be inferred (see cervical and ovarian factors). After these investigations the patients should ideally be seen together and their problems discussed. A prognosis should be given and a regime of treatment delineated. This is the time to sound their motivation, to encourage adoption if the prognosis is poor, to set a time limit on management, or to discourage further investigation or treatment if the urological, gynaecological or future obstetric problems are too great.

Management of Specific Infertility 'Factors'

Cervical factors

It is convenient but physiologically misleading to refer to a cervical *factor* or *cervical hostility* as a cause of infertility. The normal cervix produces mucus from cells lining the endocervical canal, the mucus increasing in quantity clarity and distensibility (spinnbarkeit) and reducing in cells and viscosity up to the time of ovulation. The mucus secretion is stimulated by increasing ovarian oestrogen secretion, and abnormalities may be due to anatomical or physiological causes. The mucus secreting cells may have been destroyed or grossly reduced by cervical amputation (Manchester repair), cone biopsy for diagnosis of major cervical cytological abnormalities, or extensive diathermy to reduce vaginal discharge and gross ectopic columnar epithelium on the ectocervix. The remedy is to inseminate the semen directly into the uterus. However the most important investigation is to confirm that ovulation is taking place. Anovulation or disordered follicular maturation associated with low oestrogen levels will also be characterised by cervical mucus of reduced volume, more viscous and less distensible than optimal for the preovulatory phase of the cycle. The 'infantile' cervix, small with a very narrow endocervical canal, is a reflection of the primary amenorrhoea or persistent anovulation rather than a major problem in itself. Management then revolves around the underlying diagnosis and induction of ovulation.

Excessive discharge may result from extensive outgrowth of endocervical columnar epithelium onto the ectocervix during adolescence or a previous pregnancy, with variable transformation by squamous metaplasia to non-secreting epithelium ('erosion'). This does not constitute any barrier to fertility but is frequently treated by diathermy or more often nowadays by cryosurgery, primarily because of the annoying symptom of persistent vaginal discharge. If the squamous metaplasia is atypical an abnormal cervical smear may be obtained and this should be investigated by colposcopy before further treatment.

Endocervical inflammation may be gonococcal in origin. The mucus tends to be opaque in the acute or subacute phases but the patient may be an asymptomatic carrier. The more frequent causes of vaginal discharge associated with cervical involvement are trichomonas vaginalis, vaginal candida albicans, or haemophilus vaginalis. These are not in themselves barriers to conception and may be asymptomatic, but they may also be associated with an acute vulvo-vaginitis and more important is the dyspareunia or even apareunia and so these conditions require treatment. Other causes of cervicitis are rare in this country. The diagnosis should not be used to describe the red cervix ('erosion') described more accurately above.

The clinical diagnosis should always be confirmed by culture. Candida and trichomonas can be found when 2–3 ml of sterile saline are instilled into the vaginal vault or over the cervix, and then aspirated in a pasteur pipette for examination microscopically. After the examination for trichomonas in a wet preparation, culture will confirm the candida or haemophilus vaginalis. Transport media are now available for better diagnosis of candida and trichomonas. Endocervical and urethral cultures are ideally required for diagnosis of gonococci: charcoal impregnated swabs are best for transport and slides can be prepared for later laboratory diagnosis. Trichomoniasis is treated by giving both the male and female partner metronidazole 200 mg three times daily for one week. Monilial vaginitis is treated with nystatin pessaries 1 twice daily for five days with oral nystatin, and nystatin cream application under the prepuce if the condition recurs. Nystatin cream is also useful for vulval involvement, and amphotericin B is useful in resistant cases.

Mycoplasma hominis particularly T-mycoplasma have been implicated in infertility recently (Gnarpe and Friberg, 1973) although this has been disputed (Matthews et al, 1975). Infertile couples are said to harbour the organism in from 67 to 90 per cent of cases, but Matthews et al (1975) have shown no difference in isolation rates in the vaginal wall and endocervix in fertile but non-pregnant or pregnant patients. Horne, Kundsin and Kosasa (1974) suggested that myco-plasma may be implicated as a cause of infertility where (a) the husband's ejaculate is normal but the postcoital test in good quality mucus is poor, (b) chronic cervicitis exists, (c) the wife has recurrent cystitis, (d) there is a history of one or more spontaneous abortions, (e) focal plasma cell granulomatous lesions are found in the endometrium on biopsy, or (f) there has been previous pelvic inflammatory disease. Treatment with large doses of tetracycline has been claimed to promote fertility (Gnarpe and Friberg, 1972) but the regime is not gaining adherents.

Cervical mucus may rarely be of poor quality even when ovulation appears to be taking place. Ovulation would need to be 'confirmed' by serial steroid assay of follicle maturation, and corpus luteum function either by plasma oestradiol or progesterone or urinary total oestrogen and pregnanediol during the follicular and luteal phases respectively, before this could seriously be entertained. Small doses of oestrogens have been recommended to improve the preovulatory mucus, e.g. 0.01 mg ethinyloestradiol twice daily from days 9–14, but although the mucus may become less viscid and more copious, endogenous FSH may be inhibited and further follicle maturation inhibited leading to anovulation. Pregnancies are however sometimes reported. Poor cervical mucus also occurs in some patients treated with clomiphene to induce ovulation, and if oestrogen excretion or plasma levels are compatible with normal follicular maturation ethinyloestradiol on the above regime may be used. Alternatively tamoxifen may be used or recourse had to human menopausal gonadotrophin (HMG). If poor quality semen results in a poor postcoital test then the remedy lies in treatment of the male. However, a consistently small volume ejaculate may benefit from AIH. This is very rarely applicable as small volume ejaculates are usually associated with other abnormal characteristics (see male factors).

If the postcoital test reveals immobilised sperm in the endocervical mucus and both the mucus and the ejaculated sperm are of good quality then there may be additional factors involved.

For more complete definition of a negative or poor postcoital test where the components seem satisfactory an in vitro fractional postcoital cross test has been described by Davajan and Nakamura (1975).

Mucus and separate ejaculated sperm are obtained as well as donor sperm and donor cervical mucus. Separate mixing in vitro of each of the four combinations allows localisation of the factor to a patient's mucus or her husband's sperm. An abnormal seminal plasma factor has been suggested as a result of using this technique. The *cross test* is a variation of the more widely used Miller–Kurzrok test where a drop of each of the two components is allowed to touch on the slide and is then examined microscopically (Perloff and Steinberger, 1963). In this way poor sperm penetration of the mucus might be identified more readily.

Immunological causes of sperm immobilisation may be of different types. Parish and Ward (1968) described an IgG antibody cytotoxic to spermatozoa and specific for spermatozoa coating antigens. Non-cytotoxic agglutinating antibodies of low affinity are present in the female's peripheral serum and their significance is uncertain. Shulman, Jackson and Stone (1975) tested the sera of 150 infertile and 113 fertile women using sperm agglutination methods. The former group demonstrated 23 and 16 per cent positive tests (Kibrick and Franklin–Dukes tests respectively) where the latter group showed 2.7 per cent positive results in each test, indicating that circulating antibody occurs even in some fertile women and that the incidence of positive serum tests in women is not high. Shulman and Friedman (1975) used the same methods in a few samples of extracted cervical mucus. They found that Kibrick agglutination and Franklin–Dukes immobilisation occurred when they could demonstrate reasonable amounts of IgG and serum type IgA but no IgM. Rebello, Green and Fox (1975) recently examined the female genital tract for evidence of secretory immune activity using immunofluorescence and found essentially IgA principally localised to the endocervix. As the IgA is released from plasma cells localised in the lamina propria it passes through the intercellular spaces and is linked to *secretory component* synthesised by the epithelial cells. It is then somewhat protected against proteolysis as opposed to the 7S serum IgA or IgG. This endocervical contribution to the cervical mucus would appear to be the local immune response and might be expected to be of greater contributory importance to the infertility than any peripheral serum antibodies.

Behrman (1975b) has treated 58 patients with positive serum microhaemagglutination tests (after Franklin–Dukes) by using a condom for some months to reduce antibody stimulation. Of the 24 patients whose sera became negative 13 (54 per cent) became pregnant after the condom regime was stopped. Although this is encouraging, the immunological immobilisation of sperm in the endocervix is not yet fully understood and its import is as yet uncertain.

Uterine factors

Bimanual pelvic examination may reveal a firm irregular uterus suggestive of fibromyomata uteri (fibroids) or a submucuous fibroid may be diagnosed on hysterosalpingography. This radiographic examination may demonstrate a septum of the uterus or synechiae. The number, size, location, and blood supply of the fibroids determine the likely infertility. Malone and Ingersoll (1975) described 75 patients who had myomectomy performed and 35 had associated pelvic pathology. Following myomectomy 49 per cent of those with primary sterility conceived as did 50 per cent of those with secondary sterility. Subsequent myomectomies were required in 14 of 22 patients in whom they recurred. Of those who became pregnant 59 per cent did so within one year of surgery and 70 per cent within two years. Subsequent delivery is usually by elective caesarean section to prevent the possibility of rupture of the uterine scar.

Excision of a partial mid-line uterine septum is usually undertaken after abortion or if the patient suffers from severe dysmenorrhoea. Buttrum et al (1974b) reported a postoperative fetal survival of 87 per cent in 28 patients compared to a preoperative rate of 20 per cent. A septum is rarely diagnosed except after hysterosalpingography although a broad fundus with a dimple may be seen externally at laparoscopy. Associated pathology especially endometriosis may occur in one-third hence a lost pregnancy, (i.e. abortion or premature labour) is usually the stimulus to perform the operation otherwise failure to conceive after operation may be due to pre-existing associated causes.

Intrauterine adhesions or synechiae (Asherman's syndrome) are rare but may follow curettage shortly after abortion or delivery and result in amenorrhoea or recurrent abortion. The previously poor prognosis for fertility has been strikingly improved by curettage and introduction of an intrauterine device for some months. Oelsner et al (1974) described 14 successful pregnancies in 16 patients after this procedure compared with a loss of 48 out of 57 pregnancies prior to it.

Endometrial factors

Atrophy of the endometrium, lack of secretory activity, and cystic glandular hyperplasia are reflections of ovarian activity and the primary therapy should be directed there. Infection may be part of a more general pelvic infection e.g. in gonorrhoea, although biopsy and culture of the endometrium may be the only way to make a diagnosis of tuberculosis. It is difficult to know the significance of more subtle alterations. Retardation of endometrial maturation may be a reflection of reduced ovarian progesterone production in the luteal phase or of an abnormal sequence of oestradiol/progesterone exposure (Cooke et al, 1972), and efforts have been directed to stimulation of ovarian function. However, an insensitivity of the tissue itself has been postulated (Gore and Gordon, 1974) where light microscopy showed a normal secretory pattern and electronmicroscopy revealed an absence of the nucleolar channel system thought to be a progesterone response. It is theoretically possible that changes in cytoplasmic steroid receptor activities (Davies and Ryan, 1973) could themselves be abnormal. Enzymes in the carbohydrate metabolism pathway have been described as grossly reduced (Spellman et al, 1974). It is not known how these indices of function respond to therapy.

Tubal factors

Tubal occlusion as the major cause of infertility has been estimated as occurring in 11 per cent of 900 patients (Cox, 1975). Westrom (1975) reviewed

415 women treated for laparoscopically verified pelvic inflammatory disease after nine years and found a tubal occlusion in 13 per cent after one episode of infection, 36 per cent after two and in 75 per cent after three episodes. The surprising feature of these data is really the low incidence of tubal occlusion after a single episode; the involuntary infertility in these patients was almost all due primarily to tubal occlusion which was more common after non-gonorrhoeal than after gonorrhoeal salpingitis and was related to the degree of inflammation seen at laparoscopy.

Fjallbrant (1975) reported a study of 851 patients in whom 33 per cent had evidence of tubal damage as seen on hysterosalpingography. Of these 248 patients 101 came to tubal surgery because after assessment of all factors it was felt that there was a prospect of achieving tubal patency.

Unless there is a contraindication to laparoscopy or there is palpable pelvic pathology for which a laparotomy would anyway be required, laparoscopy and instillation of dilute dye through the cervix (hydrotubation) should be performed prior to definitive surgery. Some simple procedures such as division of a few fine adhesions may be undertaken at laparoscopy making laparotomy unnecessary, although it is usually better to proceed to laparotomy for most procedures. Gomel (1975) however, reported dilatation of phimosis of tubal ostia and salpingolysis by laparoscopy. Because minimal tubal disease or peritubal adhesions may not be recognised at hysterosalpingography most gynaecologists would advise laparoscopy prior to concluding infertility investigations and particularly if there were no other demonstrable cause.

Duignan et al (1972) compared the diagnostic accuracy of laparoscopy and hysterosalpingography in 273 patients and found that similar information was only provided in 70 per cent of patients, the most notable finding being that in 22 of 70 patients in whom the hysterosalpingogram suggested bilateral tubal occlusion subsequent laparoscopy showed patent tubes. On the other hand the hysterosalpingogram showed patent tubes in 10 patients in whom it could not be demonstrated at laparoscopy. Endometriosis and other pelvic diseases may also be seen at laparoscopy (Moghissi and Sim, 1975).

A number of surgical procedures are available according to the site and degree of damage. In one study the results were computed as the probability of being pregnant with an indefinite follow-up (Umezaki et al, 1974). Salpingolysis (lysis of peritubal adhesions) was calculated as having a pregnancy rate of 66 per cent and separation of partially sealed fimbria or salpingoplasty 40 per cent. Reimplantation of the proximal ends of the tubes (cornual implantation) was associated with a pregnancy rate of 38 per cent and multiple procedures with 21 per cent. Reversal of previous sterilisation procedures such as tubal ligation, a request met with increasing frequency (Siegler and Perez, 1975), may be accomplished by mid-segment resection and anastomosis with a pregnancy rate of 50 per cent. These better results are probably a result of having normal epithelium and a lesion localised to one segment of the tube. Patients having anastomosis and cornual implantation achieve their pregnancies within the first year and although a lower pregnancy rate is achieved in the first year with the other procedures pregnancies do occur over the next three or four years. Fjallbrant's study (1975) however, distinguished the live birth rate from the conception rate and noted that the live birth rate was twice as high after salpingolysis as after salpingostomy, indicating that minor disease, particularly that not involving the tubal epithelium (Brosens and de Graef, 1975), has a substantially better prognosis. Major disease results in more ectopic gestations.

The use of the silastic prosthesis to cover the site of surgery at the distal end of the tube (hood) introduced by Mulligan, Rock and Easterday (1953) has decreased recently, a second laparotomy being required for removal, although a device that can be withdrawn through the anterior abdominal wall some months after initial surgery has recently been introduced. The use of hoods however appears to have decreased more since it has been appreciated that viable pregnancies are few after procedures that attempt to treat more than minimal damage. Polyethylene strips are used to support mid-segment resections but microsurgical techniques with polyglycollic acid sutures and no splints (Garcia, 1972) or nylon sutures and minimal splinting (Paterson and Wood, 1974; Winston, 1975) provide better histological evidence of healing. Swolin (1975) described the use of a microthermocautery for salpingostomy with good results because of his relatively atraumatic and bloodless technique; he also advocated laparoscopy at six to eight weeks to separate postoperative adhesions.

Flushing of the tubes (via the cervix) with solutions of hydrocortisone, chymotrypsin, or antibiotics (hydrotubation) is frequently used but the evidence for improved pregnancy rates is sparse (Grant, 1971). Postoperative dexamethasone to reduce fibroblast proliferation before the serosal cells can cover the damaged tissue and promethazine to reduce the histamine reaction locally can minimise early formation of fibrinous exudate. It has been used by Horne et al (1973) with good results as judged against those in the literature, but the benefit due to the additional therapy is controversial.

If tubal damage is severe or a hydrosalpinx is of moderate size no restitution of function is possible and salpingectomy may be necessary, or even hysterectomy if.both tubes need to be sacrificed or if there is extensive inflammatory or endometriotic disease because of the longer term implications.

Two developments will be watched with great interest. Steptoe and Edwards (1970) have primed ovaries with gonadotrophins and harvested preovulatory human oocytes laparoscopically (see also Berger et al, 1975). In vitro fertilisation has been followed by attempts to replace the morula in the uterus via the cervix because of the grossly damaged tubes. No successful pregnancy has yet been reported. Sillo-Seidl (1975) reported a tubal transplant following preservation of the donor tube in liquid nitrogen. No immunosuppression was used but 'a serum activator' method was employed. The tube was subsequently found to be patent but again no pregnancy has yet been reported.

Ovarian factors: amenorrhoea

Amenorrhoea is not a common mode of presentation of infertility; patients with *primary* amenorrhoea (1 per cent, Cox, 1975) tend to present earlier for gynaecological investigation. Ambiguous external genitalia are usually recognised at birth, or failure of development of secondary sexual characteristics is a reason of referral (Boczkowski, 1970). Ultimate fertility may well be an underlying anxiety of the patient or her parents, and this should be discussed fully after a diagnosis has been made giving details of proposed regimes of induction of ovulation if fertility can ultimately be achieved. Physical examination, perhaps under anaesthesia, will reveal a primary vaginal or uterine abnormality or testicular feminisation and laparoscopy will confirm the streak or absent gonads in gonadal dysgenesis. The phenotype of Turner's syndrome is only likely to be obscured in mosaic forms, and adrenogenital syndrome is also usually diagnosed in infancy or childhood although there is a pubertal form.

The full investigation and management of these problems has been described elsewhere (Shearman, 1968) and induction of ovulation in these patients is the same as that described below for secondary amenorrhoea. It depends on a potentially functional ovary with or without a potentially functional hypothalamo-pituitary axis.

Secondary amenorrhoea is a more common problem in infertility clinics (20 per cent, Cox, 1975) and demands investigation when it has lasted more than six months (Newton and Collins, 1974). Rarely does physical examination contribute to an understanding although a pregnancy in an oligoovulatory patient is always a possibility. Historically oligomenorrhoea may be elicited in patients with Stein–Leventhal syndrome or amenorrhoea during or after oral contraceptive medication (Starup, 1972; Buttram et al, 1974a; Grant, 1973) with or without galactorrhoea (Tyson et al, 1975). Stress may be a feature even without overt psychiatric disease and weight-related amenorrhoea should be recognised (Warren et al, 1975). This may be associated with obesity but is more likely to be related to weight reduction often acute and self-imposed, and a spectrum through to anorexia nervosa may be seen. These patients need to have their general health investigated. It may be inappropriate to consider pregnancy at that time or stabilisation of treatment may be required before embarking on a pregnancy. In any case the effects of pregnancy on the underlying disease need to be considered. Investigations performed are lateral skull x-ray, chest x-ray, full blood count and ESR. Adrenal and thyroid function need to be assessed and diabetes mellitus excluded, and although a peripheral leucocyte karyotype is usually done it is rarely rewarding. Plasma or urinary FSH and LH need to be assayed; 24 hour urinary values are not subject to episodic fluctuation but can still vary remarkably and two or three spaced samples are better, although Kulin et al (1975) described a good correlation between multiple plasma sample values and a three hour urinary sample value.

Urinary total oestrogen or plasma oestradiol assays are helpful in determining existing ovarian activity and most recently serum prolactin estimation has allowed identification of a separate group amenable to specific therapy.

Lunenfeld and Insler (1974) distinguish three groups. The *first* is associated with low oestrogen activity, and pathologically high gonadotrophin levels. This is due to ovarian failure and clinically the patient usually complains of hot flushes. Confirmation by laparoscopic ovarian biopsy may be useful although Starup and Sele (1973) found 2 of 26 patients had morphologically normal ovarian follicles which failed to respond to high doses of human menopausal gonadotrophin. The high endogenous levels of gonadotrophin provide a functional appraisal of the ovary and this is usually adequate for a diagnosis unless laparoscopy or laparotomy be undertaken for another purpose. It may be considered important in young patients with a premature menopause. These patients will not respond to clomiphene, releasing hormone or gonadotrophins.

A *second* group consists of patients with normal gonadotrophins and some oestrogen activity (urinary total oestrogens more than 10 μg per 24 h: 34 nmol/24 h); they may be amenorrhoeic or they may have some menstrual bleeding pattern, even regular. However, the amenorrhoeic patients may be made to bleed by giving 5–10 days of a progestagen, e.g. norethisterone acetate 5 mg three times daily. These patients then clearly have an endometrium capable of a normal response to steroids and some endogenous oestrogen activity which must be ovarian in origin. They must also have sufficient gonadotrophin releasing hormone activity to simulate some gonadotrophin release to elicit at least some ovarian follicular response. The defect in these patients must be localised to the feed-back mechanism. They will respond to clomiphene, or gonadotrophin releasing hormone as diagnostic tests and these agents may then be used therapeutically. This group may have elevated serum prolactin levels (8 of 40 patients, Franks et al, 1975) and if a pituitary tumour can be excluded by tomography of the pituatary fossa bromocriptine results in resumption of ovulation.

The *third* group of amenorrhoeic patients described by Lunenfeld and Insler (1974) is characterised by low levels of gonadotrophins and negligible oestrogen levels (urinary oestrogen of less than 10 μg/24 h: 35 nmol/24 h). These do not usually respond to progestagen alone by withdrawal bleeding and require a cyclic oestrogen/progestagen combination for up to three months. The medication may be either a combined oral contraceptive formulation or a sequential. Hyperprolactinaemia is only likely to be present in this group after hypophysectomy for pituitary tumour (Franks et al, 1975), but such patients may well be candidates for replacement gonadotrophin therapy. If prolactin levels are normal then the defect may be localised to the hypothalamus or to the pituitary using a gonadotrophin releasing hormone test. A positive response indicates hypothalamic failure, probably the most common condition and a negative response localises the lesion to the pituitary. Recent work however (Serra et al, 1975) suggests that an absent pituitary response may represent the effect of a chronic deficiency of hypothalamic secretion and after slow and prolonged treatment with the decapeptide Luteinising Hormone Releasing Hormone (LHRH) normal pituitary responsiveness could return. Neither the hypothalamic nor pituitary lesions respond to clomiphene and although at the present time replacement gonadotrophin therapy is preferred new LHRH analogues such as [Des-Gly-NH_2^{10}, Proethylamide^9-]LHRH (Nakano et al, 1974; Nakano et al, 1975), D-Lys^6-LHRH coupled to sodium polyglutamate (Amoss, Monahan and Verlander, 1974), or D-Ala^6-LHRH (de la Cruz et al, 1975), by virtue of their potency may come to be therapeutically useful.

DIAGNOSTIC TESTS AND THERAPY: FEMALES

Clomiphene

A five day test of clomiphene citrate 200 mg/day orally with assay of LH and FSH during and one day after the course has been described as a test of pituitary reserve by Newton and Dixon (1971). Shaw et al (1975) reported an oestrogen 'provocation test' as a means of predicting a response to clomiphene in amenorrhoeic women. They gave 1 mg oestradiol benzoate intramuscularly and assayed serum oestradiol, FSH and LH over the subsequent 72 h. Significant elevation of LH above the base-line demonstrated positive feed-back release of LH hence it was inferred that the hypothalamo-pituitary axis was intact and that the patients would be likely to ovulate on clomiphene. Lunenfeld and Insler (1974) also use the clomiphene test to categorise their second group with failure of the normal feed-back mechanism.

There is much to be said, however, for performing a therapeutic trial of clomiphene using 50 mg daily for five days commencing on day two or day six (Adams and Cooke, 1974). The response can be monitored by the basal temperature record and in successive months (or arbitrarily in amenorrhoeic patients) the dose may be increased by 50 mg increments to 200 mg or until a response is seen. A normal response is characterised by a sustained 12 to 14 day elevation of the basal temperature record occurring up to eight days after the last tablet. However although MacGregor et al (1968) indicated that ovulation rates were high in patients with ovarian dysfunction (Stein–Leventhal syndrome) and secondary amenorrhoea or oligo-ovulation (72 to 76 per cent), the overall pregnancy rates are lower (33 per cent). This has been highlighted by Hancock and Oakey (1973) who by measuring urinary oestrone concluded that ovulation is incorrectly assumed to occur in many patients and this is the explanation for the discrepancy between apparent ovulation and pregnancy rates.

A defective response may be represented by a poorly sustained elevation in basal temperature record or a short luteal phase (less than 10 days). When this occurs the pregnancy rates are poor and one should consider changing the therapy. There may be inadequate follicular stimulation (Strott et al, 1970) and although this may be remedied by increasing the dose it may become more marked as the clomiphene stimulates further FSH and LH output perhaps with an inappropriate ratio. These defective responses cannot really be assessed except by assay of urinary total oestrogens with findings outside a normal response of 50–150 μg/24 h (170-500 nmol/24 h) or of plasma oestradiol (200–600 pg/ml : 7–20 pmol/l) during follicular development, such as days 9–14.

Low oestrogen values suggest an increase in the dose, but if adequate preovulatory levels have been obtained the same regime should be continued for up to six months. Very high oestrogen values are usually thought to be associated with hyperstimulation, but we have seen this not infrequently in patients with defective temperature records without any evidence of enlarged or tender ovaries and the explanation is obscure. In any case the dose should be reduced to that which produces oestrogen levels in the normal preovulatory ranges.

Luteinising hormone releasing hormone (LHRH)

An intravenous bolus of 100 μg LHRH with samples obtained at $-10, 0, +30$, $+60$ and $+90$ min with assay of plasma FSH and LH is known as an LHRH test, and has been used extensively by Nillius and Wide (1972); Keller (1973); and Mortimer et al (1973) to distinguish patients with low gonadotrophin levels with hypothalamic failure who will respond and those with pituitary failure who will not respond. A response is generally considered to be an increase of 70 per cent over the basal LH value by the end of the test; the FSH levels also increase but the response is more variable. At the present time this is of academic interest as both groups need to be treated with replacement gonadotrophins but in the future, potent LHRH analogues may be available for use in patients with hypothalamic failure who have responsive pituitaries. Studies have, however, been carried out in amenorrhoeic women since Zarate et al (1974) achieved seven pregnancies following doses of 200–1000 µg daily in 27 women, although the patients seemed to have some endogenous ovarian activity. Breckwoldt et al (1974) using lower doses were unable to achieve ovarian stimulation in patients with low endogenous ovarian activity who were otherwise responsive to HMG. They also failed in their attempt to induce ovulation after HMG stimulation of follicular growth. Figueroa Cassas et al (1975) however gave graded doses of LHRH to maintain follicular maturation and induced ovulation by intravenous infusions and/or intramuscular injection of LHRH following maturation. Five pregnancies resulted from 10 ovulations in 25 treatment cycles of 15 patients. Furthermore Crosignani et al (1975) used HMG to stimulate the follicles and a preparation of LHRH in 15 per cent gelatine intramuscularly (100 µg at 08 : 00 and at 18 : 00) to induce ovulation. They claimed that LHRH used in this way as a 'retard' preparation (peak activity at 3 h) did not induce hyperstimulation even in the presence of exaggerated follicular growth and although the optimal conditions for the use and monitoring of LHRH treatment have not yet been clarified this could be an important advance.

Bromocriptine (2-bromo-α-ergocryptine)

Hyperprolactinaemia has been recognised more widely since the advent of the radioimmunoassay for human prolactin (Hwang et al, 1971). It was found in patients with galactorrhoea (Besser and Edwards, 1972) and more recently in those with amenorrhoea without galactorrhoea (Frantz et al, 1972; Franks et al, 1975). The hyperprolactinaemia may result in altered gonadotrophin dynamics (Mortimer et al, 1973) or may suppress ovarian steroidogenesis (McNatty et al, 1974). Reduction of plasma prolactin levels to normal by treatment with bromocriptine allows restoration of normal gonadal function (Besser et al, 1972; Rolland et al, 1974; Besser and Thorner, 1976). As a result of these developments plasma prolactin should be assayed routinely in all patients with amenorrhoea and a therapeutic test carried out if hyperprolactinaemia is present. Bromocriptine 2.5 mg daily, increasing to 7.5 mg twice daily, may be used but the usual dose is 2.5 mg twice daily. It should be taken initially at night with food to avoid nausea although postural hypotension may be a minor problem. The response should be monitored by a repeat plasma estimation but the precise level the treatment should achieve has not been well documented, indeed if the levels fall too low amenorrhoea may again supervene. Therapeutic combinations of bromocriptine and clomiphene or HMG have not been used much, but these regimes are being tested at present.

Bromocriptine should be used daily until pregnancy occurs and should be stopped as soon as pregnancy has been diagnosed although no fetal abnormalities have been reported in the babies delivered so far. Hyperprolactinaemia however should be investigated by pituitary fossa films before treatment if pregnancy is desired, as visual disturbances and even blindness may be precipitated by rapid pituitary tumour enlargement (Gemzell, 1975). If there is objective evidence of tumour then radiotherapy should be given and three months' bromocriptine maintained before any attempt at conception is allowed (Besser and Thorner, 1976). Replacement gonadotrophin therapy may be required if pituitary damage is extensive.

Gonadotrophins

Although PMS (pregnant mares' serum) has been used diagnostically by Shearman (1964) and Swyer et al (1968) separate diagnostic tests are not now usually performed and a therapeutic regime is initiated and used to gauge response. In fact this is also the best way of assaying the gonadotrophins themselves (Pepperell et al, 1974). Human pituitary gonadotrophins extracted from autopsy pituitary glands and used by Brown et al (1969) and Shearman (1969) and human menopausal gonadotrophins extracted from postmenopausal urine by Lunenfeld and Donini (1966) are both effective and HMG is readily available commercially. Patients with hypothalamic or pituitary failure tend to require larger doses of gonadotrophins than those with feed-back failure.

The dosage schedules may be daily and individualised according to the daily oestrogen results or according to a standardised alternate day (1, 3, 5) schedule. The relative merits of these particularly in relation to the logistics of out-patient control have been discussed by Adams and Cooke (1974), and Butler (1972) showed that the total amount of HMG used and the pregnancy rates were similar in the two regimes. It is perhaps not important in treatment of patients with feed-back failure but in those with hypothalamic/pituitary failure a pregnancy is likely to be achieved sooner with a daily regime. This regime has important implications for staff and laboratory services and is the system used in Australia and Israel.

Lunenfeld and Insler (1974) reviewed their HMG results and reported 185 pregnancies from 621 treatment cycles in hypothalamic/pituitary failure patients. They had an abortion rate of 17.3 per cent and a multiple pregnancy rate of 23.8 per cent. In the patients with feed-back failure they achieved 127 pregnancies in 784 treatment cycles. The abortion rate was 20.5 per cent and the multiple pregnancy rate 14.3 per cent. Hyperstimulation from mild (Grade I — small ovarian cysts, 5.5–10.8 per cent) to severe (Grade III — large ovarian cysts and ascites, 0.6–1.0 per cent) was uncommon but apparently not completely preventable even with meticulous patient selection and monitoring.

Brown et al (1973) described the outcome in HPG treated cycles resulting in an optimum response as shown by urinary oestrogen and pregnanediol excretion. They reported that 68 per cent of 264 cycles achieved optimum urinary oestrogens of from 50 to 100 μg (170–350 nmol) per 24 h on this daily regime. Of these ideal cycles 54 per cent resulted in pregnancies of which 22 per cent were multiple and 9 per cent ended in abortion.

The daily treatment regime (e.g. of HMG) consists of 150 IU of FSH and LH (two ampoules) given intramuscularly daily and continued for up to seven days. On the eighth day the dose of HMG is increased by 50 per cent if the 24 h urinary oestrogen excretion has not reached 50 µg (170 nmol) and continued for another seven days. Daily assays show any oestrogen increment and the dose is manipulated to achieve a graded and smooth rise in excretion values. When optimum follicular maturation has been inferred the follicle is stimulated to ovulate using HCG (e.g. 1500 IU). Brown et al (1969) use supplementary doses of HCG (500–1500 IU) to maintain the corpus luteum through the time of potential implantation according to the urinary pregnanediol which is also assayed daily. If no response has been seen by two weeks the treatment is stopped for one week and begun one week later at a higher dose.

Butler (1969) described the 1, 3, 5 regime, the object being to induce a response by day 8 so that a developed follicle may be ovulated by HCG. Increments in the next course are one-third of the previous dose. If no response is achieved another course may commence one week later. Using this regime it is possible to stimulate a patient so that an excessive oestrogen response is achieved. This may be seen by a urinary oestrogen on day 8 of more than 150 µg (500 nmol) per 24 h or a rate of rise where the urinary total oestrogen values more than double each 24 h. More than one follicle has probably been developed and so as to avoid a multiple pregnancy the ovulating dose of HCG must be withheld and coitus interdicted. Plasma oestradiol and progesterone may be monitored in preference to urinary steroids (Shaaban and Klopper, 1973; Wu, 1975) but their use is not widespread.

Unfortunately both treatment regimes require considerable experience for optimal results as the individual patient response is somewhat unpredictable and may vary from course to course at the same dose level. Small variations in doses are usually a feature of the two regimes. If ovulatory steroid levels have been achieved then patients are usually offered further courses at similar doses and may take from 1 to 12 courses to achieve a pregnancy or indeed may not do so. Patient motivation needs to be very high and elaborate explanations of the regime and possible problems must be given to each partner. Some patients will voluntarily withdraw from treatment after successive failures. Some will achieve no results even on large doses (e.g. 3×20 ampoules) on the 1, 3, 5 regime and treatment is usually stopped. Melmed et al (1969) have used higher doses but Dewhurst et al (1975) describe a patient with 'the resistant ovary syndrome' who had elevated endogenous gonadotrophins and normal follicles on ovarian biopsy. Such patients would be screened out from treatment by the above regime by their elevated basal gonadotrophin values but may perhaps respond to massive gonadotrophin dosage although this was not tried in their patient. The whole concept of resistant ovaries needs to be re-evaluated in the light of newer data on hyperprolactinaemia since specific therapy aimed at reducing the plasma prolactin level to normal may allow more normal ovarian response to gonado-trophins, endogenous or exogenous. Bromocriptine therapy is much simpler to manage than gonadotrophin therapy.

Anovulation

Although amenorrhoeic patients may be regarded as anovulatory, only 38 per cent of Cox's 386 women with ovulatory failure were amenorrhoeic, 43 per cent presented with oligomenorrhoea and 20 per cent had regular but anovulatory menstruation. Infrequent or regular menstruation signifies that there is at least some endogenous oestrogen production, but in general the same investigation of the hypothalamic/pituitary/ovarian axis is required. The contribution of small elevations of plasma prolactin to this picture is not known and the therapeutic possibilities of bromocriptine in this area, although not likely to be great, have not been fully evaluated.

Clomiphene is the initial treatment of choice although other agents for induction of ovulation have been used. Tamoxifen (Williamson and Ellis, 1973) and cyclofenil (Bernard and Beauchamps, 1971) both anti-oestrogenic have had very limited use and they seem to offer no obvious advantages. The clomiphene regime is the same as for amenorrhoeic patients. Most pregnancies occur within the first three months but a few occur after six months, and interestingly some pregnancies occur in the months after stopping therapy (Widholm, 1975; Kistner, 1975b). Perhaps this is the result of a longer term effect on pituitary gonadotrophin production. If a pregnancy does not result monitoring of steroid responses may facilitate the treatment (Hancock and Oakey, 1973). Plasma progesterone or urinary pregnanediol assays may provide data on corpus luteum function which may be supplemented by HCG during the luteal phase from 500 to 5000 IU repeated perhaps three times at intervals of two to three days, although the evidence for the success of this regime is limited (Kistner, 1975).

Before proceeding to gonadotrophin therapy a thorough re-evaluation of the diagnosis of all factors involved in the couple's infertility, and of their motivation is essential. If laparoscopy has not already been done it should be performed at this stage, primarily to view the ovaries and determine that they are normal, and ideally laparoscopic biopsy may be carried out (Black and Govan, 1972). On the other hand, it may well be considered that in the face of moderate oligospermia treatment should stop at that stage.

Polycystic ovarian disease

Goldzieher and Green when reviewing all published cases of the Stein–Leventhal syndrome in 1964 found that amenorrhoea was only present in 50 per cent and infertility in only 74 per cent of patients, and called for adoption of the term polycystic ovarian disease in place of the eponymous syndrome. The features of the syndrome were so variable and as the diagnosis was made so frequently at laparoscopy or culdoscopy in the absence of bilateral palpable ovarian enlargement, the designation *syndrome* was no longer valid. The primary defect might appear to be failure of the hypothalamic cycling centre to develop (Goldzieher, 1975). Apart from the steroid biosynthetic abnormalities in the ovary leading to excess androgen production the adrenal is involved to a variable extent; and the dynamic tests previously used to distinguish ovarian and adrenal contributions to this disease, especially when hirsutism is a problem, have been largely invalidated by the overlapping androgen production of ovary and adrenal shown by Kirschner and Jacobs (1971).

Further attempts to classify patients within the wide clinical spectrum have been made by Berger et al (1975) who describe 'typical' (Type I) histological findings of small to slightly enlarged ovaries without subcortical cysts and with thickened capsules. They had widely fluctuating but markedly elevated LH levels (also used as a discriminatory feature in the differential diagnosis of secondary amenorrhoea by Kletzky et al, 1975). The 'atypical' (Type II) cases had inconsistent histological features, occasionally with stromal hyperplasia and thecal luteinisation and had lower and less fluctuant LH levels. There was no difference in symptomatology, 17-ketosteroid, testosterone or FSH levels, but Type II was felt to represent a heterogeneous collection of disorders. Thus Givens et al (1975) put forward the concept that some cases may be due to X chromosomal factors causing an abnormal follicular apparatus. Diagnosis may not be easy and apart from clinical history and laparoscopic ovarian biopsy Kletzky et al (1975) suggest steroid and gonadotrophin assays every 15 minutes for 4 hours, whereas Givens et al (1974) assess the response of plasma androstenedione and testosterone to a three weeks' suppression by norethisterone 2 mg and mestranol 0.1 mg.

Treatment depends on the presenting symptoms and only infertility should be treated with clomiphene, initially with the smaller dose of 25 mg daily for 5 days from the fifth day of the cycle (or arbitrarily if there is amenorrhoea) because of increased patient sensitivity. Wedge resection should be avoided unless the patient is unable to take clomiphene or has failed to conceive on clomiphene. Occasionally wedge resection is performed incidentally at laparotomy but this should only be done if other infertility assessment makes it appropriate and if the patient wishes to conceive immediately. Buttram and Vaquero (1975) point out the high incidence of postwedge resection adhesive disease which was associated with persistent inability to conceive in 40 of 43 infertile patients from a group of 111 patients followed up over a 15-year period after wedge resection.

Defective ovulation

Recently it has been recognised that subtle alterations in endocrine profiles may be found in infertile patients and this has given rise to speculation that the changes may themselves be the cause of the infertility (Sherman and Korenman, 1974). The classical clinical criteria of ovulation, secretory phase endometrium, plasma progesterone (Cooke et al, 1972; Nadji et al, 1975) or urinary pregnanediol elevations, mid-cycle LH surge or even the signs of prepared follicles such as elevated plasma or urinary oestrogens prior to mid-cycle or good quality cervical mucus are all indirect parameters. It may be that ovulation occurs much less frequently than formerly supposed (Jones, 1949; Lenton and Cooke, 1974; Dodson et al, 1975).

Using the basic minimal clinical investigations, these patients are often described as having 'no abnormality', but Lenton et al (1977) recently followed up 96 such patients and found that by life-table computation at eight years their pregnancy rate was only 40 per cent of a normal fertile population, much less than the treated anovulatory group of Lamb (1972). The group contains many types of defects, single or combinations of follicular mid-cycle or luteal phase abnormalities and although clomiphene, HMG or even oestrogen and progesterone supplementation have been used, the results are poor and the area is still confused. Determination of the prime defect is time consuming and very expensive and at present can only be a research procedure.

Endometriosis

Kelly and Rock (1956) using culdoscopy found endometriosis associated with tubo-ovarian adhesions in 24 per cent of 143 infertile women. Since Ridley and Edwards (1958) showed that menstrual blood injected into the rectus sheath would produce endometriosis the implantation theory of the disease has been recognised more clearly. Laparoscopy is now used extensively in the investigation of dysmenorrhoea, dyspareunia and otherwise unexplained infertility and has led to an appreciation that many patients have some evidence of the disease. It causes its infertility effects probably by reduction of tubo-ovarian motility secondary to scarring and fibrosis. Kistner (1975a) has recently reviewed the subject.

Prolonged use of oral contraception probably reduces the incidence of the disease and suppression of ovulation is used therapeutically on the short term, particularly before or after conservative surgery. Oestrogen alone or androgens should not be used, and combined oestrogen/progestagen regimes should not use a dose of more than 50 μg of ethinyl oestradiol per day in view of the epidemiological evidence of deep vein thrombosis and pulmonary embolism (Inman and Vessey, 1968). The object of treatment where there is ovarian endometriosis without anatomical deformity of the ovary or tube is to induce a pseudopregnancy for six months, i.e. suppression of menstruation, e.g. by giving a combined preparation of norgestrel and ethinyl oestradiol continuously or by using a progestagen alone (norethisterone 20 mg daily initially). Breakthrough bleeding may be overcome by increasing the progestagen by 10 mg increments up to 50 mg per day but an increase in the oestrogenic component should be avoided. After prolonged suppression of ovulation by progestagen, induction of ovulation with clomiphene may be required.

Danazol, a 2,3,isoxozol derivative of 17α ethinyl testosterone, suppresses gonadotrophin release and has a progestational effect at high doses and has been used in the treatment of endometriosis (Greenblatt et al, 1971). The endocrine effects of 200 mg four times daily orally (Wood et al, 1975) and laparoscopic and histological improvement (Dmowski and Cohen, 1975) are impressive and have confirmed the original findings. The overall pregnancy rate of 43 per cent (Greenblatt et al, 1974) gives promise of an extremely useful agent.

Conservative surgery should be employed for disease such as ovarian endometriomata or nodules in the Pouch of Douglas palpable on pelvic examination, when excision of disease and meticulous reconstruction of normal anatomy is important. Pregnancy rates of 40 to 50 per cent are usual (see Kistner, 1975) and tend to occur within two years of operation.

Total hysterectomy may later be necessary or may even need to be performed at the primary laparotomy in older patients with extensive disease. Bilateral oophorectomy and treatment with progestagen postoperatively reduces the symptoms of endometriosis by inducing a surgical menopause and inhibits postmenopausal symptoms. Longer term oestrogen replacement therapy may be required by the patient.

The Male 'Factor'

The history in the male should cover the routine fields of enquiry with particular emphasis on the occupation (including whether or not the environment is hot), duration of involuntary infertility, frequency and adequacy of coitus as well as the nature and duration of any contraception used. Details of all previous conceptions (including extra-marital) should be sought. Relevant past medical history includes venereal disease, tuberculosis, mumps and other viral illnesses, herniorrhaphies, or testicular operations. A family history of recurrent abortions or of abnormal children may suggest chromosomal disorders. On clinical examination attention is paid to general body build, hair distribution, and the type of underclothing worn. The site of the testes is noted (whether scrotal or otherwise) as well as their size and consistency. The normality or otherwise of the remainder of the genitalia is noted, including the prostate and seminal vesicles. Hypospadias may be missed if the foreskin of the penis is not retracted. It is always necessary to have the patient stand and then the scrotal vas is palpated for a cough impulse; unless this is done a varicocoele cannot be excluded.

Investigations

Seminal analysis

There is no substitute for a properly performed seminal analysis in the assessment of fertility in the male. The sample is best collected by masturbation after a period of continence of three to five days. After collection the specimen is kept at room temperature and examined within two hours — condoms should not be used as these destroy the motility of the sperm. The volume of semen produced usually ranges from 1–4 ml and the variables measured are sperm concentration, motility, and morphology. To some extent they are interrelated in as much as if the count is normal so usually are the motility and morphology. However in general deficiencies in one parameter cannot be compensated by above average values for the others. This applies particularly where motility is impaired.

Sperm concentration can be measured in a Neubauer chamber or a Coulter counter and fertility is usually not impaired until the count falls below 20 million/ml. McLeod (1951) found only 5 per cent of conceptions occurring with a sperm concentration less than 20 millions/ml as did Rehan et al (1975) but counts below this are not incompatible with fertility provided motility is good. There is no evidence that fertility is improved by an increase in the sperm concentration, once a certain minimum has been reached. The count can also vary quite substantially in any individual over relatively short periods of time.

Motility (speed of forward progression) is by far the most important measure of semen quality and can compensate for a low sperm concentration. An experienced eye can assess motility as accurately as is required for routine analysis. Fertility is severely impaired once the proportion of actively motile sperm falls below 40 per cent.

Sperm morphology is an index of the state of the germinal epithelium and tends to remain constant for each individual. The smears are usually stained according to the method of Papanicolaou and the oval cell is regarded as the normal form. Most fertile men have at least 60 per cent of their cells morphologically normal. An increase in the number of spermatids and other immature forms has been described as a stress pattern (McLeod, 1970a) and is seen with varicocoele or after allergic reactions or viral illnesses.

Chemical analysis of the seminal fluid is not usually helpful in routine clinical practice, except for the presence of fructose in azoospermic patients. If this is present obstruction of the ejaculatory ducts is excluded.

Hormonal investigations

Urinary 24 hour excretion of FSH and LH, 17 oxo and oxogenic steroids and plasma testosterone as well as thyroid function tests should be done to assess the prognosis as well as excluding more subtle causes of oligospermia. FSH and LH are both necessary for spermatogenesis and where there is severe damage to the germinal epithelium, the FSH levels particularly tend to be well above the normal range (de Kretser, 1974). The exact mechanism by which FSH secretion is controlled is not known, but the process of sperm maturation probably produces a substance ('inhibin') which inhibits FSH secretion directly or via intermediates. It seems likely that the Sertoli cells play a role in this process as well. Testosterone, which inhibits LH secretion, does not directly influence FSH secretion, although it is necessary for spermatogenesis.

Immunological investigations

Theoretically, azoospermia or oligospermia may result from auto-immune destruction of the testes. There has however been no definite evidence to implicate either humoral or cell mediated immune mechanisms in the aetiology of human azoospermia (Wall et al, 1975; Rumke, 1975). On the other hand there is quite good evidence that antibodies to spermatozoa play a part in the pathogenesis of infertility. Antibodies may be agglutinating (Kibrick et al, 1952, Franklin and Dukes, 1964) immobilising (Isojima et al, 1968) or fluorescent (Husted, 1975). Rumke et al (1974) in a study of 254 patients found an inverse correlation between fertility and the titre of sperm agglutinins in the serum as determined by the Kibrick method, and similar findings was reported by Fjallbrant (1965). Ansbacher et al (1973) found the presence of immobilising antibodies to be a more potent barrier to fertility than agglutinins. This was consistent with the findings of Isojima et al (1972) who studied infertile women. Immunofluorescent antibody techniques are relatively new, but they are unlikely to play a significant role in the diagnosis of infertility (Husted, 1975; Husted and Hjort, 1975).

Cytogenetic factors

Genetic factors may influence reproduction either by interfering adversely with gamete production or by elimination of genetically abnormal zygotes. Genetic factors may be clinically recognisable, in the form of an abnormal phenotype, such as Klinefelter's syndrome. Alternatively abnormal chromosomes may preclude the germ cells from entering or completing meiosis, although the phenotype appears normal. Recent progress in cytogenetics, particularly the use of 'C' and 'Q' banding, has made a significant contribution to the understanding of male infertility, and it is now possible to identify accurately almost all chromosome abnormalities (Robinson, 1976).

A peripheral blood karyotype is an essential investigation of an infertile male. The reported incidence of abnormal karyotypes varies from 2 to 6 per cent (Kjessler, 1972; Chandley et al, 1975). The most common abnormality found constituting about half the number is 47XXY (Klinefelter's syndrome). Other abnormalities found include other sex chromosome abnormalities, for example 47XYY as well as autosomal translocations, particularly in the D group (Plymate et al, 1976) and extra marker chromosomes. The incidence of chromosomal abnormalities increases markedly in patients with severe oligospermia and has been reported as high as 20 per cent (Kjessler, 1972). Abnormal sperm morphology has also been found to be increased in these patients, when compared to chromosomally normal infertile men (Chandley et al, 1975).

Meiotic studies

Meiotic studies on testicular biopsy material are becoming less important from the diagnostic aspect since the introduction of the new banding techniques; however some abnormalities cannot be recognised with mitotic karyotypes, for example a reciprocal translocation reported by Chandley et al (1975). Meiotic studies are probably of greater value in furthering our understanding of human male meiosis and the derangements which can occur in this in the presence of abnormal chromosome patterns. They may also be of some value in predicting response to treatment as if there is severe disorganisation of the meiotic process, treatment will probably be of little benefit.

The mechanism by which chromosomal abnormalities gives rise to breakdown of spermatogenesis is not known, but the male seems more susceptible to these than is the female. Reciprocal translocations have been reported which give rise to human male but not female sterility (Chandley et al, 1972).

Testicular biopsy

The value of testicular biopsy in the management of infertile men is now becoming more widely appreciated. It is easy to perform, takes only a few minutes, and has virtually no complications, although a transient fall in sperm count has been noted (Paulsen, 1970). The procedure is usually undertaken on a day case basis under general anaesthesia. It is not necessary to biopsy both testes as the changes seen are bilateral (Hendry et al, 1973). The material is fixed in Bouin's solution and stained with haemotoxylin and eosin in the usual manner. It is also valuable to have meiotic chromosome analysis undertaken as well as electron microscopy if facilities for these procedures exist. Histopathological descriptions of the sections vary from author to author, but in general the appearances range from a normal or near-normal appearance through disorganised or arrested spermatogenesis to Sertoli cell only tubules and tubular hyalinisation. Almost certainly the picture of Sertoli cell only and hyalinised tubules represents a progression in the disease process from other less severe abnormalities. Because of differing histopathological descriptions comparison of the findings of one group with another has been extremely difficult. However a semi-quantitative method, the score count method (Johnsen, 1970), is being used more frequently and biopsy results are now more comparable. The method is an index of the stage of maturation of the germinal epithelium. Histological appearances do not correlate with the clinical findings (Meinhard et al, 1973) but the biopsy score is useful in predicting which patients are likely to respond to treatment — hence the value of biopsy. Those patients with a low score, indicating the absence of spermatids, have a bad prognosis (Hendry et al, 1973, Aafes et al, 1974). A biopsy is also indicated in those patients who have obstructive azoospermia and in whom reanastomosis is contemplated — where the lesion is severe this operation would have virtually no chance of success.

Reassessment

It is customary to review the male partner's data two to three months after the initial consultation. This enables a proper assessment of the case to be made in the light of the results of the investigations, as well as the effect of the general measures outlined below. Most of the oligospermic patients have no demonstrable abnormality so testicular biopsy is then undertaken.

Treatment

General measures

Too frequent intercourse can further deplete a low sperm count, as can the wearing of tight underpants which raise the scrotal temperature. Advice on these measures as well as the limitation of smoking and alcohol intake produced significant improvements in the sperm count in a proportion of cases (Hendry et al, 1973) with only mild degrees of oligospermia. Orthodox Jewish patients may have problems with the nidah but dispensation can be obtained.

Coital difficulties

Impotence is most often due to psychosexual disorders but these should not be diagnosed until organic causes such as diabetes or other neuropathies have been excluded. Hyperprolactinaemia has recently been recognised as an uncommon cause of impotence (Besser and Thorner, 1976). Antihypertensive sympathetic blocking drugs, such as guanethidine, phenothiazines and many others may also cause it (Cooper, 1974). Pituitary tumours have been found in patients with aspermia (orgasm without ejaculation of semen) and loss of libido (Kjessler and Lundberg, 1974). In certain couples extensive investigation may produce or exacerbate impotence (Bullock, 1974). Retrograde ejaculation has usually been managed by insemination with sperm recovered from the urine and successful results have been reported (Bourne et al, 1971), although adrenergic drugs have been reported as successfully correcting this disorder in some patients (Stockamp et al, 1974; Stewart and Bergant, 1974).

Mycoplasma

T-Mycoplasma infections have been implicated in the aetiology of infertility (Friberg and Gnarpe, 1974). This work needs to be confirmed although impaired semen morphology and motility have been demonstrated in men with cultures positive for Mycoplasma (Fowlkes et al, 1975). The recommended treatment is doxycycline 200 mg daily for eight days.

Varicocoele

A varicocoele is found in approximately 10 per cent of the normal population and up to 40 per cent of an infertility clinic (Johnson et al, 1970; Dubin and Amelar, 1971). It results from incompetence or absence of the valves in the internal spermatic vein leading to reflux. Initially only the spermatic vein is involved but secondary incompetence of the cremasteric system may develop in more advanced cases. The effect of a varicocoele on spermatogenesis has been thought to be due to a raised scrotal temperature resulting from interference with the heat exchange of the spermatic artery and vein. However, recent work has suggested that other factors may be involved. A higher tympanic membrane temperature (representing whole body temperature) has been found in vari-cocoele patients (Zorgionotti and McLeod, 1973). Catecholamines have been found in higher concentration in the spermatic vein of varicocoele patients, suggesting that chronic vasoconstriction may be an important aetiological factor (Comhaire and Vermeulen, 1974).

A varicocoele should be ligated and at the same time a testicular biopsy can be taken. Usually only the internal spermatic vein need be ligated and the most common site of ligation is at the level of the inguinal canal; in some cases the cremasteric system needs ligation as well. The pregnancy rate varies from 40 to 55 per cent (McLeod, 1969; Dubin and Amelar, 1975). Since the main effect of treatment is to improve motility the prognosis for pregnancy is much more favourable if the initial sperm count is greater than 10 million/ml. McLeod noted no pregnancies where only the count or the morphology or both improved. Most pregnancies occur six to eight months postoperatively. Ligation may be followed with medical treatment and an improvement in the pregnancy rate has been noted in patients treated with postoperative HCG (Dubin and Amelar, 1975).

Specific Treatment

General

Treatment for the infertile male remains, in general, empirical. When all investigations have been completed usually no definite diagnosis is reached. Therapy therefore has to be administered as a therapeutic trial; however, those patients with evidence on testicular biopsy of early maturation arrest are most unlikely to respond to any form of medical treatment and there seems little point in pursuing this. Similarly patients with Sertoli cells only in the tubules or tubular hyalinisation are beyond therapy, as are those azoospermic patients without a demonstrable blockage. These couples should be informed of this and the alternatives of adoption or artificial insemination discussed.

Hormone therapy

HCG and HMG combined have been shown to be effective in restoring spermatogenesis in parients suffering from hypopituitarism (McLeod, 1970b). However, where gonadotrophin excretion is normal and the defect is thought to be primarily in the testis neither HCG nor HMG alone or in combination has been shown consistently to be of benefit. Success has been claimed in some patients (Schwarzstein, 1974) but the majority show no improvement (Schirren and Toyosi, 1970; Lunenfeld and Shalkovsky-Weissenberg, 1970). More recently LHRH has been used with some benefit (Schwarzstein et al, 1975) but the treatment cannot be considered practicable until a long acting preparation is available.

Testosterone therapy has been used to achieve a 'rebound' phenomenon after producing an initial azoospermia (Rowley and Heller, 1972) but there is a risk of permanent azoospermia and this mode of therapy has generally been abandoned. More recently a new androgen, mesterolone (1α-methyl-5α-androstan-17β-ol-3-one) has been claimed to be useful in the treatment of patients with moderate degrees of oligospermia (but not severe oligospermia or azoospermia) (Schellen and Beck, 1972; Hendry et al, 1973). Its mode of action is uncertain but it may bypass certain metabolic steps necessary for spermatogenesis. Treatment (25 mg four times daily) needs to be continued for at least six months before a satisfactory response is obtained but better data are required to confirm this. A more potent oral androgen fluoxymesterone (9α-fluoro-11β-hydroxy-17α-methyltestosterone) has been advocated where the count is normal but motility is impaired (Brown, 1975). Clomiphene citrate 50 mg daily for three months has been reported as improving the count in some patients (Paulson et al, 1975; Halim et al, 1973).

Surgery

Infertility surgery is limited to bypassing mechanical obstruction. In most cases this involves either epididymovasostomy or vasovasostomy. In recent reviews the pregnancy rate for epididymovasostomy has varied between 5 and 48 per cent (Kar and Phadke, 1975) and for vasovasostomy 10 to 60 per cent (Hulka and Davis, 1972). In the presence of a normal sperm count, failure to achieve pregnancy may be due to immature forms in the ejaculate or the development of antibodies.

Artificial Insemination

Where it seems that the male is the major contributor to a couple's infertility and medical treatment has failed or is inappropriate the question of artificial insemination should be discussed with the couple. (Artificial Insemination may be undertaken with the Husband's semen (AIH) or with Donor semen (AID).

AIH can be undertaken with husband's semen when there are physical abnormalities preventing coitus. Psychosexual difficulties resulting in consummation or impotence must be looked at extremely carefully as pregnancy may not necessarily be a solution to the problem (Cooper, 1974). Recovery of sperm from the urine in cases of retrograde ejaculation has already been described. It is also possible to separate two components of the ejaculate — the first or prostatic component is usually rich in sperm, while the second or vesicular portion contains considerably fewer sperm whose motility is considerably impaired (Eliasson and Lindholmer, 1972). Attempts have, therefore, been made to use the first half of the ejaculate to achieve insemination with a high concentration of ejaculate, but the pregnancy rate has not been consistently high. An alternative would be to store and concentrate oligospermic ejaculates and subsequently inseminate the wife, but poor quality semen does not survive the storage process to a satisfactory degree and, in general, the success rate with this has been low. However, one recent experience with 20 patients has reported a pregnancy rate of 55 per cent (Barwin, 1974). Caffeine has been shown to stimulate sperm motility (Schoenfield et al, 1975) while albumin restored motility in the vesicular component of a split ejaculate (Lindholmer and Eliasson, 1974). These findings may prove beneficial to those patients with a normal sperm count but low motility. In those patients with sperm agglutinins, insemination with washed (to remove the antibodies) and concentrated sperm has been used with some degree of success (Halim et al, 1973).

Where AIH has either failed or is not possible, AID remains the only alternative for the couple. Many couples who would not have previously considered AID are now forced to do so if they are not to remain childless because of the difficulties in obtaining babies for adoption. There are, however, many legal and ethical aspects of AID which must be considered carefully before embarking upon this procedure.

Considerable discussion between the doctor performing AID and both the husband and wife must take place before the decision to proceed is taken. It is important that the degree of rapport between the partners is assessed, although the incidence of divorce in these marriages is low (Behrman, 1975a). The husband's ego may be threatened or there may be conflicts in one or both partners about the desirability of undertaking the procedure. Confidentiality of donor and recipient is essential.

Donors should be matched with the husband as closely as possible and at least in respect of blood group; some practitioners attempt to match physical characteristics as well. The donors are usually medical personnel who are known to the doctor responsible for the insemination — a minimum intelligence is guaranteed, their background is usually known, and they should be responsible enough to declare any family history of disease which would make them unsuitable as donors. Fresh semen or semen which has been stored may be used. Donors however are difficult to recruit even if they are paid and candidates for vasectomy with normal reproductive histories may also be suitable.

Legal and ethical problems

In the United Kingdom children born as a result of AID are technically illegitimate. However since paternity can never be proven, only inferred (in contrast to maternity), registration of the child as the legitimate offspring of the parents involves no act of perjury.

Thus although it may be unlikely that the husband is the genetic father of the child, this can never be proven and a court would assume that a child born to the family was legitimate unless evidence was produced to the contrary. The act of AID is not illegal and the husband's consent is not legally required although it is obviously wise to obtain it. If it is not obtained, the treatment does not constitute adultery by the wife.

In the United States the law varies from state to state but in some states, for example California and Oklahoma, AID is legal and children born of AID are regarded as legitimate provided there has been written consent by both partners.

The doctor has a legal responsibility to exercise a proper degree of care and skill in discharging his duties with AID, no less than any other medical or surgical procedure. It is thus essential that the doctor satisfies himself that the couple are emotionally capable of coping with the problems of AID and child bearing in general, having already warned them of these possibilities. Certain diseases such as gonorrhoea or syphilis or Australia antigen may be transmitted in semen and care should be taken to exclude these. Similarly donor selection is important and reasonable care needs to be shown in excluding a family history of any disease, e.g. diabetes, where a hereditary factor is involved. The possibility exists that a child born of AID might have a right of action against a doctor where it was felt that reasonable care had not been taken. An accidental incestuous relationship between two offspring of the same donor is a possibility if the same donor is used on a number of occasions. Although this is not likely to be a problem at present, it is possible that with more widespread use of AID it could become so.

Ethically, AID raises many problems. The possibility of genetic manipulation by the non-random union of genetic pools needs to be considered, but more fundamental is the physical separation of the act of love between husband and wife from the act of procreation. Such separation could influence the subsequent parent-child relationship, especially that of the father.

Storage of semen

Semen is stored according to the method described by Sherman (1973). Glycerol is added to the specimen and it is then transferred to sterilised ampoules or plastic straws, 1 ml of semen being placed in each ampoule which is then sealed with a gas flame. The ampoules are then cooled in nitrogen vapour and subsequently transferred to a liquid nitrogen tank for storage at $-196°C$. Adequate identification of each specimen is essential and the rate of cooling must be carefully controlled as this has a considerable effect on sperm survival. A typical nitrogen semen tank accommodates approximately 1000 ampoules.

Although sperm banking slightly reduces the fertilising capacity of the sperm there is no evidence of genetic damage induced by freezing and thawing and normal births have been reported with semen preserved for up to 10 years (Sherman, 1973).

Technical aspects

There are relatively few technical problems with AID. The main difficulty is in predicting ovulation in the woman. To circumvent this problem, basal temperature records are used as a guide and confirmed by steroid assays. Most centres use two to four inseminations per cycle to cover the period of ovulation. Where a cycle is irregular, ovulation may be induced. The semen may be injected into the cervix, or placed in a small cup which is left in contact with the cervix for about eight hours; intra-uterine insemination is not often used. The pregnancy rate varies between 50 and 80 per cent and most of the conceptions will have occurred within six months of commencing treatment (Dixon and Buttram, 1976; Chong and Taymor, 1975).

CONCLUSION

Aspect of infertility investigations and treatment of both male and female partners have been described in some detail. The question of abortion has not been discussed but was recently reviewed by Stewart and Cooke (1974) where both the effects of spontaneous and therapeutic abortion in subsequent pregnancy were referred to.

The subsequent obstetric management of any patient conceiving after experiencing infertility requires expert supervision. The pregnancy should be regarded as high risk with delivery in a Consultant unit.

Those patients who do not conceive after perhaps 18 months of investigations and treatment and in whom there is a significant barrier to conception should be given their prognosis as clearly as possible and given an alternative of seeking discussion regarding adoption. It seems inadvisable to have patients returning to the clinic for prolonged periods of time as indicated in the introduction. An early reference to a concluding date for investigations and treatment is a realistic and humane way to manage the couple's problem.

REFERENCES

Aafjes, J. H. & Van Der Vijver, J. C. M. (1974) A relationship between testicular biopsy score count and fertility of men treated for oligospermia. *Fertility and Sterility*, **25**, 809–812.
Adams, M. & Cooke, I. D. (1974) Management of ovulation. *Clinics in Obstetrics and Gynaecology*, **1**, 285–311.
Amoss, M. S. Jr., Monahan, M. W. & Verlander, M. S. (1974) A long-acting polymer-coupled LRF analog. *Journal of Clinical Endocrinology and Metabolism*, **39**, 187–190.
Ansbacher, R., Keung-Yeung, K. & Behrman, S. J. (1973) Clinical significance of sperm antibodies in infertile couples. *Fertility and Sterility*, **24**, 305–308.
Barwin, B. N. (1974) Intrauterine insemination of husband's semen. *Journal of Reproduction and Fertility*, **36**, 101–106.
Behrman, S. J. (1975a) In *Progress in Infertility*, 2nd edn, ed. Behrman, S. J. & Kistner, R. W. p. 779. Boston: Little Brown.
Behrman, S. J. (1975b) In *Progress in Infertility*, 2nd edn, ed. Behrman, S. J. & Kistner, R. W., p. 793. Boston: Little Brown.
Berger, M. J., Smith, D. M., Taymor, M. L. & Thompson, R. S. (1975) Laparoscopic recovery of mature human oocytes. *Fertility and Sterility*, **26**, 513–522.
Berger, M. J., Taylor, M. L. & Patton, W. C. (1975) Gonadotrophin levels and secretory patterns in patients with typical and atypical polycystic ovarian disease. *Fertility and Sterility*, **26**, 619–626.
Bernard, I. & Beauchamps, G. (1971) Notre experience du cyclofenil dans la stimulation de l'ovulation. *Gynecologie et Obstetrique*, **70**, 207–214.
Besser, G. M. & Edwards, C. R. W. (1972) Galactorrhoea. *British Medical Journal*, **ii**, 280–282.
Besser, G. M., Parkes, L., Edwards, C. R. W., Forsyth, I. A. & McNeilly, A. S. (1972) Galactorrhoea: successful treatment with reduction of plasma prolactin levels by Brom-ergocryptine. *British Medical Journal*, **iii**, 669–672.
Besser, G. M. & Thorner, M. O. (1976) Bromocriptine in the treatment of the hyperprolactinaemia — hypogonadism syndromes. *Postgraduate Medical Journal*, **52**, suppl. 1, 64–70.
Black, W. P. & Govan, A. D. T. (1972) Laparoscopy and ovarian biopsy for the investigation of secondary amenorrhoea. *American Journal of Obstetrics and Gynecology*, **114**, 739–747.
Boczkowski, K. (1970) Further observations on the syndrome of pure gonadal dysgenesis. *American Journal of Obstetrics and Gynecology*, **106**, 1177–1183.
Bourne, R. B., Kretzchmar, W. A. & Esser, J. H. (1971) Successful artificial insemination in a diabetic with retrograde ejaculation. *Fertility and Sterility*, **22**, 275–277.

Breckwoldt, M., Czygan, P-J., Lehmann, F. & Bettendorf, G. (1974) Synthetic LHRH as a therapeutic agent. *Acta endocrinologica,* **75,** 209–220.

Brosens, I. A. & de Graef, R. (1975) Microbiopsy of the fallopian tube as a method for clinical investigation of tubal function in infertility. *International Journal of Fertility,* **20,** 55–60.

Brown, J. B., Evans, J. H., Adey, F. D., Taft, H. P. & Townsend, L. (1973) In *Endocrinology,* ed. Scow, R. O., Ebling, F. J. G. and Henderson, I. W. *International Congress series,* pp. 891–896. Amsterdam: Excerpta Medica.

Brown, J. B., Evans, J. H., Adey, F. D., Taft, H. P. & Townsend, S. L. (1969) Factors involved in clinical induction of fertile ovulation with human gonadotrophins. *Journal of Obstetrics and Gynaecology of the British Commonwealth,* **76,** 289–307.

Brown, J. S. (1975) The effect of orally administered androgens on sperm motility. *Fertility and Sterility,* **26,** 305–308.

Bullock, J. L. (1974) Iatrogenic impotence in an infertility clinic: illustrative case. *American Journal of Obstetrics and Gynecology,* **20,** 476–478.

Butler, J. K. (1969) Time course of urinary oestrogen excretion after various schemes of therapy with human follicle stimulating hormone (Pergonal). *Proceedings of the Royal Society of Medicine,* **62,** 34–37.

Butler, J. K. (1972) Clinical results with human gonadotrophins in anovulation using two alternative dosage schemes. *Postgraduate Medical Journal,* **48,** 27–32.

Buttram, V. C. Jr., Vanderheyden, J. D., Besch, P. K. & Acosta. A. A. (1974) Post 'pill' amenorrhoea. *International Journal of Fertility,* **19,** 37–44.

Buttram, V. C. & Vaquero, C. (1975) Postovarian wedge resection adhesive disease. *Fertility and Sterility,* **26,** 874–876.

Buttram, V. C. Jr., Zanotti, L., Acosta, A. A., Vanderheyden, J. S., Besch, P. K. & Franklin, R. R. (1974) Surgical correction of the septate uterus. *Fertility and Sterility,* **25,** 373–379.

Chandley, A. C., Christie, S., Fletcher, J., Freckiewicz, A. & Jacobs, P. S. (1972) Translocation heterozygosity and associated infertility in man. *Cytogenetics,* **11,** 516–533.

Chandley, A. C., Edmond, P., Christie, S., Gowans, L., Fletcher, J., Frackiewicz, A. & Newton, M. (1975) Cytogenetics and infertility in man: I. Karyotype and seminal analysis. *Annals of Human Genetics,* **39,** 231–252.

Chong, A. P. & Taymor, M. L. (1975) Sixteen years' experience with therapeutic donor insemination. *Fertility and Sterility,* **26,** 791–795.

Cooke, I. D., Morgan, C. A. & Parry, T. W. (1972) Correlation of endometrial biopsy and plasma progesterone levels in infertile women. *Journal of Obstetrics and Gynaecology of the British Commonwealth,* **79,** 647–650.

Comhaire, F. & Vermeulen, A. (1974) Varicocele sterility: cortisol and catecholamines. *Fertility and Sterility,* **25,** 88–95.

Cooper, A. J. (1974) Psychosocial factors in infertility. *Clinics in Obstetrics and Gynaecology,* **1,** 429–447.

Cox, L. W. (1975) Infertility — a comprehensive programme. *British Journal of Obstetrics and Gynaecology,* **82,** 2–6.

Crosignani, P. G., Trojsi, L., Attanasio, A., Tonani, E. & Donini, P. (1975) Hormonal profiles in anovulatory patients treated with gonadotrophins and synthetic luteinizing releasing hormone. *Obstetrics and Gynecology,* **46,** 15–22.

de la Cruz, A., de la Cruz, K. G., Arimura, A., Coy, D. H. Vilchez-Martinez, J. A., Coy, E. J. & Schally, A. V. (1975) Gonadotrophin-releasing activity of two highly active and long acting analogues of luteinising hormone releasing hormone after subcutaneous intravaginal and oral administration. *Fertility and Sterility,* **26,** 894–900.

Davajan, V. & Nakamura, R. M. (1975) In *Progress in Infertility,* 2nd edn, ed. Behrman, S. J. and Kistner, R. W., p. 17. Boston: Little Brown.

Davies, I. J. & Ryan, K. J. (1973) The modulation of progesterone concentration in the myometrium of the pregnant rat by changes in cytoplasmic 'receptor' protein activity. *Endocrinology,* **92,** 394–401.

Dewhurst, C. J., de Koos, E. B. & Ferreira, H. P. (1975) The resistant ovary syndrome. *British Journal of Obstetrics and Gynaecology,* **82,** 615.

Dixon, R. E. & Buttram, V. C. Jr. (1976) Artificial insemination using donor semen. A report of 171 cases. *Fertility and Sterility,* **27,** 130–134.

Dmowski, W. P. & Cohen, M. R. (1975) Treatment of endometriosis with an antigonadotrophin, Danazol. A laparoscopic and histologic evaluation. *Obstetrics and Gynecology,* **46,** 147–154.

Dodson, K. S., McNaughton, M. C. & Coutts, J. R. T. (1975) Infertility in women with apparently ovulatory cycles. *British Journal of Obstetrics and Gynaecology,* **82,** 615–624.

Dubin, L. & Amelar, R. D. (1971) Etiologic factors in 1294 consecutive cases of male infertility. *Fertility and Sterility,* **22,** 469–474.

Dubin, L. & Amelar, R. D. (1975) Varicocelectomy as therapy in male infertility: a study of 504 cases. *Fertility and Sterility*, **26**, 217–220.

Duignan, N. M., Jordan, J. A., Coughlan, B. M. & Logan-Edwards, R. (1972) One thousand consecutive cases of diagnostic laparoscopy. *Journal of Obstetrics and Gynaecology of the British Commonwealth*, **79**, 1016–1024.

Eliasson, R. & Lindholmer, C. (1972) Distribution and properties of spermatozoa in different fractions of split ejaculates. *Fertility and Sterility*, **23**, 252–256.

Figueroa Casas, P. R., Badano, A. R., Aparicio, N., Lencioni, L. J., Berli, R. R., Badano, H., Biccoca, C. & Schally, A. V. (1975) Luteinising hormone-releasing hormone in the treatment of anovulatory infertility. *Fertility and Sterility*, **26**, 549–553.

Fjallbrant, B. (1965) Immunoagglutination of sperm in cases of sterility. *Acta obstetrica et gynecologica Scandinavica*, **44**, 474–490.

Fjallbrant, B. (1975) Tubal Surgery. Report of 101 cases with special reference to the experience of the surgeon. *Acta obstetrica et gynecologica Scandinavica*, **54**, 463–467.

Fowlkes, D. M., Macleod, J. & O'Leary, W. M. (1975) T-Mycoplasmas and human infertility. Correlation of infection with alterations in seminal parameters. *Fertility and Sterility*, **26**, 1212–1218.

Franklin, R. R. & Dukes, C. D. (1964) Further studies on sperm agglutinating antibody and unexplained fertility. *Journal of the American Medical Association*, **190**, 682–683.

Franks, S., Murray, M. A. F., Jequier, A. M., Steele, S. J., Nabarro, J. D. N. & Jacobs, H. S. (1975) Incidence and significance of hyperprolactinaemia in women with amenorrhoea. *Clinical Endocrinology*, **4**, 597–603.

Frantz, A. G., Kleinberg, D. L. & Noel, G. L. (1972) Studies on prolactin in man. *Recent Progress in Hormone Research*, **28**, 527–590.

Friberg, J. & Gnarpe, H. (1974) Mycoplasma infections and infertility. In *Male Fertility and Sterility*, ed. Mancini R. E. and Martini, L. pp. 327–336. London: Academic Press.

Garcia, C. R. (1972) Regaining fertility via microsurgery. Presented at *Eleventh Annual Meeting of the American Fertility Society*, April 1972, New York. Cited in *Progress in Infertility*, 2nd edn, ed. Behrman, S. J. and Kistner, R. W., p. 261. Boston: Little Brown.

Gemzell, C. (1975) Induction of ovulation in infertile women with pituitary tumors. *American Journal of Obstetrics and Gynecology*, **121**, 311–315.

Givens, J. R., Andersen, R. N., Wiser, W. L. & Fish, S. A. (1974) Dynamics of suppression and recovery of plasma FSH, LH, androstenedione and testosterone in polycystic ovarian disease using an oral contraceptive. *Journal of Clinical Endocrinology and Metabolism*, **38**, 727–735.

Givens, J. R., Wilroy, S., Summitt, R. L., Andersen, R. N., Wiser, W. L. & Fish, S. A. (1975) Features of Turner's syndrome in women with polycystic ovaries. *Obstetrics and Gynecology*, **45**, 619–624.

Gnarpe, H. & Friberg, J. (1972) Mycoplasma and human reproductive failure. 1. The occurrence of different mycoplasmas in couples with reproductive failure. *American Journal of Obstetrics and Gynecology*, **114**, 727–731.

Gnarpe, H. & Friberg, J. (1973) T-Mycoplasmas as a possible cause for reproductive failure. *Nature*, **242**, 120–121.

Goldzieher, J. W. (1975) In *Progress in Infertility*, 2nd edn, ed. Behrman, S. J. and Kistner, R. W., p. 325. Boston: Little Brown.

Goldzieher, J. W. & Green, J. A. (1964) The polycystic ovary. I. Clinical and histologic features. *Journal of Clinical Endocrinology and Metabolism*, **22**, 325–338.

Gomel, V. (1975) Laparoscopic tubal surgery in infertility. *Obstetrics and Gynecology*, **46**, 47–48.

Gore, B. L. & Gordon, M. (1974) Fine structure of epithelial cell of secretory endometrium in unexplained primary infertility. *Fertility and Sterility*, **25**, 103–107.

Grant, A. (1971) Infertility surgery of the oviduct. *Fertility and Sterility*, **22**, 496–503.

Grant, A. (1973) Infertility due to anovulation before and after the 'Pill era'. *International Journal of Fertility*, **18**, 44–48.

Greenblatt, R. B., Smowski, W. P., Mahesh, V. B. & Scholer, H. F. L. (1971) Clinical studies with an antigonadotrophin — Danazol. *Fertility and Sterility*, **22**, 102–112.

Greenblatt, R. B., Borenstein, R. & Hernandez-Ayup, S. (1974) Experiences with Danazol (an antigonadotrophin) in the treatment of infertility. *American Journal of Obstetrics and Gynecology*, **118**, 783–787.

Halim, A., Antoniou, D., Leedham, P., Blandy, J. P., Tresidder, G. C. (1973) Investigations and treatment of the infertile male. *Proceedings of the Royal Society of Medicine*, **66**, 373-378.

Hancock, K. W. & Oakey, R. E. (1973) The low incidence of pregnancy following clomiphene therapy. *International Journal of Fertility*, **18**, 49–54.

Hendry, W. F., Sommerville, I. F., Hall, R. R. & Pugh, R. C. B. (1973) Investigation and treatment of the subfertile male. *British Journal of Urology*, **45**, 684–692.

Horne, H. W. Jr., Clyman, M., Debrovner, C., Griggs, G., Kistner, R., Kosasa, T., Stevenson, C. S. & Taymor, M. (1973) The prevention of postoperative pelvic adhesions following conservative operative treatment for human infertility. *International Journal of Fertility*, **18**, 109–115.

Horne, H. W. Jr., Kundsin, R. B. & Kosasa, T. A. (1974) The role of mycoplasma infection in human reproductive failure. *Fertility and Sterility*, **25**, 380–389.

Hulka, J. F. & Davis, J. E. (1972) Vasectomy and reversible vasocclusion. *Fertility and Sterility*, **23**, 683–696.

Husted, S. (1975) Sperm antibodies in men from infertile couples. *International Journal of Fertility*, **20**, 113–121.

Husted, S. & Hjort, T. (1975) Sperm antibodies in serum and seminal plasma. *International Journal of Fertility*, **20**, 97–105.

Hwang, P., Guyda, H. & Friesen, H. (1971) A radioimmunoassay for human prolactin. *Proceedings of the National Academy of Sciences of the USA*, **68**, 1902–1906.

Inman, J. I. & Vessey, M. P. (1968) Investigation of deaths from pulmonary coronary and cerebral thrombosis and embolism in women of child bearing age. *British Medical Journal*, **ii**, 193–199.

Isojima, S., Li, T. S. & Ashitaka, Y. (1968) Immunologic analysis of sperm immobilization factor found in sera of women with unexplained sterility. *American Journal of Obstetrics and Gynecology*, **101**, 677–683.

Isojima, S., Tsuchiya, K., Koyama, K., Tanaka, C., Naka, O. & Adachi, H. (1972) Further studies on sperm immobilising antibody found in sera of unexplained cases of sterility in women. *American Journal of Obstetrics and Gynecology*, **112**, 199–207.

Johnson, D. E., Pohl, D. R. & Rivera-Correa, H. (1970) Varicocoele: an innocuous condition? *Southern Medical Journal*, **63**, 34–36.

Johnsen, S. G. (1970) Testicular biopsy score count — a method for registration of spermatogenesis in human testes: normal values and results in 335 hypogonadal males. *Hormones*, **1**, 2–25.

Jones, G. E. S. (1949) Some newer aspects of the management of infertility. *Journal of the American Medical Association*, **141**, 1123–1127.

Kar, J. K. & Phadke, A. M. (1975) Vaso-epididymal anastomosis. *Fertility and Sterility*, **26**, 743–756.

Keller, P. J. (1973) A pituitary function test with synthetic LH releasing hormone. *Journal of Obstetrics and Gynaecology of the British Commonwealth*, **80**, 72–74.

Kelly, J. V. & Rock, J. (1956) Culdoscopy for diagnosis in infertility: report of 492 cases. *American Journal of Obstetrics and Gynecology*, **72**, 523–527.

Kibrick, S., Belding, D. L. & Merrill, B. (1952) Methods for the detection of antibodies against mammalian spermatozoa. II. A gelatin agglutination test. *Fertility and Sterility*, **3**, 430–438.

Kirschner, M. A. & Jacobs, J. B. (1971) Combined ovarian and adrenal vein catheterisation to determine the site(s) of androgen overproduction in hirsute women. *Journal of Clinical Endocrinology and Metabolism*, **33**, 199–209.

Kistner, R. W. (1975a) The management of endometriosis in the infertile patient. *Fertility and Sterility*, **26**, 1151–1166.

Kistner, R. W. (1975b) In *Progress in Infertility*, 2nd edn, ed. Behrman, S. J. & Kistner, R. W., p. 509. Boston: Little Brown.

Kjessler, B. (1973) Genic and chromosomal factors in male infertility. In *Endocrinology*, ed. Scow, R. O., Ebling, F. J. G. and Henderson, I. W. International Congress series, 273, pp. 965–962. Amsterdam: Exerpta Medica.

Kjessler, B. & Lundberg, P. O. (1974) Dysfunction of the neuroendocrine system in nine males with aspermia. *Fertility and Sterility*, **25**, 1007–1017.

Kletzky, O. A., Davajan, V., Nakamura, R. M. & Mishell, D. R. Jr. (1975) Classification of secondary amenorrhoea based on distinct hormonal patterns. *Journal of Clinical Endocrinology and Metabolism*, **41**, 660–668.

Kulin, H., Bell, P. M., Santer, R. J. & Ferber, A. J. (1975) Integration of pulsatile gonadotrophin secretion by timed urinary measurements: an accurate and sensitive 3-hour test. *Journal of Clinical Endocrinology and Metabolism*, **40**, 783–789.

de Kretser, D. M. (1974) The management of the infertile male. *Clinics in Obstetrics & Gynaecology*, **1**, 409–427.

Lamb, E. J. (1972) Prognosis for the infertile couple. *Fertility and Sterility*, **23**, 320–325.

Lenton, E. & Cooke, I. D. (1974) Other disorders of ovulation. In *Clinics in Obstetrics and Gynaecology*, **1**, 313–344.

Lenton, E., Weston, G. & Cooke, I. D. (1977) *Fertility and Sterility*, in press.

Lindholmer, C. & Eliasson, R. (1974) The effects of albumin magnesium and zinc on human sperm survival in different fractions of split ejaculates. *Fertility and Sterility*, **25**, 424–431.

Lunenfeld, B. & Donini, P. (1966) In *Ovulation*, ed. R. B. Greenblatt, p. 105. Philadelphia: Lippincott.

Lunenfeld, B. & Shalkovsky-Weissenberg, R. (1970) Assessment of gonadotrophin therapy in male infertility. *The Human Testis*, ed. Rosemberg, E. and Paulsen, C. A. pp. 613–629. New York: Plenum Press.

Lunenfeld, B. & Insler, V. (1974) Classification of amenorrhoeic states and their treatment by ovulation induction. *Clinical Endocrinology*, **3**, 223–237.

Macleod, J. (1951) Semen quality in one thousand men of known fertility and eight hundred cases of infertile marriage. *Fertility and Sterility*, **2**, 115–139.

Macleod, J. (1969) Further observations on the role of varicocoele in male infertility. *Fertility and Sterility*, **20**, 545–563.

Macleod, J. (1970a) The significance of deviations in human sperm morphology. In *The Human Testis*, ed. Rosemberg, E. and Paulsen, C. A. pp. 481–494. New York: Plenum Press.

Macleod, J. (1970b) The effects of urinary gonadotrophins following hypophysectomy and in hypogonadotrophic eunuchoidism. In *The Human Testis*, ed. Rosemberg, E. and Paulsen, C. A. pp. 577–588. New York: Plenum Press.

MacGregor, A. H., Johnson, J. E. & Bunch, C. A. (1968) Further clinical experience with clomiphene citrate. *Fertility and Sterility*, **19**, 616–622.

McNatty, K. P., Sawers, R. S. & McNeilly, A. S. (1974) A possible role for prolactin in control of steroid secretion by the human Graafian follicle *Nature*, **250**, 653–655.

Malone, L. J. & Ingersoll, F. M. (1975) In *Progress in Infertility*, 2nd edn, ed. Behrman, S. J. & Kistner, R. W., p. 85. Boston: Little Brown.

Matthews, C. D., Elmslie, G., Clapp, K. H. & Svigos, I. M. (1975) The frequency of genital mycoplasma injection in infertility. *Fertility and Sterility*, **26**, 988–990.

Meinhard, E., McRae, C. U. & Chisholm, G. D. (1973) Testicular biopsy in evaluation of male infertility. *British Medical Journal*, **iii**, 577–581.

Melmed, H., Mashiad, S., Insler, V., Lunenfeld, B. & Rabau, E. (1969) The response of the hyposensitive ovary to massive stimulation with human gonadotrophins. *Journal of Obstetrics and Gynaecology of the British Commonwealth*, **76**, 437–443.

Moghissi, K. S. & Sim, G. S. (1975) Correlation between hysterosalpingography and pelvic endoscopy for the evaluation of the tubal factor. *Fertility and Sterility*, **26**, 1178–1181.

Mortimer, C. H., Besser, G. M., McNeilly, A. S., Marshall, J. C., Harsoulis, P., Tunbridge, W. M. G., Gomez-Pan, A. & Hall, R. (1973) Luteinizing hormone and follicle stimulating hormone releasing hormone test in patients with hypothalamic pituitary dysfunction. *British Medical Journal*, **iv**, 73–77.

Mulligan, W. J., Rock, J. & Easterday, C. L. (1953) Use of polyethylene in tuboplasty. *Fertility and Sterility*, **4**, 428–435.

Nadji, P., Reyniak, V., Sedlis, a., Szarowski, D. H. & Bartosik, D. (1975) Endometrial dating correlated with progesterone levels. *Obstetrics and Gynecology*, **45**, 193–194.

Nakano, R., Takekida, H., Kotsuji, F., Miyazaki, Y. & Tojo, S. (1974) Gonadotropin response to a new analogue of luteinizing hormone-releasing factor [Des-Gly-NH$_2^{10}$, Proethylamide^9] — LRF, in man. *Journal of Clinical Endocrinology and Metabolism*, **39**, 802–804.

Nakano, R., Takekida, H., Kotsuji, F. & Tojo, S. (1975) Pituitary response to a new analog of luteinizing hormone-releasing factor during the menstrual cycle. *Obstetrics and Gynecology*, **45**, 263–266.

Newton, J. R. & Dixon, P. F. (1971) Site of action of clomiphene and its use as a test of pituitary function. *Journal of Obstetrics and Gynaecology of the British Commonwealth*, **78**, 812–821.

Newton, J. & Collins, W. (1974) Investigation of hypothalamic pituitary function. *Clinics in Obstetrics and Gynaecology*, **1**, 269–284.

Nillius, S. J. & Wide, L. (1972) The LH releasing hormone test in 31 women with secondary amenorrhoea. *Journal of Obstetrics and Gynaecology of the British Commonwealth*, **79**, 874–882.

Oelsner, G., David, A., Insler, V., Serr, D. M. (1974) Outcome of pregnancy after treatment of intrauterine adhesions, *Obstetrics and Gynecology*, **44**, 341–344.

Parish, W. E. & Ward, A. (1968) Studies of cervical mucus and serum from infertile women. *Journal of Obstetrics and Gynaecology of the British Commonwealth*, **75**, 1089–1100.

Paterson, P., Wood, C. (1974) The use of microsurgery in the reanastomosis of the rabbit fallopian tube. *Fertility and Sterility*, **25**, 756–761.

Paulsen, C. A. (1970) In *The Human Testis*, ed. Rosemberg, E. and Paulsen, C. A., p. 542. New York: Plenum Press.

Paulson, D. F., Wacksman, J., Hammond, C. B. & Wiebe, H. R. (1975) Hypofertility and clomiphene citrate therapy. *Fertility and Sterility*, **26**, 982–987.

Pepperell, R. J., Rennier, G. C., Brown, J. B., Evans, J. H., Taft, H. P., Schiff, P., Burger, H. G. & de Kretser, D. M. (1974) The use of human ovarian responsiveness in a new bioassay for follicle stimulating hormone. *Journal of Clinical Endocrinology and Metabolism*, **39**, 1081–1089.

Perloff, W. H. S., Steinberger, E. (1963) In vitro penetration of cervical mucus by spermatozoa. *Fertility and Sterility*, **14**, 231–236.

Plymate, S. R., Bremner, W. J. & Paulsen, C. A. (1976) The association of D group chromosomal translocations and defective spermatogenesis. *Fertility and Sterility*, **27**, 139–144.

Potter, R. G. & Parker, M. P. (1964) Predicting the time required to conceive. *Population Studies*, **18**, 99–116.

Rebello, R., Green, F. H. Y. & Fox, H. (1975) A study of the secretory immune system of the female genital tract. *British Journal of Obstetrics and Gynaecology*, **82**, 812–816.

Rehan, N. E., Sobrero, A. J. & Fertig, J. W. (1975) The semen of fertile men: statistical analysis of 1300 men. *Fertility and Sterility*, **26**, 492–502.

Ridley, J. H. & Edwards, I. K. (1958) Experimental endometriosis in the human. *American Journal of Obstetrics and Gynecology*, **76**, 783–790.

Robinson, J. A. (1976) Recent advances in cytogenetics and their relevance to medicine. *Proceedings of the Royal Society of Medicine*, **69**, 33–38.

Rolland, R., Schellekens, L. A. & Lequin, R. M. (1974) Successful treatment of galactorrhoea and amenorrhoea and subsequent restoration of ovarian function by a new ergot alkaloid 2-brom-alpha-ergocryptine. *Clinical Endocrinology*, **3**, 155–166.

Rowley, M. J. & Heller, C. G. (1972) The testosterone rebound phenomenon in the treatment of male infertility. *Fertility and Sterility*, **23**, 498–504.

Rumke, P. H. (1975) In *Clinical Aspects of Immunology*, ed. Gell, P. G. H., Coombs, R. R. and Lachman, P. J., p. 1518. Oxford: Blackwell Scientific Publications.

Rumke, P., Van Amstel, N., Messer, E. N. & Bezemer, P. D. (1974) Prognoses of fertility of men with sperm agglutinins in the serum. *Fertility and Sterility*, **25**, 393–398.

Santomauro, A. G., Sciarra, J. J. & Varma, A. O. (1972) A clinical investigation of the role of the semen analysis and postcoital test in the evaluation of male infertility. *Fertility and Sterility*, **23**, 245–251.

Schellen, T. M. C. M. & Beek, J. M. J. H. A. (1972) The influence of high doses of mesterolone on the spermogram. *Fertility and Sterility*, **23**, 712–714.

Schirren, C. & Toyosi, J. O. (1970) Assessment of gonadotrophin therapy in male infertility. In *The Human Testis*, ed. Rosemberg, E. & Paulsen, C. A., p. 605. New York: Plenum Press.

Schoenfeld, C. Y., Amelar, R. D. & Dubin, L. (1975) Stimulation of ejaculated human spermatozoa by caffeine. *Fertility and Sterility*, **26**, 158–161.

Schwarzstein, L. (1974) Human menopausal gonadotrophins in the treatment of patients with oligospermia. *Fertility and Sterility*, **25**, 813–816.

Schwarzstein, L., Aparicio, N. J., Turner, D., Calamera, J. C., Mancini, R. & Schally, A. V. (1975) Use of synthetic luteinizing hormone — releasing hormone in treatment of oligospermic men: a preliminary report. *Fertility and Sterility*, **26**, 331–336.

Serra, G. B. Muscatello, P., Menini, E., Lafuenti, G. & Caniglia, R. (1975) Enhancement of deficient pituitary response to Luteinizing hormone releasing hormone in patients with primary amenorrhoea. *Obstetrics and Gynecology*, **45**, 523–526.

Shaaban, M. & Klopper, A. (1973) A study on the monitoring of gonadotrophin therapy by the assay of plasma oestradiol and progesterone. *Journal of Obstetrics and Gynaecology of the British Commonwealth*, **80**, 783–793.

Shaw, R. W., Butt, W. R., London, D. R. & Marshall, J. C. (1975) The oestrogen provocation test; a method of assessing the hypothalamic-pituitary axis in patients with amenorrhoea. *Clinical Endocrinology*, **4**, 267–276.

Shearman, R. P. (1964) Diagnostic ovarian stimulation with heterologous gonadotrophin. *British Medical Journal*, **ii**, 1115–1116.

Shearman, R. P. (1968) A physiological approach to the differential diagnosis and treatment of primary amenorrhoea. *Journal of Obstetrics and Gynaecology of the British Commonwealth*, **75**, 1101–1107.

Shearman, R. P. (1969) Progress in the investigation and treatment of anovulation. *American Journal of Obstetrics and Gynecology*, **103**, 444–463.

Sherman, B. M. & Korenman, S. G. (1974) Measurement of serum LH, FSH, estradiol and progesterone in disorders of the human menstrual cycle: the inadequate luteal phase. *Journal of Clinical Endocrinology and Metabolism*, **39**, 145–149.

Sherman, J. K. (1973) Synopsis of the uses of frozen human semen since 1964. State of the art of human semen banking. *Fertility and Sterility*, **24**, 397–412.

Shulman, S. & Friedman, M. R. (1975) Antibodies to spermatozoa. V Antibody activity in human cervical mucus. *American Journal of Obstetrics and Gynecology*, **122**, 101–105.

Shulman, S., Jackson, H. & Stone, M. L. (1975) Antibodies to spermatozoa. VI. Comparative studies of sperm agglutinating activity in groups of infertile and fertile women. *American Journal of Obstetrics and Gynecology*, **123**, 139–146.

Siegler, A. M. & Perez, R. J. (1975) Reconstruction of fallopian tubes in previously sterilized patients. *Fertility and Sterility*, **26**, 383–392.

Sillo-Seidl, I. G. (1975) The first transplantation of a fallopian tube of frozen material in woman. *International Journal of Fertility*, **20**, 106–108.

Spellman, C. M., Fottrell, P. F., O'Dwyer, E. M. & Clinch, J. D. (1974) Abnormal endometrial enzyme levels in primary infertility. *Fertility and Sterility*, **25**, 774–777.

Starup, J. (1972) Amenorrhoea following oral contraception. *Acta obstetrica et gynecologica Scandinavica*, **51**, 341–345.

Starup, J. & Sele, V. (1973) Premature ovarian failure. *Acta óbstetrica et gynecologica Scandinavica*, **52**, 259–268.

Steptoe, P. C. & Edwards, R. G. (1970) Laparoscopic recovery of preovulatory human oocytes after priming of ovaries with gonadotrophins. *Lancet*, **i**, 683–689.

Stewart, B. H. & Bergant, J. A. (1974) Correction of retrograde ejaculation by sympathomimetic medication. *Fertility and Sterility*, **25**, 1073–1074.

Stewart, C. R. & Cooke, I. D. (1974) Pregnancy following infertility. *Clinics in Obstetrics and Gynaecology*, **1**, 454–475.

Stockamp, K., Schreiter, F. & Altwein, J. E. (1974) Alpha-adrenergic drugs in retrograde ejaculation. *Fertility and Sterility*, **25**, 817–820.

Strott, C. A., Cargille, C. M., Ross, G. T. & Lipsett, M. B. (1970) The short luteal phase. *Journal of Clinical Endocrinology and Metabolism*, **30**, 246–251.

Swolin, K. (1975) Electromicrosurgery and salpingostomy: long-term results. *American Journal of Obstetrics and Gynecology*, **121**, 418–419.

Swyer, G. I. M., Little, V., Lawrence, D. & Collins, J. (1968) Gonadotrophin stimulation test of ovarian function. *British Medical Journal*, **i**, 349–352.

Tyson, J. E., Andreasson, B., Huth, J., Smith, B. & Zacur, H. (1975) Neuroendocrine dysfunction in galactorrhoea — amenorrhoea after oral contraceptive use. *Obstetrics and Gynecology*, **46**, 1–11.

Umezaki, C., Katayama, K. P. & Jones, H. W. (1974) Pregnancy rates after reconstructive surgery on the fallopian tubes. *Obstetrics and Gynecology*, **43**, 418–424.

Wall, J. R., Stedronska, J., David, R. D. Harrison, R. F., Goriup, D. & Lessof, M. B. (1975) Immunologic studies of male infertility. *Fertility and Sterility*, **26**, 1035–1041.

Warren, W. P., Jewelewicz, R., Dyrenforth, I., Ans, R., Khalaf, S. & Vande Wiele, R. L. (1975) The significance of weight loss in the evaluation of pituitary response to LHRH in women with secondary amenorrhoea. *Journal of Clinical Endocrinology and Metabolism*, **40**, 601–611.

Weström, L. (1975) Effect of acute pelvic inflammatory disease on fertility. *American Journal of Obstetrics and Gynecology*, **121**, 707–713.

Widholm, O. (1973) Clomifen in the treatment of anovulatory women. *International Journal of Fertility*, **18**, 81–84.

Williamson, J. G. & Ellis, J. D. (1973) The induction of ovulation by tamoxifen. *Journal of Obstetrics and Gynaecology of the British Commonwealth*, **80**, 844–847.

Winston, R. M. L. (1975) Microsurgical reanastomosis of rabbit oviduct and its functional and pathological sequelae. *British Journal of Obstetrics and Gynaecology*, **82**, 513–522.

Wood, G. P., Wu, C.-H., Flickinger, G. L. & Mikhail, G. (1975) Hormonal changes associated with Danazol therapy. *Obstetrics and Gynecology*, **45**, 302–304.

Wu, C.-H. (1975) Plasma estrogen monitoring of ovulation induction. *Obstetrics and Gynecology*, **46**, 294–298.

Zarate, A., Canales, E. S., Soria, J., Kastin, A. J., Schally, A. V. & Gonzalez, A. (1974) *Proceedings of the Workshop and Congress on Gonadotrophins and Gonadal steroids*, Milan, 24–26 May, 1973.

Zorgionotti, A. W. & Macleod, J. (1973) Studies in temperature, human semen quality and varicocele. *Fertility and Sterility*, **24**, 854–863.

18
ENDOCRINOLOGY OF THE HYPOTHALAMUS

C. H. Mortimer   G. M. Besser

Since the experiments of Green and Harris (1947) and Scharrer and Scharrer (1954) it has been recognised that the hypothalamus is concerned with the modulation of anterior pituitary function by the secretion of regulatory hormones into the hypothalamic-pituitary capillary portal system. Prior to this it had been established that hypothalamic nuclei synthesise vasopressin, neurophysin and oxytocin which are then transferred to the posterior pituitary to be stored there until required. The implications of the recent synthesis and availability of these hypothalamic hormones together with a review of the rapidly changing field of clinical neuroendocrinology will be considered in this chapter.

THE HYPOTHALAMUS AND ANTERIOR PITUITARY GLAND

Although there was much experimental evidence to suggest that hypophysiotropic substances were synthesised in the hypothalamus, stored in the median enimence and then released into the portal capillaries to control the secretion of anterior pituitary hormones, it was not until 1969 that the structure of such a material was characterised (Folkers et al, 1969; Burgus et al, 1970). This substance was isolated from many hundreds of thousands of pig hypothalami and was shown to be a tripeptide with thyrotrophin (TSH) releasing properties and has been subsequently synthesised by many laboratories. This work provided a major breakthrough in the exploration of hypothalamic–pituitary-target organ function. Previous physiological experiments had been carried out with crude hypothalamic extracts which had been shown either to stimulate or inhibit the release of individual pituitary hormones.

Since the availability of thyrotrophin releasing hormone (TRH), the gonadotrophin releasing hormone (Gn-RH or LH/FSH-RH) and growth hormone release inhibiting hormone (GH-RIH or somatostatin) have been isolated and synthesised (Table 18.1). Since initially these were not available in a pure form the term '*factor*' was applied to these extracts, and the term '*hormone*' has been restricted more recently to substances with a known structure which have been synthesised and their physiological properties validated.

Thyrotrophin Releasing Hormone

The administration of TRH intravenously in doses ranging from 15 to 500 µg results in a dose related secretion of TSH with the peak response occurring at

Table 18.1 Hypothalamic regulatory hormones and factors

		Hormones affected
Releasing hormones (H) or factors (F) for anterior pituitary hormones		
TRH	(pyro-Glu-His-Pro-NH₂)	TSH, prolactin, FSH*, LH*, GH*
Gn-RH	(pyro-Glu-His-Trp-Ser-Tyr-Gly-Leu-Arg-Pro-Gly-NH₂)	LH, FSH, GH*
GH-RF	structure unknown	GH
PRF	,, ,,	Prolactin
CRF	,, ,,	ACTH
MRF	,, ,,	MSH‡
Release inhibiting hormones (H) or factors (F) for anterior pituitary hormones		
GH-RIH	H-Ala-Gly-Cys-Lys-Asn-Phe-Phe-Trp-Lys-Thr-Phe-Thr-Ser-Cys-OH	GH, TSH, FSH, insulin, glucagon, gastrin, VIP, GIP, renin, platelet function.
PIF	Structure unknown ? dopamine	Prolactin
MIF	Structure unknown	MSH‡
Hypothalamic hormones and the posterior pituitary†		
Vasopressin	Cys-Tyr-Phe-Glu-Asp-Cys-Pro-Arg-Gly-NH₂	
Oxytocin	Cys-Tyr-Ileu-Glu-Asp-Cys-Pro-Leu-Gly-NH₂	
Neurophysin	Structure(s) unknown	

* Anterior pituitary hormones which may be released under particular circumstances (see text)
† See text for details of actions
‡ Existence doubtful in man

approximately 20 minutes. This is followed some hours later by an increase in the secretion of triiodothyronine (T_3) and then of thyroxine (T_4) (Lawton, 1972). The TSH responses are greater at night, and in women and in oestrogen-treated men (Weeke, 1974; Mortimer et al, 1974a).

TRH stimulation tests

A standard intravenous TRH test has been developed which will differentiate both hyperthyroidism and hypothyroidism from euthyroid patients. In this test serum immunoreactive TSH is measured before and 20 and 60 minutes after the intravenous injection of 200 μg TRH (Fig. 18.1).

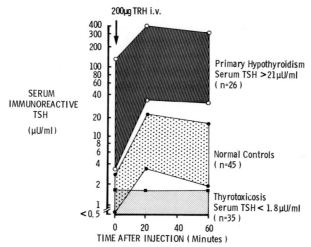

Figure 18.1 TSH responses to TRH (200 μg i.v.) in euthyroid, hyperthyroid, and primary hypothyroid patients. (Reproduced, with permission, from Besser and Mortimer, 1974, *Journal of Clinical Pathology*, **27**, 173)

In hyperthyroidism the high circulating T_3 and T_4 levels inhibit the action of TRH on the pituitary thyrotroph cell and suppress the TSH response. Using the 200 μg test a significant rise (>1 μU/ml) in TSH does not occur in thyrotoxicosis although with larger doses of TRH some TSH secretion may occur. This test provides confirmatory evidence of clinically suspected thyrotoxicosis even when other thyroid function tests are normal or equivocal especially in T_3-toxicosis or borderline T_4-toxicosis. Before this test had been developed the T_3 suppression test was used which required a radioactive iodine uptake study before and seven days after treatment with supraphysiological dose of T_3 (80–120 μg/day). Not only was this test time-consuming, it was also potentially dangerous since it could exacerbate the thyrotoxicosis. The TRH test can be used on an outpatient basis and is without side-effects except for transient flushing or nausea and a desire to micturate. However, few of these symptoms are troublesome. Apart from thyrotoxicosis an absent TSH response may be found in some clinically euthyroid patients on replacement therapy with T_3 or T_4, Cushing's syndrome, corticosteroid therapy, multinodular goitres and Graves' disease despite clinical euthyroidism.

In primary hypothyroidism (due to hypofunction of the thyroid itself) basal TSH levels are usually elevated but in mild cases there may be overlap with the normal range. The TRH test, however, enables hypothyroid patients to be distinguished from normal since the TSH response is excessive in the former group. Occasionally patients are seen who are clinically euthyroid with normal circulating T_3 and T_4 levels, but who have elevated basal serum TSH levels with an excessive response to TRH. These patients may not have objective clinical evidence of thyroid hormone insufficiency and are in a compensated state in which the thyroid gland produces normal amounts of T_3 and T_4 under the stimulation of the increased TSH drive. These patients may require replacement therapy in the future should they become clinically hypothyroid.

In patients developing hypothyroidism due to disorders of the pituitary (secondary hypothyroidism) or hypothalamus (tertiary hypothyroidism) the results of the TRH test are less clearly defined. However, if the patient is clinically hypothyroid, with decreased T_4 levels but with an absent, impaired or normal response to TRH (that is less than excessive), then hypothalamic or pituitary disease should be suspected. If the 20 minute value is normal but is followed by a further increase, so that the 60 minute value is higher than at 20 minutes, this is abnormal and indicates hypothalamic or pituitary disease.

Other hormonal effects

Apart from releasing TSH, TRH stimulates the release of prolactin in both sexes (Jacobs et al, 1971), and follicle stimulating hormone (FSH) in the male only (Mortimer et al, 1974). The latter effect can be suppressed by ethinyl oestradiol, 30 µg daily for three days. Luteinising hormone (LH) is usually unaffected by TRH although Franchimont (1972) reported a rise in some normal women at midcycle. In acromegaly TRH may stimulate growth hormone (GH) release (Irie and Tsushima, 1972). However, this response and the TSH and FSH responses (but not the prolactin response) are inhibited by GH-RIH. This suggests that there is a lack of receptor specificity in acromegaly although not all hormones may be affected.

Gonadotrophin Releasing Hormone

Although it had been expected that there were separate releasing hormones for LH and FSH (McCann, 1962; McCann and Dhariwal, 1966) it proved possible to isolate only a single gonadotrophin releasing hormone (Schally et al, 1971). This decapeptide releases both gonadotrophins in a dose related manner when administered intravenously in doses between 25 and 500 µg (Besser et al, 1972a). Although there is usually a simultaneous increase in circulating LH and FSH levels following an intravenous bolus injection, infusions of Gn-RH have shown that in normal men FSH secretion precedes that of LH by a few minutes, that circulating levels are pulsatile and that the LH and FSH fluctuations are asynchronous (Mortimer et al, 1973b). This suggests that there are times when the pituitary gonadotrophic cells are refractory to the action of the releasing hormone. As well as the different time course of release of the gonadotrophins, the pattern of response alters with age. In prepubertal children the FSH response is similar to that of the adult, but the LH response is slight and smaller than that of FSH; as the patient passes through puberty, the LH response increases to reach the adult pattern with a greater LH than FSH release (Franchimont et al, 1974). In women with a normal menstrual cycle pituitary sensitivity alters with the phase of the cycle. The greatest gonadotrophin response to Gn-RH is seen at the time of ovulation, and is greater in the luteal than the follicular phase (Nillius and Wide, 1972; Yen, VandenBerg, Rebar and Ehara, 1972). These changes in pituitary responsiveness appear to be the result of feed-back effects of changes in circulating oestrogen and progesterone levels. Apart from alteration in pituitary responsiveness there is also evidence of an increase in hypothalamic secretion of endogenous Gn-RH and this may be measured in the circulation at midcycle by radioimmunoassay (Arimura et al, 1974). Our own observations show that secretion of immunoreactive Gn-RH occurs in brief pulses, producing circulating levels which range between <0.2 and 2.5 pg/ml. The effect of oestrogen in combination with progesterone in the second half of the cycle diminishes pituitary responsiveness.

Feedback pathways in males

In men, the effect of oestrogen is different in that there is no clear evidence of positive feed-back at either the pituitary or hypothalamic level. Instead the administration of oestrogen in normal males results in the suppression of basal gonadotrophin levels and of the pituitary response to Gn-RH (Mortimer et al, 1973a). The effect of testosterone on hypothalamic-pituitary function is not clear in the male since there is in vivo conversion to oestrogen (Von zur Mühlen and Köbberling, 1973). However, it would appear that any feed-back effects of testosterone are less suppressive on pituitary function than for a similar increase in oestrogen levels. Dihydrotestosterone probably has little if any inhibitory effect on pituitary function. Gn-RH does not affect the secretion of other pituitary hormones although it may cause GH release in some acromegalics (Faglia et al, 1973).

Gn-RH stimulation tests

Gonadotrophin releasing hormone, as well as TRH, may be used as a test of pituitary function. A standard test has been devised in which serum immunoreactive LH and FSH levels are measured before and 20 and 60 minutes after the intravenous injection of 100 µg Gn-RH. This test is without any side-effects. There is a condition of so called 'isolated gonadotrophin deficiency', in which patients show absent or partial puberty, low or absent circulating gonadotrophin levels with no response to clomiphene, but a normal gonadal steroid response to exogenous gonadotrophins and no other evidence of pituitary deficiency. In this disorder, patients show clear gonadotrophin responses to Gn-RH. This suggests that there is a hypothalamic deficiency of the gonadotrophin releasing hormone, rather than a primary abnormality at the pituitary level (Marshall, et al, 1972; Mortimer et al, 1973c). The administration of Gn-RH to 155 patients with a variety of hypothalamic-pituitary-gonadal defects showed that despite clinical hypogonadism in 137 at the time of testing, only nine had an absent response to the releasing hormone. Normal responses were seen in patients with organic diseases of the hypothalamus (craniopharyngioma) or pituitary (chromophobe adenomas, acromegaly). A normal gonadotrophin response therefore to Gn-RH does not exclude hypothalamic or pituitary disease. Conversely an absent or impaired response indicates the presence of dysfunction and requires further investigation. The test merely indicates the functional reserve capacity of the pituitary for gonadotrophin secretion at the time of testing.

Patients who are postmenopausal or who have primary gonadal failure after the age of normal puberty and therefore deficient in the feed-back effects of gonadal steroids at the hypothalamic or pituitary level (such as Turner's syndrome or patients with Klinefelter's syndrome and low circulating testosterone levels) have excessive gonadotrophin responses to the releasing hormone. Patients with apparent primary gonadal failure who do *not* have an excessive response should be suspected of hypothalamic or pituitary disease. Although gonadal steroids clearly affect gonadotrophin feed-back mechanisms it appears that a further substance, 'inhibin' produced during spermatogenesis, may also be involved in the regulation of FSH secretion. Patients with oligo- or azöospermia but normal testosterone levels and virilisation will often show a normal LH response to Gn-RH but an excessive FSH response indicating the diminished negative feed-back effect of inhibin at the pituitary level. Patients who have azöospermia with normal testosterone levels and LH and FSH responses to the releasing hormone may have blocked vasa deferentia and require investigation.

Therapeutic uses

Since patients with impaired or absent gonadotrophin responses to initial testing with 100 μg of the releasing hormone may be made to release gonadotrophins after repeated stimulation with higher, repeated doses, Gn-RH has been used in the treatment of hypogonadotrophic hypogonadism. Studies of

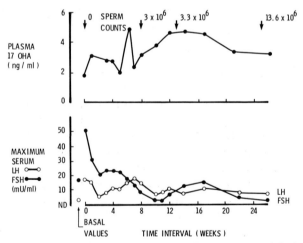

Figure 18.2   Top Plasma 17β-hydroxyandrogen levels (mainly testosterone) during Gn-RH therapy (normal range 5–22.5 ng/ml). Increasing total sperm counts are shown at the top. *Bottom* Maximum serum LH and FSH levels following a therapeutic dose of Gn-RH 500 μg s.c. every 8 h during therapy in a male with acromegaly. (Reproduced, with permission, from Mortimer et al, 1974d, *British Medical Journal*, **4**, 617)

the time course of action of the synthetic decapeptide have shown that it is equally effective in promoting gonadotrophin secretion whether given intravenously, intramuscularly or subcutaneously, although the intranasal route is far less effective (London et al, 1973; Mortimer et al, 1974b). When sufficient supplies of the material became available doses of 500 μg were given subcutaneously, eight hourly to four infertile males with craniopharyngioma, acromegaly or 'isolated gonadotrophin deficiency'. All these patients were treated for up to 18 months. Potency increased within 3–16 days of starting treatment despite only small changes in testosterone levels. During therapy sperm counts increased from zero (or 600 000 dead sperms in the craniopharyngioma patient who had received intramuscular gonadotrophin therapy four months earlier) to maximum total counts of 432, 170, 66 and 7.8 millions with 40 to 75 per cent motility. The initial results in the acromegalic patient are shown in Figure 18.2. This patient's wife became pregnant after he had been on therapy for 16 months when the total sperm count was in the region of 132 millions, and has since delivered a normal boy (Mortimer et al, 1974d). It remains to be seen whether patients with oligospermia due to primary gonadal disease or FSH deficiency can be made fertile. However, since LH and FSH release can be promoted and maintained over long periods in patients who may show no gonadotrophin secretion before treatment, it is clear that Gn-RH stimulates the synthesis as well as the release of gonadotrophins.

Ovulation induction

Subcutaneous Gn-RH in a dose of 500 μg eight hourly has also been used to induce ovulation (Mortimer, Besser and McNeilly, 1975). Four patients with anorexia nervosa and clomiphene unresponsive secondary amenorrhoea of 5–7 years' duration were treated. Two were at their ideal body weight and two of them 3.8 kg and 5.8 kg below this. During initial treatment for 1–7 and then 12–14 days each showed a rise in 24 h urine oestrogens to between 62 and 135 μg/24 h and one patient menstruated although none ovulated. There was evidence of spontaneous LH and FSH release on days 18–28 despite being off therapy indicating that there had been positive feed-back of the rise in circulating oestrogens at the hypothalamic-pituitary level. It seemed that the hypothalamus, pituitary and gonads were no longer functioning in isolation but the normal feed-back cycle of gonadal steroids on the hypothalamic-pituitary system was operating. Two of these patients were then retested with clomiphene 12–14 weeks later and both had now become responsive with a rise in serum gonadotrophins and 24 h urinary oestrogens together with ovulation and menstruation. The other two patients were not retested with clomiphene but received a further course of 14 days' Gn-RH therapy (Fig. 18.3). Both showed a rise in 24 h urinary oestrogens and a rise in plasma progesterone before 4500 units human chorionic gonadotrophin (HCG) had been given, suggesting ovulation had occurred before the HCG. One of these patients then received 28 days of continuous Gn-RH therapy together with HCG on day 14 and became pregnant. Ovulation has also been achieved by other workers with Gn-RH (Zanartu et al, 1973). It may be that Gn-RH therapy will become the treatment of choice replacing gonadotrophin therapy: the gonadotrophin and oestrogen levels

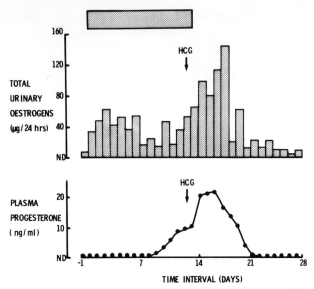

Figure 18.3   Gn-RH therapy, 500 µg s.c. every 8 h for 14 days in a female with anorexia nervosa. Human chorionic gonadotrophin (HCG) 4500 units i.m. was given on day 14. (Reproduced, with permission, from Mortimer et al, 1976, *Annales de Biologie Animale, Biochemie, Biophysique,* **16**, 235)

produced during treatment remain within the physiological range because the normal gonadal-pituitary feed-back mechanisms and cyclicity operate, therefore hyperstimulation and multiple births should be avoided.

Other hormonal effects

Gn-RH may have other effects apart from stimulating secretion of pituitary gonadotrophins. Moss and McCann (1973) and Pfaff (1973) have noted a marked increase in sexual activity in ovariectomised and hypophysectomised rats. This work indicated that Gn-RH was exerting a direct central stimulatory effect on sexual behaviour which was independent of gonadotrophin or gonadal steroid secretion. The implication of these effects in psychogenic impotence in men requires further investigation.

Further analogues more resistant to enzymatic degradation are currently being developed and assessed in order to provide satisfactory and possibly intranasal therapy for male and female infertility.

Growth Hormone Releasing Factor

Growth retardation following the destruction of the ventral hypothalamus in rats was first demonstrated by Hetherington and Ranson (1940). However, an extractable hypothalamic factor responsible for GH release in rats was not isolated until 1964 (Deubin and Meites). Similar releasing factors have been identified in hypophysial portal blood (Wilber and Porter, 1970), and rat stalk median eminence extracts cause the secretion of GH. Although there is clear experimental evidence for the existence of GH-RF this substance remains to be isolated and its amino acid sequence identified.

Growth Hormone Release Inhibiting Hormone

The latest hypothalamic hormone to be isolated is GH-RIH (Brazeau et al, 1973). This hormone has 14 amino acids and was isolated from ovine hypothalami. Preliminary studies showed that it inhibited GH release in animals and man during insulin induced hypoglycaemia, arginine and L-dopa administration, and during sleep and exercise (Hall et al, 1973; Prange Hansen et al, 1973; Siler et al, 1973). In addition it also inhibits TSH and FSH secretion (and GH secretion in acromegaly), but not prolactin secretion after TRH. The gonadotrophin responses after Gn-RH are not affected. Basal TSH levels are suppressed (Weeke, Hansen and Lundbaek, 1975).

As well as suppressing the release of pituitary hormones GH-RIH suppresses pancreatic secretion of insulin (Alberti et al, 1973) and glucagon from the normal pancreas and in a patient with a glucagonoma (Mortimer et al, 1974c), gastrin and gastric acid (Bloom et al, 1974), vasoactive intestinal polypeptide, gastric inhibitory polypeptide, motilin and renin secretion (Besser, Hall, Bloom, Mortimer, Gomez-Pan, unpublished data) and impairs platelet function in baboons, and humans (Koerker, Harker and Goodner, 1975; Besser et al, 1975). Although TRH and Gn-RH may be found outside the hypothalamus, they have not been reported to occur in tissues outside the central nervous system. However, GH-RIH has been localised by immunofluorescent techniques and radioimmunoassay in the stomach and in the pancreatic islets where it may play an important role in the regulation of the secretion of other hormones (Arimura et al, 1975; Polak et al, 1975; Hökfelt et al, 1975).

Therapeutic uses

Since it has such a multiplicity of actions the use of GH-RIH in the treatment of conditions such as acromegaly, diabetes mellitus, Zollinger Ellison syndrome, glucagonoma, and insulinoma, has been contemplated. However, it is likely that the suppression of so many hormones will decrease its therapeutic value unless analogues prove more selective.

Its value in acromegaly has been superseded by the use of the ergot alkaloid, bromocriptine. This dopaminergic drug was shown to lower GH levels in this condition in 1972 (Liuzzi et al, 1972). Subsequently it was used as long-term therapy with clinical as well as biochemical improvement in acromegalic patients (Thorner et al, 1975b). Dopamine is found in the hypothalamus as well as throughout the central nervous system and may play an important role in the regulation of pituitary function.

Prolactin Releasing Factor

Evidence for a prolactin releasing hormone has been provided following injections of crude rat hypothalamic extracts into oestrogen primed rats which showed an increase in circulating levels of prolactin. However, although TRH produces prolactin secretion it is not thought to be the physiologically important prolactin releasing hormone. The actions of TRH on prolactin and TSH secretion may be dissociated, e.g. in isolated TSH deficiency (Sachson et al, 1972). The secretion of PRF, probably a polypeptide, may be dependent on serotonin as the intrahypothalamic transmitter. However, the nature of this hormone remains to be elucidated.

Prolactin Release Inhibiting Factor

Prolactin was the first hormone shown to be predominantly under the control of a hypothalamic inhibitory influence (Desclin, 1950; Everett, 1954). It was observed that removal of the pituitary and transplantation to the renal capsule resulted in the maintenance of the function of corpora lutea and mammary glands. Later it was shown that median eminence or pituitary stalk lesions would result in continuous release of prolactin in rats in vivo (Meites, Nicoll and Talwalker, 1963). Similarly patients with pituitary stalk lesions will continue to secrete prolactin. This may also occur with pituitary cell tumours secreting prolactin autonomously. Although the exact nature of prolactin release inhibiting factor (PIF) is not known, recent work (Schally et al, 1974), suggested that the most active purified hypothalamic extracts contained no peptide, only catecholamines including dopamine. It has been shown subsequently that dopamine itself can suppress prolactin levels by a direct action at the pituitary level. Although a polypeptide hormone has been sought there is as yet no evidence of its identity, and it seems likely that dopamine itself is an important PIF.

In the clinical situation, dopaminergic agonists have been used to lower normal or elevated prolactin levels. Dopamine infusions (or its precursor L-dopa) lower prolactin levels although the effects are only transient (Malarky, Jacobs and Daughaday, 1971). More recently an ergot alkaloid, 2-bromergocriptine (bromocriptine, CB154) has been shown to be a long acting dopaminergic agent and it is highly effective in lowering prolactin levels (Besser et al, 1972b).

Hyperprolactinaemia

The majority of patients with hyperprolactinaemia whether male or female are hypogonadal and may have galactorrhoea. There is no evidence in humans for a reciprocal relationship between gonadotrophins and prolactin and there does not appear to be competition for their release (Mortimer et al, 1973d). The action of prolactin in inducing hypogonadism may be to interfere directly at the gonadal level by inhibiting the action of gonadotrophins (McNatty, Sawers, and McNeilly, 1974; Thorner et al, 1974), although an effect at the hypothalamic level cannot be ruled out.

Treatment of hyperprolactinaemia with bromocriptine results in a rapid return of libido and regular menstruation and fertility and has not been shown to be associated with teratogenicity. However, patients are told to stop taking the drug if a period is missed so that there is minimum exposure of the foetus to the drug. So far in our series 13 patients with hyperprolactinaemia, 5 with proven or suspected pituitary tumours, have conceived and have to date delivered 12 normal children (Thorner et al, 1975a).

Corticotrophin Releasing Factor

The identity of CRF is still not known although evidence for the release of adrenocorticotrophic hormone (ACTH) by crude median extracts has been demonstrated (Saffran, Schally, and Benfey, 1955). This activity was differentiated from vasopressin (which has CRF activity) by bioassay (Anderson, 1966) although the structure of the hormone remains to be determined.

Melanocyte Releasing Factor and Melanocyte Release Inhibiting Factor

Melanocyte stimulating hormone (MSH) is a pigment-regulating hormone in lower animals although its existence in man has recently been placed in doubt (Bloomfield et al, 1974). However, in other animals it has been demonstrated that MSH is under the control of two agents melanocyte releasing factor (MRF) and melanocyte release inhibiting factor (MIF) (Kastin, Miller and Schally, 1968; Kastin et al, 1969). Although MRF and MIF appear to be active in lower animals they have not been shown to be active in man.

THE HYPOTHALAMUS AND POSTERIOR PITUITARY GLAND

As early as 1895 it had been demonstrated that extracts of the posterior lobe of the pituitary caused transient peripheral vasoconstriction and an increase in blood pressure. A further active material was shown to stimulate uterine muscle and was named oxytocin. A third was then described with a molecular weight of approximately 30 000 and was called neurophysin, which appeared to be a carrier protein for both the other active substances (Van Dyke, 1968; Acher, 1968). Although these hormones were thought of as posterior pituitary hormones they are in fact synthesised in the hypothalamus before being transported, viâ the axons leading from the cell bodies of the hypothalamic nuclei ('neurosecretion'), to the posterior pituitary for storage and release.

The release of the antidiuretic hormone (ADH) is under neural rather than humoral control. Stimuli for its release arrive from both the peripheral and central nervous system and are transmitted to the posterior pituitary via the hypothalamus. Osmolar and plasma volume mediated control are the most important, but stress is also effective. Vasopressin release is stimulated by acetylcholine and nicotine.

Syndrome of Inappropriate ADH Secretion

Apart from the physiological control of ADH, the syndrome of inappropriate ADH secretion has been described and is a common clinical problem (Schwartz et al, 1957). This is characterised by hyponatraemia and may be accompanied by anorexia and vomiting with bizarre mental behaviour. Serum chloride and urea concentrations also fall and although the total body water concentration is increased, oedema is unusual. It is associated with many conditions including ectopic hormone production from malignant tumours, hypothyroidism, pneumonia, pulmonary tuberculosis, lung abscess and trauma as well as inflammatory diseases of the central nervous system (Chard and Edwards, 1972). Except when there is ectopic production from tumours, it is assumed that the excess ADH comes from the hypothalamus but the mechanisms involved are unknown. Treatment consists of water restriction to under one litre per day and of therapy of the causative lesion.

Diabetes Insipidus

Patients with hypothalamic lesions such as craniopharygiomas, or conditions such as histiocytosis or other tumours may have a varying deficiency of ADH resulting in cranial diabetes insipidus. Until recently such patients were treated with intramuscular injections of an impure pituitary extract, pitressin. Recently an analogue of vasopressin, DDAVP (desamino′-d-arg⁸-vasopressin, Desmopressin) has been developed with a longer action and negligible pressor effects. This preparation is now available and is usually given intranasally (Edwards et al, 1973): 10 to 20 μg given intranasally works for about 12 hours. However, it should be remembered that a few patients may recover hypothalamic function and therefore be able to stop continuous medication.

Oxytocin

Oxytocin-stimulating pathways arise from the nipple and cervix before ending in the hypothalamus; other endings within the cerebrum may have inhibitory effects.

The role of oxytocin in the human in labour is far from established since normal deliveries occur in patients with posterior pituitary disease (Chau, Fitzpatrick and Jamieson, 1969). However, it has been suggested that oxytocin from the fetal posterior pituitary gland may play an important part in labour (Chard et al, 1971).

Ectopic production of oxytocin has been described in a pancreatic tumour (Marks et al (1968).

Neurophysins

Since the discovery of carrier proteins for oxytocin and vasopressin, these have been shown in several species. There are at least two which have molecular weights of between 9000 to 30 000 and there may be species specificity (Ginsberg, Jayasena and Thomas, 1966; Hope and Hollenberg, 1968). The vasopressin-related neurophysin also appears to be released into the peripheral circulation and may provide an indication of neurohypophysial function.

SUMMARY

It is clear that there have been many major advances in the understanding of the endocrinology of the hypothalamus since the availability of the purified hormones and the ability to assay them. It is therefore expected that further basic physiological information on the complex interactions of the hypothalamic-pituitary-target organ system will be clarified in the near future possibly leading to earlier recognition and treatment of as yet obscure disease syndromes.

ACKNOWLEDGEMENTS

We wish to thank the editor of the *Journal of Clinical Pathology* for permission to reproduce Figure 18.1, the editor of the *British Medical Journal* for Figure 18.2, and the editor of *Annales de Biologie Animale, Biochimie, Biophysique* for Figure 18.3.

REFERENCES

Acher, R. (1968) Neurophysin and neurohypophysial hormones. *Proceedings of the Royal Society, (Biol)*, **170**, 7–16.

Alberti, K. G. M. M., Christensen, N. J., Christensen S. E., Prange Hansen, Aa., Iversen, J., Lundbaek, K., Seyer-Hansen, K. & Ørskov, H. (1973) Inhibition of insulin secretion by somatostatin. *Lancet*, **ii**, 1299–1300.

Anderson, E. (1966) Adrenocorticotrophin-releasing hormone in peripheral blood: increase during stress. *Science*, **152**, 379–380.

Arimura, A., Kastin, A. J., Schally, A. V., Saito, M., Kumasaka, T., Yaoi, Y., Nishi, N. & Ohjura, K. (1974) Immunoreactive LH-releasing hormone in plasma: mid-cycle elevation in women. *Journal of Clinical Endocrinology and Metabolism*, **38**, 510–513.

Arimura, A., Sato, H., Dupont, A., Nishi, N. & Schally, A. V. (1975) Abundance of immunoreactive GH-release inhibiting hormone in the stomach and the pancreas of rat. *Federation Proceedings*, **34**, 273.

Besser, G. M., McNeilly, A. S., Anderson, D. C., Marshall, J. C., Harsoulis, P., Hall, R., Ormston, B. J., Alexander, L. & Collins, W. P. (1972a) Hormonal responses to synthetic luteinising hormone and follicle stimulating hormone releasing hormone in man. *British Medical Journal*, **3**, 267–271.

Besser, G. M., Parke, L., Edwards, C. R. W., Forsyth, I. A. & McNeilly, A. S. (1972b) Galactorrhoea: successful treatment with reduction of plasma prolactin levels by bromoergocryptine. *British Medical Journal*, **3**, 669–672.

Besser, G. M., Paxton, A. M., Johnson, S., Moody, E., Mortimer, C. H., Hall, R., Gomez-Pan, A., Schally, A. V., Kastin, A. J. & Coy, D. H. (1975) Impairment of platelet function by growth-hormone release-inhibiting hormone. *Lancet*, **ii**, 1166–1168.

Bloom, S. R., Mortimer, C. H., Besser, G. M., Hall, R., Gomez-Pan, A., Russell, R. C. G., Coy, D. H., Kastin, A. J. & Schally, A. V. (1974) Inhibition of gastrin and gastric acid secretion by growth-hormone release inhibiting hormone. *Lancet*, **ii**, 1106–1113.

Bloomfield, G. A., Scott, A. P., Lowry, P. J., Gilkes, J. J. H. & Rees, L. H. (1974) A reappraisal of human β MSH. *Nature*, **252**, 492–493.

Brazeau, P., Vale, W., Burgus, R., Ling, N., Butcher, M., Rivier, J. & Guillemin, R. (1973) Hypothalamic polypeptide that inhibits the secretion of immunoreactive pituitary growth hormone. *Science*, **179**, 77–79.

Burgus, R., Dunn, T. F., Desiderio, D., Ward, D. N., Vale, W. & Guillemin, R. (1970) Characterisation of ovine hypothalamic hypophysiotropic TSH-releasing factor. *Nature*, **226**, 321–325.

Chard, T. & Edwards, C. R. W. (1972) The hypothalamus and posterior pituitary. In *Modern Trends in Endocrinology*, vol. 4, ed. Prunty, F. T. G. and Gardiner-Hill, H. p. 102. Butterworth.

Chard, T., Hudson, C. N., Edwards, C. R. W. & Boyd, N. R. H. (1971) Release of oxytocin and vasopressin by the human fetus during labour. *Nature*, **234**, 352–354.

Chau, S. S., Fitzpatrick, R. J. & Jamieson, B. (1969) Diabetes insipidus and parturition. *Journal of Obstetrics and Gynaecology in the British Commonwealth*, **76**, 444–450.

Edwards, C. R. W., Kitau, M. J., Chard, T. & Besser, G. M. (1973) Vasopressin analogue DDAVP in Diabetes Insipidus: clinical and laboratory studies. *British Medical Journal*, **3**, 375–378.

Everett, J. W. (1954) Luteotrophic function of autografts of the rat hypophysis. *Endocrinology*, **54**, 685–690.

Faglia, G., Beck-Peccoz, P., Ferrari, C., Travaglini, P., Parrachi, A., Spada, A. & Lewin, A. (1973) Plasma growth hormone response to gonadotrophin releasing hormone in patients with active acromegaly. *Journal of Clinical Endocrinology and Metabolism*, **36**, 1259–1262.

Folkers, K., Enzman, F., Boler, J., Bowers, C. Y. & Schally, A. V. (1969) Discovery of modification of the synthetic tripeptide sequence of the thyrotropin releasing hormone having activity. *Biochemical and Biophysical Research Communications*, **37**, 123–126.

Franchimont, P. (1972) Thyrotrophin releasing hormone. In *Frontiers in Hormone Research*, 1972, vol. 1, ed. Hall, R., Werner, I. and Holgate, H. p. 139. Basel: Karger.

Franchimont, P., Becker, H., Ernould, G., Thys, C., Demoulin, A., Bourguignon, J. P., Legros, J. J. & Valcke, J. C. (1974) The effect of hypothalamic luteinising hormone releasing hormone (LH-RH) on plasma gonadotrophin levels in normal subjects. *Clinical Endocrinology*, **3**, 27–39.

Ginsburg, M. O., Jayasena, K. & Thomas, P. J. (1966) Preparation and properties of porcine neurophysin and the influence of calcium on hormone — neurophysin complex. *Journal of Physiology*, **184**, 387–401.

Green, J. D. & Harris, G. W. (1947) The neurovascular link between the neurohypophysis and adenohypophysis. *Journal of Endocrinology*, **5**, 136.

Hall, R., Besser, G. M., Schally, A. V., Coy, D. H., Evered, D., Goldie, D. J., Kastin, A. J., McNeilly, A. S., Mortimer, C. H., Tunbridge, W. M. G., Phenekos, C. & Weightman, D. (1973) Action of growth-hormone release-inhibiting hormone in healthy men and in acromegaly. *Lancet*, **ii**, 581–584.

Hökfelt, T., Etendić, S., Hellerström, C., Johansson, O., Luft, R. & Arimura, A. (1975) Cellular localisation of somatostatin in endocrine-like cells and neurones of the rat with special references to the A₁-cells of the pancreatic islets and to the hypothalamus. *Acta Endocrinologica*, **80** (Suppl. 200).

Hope, D. B. & Hollenberg, M. D. (1968) Crystallisation of complexes of neurophysins with vasopressins and oxytocin. *Proceedings of the Royal Society*, **170**, 37–47.

Irie, M. & Tsushima, T. (1972) Increase in serum growth hormone concentration following thyrotrophin-releasing hormone injection in patients with acromegaly or gigantism. *Journal of Clinical Endocrinology and Metabolism*, **35**, 97–100.

Jacobs, L. S., Snyder, P. J., Wilber, J. F., Utiger, R. D. & Daughaday, W. H. (1971) Increased serum prolactin after administration of synthetic TRH in man. *Journal of Clinical Endocrinology and Metabolism*, **33**, 996–998.

Kastin, A. J., Miller, M. C. & Schally, A. V. (1968) MSH activity in the rat pituitary after treatment with nembutal and morphine: a new bioassay for MSH-release inhibiting factor (MIF). *Endocrinology*, **83**, 137–140.

Kastin, A. J., Schally, A. V., Viasca, S. & Miller, M. C. (1969) MSH activity in plasma and pituitaries of rats after various treatments. *Endocrinology*, **84**, 20–29.

Koerker, D. J., Harker, L. A. & Goodner, C. H. (1975) Effects of somatostatin on hemostasis in baboons. *New England Journal of Medicine*, **293**, 476–479.

Lawton, N. F. (1972) Effects of TRH on thyroid hormone release: In *Frontiers in Hormone Research*, vol. 1, ed. Hall, R., Werner, I. and Holgate, H., pp. 91–113. Basel: Karger.

Liuzzi, A., Chiodini, P. G., Botalla, L., Cremoscoli, G. & Silverstrini, F. (1972) Inhibitory effect of l-dopa on GH release in acromegalic patients. *Journal of Clinical Endocrinology and Metabolism*, **35**, 941–943.

London, D. R., Butt, W. R., Lynch, S. S., Marshall, J. C., Owusu, S., Robinson, W. R. & Stephenson, J. M. (1973) Hormonal responses to intranasal luteinising hormone-releasing hormone. *Journal of Clinical Endocrinology and Metabolism*, **31**, 829–831.

Malarky, W. B., Jacobs, L. S. & Daughaday, W. H. (1971) Levo-dopa suppression of prolactin in non-puerperal galactorrhoea. *New England Journal of Medicine*, **285**, 1160–1163.

Marks, L. J., Berde, B., Klein, C. A., Roth, J., Goonan, S. R., Blumen, D. & Nabseth, D. C. (1968) Inappropriate vasopressin secretion and carcinoma of the pancreas. *American Journal of Medicine*, **45**, 967–982.

Marshall, J. C., Harsoulis, P., Anderson, D. C., McNeilly, A. S., Besser, G. M. & Hall, R. (1972) Isolated pituitary gonadotrophin deficiency: gonadotrophin secretion after synthetic luteinising hormone and follicle stimulating hormone. *British Medical Journal*, **4**, 643–645.

McCann, S. M. (1962) A hypothalamic luteinising releasing factor. *American Journal of Physiology*, **202**, 395–400.

McCann, S. M. and Dhariwal, A. P. S. (1966) Hypothalamic releasing factors and the neurosecretory link between the brain and anterior pituitary. *Neuroendocrinology*, **1**, 261–296.

McNatty, K. P., Sawers, R. S. & McNeilly, A. S. (1974) A possible role for prolactin in control of steroid secretion by the human graafian follicle. *Nature New Biology*, **250**, 653–655.

Meites, J., Nicoll, C. S. & Talwalker, P. I. C. (1963) The central nervous system and the secretion and release of prolactin. In *Advances in Neuroendocrinology*, ed. Nalbandov, A. V. Urbana: University of Illinois Press.

Moss, R. L. & McCann, S. M. (1973) Induction of mating behaviour in rats by luteinising hormone-releasing factor. *Science*, **181**, 177–179.

Mortimer, C. H., Besser, G. M., Goldie, D. J., Hook, J. & McNeilly, A. S. (1974a) The TSH and prolactin responses to continuous infusions of TRH and the effects of oestrogen administration in normal males. *Clinical Endocrinology*, **3**, 97–103.

Mortimer, C. H., Besser, G. M., Hook, J. & McNeilly, A. S. (1974b) Intravenous intramuscular subcutaneous and intranasal administration of LH/FSH-RH: the duration of effect and occurrence of asynchronous pulsatile release of LH and FSH. *Clinical Endocrinology*, **3**, 19–25.

Mortimer, C. H., Besser, G. M., McNeilly, A. S. & Goldie, D. (1973a) Asynchronous pulsatile LH and FSH responses during LH/FSH-RH. *Journal of Endocrinology*, **59**, 12–13.

Mortimer, C. H., Besser, G. M., McNeilly, A. S., Goldie, D. H. & Hook, J. (1973b) Asynchronous changes in circulating LH and FSH after the gonadotrophin releasing hormone. *Nature*, **246**, 22–23.

Mortimer, C. H., Besser, G. M. & McNeilly, A. S. (1975) Gonadotrophin releasing hormone therapy in the induction of puberty, potency, spermatogenesis and ovulation in patients with hypothalamic pituitary gonadal dysfunction. In *Hypothalamic Hormones, Chemistry, Physiology, Pharmacology, and Clinical Uses*. New York: Academic Press.

Mortimer, C. H., Besser, G. M., McNeilly, A. S., Marshall, J. C., Harsoulis, P., Tunbridge, W. M. G., Gomez-Pan, A. & Hall, R. (1973c) The LH and FSH releasing hormone test in patients with hypothalamic-pituitary-gonadal dysfunction. *British Medical Journal*, **4**, 73–77.

Mortimer, C. H., Besser, G. M., McNeilly, A. S., Tunbridge, W. M. G., Gomez-Pan, A. & Hall, R. (1973d). Interaction between secretion of the gonadotrophins, prolactin, growth hormone, thyrotrophin and corticosteroids in man: the effects of LH/FSH-RH, TRH and hypoglycaemia alone and in combination. *Clinical Endocrinology*, **2**, 317–326.

Mortimer, C. H., Carr, D., Lind, T., Bloom, S. R., Mallinson, C. N., Schally, A. V., Tunbridge, W. M. G., Yeomans, L., Coy, D. H., Kastin, A. J., Besser, G. M. & Hall, R. (1974c) Growth hormone release inhibiting hormone: effects on circulating glucagon, insulin and growth hormone in normal diabetic, acromegalic and hypopituitary patients. *Lancet*, **i**, 697–701.

Mortimer, C. H., McNeilly, A. S., Murray, M. A. F., Fisher, R. A. F. & Besser, G. M. (1974d) Gonadotrophin releasing hormone therapy in hypogonadal males with hypothalamic pituitary dysfunction. *British Medical Journal*, **4**, 617–621.

Nillius, S. J. & Wide, L. (1972) Variation in LH and FSH response to LH-releasing hormone during the menstrual cycle. *Journal of Obstetrics and Gynaecology in the British Commonwealth*, **79**, 865.

Pfaff, D. W. (1973) Luteinising hormone-releasing factor potentiates lordosis behaviour in hypophysectomised, ovariectomised female rats. *Science*, **182**, 1148–1149.

Polak, J. M., Grimelius, L., Pearse, A. G. E., Bloom, S. R. & Arimura, A. (1975) Growth hormone release-inhibiting hormone in gastrointestinal and pancreatic D cells. *Lancet*, **i**, 1220–1222.

Prange Hansen, Aa., Ørskov, H., Seyer-Hansen, K. & Lundbaek, K. (1973) Some actions of growth hormone release inhibiting factor. *British Medical Journal*, **3**, 523–524.

Sachson, R., Rosen, S. W., Cuatrecasas, P., Roth, J. & Frantz, A. G. (1972) Prolactin stimulation by thyrotrophin-releasing hormone in a patient with isolated thyrotrophin deficiency. *New England Journal of Medicine*, **287**, 972–973.

Saffran, M., Schally, A. V. & Benfey, B. G. (1955) Stimulation of the release of corticotropin from the adenohypophysis by a neurohypophysial factor. *Endocrinology*, **57**, 439–444.

Schally, A. V., Arimura, A., Baba, Y., Nair, R. M. G., Matsuo, A., Redding, T. W., Debeljuk, L. & White, M. F. (1971) Isolation and properties of the FSH and LH releasing hormone. *Biochemical and Biophysical Research Communications*, **43**, 393–399.

Schally, A. V., Arimura, A., Takahara, J., Redding, T. W. & Dupont, A. (1974) Inhibition of prolactin release in vitro and in vivo by catecholamines. *Federation Proceedings*, **33**, 237.

Scharrer, E. & Scharrer, B. (1954) Hormones produced by neurosecretory cells. *Recent Progress in Hormone Research*, **10**, 183.

Schwartz, W. B., Bennett, W., Curelop, S. & Bartter, F. C. (1957) A syndrome of renal sodium loss and hyponatremia probably resulting from inappropriate secretion of antidiuretic hormone. *American Journal of Medicine*, **23**, 529–542.

Siler, T. M., VandenBerg, G., Yen, S. S. C., Brazeau, P., Vale, W. & Guillemin, R. (1973) Inhibition of growth hormone release in humans by somatostatin. *Journal of Clinical Endocrinology and Metabolism*, **37**, 632–634.

Thorner, M. O., Besser, G. M., Jones, A., Dacie, J. & Jones, A. E. (1975a) Bromocriptine therapy of female infertility: a report of 13 pregnancies. *British Medical Journal*, **4**, 694–697.

Thorner, M. O., Chait, A., Aitken, M., Benker, G., Bloom, S. R., Mortimer, C. H., Sanders, P., Stuart Mason, A. & Besser, G. M. (1975b) Bromocriptine treatment of acromegaly. *British Medical Journal*, **1**, 299–303.

Thorner, M. O., McNeilly, A. S., Hagen, C. & Besser, G. M. (1974) Long term treatment of galactorrhoea and hypogonadism with bromocriptine. *British Medical Journal*, **2**, 419–427.

Van Dyke, H. B. (1968) Isolation from the posterior lobe of the pituitary gland of a protein specifically but loosely binding oxytocin and vasopressin. *Proceedings of the Royal Society (Biol)*, **170**, 3–5.

Von zur Mühlen, A. & Kobberling, J. (1973) Effects of testosterone on the LH and FSH release induction by LH releasing factor (LRF) in normal subjects. *Hormone and Metabolic Research*, **5**, 266.

Weeke, J., Hansen, A. P. & Lundbaek, K. (1975) Inhibition of somatostatin of basal levels of serum thyrotropin (TSH) in normal men. *Journal of Clinical Endocrinology and Metabolism*, **41**, 168–171.

Wilber, J. F. & Porter, J. C. (1970) Thyrotropin and GH activity in hypophysial portal blood. *Endocrinology*, **87**, 807–811.

Yen, S. S. C., VandBerg, G., Rebar, R. & Ehara, Y. (1972) Variation of pituitary responsiveness to synthetic LRF during different phases of the menstrual cycle. *Journal of Clinical Endocrinology and Metabolism*, **35**, 931–934.

Zanartu, J., Dabancens, A., Rodriguez-Bravo, R. & Schally, A. V. (1973) Induction of ovulation with synthetic gonadotrophin releasing hormone in women with constant anovulation induced by contraceptive steroids. *British Medical Journal*, **1**, 605–608.

INDEX

Norleucine
synthesis of motilin, 374

Obesity
association with cholelithiasis, 342
Obsessional neurosis, 200–202
choice of treatment, 216–218
combination of drug and behaviour therapy,
213–214
measurement of symptoms, 201–202
obsessional ruminations, 209–210
psychosurgery, 214–216
psychotropic drugs, 210–213
treatment of obsessional rituals, 206–209⁻
Oesophageal carcinoma, 2–4
incidence, 2–3
Oesophagitis, 329–330
Oligomenorrhoea, 407, 416
Oligo-ovulation, 408
Oligospermia, 422, 426, 447
Oncovin
treatment of Hodgkin's disease, 32
Ophthalmia neonatorum, 158
Oral contraceptives
and adenoma of the liver, 10
high-oestrogen
causes of secondary hyperlipidaemias, 264
reduction of endometriosis, 424
Ovarian disease, polycystic, 422
Ovarian endometriomata, 424
Overnutrition and diet, 346
Ovulation
defective, 423–424
effect of prostaglandins, 396
induction by Gn-RH, 447
in management of infertility, 407
Oxygen consumption
following exposure to cold, 314
Oxyphenisatin
hepatocellular damage, 130
Oxyphenylbutazone
treatment of Reiter's disease, 164
Oxytocin
role in labour, 452

Pain
action of prostaglandins, 400
Palmar erythema
feature of alcoholic hepatitis, 124
Pancreatic glucagon, 368–369
Pancreatic polypeptide, 366–368
chemistry and distribution, 366
pharmacology and physiology, 367
tumour production, 368
Pancreatic tumour
feature of glucagonoma, 369
Pancreatitis
acute, 330
alcoholic, 125
Pancreatone, 380
Pancytopenia, 106

Panencephalitis, subacute sclerosing, 84, 91–93,
103
Papulosis atrophicans maligna, 105
Paracetamol
hepatocellular damage, 130
Parkinsonian dementia (PD), 101
Parkinson's disease, 100
Parturition
action of prostaglandins, 394
Pellagra
feature of alcoholic hepatitis, 124
Penicillins, 181–183
control of anaerobic infections, 192
control of streptococcal infections, 191
treatment of gonococcal disease, 157
treatment of syphilitic hepatitis, 154
Peptic ulceration
feature of alcoholic hepatitis, 124
Pericardial effusion
complication of treatment of Hodgkin's
disease, 36
Pericarditis
acute, 34
feature of disseminated gonococcal disease,
156
feature of lupoid hepatitis, 135
in Reiter's disease, 162
Perimacular pigmentation
feature of rubella, 96
Peripheral neuropathy
feature of alcoholic hepatitis, 125
Peritoneoscopy
investigation of Hodgkin's disease, 26
Peroxidase
conversion to prostaglandins, 389
Pharmacokinetics, 173–177
absorption, 173
distribution, 175
excretion, 175
metabolism, 176
Pharyngitis
feature of disseminated gonococcal disease,
156
Phenelzine
treatment of obsessional states, 212
Phenobarbitone
in cholestasis, 332
Phenoxymethylpenicillin
antibiotic activity, 173
Phenylbutazone
treatment of Reiter's disease, 164
Phobias, 199–200
symptoms, 201
treatment, 202–206
Phospholipid
output and secretion of bile salts, 325
Pituitary gland
and the hypothalamus, 441–453
adrenocorticotrophic hormone (ACTH),
451
corticotrophin releasing factor (CRF), 451
diabetes insipidus, 452

World Health Organization/Frederickson classification of hyperlipidaemias, 253

Xanthomas
   feature of hypercholsterolaemia, 256, 263

Yellow fever
   cause of acute hepatitis, 113

Zieve's syndrome, 125
Zollinger–Ellison (ZE) syndrome, 361–362
   treatment with GH-RIH, 449